MAGNETIC RESONANCE IMAGING OF THE BRAIN

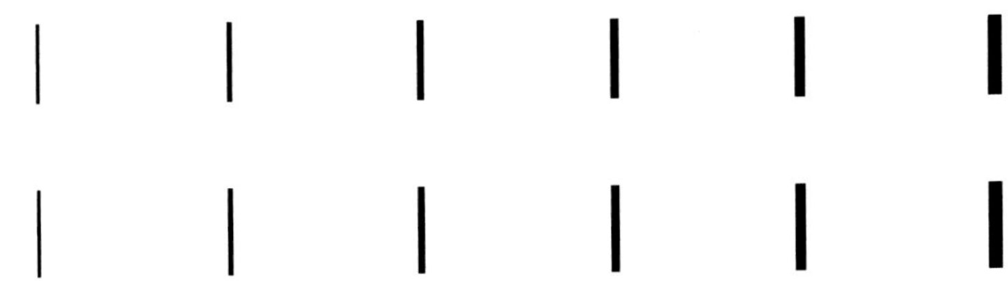

MAGNETIC RESONANCE IMAGING OF THE BRAIN

Val M. Runge, MD
Rosenbaum Professor of Diagnostic Radiology and
Professor of Biomedical Engineering
Director of the Magnetic Resonance Imaging and Spectroscopy Center
University of Kentucky
Lexington, Kentucky

Contributors

Mitchell A. Brack, MD
Watauga Radiology Associates, PC
Johnson City, Tennessee

Robert A. Garneau, MD
Radiology Group of Paducah
Paducah, Kentucky

John E. Kirsch, PhD
Assistant Professor of Diagnostic Radiology and Assistant Professor of Biomedical Engineering
Director of Research for the Magnetic Resonance Imaging and Spectroscopy Center
University of Kentucky
Lexington, Kentucky

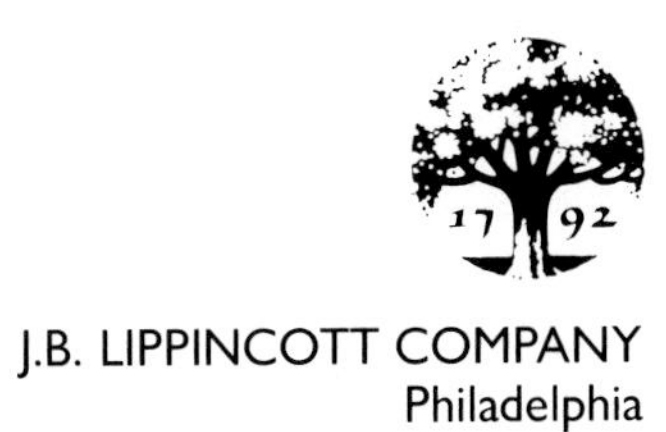

J.B. LIPPINCOTT COMPANY
Philadelphia

Sponsoring Editor: Delois Patterson
Associate Managing Editor: Grace R. Caputo
Indexer: Alexandra Weir Nickerson
Designer: Doug Smock
Cover Designer: Mark James
Production Manager: Caren Erlichman
Senior Production Coordinator: Kevin P. Johnson
Compositor: Compset Inc.
Prepress: Jay's Publisher's Service
Printer/Binder: Arcata/Kingsport

6 5 4 3 2 1

Library of Congress Cataloging-in-Publication Data

Runge, Val M.
Magnetic resonance imaging of the brain. / Val M. Runge;
contributors Mitchell A. Brack, Robert A. Garneau, John E. Kirsch.
p. cm.
Includes bibliographical references and index.
ISBN 0-397-51244-0
1. Brain—Magnetic resonance imaging—Atlases. 2. Head—Magnetic resonance imaging—Atlases. 3. Neck—Magnetic resonance imaging—Atlases. I. Title.
[DNLM. 1. Head—pathology—atlases. 2. Brain—pathology—atlases. 3. Neck—pathology—atlases. 4. Magnetic Resonance Imaging—methods—atlases. WE 17 R942m 1994]
RC386.6.M34R85 1994
617.5′107′548—dc20
DNLM/DLC
for Library of Congress 93-24586
CIP

Every effort has been made to ensure drug selections and dosages are in accordance with current recommendations and practice. Because of ongoing research, changes in government regulations, and the constant flow of information on drug therapy, reactions, and interactions, the reader is cautioned to check the package insert for each drug for indications, dosages, warnings, and precautions, particularly if the drug is new or infrequently used.

To Valerie and Sadie,
that they and their generation may have the opportunities
with which my wife and I have been blessed

and

to John Wells,
whose hard work—along with that of many others—
made this textbook possible

PREFACE

Although still early in the decade of the brain (the 1990s), magnetic resonance (MR) imaging has become firmly established as the premier diagnostic modality for the head. *Magnetic Resonance Imaging of the Brain* is designed to serve both as a primary text and as a reference source, covering in depth the diseases encountered in the clinical practice of MR today. New developments in imaging technique and contrast media have fueled the growth of MR, with continued rapid advancement anticipated. Recent advances, including MR angiography and fast spin echo imaging, have been approached in the context in which they are used today—as standards tools of the trade. Techniques that will likely become standard in the future, including diffusion, perfusion, and magnetization transfer imaging, have also been discussed in depth.

For ease of reference and continuity, *Magnetic Resonance Imaging of the Brain* is organized according to the pathology code of the *Index for Radiological Diagnoses,* 3rd edition, as published by the American College of Radiology. The atlas begins with a discussion of MR technique, normal anatomy, and congenital disease (.1). The physics of MR continue to challenge even the most technically inclined physician. Thus, substantial effort has been made to deal with this subject in a practical and clinically relevant fashion. The sections that follow cover inflammatory disease (.2), neoplasia (.3), the effect of trauma (.4), generalized systemic disorders (.5 and .6), vascular disease (.7), and miscellaneous conditions (.8 and .9). This part of the atlas, which discusses diseases of the skull and its contents (1.), is followed in logical progression by a second section, which discusses diseases of the face, mastoids, and neck (2.).

Each case begins with a short history, drawn from the patient's chart, that highlights clinical information important for film interpretation. The film findings are discussed in a succinct manner. MR images are correlated with conventional radiographs, CT scans, and angiograms where applicable. The diagnosis is then provided, followed by an in-depth discussion of the disease entity and its appearance on MR. Three special sections are included within the discussion to highlight important information with regard to MR technique, pitfalls in image interpretation, and correlative pathology. Current references are provided to further guide the interested reader.

MR—with its multiplanar imaging capability, high sensitivity to pathologic processes, and excellent anatomic detail—has had a major impact on routine clinical care over the past decade. Our knowledge base with regard to normal and pathologic brain processes has also been substantially increased. The future of MR continues to be bright, with the advent of routine second and subsecond imaging anticipated with the next generation of scanners in the mid- to late 1990s.

Val M. Runge, MD

CONTENTS

MAGNETIC RESONANCE IMAGING OF THE BRAIN

LIST OF ABBREVIATIONS AND ACRONYMS

ACA anterior cerebral artery
AD Alzheimer's disease
AICA anteroinferior cerebellar artery
AIDS acquired immunodeficiency syndrome
AP anteroposterior
AVM arteriovenous malformation
CE-FAST contrast-enhanced fourier acquired steady state
CHESS chemical shift selective suppression
CMV cytomegalovirus
C/N contrast-to-noise ratio
CNS central nervous system
CPA cerebellopontine angle
CSF cerebrospinal fluid
CSP cavum septum pellucidum
CT computed tomography
CVI cavum velum interpositum
DAI diffuse axonal injury
DPVS dilated perivascular spaces
ECG electrocardiographic
FA flip angle
FAST fourier acquired steady state
FID free induction decay
FISP fast imaging with steady precession
FLASH fast low-angle shot
FOV field of view
FSE fast spin echo
GBM glioblastoma multiforme
GMH germinal matrix hemorrhage
GMR gradient moment refocusing (or nulling)
GRASS gradient recalled acquisition in the steady state
GRE gradient echo
Hf free hydrogen (pool)
HIV human immunodeficiency virus
Hr restricted hydrogen (pool)
HSD Hallervorden-Spatz disease
IAC internal auditory canal
IR inversion recovery
IV intravenous
IVH intraventricular hemorrhage
MAST motion artifact suppression technique
MCA middle cerebral artery
MIP maximum intensity projection
MPR multiplanar reformatting
MP-RAGE magnetization-prepared rapid gradient echo
MR magnetic resonance
MRA magnetic resonance angiography
MS multiple sclerosis
MT magnetization transfer
NAA *N*-acetylaspartate
NEX number of excitations
NMR nuclear magnetic resonance
PA posteroanterior
PC phase contrast
PCA posterior cerebral artery
PICA posteroinferior cerebellar artery
PML progressive multifocal leukoencephalopathy
PNET primitive neuroectodermal tumor
PSIF time-reversed FISP
PVH periventricular hyperintensity
PVL periventricular leukomalacia
RARE rapid acquisition with relaxation enhancement
rCBF regional cerebral blood flow
rCBV regional cerebral blood volume
RF radiofrequency
SAR specific absorption rate
SE spin echo
S/N signal-to-noise ratio
SNE subacute necrotizing encephalomyelopathy
SP-GRASS spoiled gradient recalled acquisition in the steady state
SSFP steady-state free precession
STIR short tau inversion recovery
TE echo time
TI inversion time
TOF time-of-flight
TPP thiamine pyrophosphate
TR repetition time
TTP thiamine triphosphate
2D two-dimensional
3D three-dimensional
χ magnetic susceptibility (symbol for)

CHAPTER

ONE

Magnetic Resonance Imaging of the Brain,
edited by Val M. Runge.
J. B. Lippincott Company, Philadelphia © 1994.

Physics for Head Magnetic Resonance

John E. Kirsch

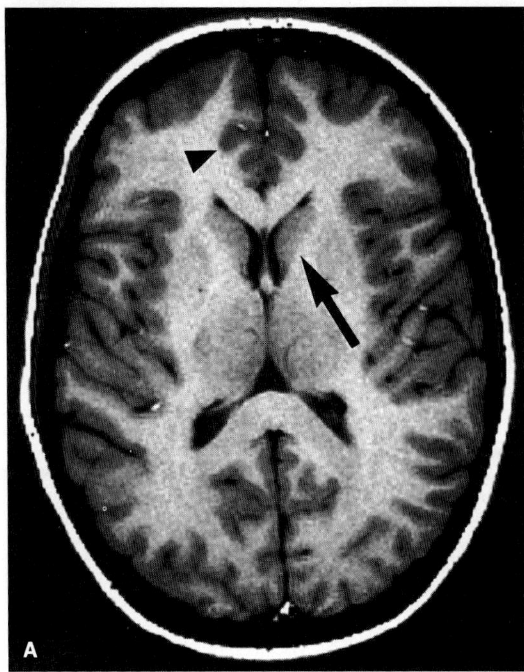

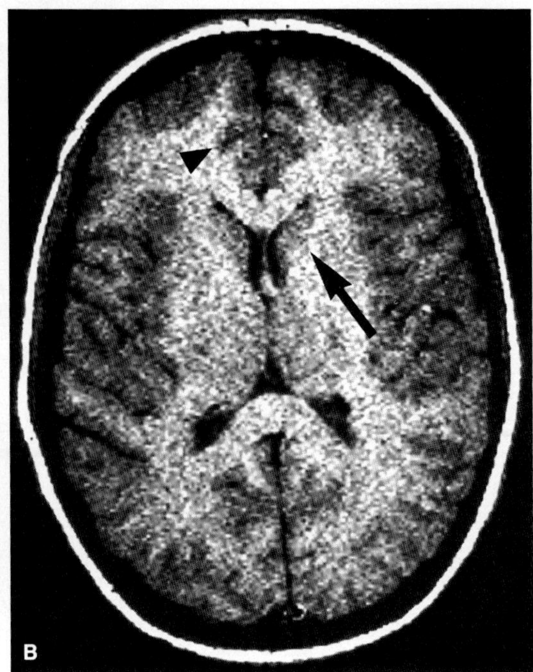

IMAGE QUALITY

Signal-to-noise ratio and contrast-to-noise ratio

FINDINGS

Axial T1-weighted spin echo (TR/TE = 400/10 msec) scans of a normal brain were obtained at high S/N (*A*) and low S/N (*B*). Difference was 4.3:1, and total scan times were 13:41 and 0:53 minutes, respectively. Inherent MR tissue contrast between *A* and *B* is identical. Loss in tissue differentiation as a result of reduced C/N is seen in *B,* particularly between gray and white matter (*arrowhead*), caudate nucleus (*arrow*), putamen, and thalamus.

CONCLUSION

Good image quality, C/N, and low tissue-contrast differentiation depend on high S/N.

DISCUSSION

In magnetic resonance (MR), the ability of a reader to differentiate between specific tissue regions of different signal levels depends on a number of parameters.[1,2] A significant factor that determines lesion conspicuity and establishes reader confidence is the noise level of the image.[3–5] Varying the MR technique and protocol can increase inherent differences in the signal of two adjacent tissues, but signal intensities are generally weak and the intrinsic contrast can be relatively small. Therefore, it is critical to minimize the amount of noise that contributes to an image whenever possible.

Although increased contrast can potentially lead to better delineation, detection of tissue differences and contrast resolution of the image are governed by the C/N given a specific spatial resolution. If the image noise is high (low C/N), signal levels of a given tissue vary greatly. Two adjacent tissues with close signal intensities that fluctuate largely as a result of noise are difficult to resolve. Conversely, if the noise is low (high C/N), even small differences in signal can be distinguished since the intensity levels do not vary widely.

Relative to a given contrast between tissue regions, C/N depends on the S/N. However, high S/N does not necessarily lead to high C/N and good differentiation. Intrinsic contrast must fundamentally exist among tissues. Less contrast requires increased S/N to maintain contrast resolution.

Advantages

Increased contrast resolution and good tissue differentiation are achieved with increased S/N.

Disadvantages

Higher S/N typically requires long scan times.

Technical References

1. Owen RS, Wehrli FW. Predictability of SNR and reader preference in clinical MR imaging. Magn Reson Imaging 1990;8:737–745.
2. Runge VM, Wood ML, Kaufman DM, et al. The straight and narrow path to good head and spine MRI. Radiographics 1988;8:507–531.
3. Edelstein WA, Bottomley PA, Hart HR, Smith LS. Signal, noise, and contrast in nuclear magnetic resonance imaging. J Comput Assist Tomogr 1983;7:391–401.
4. Constable RT, Henkelman RM. Contrast, resolution, and detectability in MR imaging. J Comput Assist Tomogr 1991; 15:297–303.
5. Hendrick RE, Raff U. Image contrast and noise. In: Stark DD, Bradley WG, eds. Magnetic resonance imaging, 2nd ed, vol 1. St Louis, Mosby–Year Book, 1992.

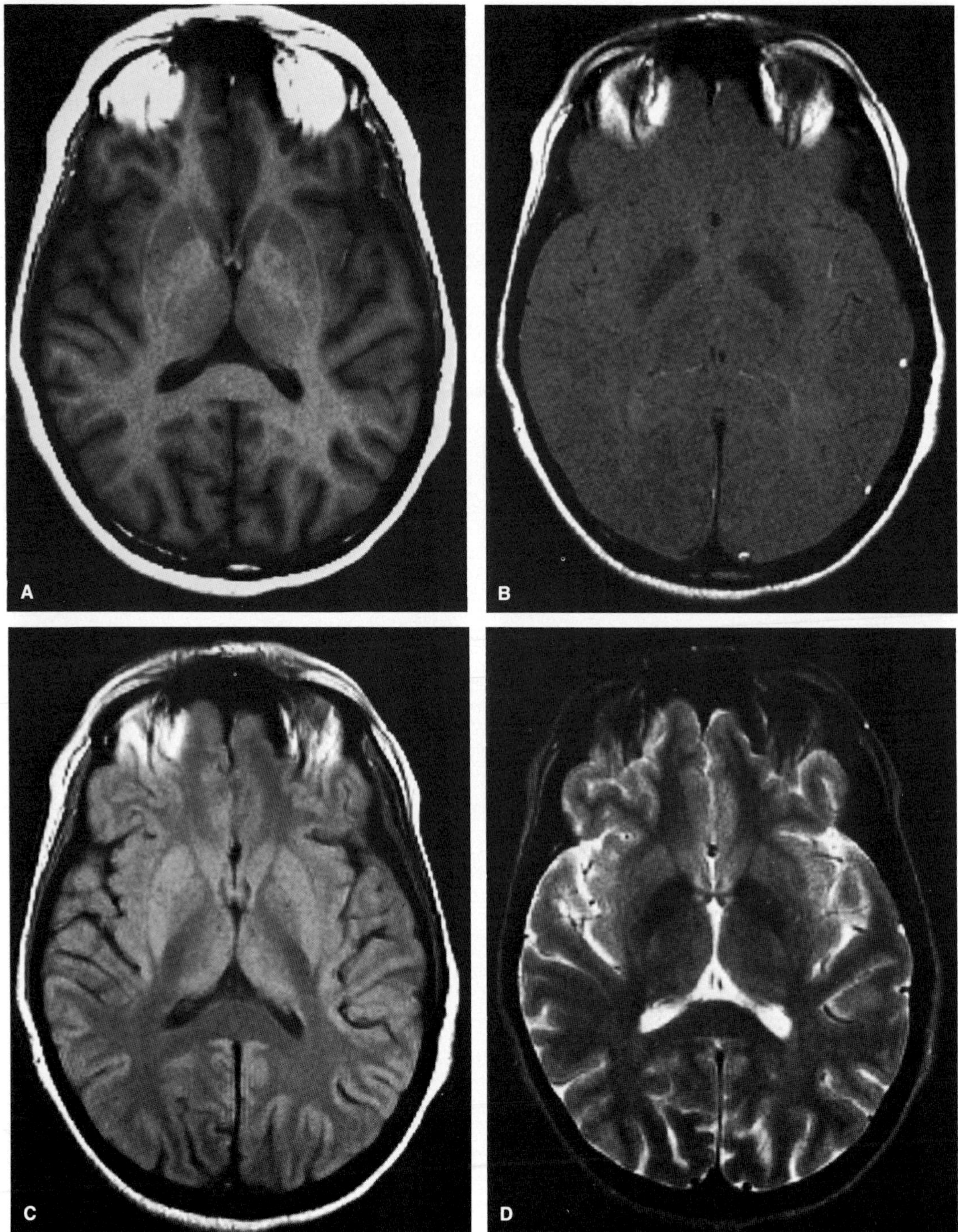

TECHNIQUE

Spin echo as a function of repetition time and echo time

FINDINGS

(*A*) On a T1-weighted SE scan (TR/TE = 300/10), fat is bright, cerebrospinal fluid (CSF) is dark, cortical gray matter is hypointense relative to white matter, and the putamen is well depicted. (*B*) Mixed weighting (TR/TE = 300/90) yields poor contrast and S/N with hypointensity seen in the globus pallidus. (*C*) With proton density weighting (TR/TE = 3000/10), high S/N is obtained but with poor overall intrinsic contrast. Gray matter is hyperintense relative to white matter. (*D*) T2 weighting (TR/TE = 3000/90) demonstrates high contrast with dark fat, bright CSF, and good differentiation among internal structures.

CONCLUSION

Optimal contrast is associated with short TR/short TE (T1 weighted) or long TR/long TE (T2 weighted), and high signal is achieved with long TR/short TE (proton density weighted).

DISCUSSION

SE has been the mainstay of MR, particularly in the brain, because of its generally high signal and contrast compared with other techniques. It is characterized by a 90° radiofrequency (RF) pulse followed by a 180° RF pulse, and generates a signal "echo" at time TE. This pulsing is repeated at intervals of TR. Tissue signal and relative contrast are derived from the user-selectable parameters TR and TE and from the differences in the intrinsic nuclear magnetic resonance (NMR) properties of hydrogen density, T1 and T2.[1–4]

Hydrogen (or spin) density, the number of hydrogen nuclei per unit volume of tissue, is linearly proportional to the MR signal. Although the amount of hydrogen present in the body is large (60% to 90% of the body is water by weight), the difference between tissues is small (ranging from 0% to 10% differential between gray and white matter). Spin density in itself is a poor parameter for contrast.

T1, also called longitudinal or spin-lattice relaxation time, is a characteristic property of tissues and refers to the amount of time it takes for the magnetization of a tissue to return to thermal equilibrium (relaxation). This indicates the state in which the magnetization in the tissue no longer changes and lies in the longitudinal direction of the external magnetic field. Tissues with short T1 values have faster magnetization recovery and return to equilibrium. In general, the value of T1 for a given tissue increases with field strength.

TR defines the time interval between successive 90°/180° RF pulse pairs and determines the degree of T1 relaxation of a tissue. MR signal increases with increasing TR. At short TR, few tissues possess fully recovered magnetization. Therefore, contrast is weighted by T1 differences and the overall signal is relatively low. At long TR, most of the magnetization recovers to equilibrium, resulting in high signal but little T1-weighted contrast.

T2, also called transverse or spin–spin relaxation time, is another intrinsic property of tissues and refers to the amount of time it takes for magnetization lying in the transverse plane to dephase and lose coherence (relaxation). Tissues with short T2 values have faster dephasing of their magnetization. T2 is generally considered to be relatively independent of field strength.

TE defines the time between the 90° RF pulse and the spin echo signal, and determines the degree of T2 relaxation of a tissue. MR signal decreases with increasing TE. At short TE, a large signal is generated because of little T2 dephasing in the tissues, and contrast from T2 differences is small. At long TE, sufficient time is allowed for T2 relaxation to occur and T2-weighted contrast is high, although the overall signal is low.

SE contrast is usually discussed in terms of the relative weighting of the intrinsic differences between hydrogen density, T1, and T2.[5] T1 signal differences are maximized at short TR and minimized at long TR. T2 differences are minimized at short TE and maximized at long TE. Therefore, short TR/short TE is called *T1 weighting,* and long TR/long TE is designated *T2 weighting.* The former tends to be used for obtaining good anatomic detail and contrast-enhanced information, whereas the latter generally provides more pathologic detail.[6,7] Images acquired at long TR/short TE minimize both T1 and T2 differences and are considered *proton weighted,* or *spin density weighted.* These images tend to be high in signal but low in contrast. The fourth possibility, short TR/long TE, is denoted *mixed weighting.* In general, contrast as well as signal tends to be low, and this approach is seldom used in standard SE protocols.

Advantages

High tissue contrast of variable weighting is achieved. Magnetic field–related artifacts are minimized (see 1.1214-26 through 1.1214-28).

Disadvantages

Moderately long scan times are required, particularly for T2-weighted studies and to obtain high spatial resolution.

Technical References

1. Wehrli FW, MacFall JR, Glover GH, et al. The dependence of nuclear magnetic resonance (NMR) image contrast on intrinsic and pulse sequence timing parameters. Magn Reson Imaging 1984;2:3–16.
2. Wehrli FW, MacFall JR, Shutts D, et al. Mechanisms of contrast in NMR imaging. J Comput Assist Tomogr 1984;8:369–380.
3. Perman WH, Hilal SK, Simon HE, Maudsley AA. Contrast manipulation in NMR imaging. Magn Reson Imaging 1984; 2:23–32.
4. Bradley WG. Effect of relaxation times on magnetic resonance image interpretation. Noninv Med Imaging 1984;1 193–204.
5. Hendrick RE, Raff U. Image contrast and noise. In: Stark DD, Bradley WG, eds. Magnetic resonance imaging, 2nd ed, vol 1. St Louis, Mosby–Year Book, 1992.
6. Feinberg DA, Mills CM, Posin JP, et al. Multiple spin-echo magnetic resonance imaging. Radiology 1985;155:437–442.
7. Posin JP, Ortendahl DA, Hylton NM, et al. Variable magnetic resonance imaging parameters: effect on detection and characterization of lesions. Radiology 1985;155:719–725.

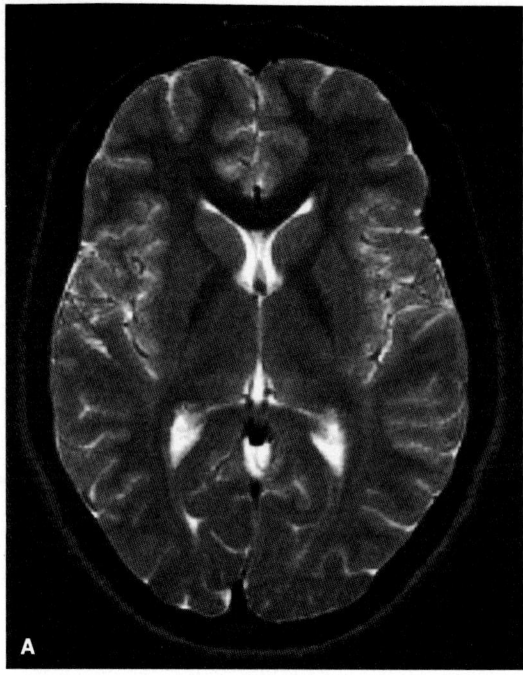

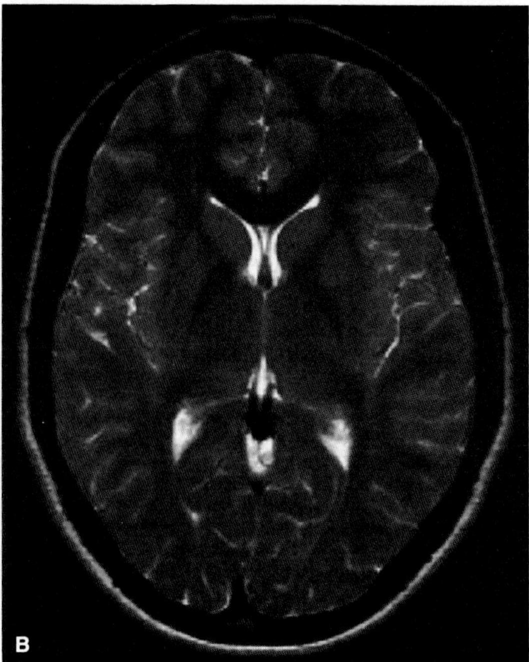

TECHNIQUE

Fast spin echo in comparison with conventional spin echo

FINDINGS

Comparison between a conventional T2-weighted SE scan (*A*) (TR/TE = 3000/90) and an eight-echo FSE scan (*B*) (TR/TE_{eff} = 3000/90) reveals similar tissue contrast. Acquisition times were 12:51 and 1:47 minutes, respectively. The most noticeable characteristic of FSE is that fat is hyperintense. A slight decrease in brain matter signal is also apparent. Less contrast effect from intrinsic tissue diffusion and susceptibility is also observed with FSE (*not shown*).

CONCLUSION

FSE is achieved in substantially reduced scan times and has similar contrast characteristics to SE techniques.

DISCUSSION

FSE is a technique that uses the characteristics of the SE technique while maximizing the efficiency of the data collection. It was first introduced as rapid acquisition with relaxation enhancement (RARE).[1] In conventional two-dimensional (2D) MR, each phase-encoding step is acquired by repeating the RF pulsing of the technique. In the SE technique, this pulsing is a 90°/180° pair that generates the spin echo at echo time TE. The repetition time is TR. In FSE, multiple echoes are generated by repeating the 180° pulse. Each echo is used to acquire additional phase-encoding steps within the same TR interval. For example, if 16 echoes are produced, one TR interval yields 16 phase encoding steps instead of 1 as in a conventional SE technique. Therefore, the total scan time is reduced in principle by a factor of 16. FSE is typically used to reduce the scan time of a T2-weighted SE study. However, it can also be used to obtain T1-weighted images. With the substantial decrease in imaging time, protocols can be combined with multiple acquisitions to improve image quality of thin-section or high-spatial-resolution scans.

The contrast in the FSE technique is similar to that in the SE technique.[2,3] However, by producing an image based on multiple spin echoes that are used for acquiring the phase encoding steps, the FSE image yields several fundamental differences. Fat, which is normally dark on T2-weighted SE images, has high signal intensity with FSE. Brain tissue intensity tends to be slightly reduced with FSE; this is believed to be partially due to magnetization transfer effects (see 1.1214-19). FSE techniques are also characterized by less signal loss associated with molecular diffusion and tissue susceptibility.[4]

Advantages

Tissue contrast approximates that in the SE technique (see 1.1214-2) in substantially less scan time.

Disadvantages

Fat signal is bright on T2-weighted images. Other aspects of contrast are slightly different from the SE technique. There is increased RF exposure to the patient.

Technical References

1. Hennig J, Naureth A, Friedburg H. RARE imaging: a fast imaging method for clinical MR. Magn Reson Med 1986;3:823–833.
2. Melki PS, Mulkern RV, Panych LP, Jolesz FA. Comparing the FAISE method with conventional dual-echo sequences. J Magn Reson Imaging 1991;1:319–326.
3. Jones KM, Mulkern RV, Schwartz RB, et al. Fast spin-echo MR imaging of the brain and spine: current concepts. AJR 1992;158:1313–1320.
4. Jones KM, Mulkern RV, Mantello MT, et al. Brain hemorrhage: evaluation with fast spin-echo and conventional dual spin-echo images. Radiology 1992;182:53–58.

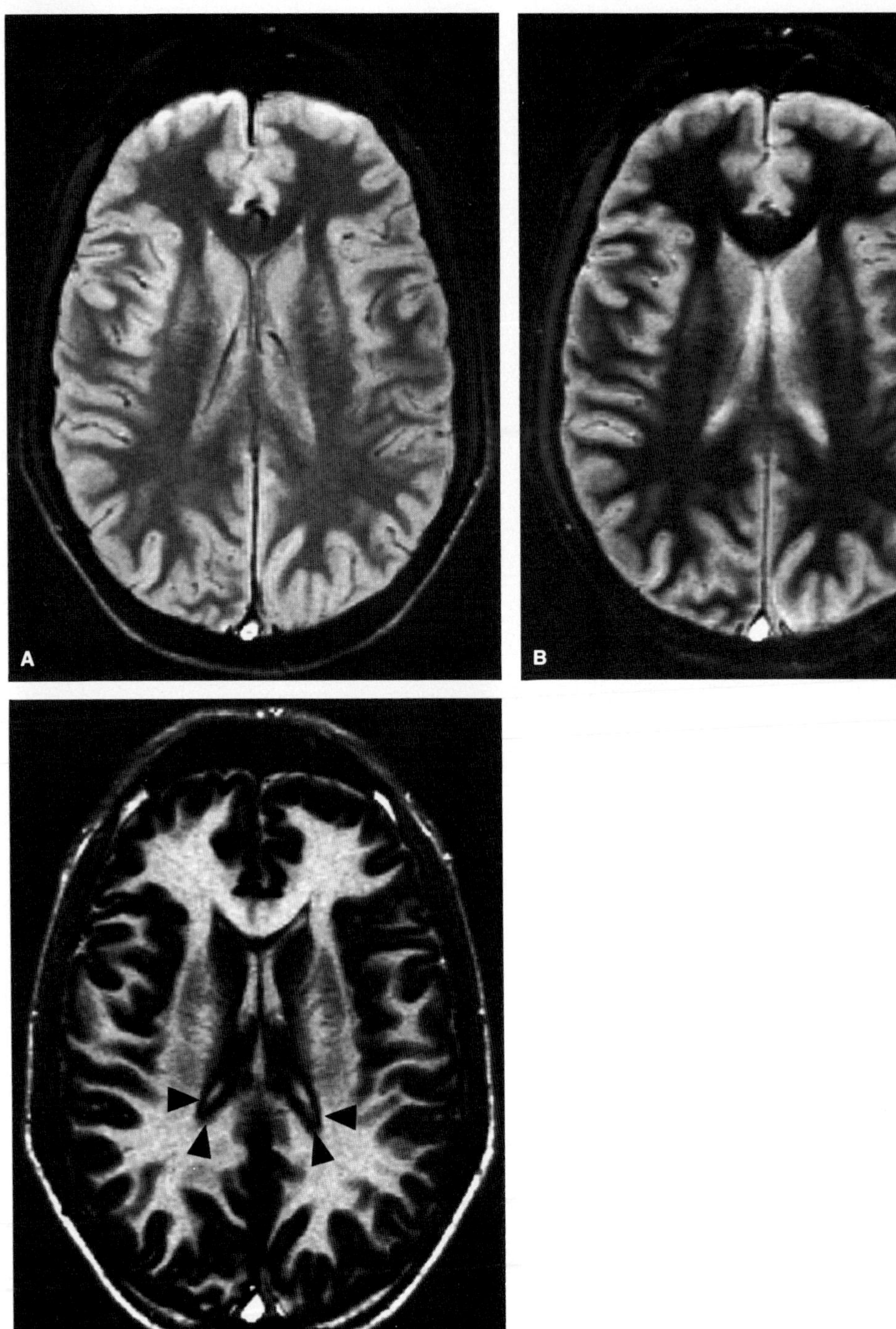

TECHNIQUE

Magnitude inversion recovery as a function of inversion time

FINDINGS

Axial magnitude reconstructed IR images (TR/TE = 2600/20) were acquired at a TI of 100 (*A*), 300 (*B*), and 600 msec (*C*). (*A*) Moderately strong T1 weighting with inverted contrast is observed at a short T1. (*B*) At intermediate TI, increased T1 weighting is seen while inverted contrast persists. (*C*) Correct tissue magnitudes and heavy T1-weighted contrast are seen at a sufficiently long TI except in the CSF of the lateral ventricles, where inverted contrast still remains. Boundary artifacts are evident between the CSF and deep white matter (*arrowheads*).

CONCLUSION

Magnitude IR possesses strong T1 weighting with superb anatomic detail, and displays anomalous inverted contrast at short and moderately short TI.

DISCUSSION

Certain MR techniques are designed to be well suited for enhancing contrast related specifically to either T1 or T2 differences in tissues. IR is inherently a technique that offers exceptional T1 weighting and superb anatomic detail.[1–3] In general head screening, IR has received less attention than SE (see 1.1214-2) because in many cases pathology is better visualized on T2-weighted studies. T1 contrast as well, which is favored for anatomic depiction, can be achieved with SE in substantially less scan time. Nevertheless, IR offers an advantage in certain clinical situations.

The IR pulse sequence is characterized by a 180°/90° RF pulsing. The initial 180° pulse inverts the longitudinal magnetization. Because no signal can be detected in MR until magnetization lies in the transverse plane, this is followed by a 90° RF pulse at inversion time TI. The signal is then collected as a spin echo or gradient echo. By initially inverting the magnetization, the time it takes for full T1 recovery is longer than in the SE technique, thereby allowing a much greater degree of T1 contrast to be obtained. TE is typically kept as short as possible to minimize introduction of T2-related contrast.

By varying TI, the degree of T1 contrast in the tissues can be altered. When the TI is chosen to be on the order of the T1 values of the tissues, the T1 contrast is maximized provided TR is long enough to allow full longitudinal recovery before the next TR interval. If TI is chosen to be extremely large, the effect of the 180° pulse becomes negligible, and the T1 contrast vanishes.

At very short TI, most signals from tissue are negative because little time is allowed for the inverted magnetization residing in the $-Z$ axis to recover to the $+Z$ axis. An absolute or magnitude reconstruction of the image actually inverts all negative signals to positive values and produces reversed tissue contrast leading to a potentially confusing display.[4] Contrast in the brain can mimic T2 weighting even though it is simply inverted T1 contrast. Absolute display can also actually reduce contrast significantly since large differences between a negative signal and a positive signal from two different tissues are both shown as positive and possibly similar intensities.[5] This type of situation leads as well to boundary artifacts at the interface between two such tissues.[6,7]

A unique aspect of IR is that because the magnetization becomes inverted ($-Z$), it must cross through a null point, or "bounce point," as it grows along the positive longitudinal ($+Z$) direction. The TI can be strategically chosen so that the signal is acquired precisely when a specific tissue of a given T1 value possesses zero longitudinal magnetization. This results in little signal output and suppression of those tissues. This phenomenon is exploited at times to suppress fat signal, particularly in the orbit (see 1.1214-15).

Advantages

Strong T1-weighted contrast and good anatomic detail are achieved. At specific TI values, specific tissue signals can be nulled (see 1.1214-15).

Disadvantages

Long scan times are required to achieve good contrast and S/N. The magnitude signal display yields inverted contrast at short TI that can be difficult to interpret. Boundary artifacts occur at tissue interfaces between inverted and uninverted signal (see 1.1214-15).

Technical References

1. Wehrli FW, MacFall JR, Shutts D, et al. Mechanisms of contrast in NMR imaging. J Comput Assist Tomogr 1984;8:369–380.
2. Wehrli FW, MacFall JR, Glover GH, et al. The dependence of nuclear magnetic resonance (NMR) image contrast on intrinsic and pulse sequence timing parameters. Magn Reson Imaging 1984;2:3–16.
3. Bydder GM, Young IR. MR imaging: clinical use of the inversion recovery sequence. J Comput Assist Tomogr 1985; 9:659–675.
4. Young IR, Bailes DR, Bydder GM. Apparent changes of appearance of inversion-recovery images. Magn Reson Med 1985;2:81–85.
5. Hendrick RE, Nelson TR, Hendee WR. Phase detection and contrast loss in magnetic resonance imaging. Magn Reson Imaging 1984;2:279–283.
6. Hearshen DO, Ellis JH, Carson PL, et al. Boundary effects from opposed magnetization artifact in IR images. Radiology 1986;160:543–547.
7. Droege RT, Adamczak SM. Boundary artifact in inversion-recovery images. Magn Reson Med 1986;3:126–131.

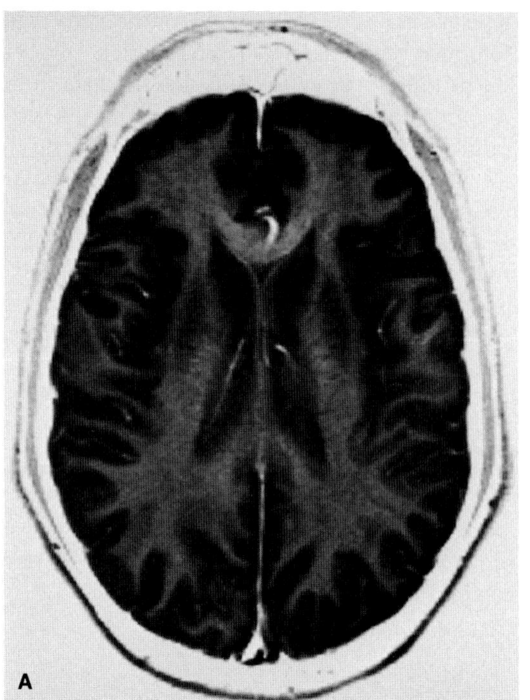
A

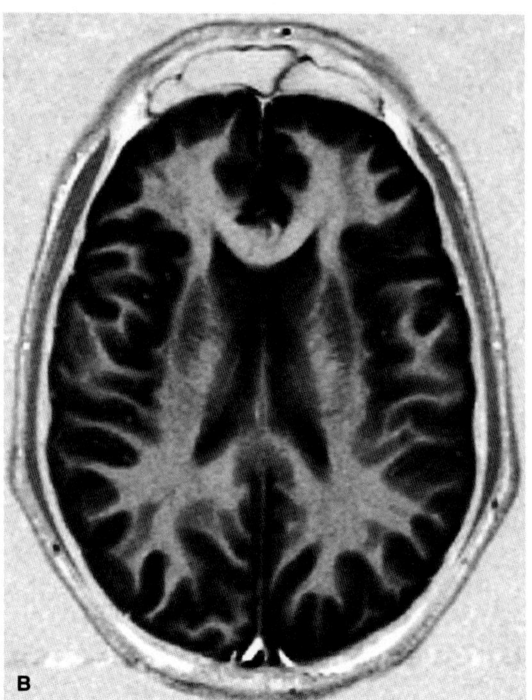
B

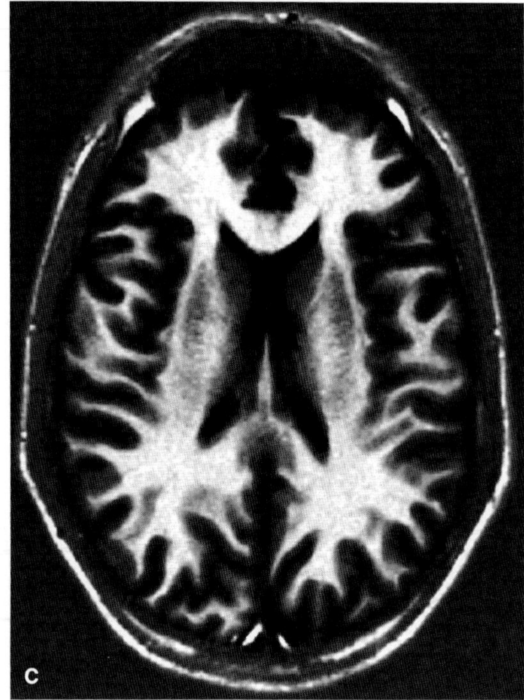
C

TECHNIQUE

Phase-sensitive inversion recovery as a function of inversion time

FINDINGS

Axial phase-sensitive IR images (TR/TE = 2600/20) were acquired at a TI of 100 (*A*), 300 (*B*), and 600 msec (*C*). T1-weighted contrast increases with TI and superb gray and white matter differentiation is apparent. In comparison with magnitude reconstruction (see 1.1214-4), correct tissue magnitudes at all TIs are observed with phase-sensitive reconstruction. Characteristically, negative tissue signal appears darker than background noise, most notable at short and intermediate TI (*A and B*).

CONCLUSION

Phase-sensitive IR has exceptional anatomic detail and strong T1 weighting with no artificial contrast reversal at short TI.

DISCUSSION

IR is a technique that offers strong T1 weighting and superb anatomic detail[1] and is described elsewhere (see 1.1214-4). By varying TI, the degree of T1 weighting in the tissues can be altered. If the TI is chosen to be on the order of the T1 values of the tissues, the T1 contrast is maximized. If TI is chosen to be extremely large, the effect of the 180° inversion RF pulse becomes negligible, and the T1 contrast vanishes.

An absolute or magnitude reconstruction of the image inverts any signals that are negative to positive values. This produces reversed tissue contrast leading to a potentially confusing display, particularly when a short TI is used.[1,2] All tissues have negative signals at extremely short TI, and the contrast can mimic T2 weighting even though it is simply inverted T1 contrast. Absolute display may also significantly reduce contrast[3] and produce boundary artifacts at interfaces[4,5] if a TI is used that yields a combination of both positive and negative tissue signals in the image.

Phase-sensitive methods exist that allow the sign (positive or negative) of the IR signals to be preserved on reconstruction thereby producing true T1-weighted IR contrast.[5–7] At very short TI when all tissues exhibit negative signals, background noise has the highest pixel intensity. At TI values when signals and pixel intensities are both positive and negative, tissue contrast is maintained at a maximum without boundary artifacts. At moderately long TI when most signals are positive, image contrast is similar to that of magnitude-reconstructed IR except for tissues such as CSF that possess very long T1.

Advantages

Strong T1-weighted contrast and good anatomic detail are achieved. True IR contrast is preserved at short TI. No boundary artifacts are produced. At specific TI values, specific tissue signals can be nulled (see 1.1214-15).

Disadvantages

Long scan times are typically required to achieve good contrast and S/N.

Technical References

1. Bydder GM, Young IR. MR imaging: clinical use of the inversion recovery sequence. J Comput Assist Tomogr 1985; 9:659–675.
2. Young IR, Bailes DR, Bydder GM. Apparent changes of appearance of inversion-recovery images. Magn Reson Med 1985;2:81–85.
3. Hendrick RE, Nelson TR, Hendee WR. Phase detection and contrast loss in magnetic resonance imaging. Magn Reson Imaging 1984;2:279–283.
4. Hearshen DO, Ellis JH, Carson PL, et al. Boundary effects from opposed magnetization artifact in IR images. Radiology 1986;160:543–547.
5. Droege RT, Adamczak SM. Boundary artifact in inversion-recovery images. Magn Reson Med 1986;3:126–131.
6. Park HW, Cho MH, Cho ZH. Real-value representation in inversion-recovery NMR imaging by use of a phase-correction method. Magn Reson Med 1986;3:15–23.
7. Moran PR, Kumar NG, Karstaedt N, Jackels SC. Tissue contrast enhancement: image reconstruction algorithm and selection of TI in inversion recovery MRI. Magn Reson Imaging 1986;4:229–235.

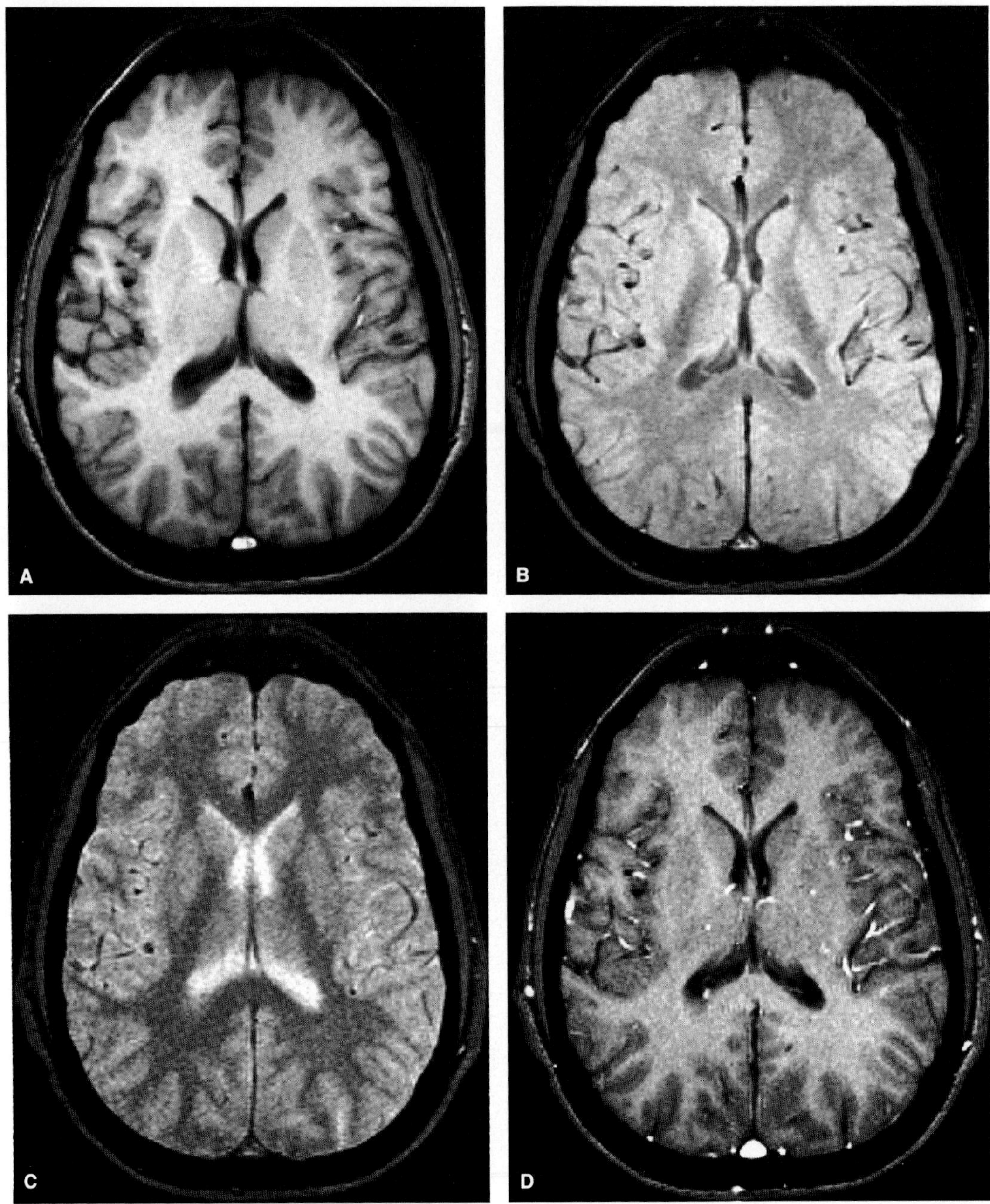

TECHNIQUE

Spoiled gradient echo as a function of repetition time and RF flip angle

FINDINGS

(*A*) Spoiled GRE with a high RF flip angle (TR/TE/FA = 300/10/90°) demonstrates similar T1 weighting to conventional SE (*not shown*) using identical short TR and short TE. By reducing the flip angle, tissue contrast approaches spin density weighting (FA = 30°) (*B*) and T2 weighting (FA = 10°) (*C*), normally observed in SE with longer TR and TE. S/N also decreases with flip angle. (*D and E*) Similar contrast behavior can also be obtained at very short TR with further reduction in flip angles. T1-weighted contrast in *D* (TR/TE/FA = 30/10/30°) is similar to *A*, and spin density weighting in *E* (TR/TE/FA = 30/10/10°) is similar to *B*. However, overall S/N is further reduced due to the shorter TR. (*F*) At very short TR and large flip angle (TR/TE/FA = 30/10/90°), S/N is decreased with characteristically large signal in the vasculature from time-of-flight inflow effects (*arrows*).

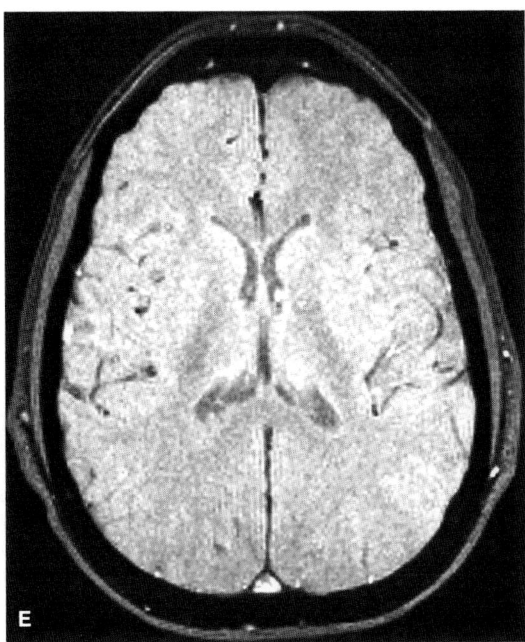

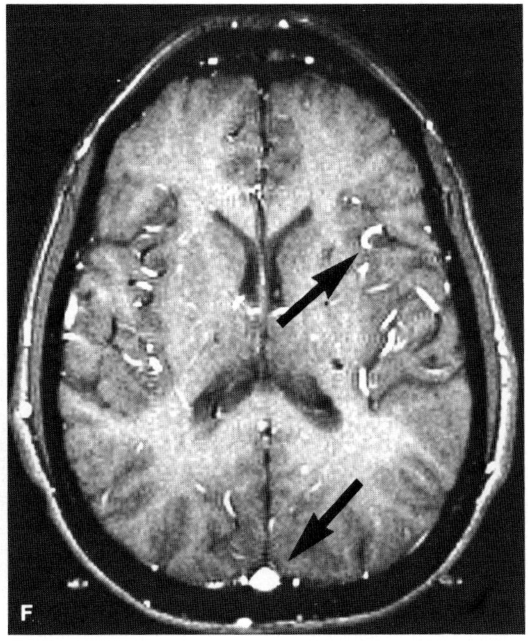

CONCLUSION

Spoiled GRE possesses similar contrast behavior to spin echo at 90° flip angle or at a shorter TR with a reduced flip angle, and S/N advantages at very short TR using low flip angles.

DISCUSSION

GRE techniques, a valuable adjunct to SE imaging (see 1.1214-2), are steady-state imaging methods that are primarily grouped into three categories: spoiled, rephased (see 1.1214-7), and contrast-enhanced (see 1.1214-8). The spoiled GRE technique, also called fast low-angle shot (FLASH) or spoiled gradient recalled acquisition in the steady state (SP-GRASS), is based on T1 recovery and the free induction decay (FID) signal. It is characterized by the fact that only longitudinal magnetization is allowed to approach a steady state. Transverse magnetization is "spoiled" away before subsequent RF pulsing and therefore does not contribute to the FID signal.

Spoiled GRE is similar to SE with respect to signal generation and contrast. Unlike SE, however, there is no 180° RF pulse that normally produces the echo, which must be created by the use of gradients. In addition to TR and TE, the tissue contrast is complicated by a dependence on the RF flip angle.[1] Furthermore, because of the absence of the 180° pulse the signal decays faster with larger TE according to T2* instead of T2.

At an RF flip angle of 90°, the contrast behavior is the same as in SE except for the differences between T2* and T2 with TE.[2,3] At a reduced flip angle, less time is taken for recovery of the magnetization. Therefore, similar contrast can be achieved at a shorter TR using small flip angles. If the TR is short enough, the S/N exceeds that for a 90° pulsing at the same TR. However, because only a portion of the magnetization becomes transverse after a small flip angle pulse, the maximum achievable signal at a long TR is less than at 90°. Thus the only advantage of spoiled GRE is at short TR using reduced flip angles.

Since the origin of the FID signal is based on T1 recovery, spoiled GRE provides good T1-weighted contrast. At reduced flip angles, T1 contrast can be maintained with a shorter TR thereby reducing scan time, provided TE is kept shorter than for SE because of the faster T2* decay of the signal.[4,5] With smaller flip angles, a very short TR can be used and still achieve T1-weighted contrast. In 2D MR, this enables rapid imaging for breathhold or perfusion techniques (see 1.1214-17), and allows three-dimensional (3D) data to be acquired in reasonable scan times (see 1.1214-9).[6–8] With very small flip angles, a TR that normally is used in SE for T1 weighting can provide proton density weighting. In conjunction with a moderately long TE, T2* weighting similar to T2 weighting can be obtained.[4,5,9]

Without a 180° pulse, the spoiled GRE signal is subject to dephasing based on all field inhomogeneities in addition to T2 and susceptibility that comprise T2*. This includes chemical shift differences between fat and water that cause signal modulation with TE (see 1.1214-16), bulk susceptibility artifacts (see 1.1214-26), and accentuated artifacts from metal (see 1.1214-27). Normally, the 180° pulse in SE minimizes these effects, but in GRE techniques they can substantially reduce tissue signal, cause image distortions, and change contrast particularly as a result of intrinsic tissue susceptibility differences.

Advantages

The spoiled GRE technique provides approximate T1- and T2-weighted contrast with shorter TR and faster scan time than SE (see 1.1214-2) when using RF flip angles less than 90°. Very short TR at small flip angles enables rapid 2D imaging and practical 3D imaging with flexible contrast.

Disadvantages

Absence of the 180° RF pulse in spoiled GRE imaging can accentuate magnetic field errors not seen in SE images (see 1.1214-2). This includes signal modulation (see 1.1214-16), susceptibility artifact (see 1.1214-26), and increased metal artifact (see 1.1214-27).

Technical References

1. Buxton RB, Edelman RR, Rosen BR, et al. Contrast in rapid MR imaging: T1- and T2-weighted imaging. J Comput Assist Tomogr 1987;11:7–16.
2. Bydder GM, Young IR. Clinical use of the partial saturation and saturation recovery sequences in MR imaging. J Comput Assist Tomogr 1985;9:1020–1032.
3. Schorner W, Sander B, Henkes H, et al. Multiple slice FLASH imaging: an improved pulse sequence for contrast enhanced MR brain studies. Neuroradiology 1990;32:474–480.
4. Stadnik TW, Luypaert RR, Neirynck EC, Osteaux M. Optimization of sequence parameters in fast MR imaging of the brain with FLASH. Am J Neuroradiol 1989;10:357–362.
5. Mills TC, Ortendahl DA, Hylton NM, et al. Partial flip angle MR imaging. Radiology 1987;162:531–539.
6. Van der Meulen P, Groen JP, Cuppen JJM. Very fast MR imaging by field echoes and small angle excitation. Magn Reson Imaging 1985;3:297–299.
7. Frahm J, Haase A, Matthaei D. Rapid three-dimensional MR imaging using the FLASH technique. J Comput Assist Tomogr 1986;10:363–368.
8. Shogry MEC, Elster AD. Cerebrovascular enhancement in spoiled GRASS (SPGR) images: comparison with spin-echo technique. J Comput Assist Tomogr 1992;16:48–53.
9. Bydder GM, Payne JA, Collins AG, et al. Clinical use of rapid T2 weighted partial saturation sequences in MR imaging. J Comput Assist Tomogr 1987;11:17–23.

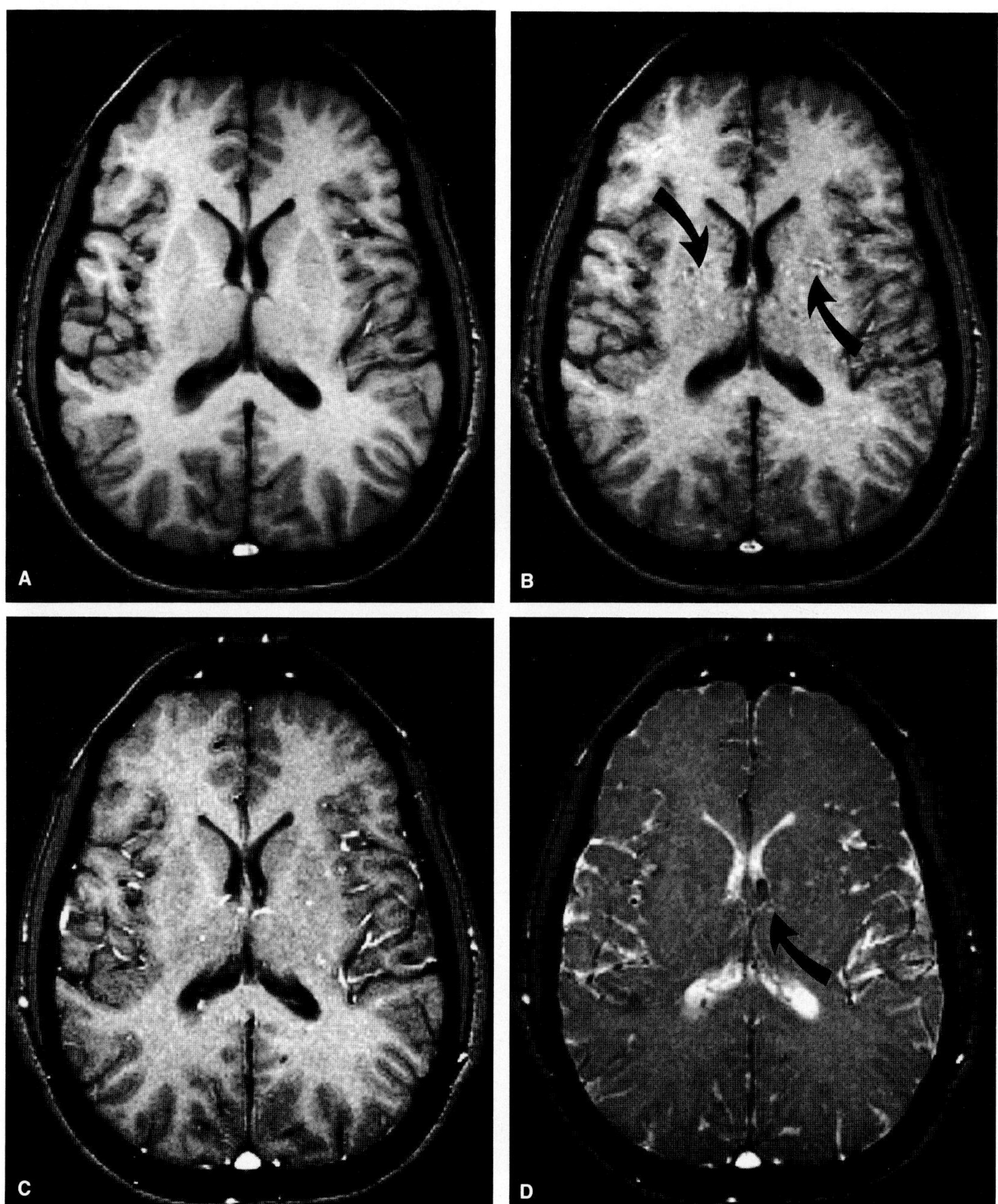

TECHNIQUE

Rephased gradient echo as a function of repetition time and RF flip angle in comparison with spoiled gradient echo

FINDINGS

At longer TR (TR/TE/FA = 300/10/90°), contrast behavior in spoiled GRE (*A*) is nearly identical to rephased GRE (*B*), regardless of flip angle. The additional echo component of rephased GRE may produce increased pulsation artifacts (*arrows*). At very short TR (TR/TE/FA = 30/10/30°), spoiled GRE shows similar T1-weighted contrast at reduced flip angle (*C*), but rephased GRE demonstrates T2/T1 weighting with a loss in gray–white matter differentiation and high signal from water components (*D*). Signal voids from flow and pulsation artifacts may be pronounced (*arrow*). (*E*) Large flip angle and very short TR with rephased GRE (TR/TE/FA = 30/10/90°) can yield an extremely large signal from CSF producing a myelographic effect as seen on a sagittal midline section.

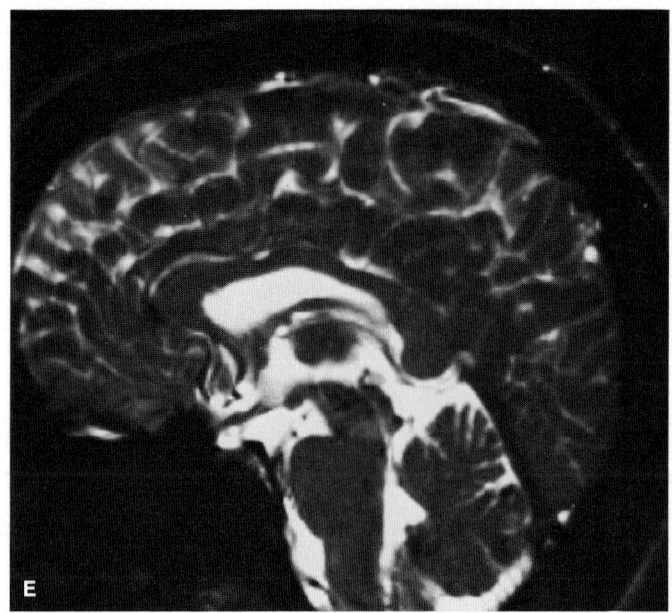

CONCLUSION

Rephased GRE has similar contrast behavior to spoiled GRE at long TR, and high water signal at very short TR using large flip angles.

DISCUSSION

The rephased GRE technique, also called fast imaging with steady precession (FISP), fourier acquired steady state (FAST), and gradient recalled acquisition in the steady state (GRASS), is a steady-state free precession (SSFP) method based on T1 and T2 recovery and the SSFP-FID signal. It is characterized by the fact that both longitudinal and transverse magnetization are allowed to approach a steady state. In contrast to spoiled GRE (see 1.1214-6), the transverse magnetization coherency is maintained before subsequent RF pulsing and therefore contributes an additional component to the FID signal.[1]

When the transverse magnetization is preserved during pulsing, it can survive through multiple TR intervals. Every pair of adjacent RF pulses that constitutes a time of 2*TR generates a spin echo based on the transverse magnetization called the SSFP-echo. Its strength depends on T2 and the "echo time" of 2*TR. This signal adds to the FID signal created by each individual RF pulse which is based on the longitudinal magnetization and whose strength depends on T1 and TR. Unlike the FID in spoiled GRE, the combined signal is therefore additionally based on T2 and is called the SSFP-FID. Being a GRE technique, however, the signal decays faster with TE according to T2* instead of T2 because of the absence of the 180° pulse.

The difference in contrast between spoiled GRE and rephased GRE is simply the degree to which the SSFP-echo contributes to the signal. At long TR, little or no transverse magnetization survives through two TR intervals even from tissues with long T2. In effect, T2 decay behaves like a "spoiling" mechanism. Therefore, the SSFP-echo is negligible and rephased GRE produces the same contrast as spoiled GRE. As TR is reduced, however, the contribution of the SSFP-echo increases with the highest signal coming from tissues with the longest T2. Furthermore, higher RF flip angles generate greater SSFP-echo signal as well. Thus, the largest differences in tissue contrast between spoiled GRE and rephased GRE occur when a short TR and large flip angle are used. This is seen primarily as a combined T1 and T2 mixed weighting and is more precisely a T2/T1 weighting.[1] Because free water such as CSF has the longest T2 and generates the largest SSFP-echo signal, rephased GRE contrast is sometimes called *water weighting*.

With its largest difference in tissue contrast being produced at very short TR, rephased GRE has been primarily used in rapid 2D imaging for breathhold or perfusion studies (see 1.1214-17) and in 3D acquisitions.[2–4] However, with the absence of a 180° pulse, the rephased GRE technique is subject to the same magnetic field errors as spoiled GRE (see 1.1214-6). This includes chemical shift differences between fat and water that cause signal modulation with TE (see 1.1214-16), bulk susceptibility artifacts (see 1.1214-26), and accentuated artifacts from metal (see 1.1214-27).

Advantages

The rephased GRE technique provides a T2/T1 or mixed tissue contrast at very short TR and water weighting when combined with a large flip angle. Very short TR enables rapid 2D imaging and practical 3D imaging with flexible contrast.

Disadvantages

Absence of the 180° RF pulse in rephased GRE imaging can accentuate magnetic field errors not seen in SE images (see 1.1214-2). This includes signal modulation (see 1.1214-16), susceptibility artifact (see 1.1214-26), and increased metal artifact (see 1.1214-27).

Technical References

1. Tkach JA, Haacke EM. A comparison of fast spin echo and gradient field echo sequences. Magn Reson Imaging 1988;6:373–389.
2. Gyngell ML. The application of steady-state free precession in rapid 2DFT NMR imaging: FAST and CE-FAST sequences. Magn Reson Imaging 1988;6:415–419.
3. Steinberg PM, Ross JS, Modic MT, et al. The value of fast gradient-echo MR sequences in the evaluation of brain disease. Am J Neuroradiol 1990;11:59–67.
4. Hesselink JR, Martin JF, Edelman RR. Fast imaging. Neuroradiology 1990;32:348–355.

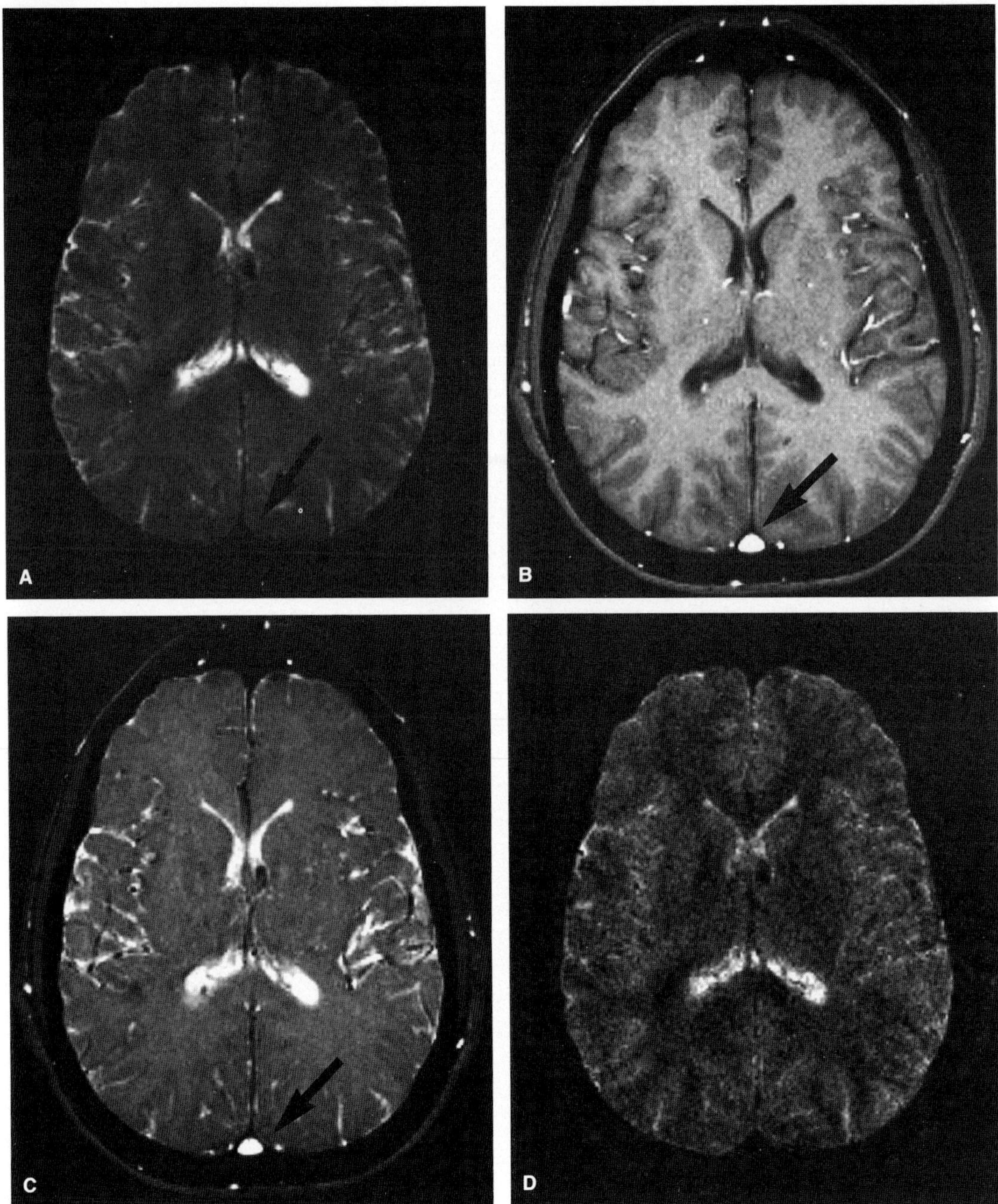

TECHNIQUE

T2-enhanced gradient echo in comparison with spoiled and rephased GRE

FINDINGS

T2-weighted contrast is observed with T2-enhanced GRE at very short TR and relatively large flip angle (TR/TE/FA = 30/50/30°) when the SSFP echo (*A*) is isolated from the FID signal (*B*) of a spoiled GRE. (*C*) The combined signal from the two produces the SSFP-FID signal of rephased GRE. A large signal from the vasculature is generated with the spoiled GRE component due to inflow effects (*B and C*), and vessel voids are observed in T2-enhanced GRE (*arrows*). (*D*) Lower S/N is associated with longer TR (*not shown*) and smaller flip angle (TR/TE/FA = 30/50/10°).

CONCLUSION

T2-enhanced GRE possesses T2-weighted contrast at short TR, and higher S/N at very short TR and large flip angle.

DISCUSSION

The T2-enhanced GRE technique, also known as contrast-enhanced fourier acquired steady state (CE-FAST) and time-reversed FISP (PSIF), is an SSFP method primarily based on T2 recovery and the SSFP-echo signal. It is characterized by maintaining transverse magnetization in a steady state. In contrast to other GRE techniques (see 1.1214-6 and 1.1214-7), the FID is not acquired but rather the SSFP-echo is isolated and used as a gradient echo for imaging.[1]

During short TR pulsing, the transverse magnetization is preserved and survives through multiple TR intervals. Every pair of adjacent RF pulses that constitutes a time of 2*TR will generate a spin echo based on the transverse magnetization called the SSFP-echo. Its strength is primarily dependent on T2 and the "echo time" of 2*TR. Unlike the FID in spoiled GRE or the SSFP-FID signal in rephased GRE, the SSFP-echo signal in T2-enhanced GRE is largely associated with T2. Like all GRE techniques, however, the signal decays faster with TE according to T2* instead of T2 because of the absence of the 180° pulse.

T2-enhanced GRE contrast is based on the intensity of the SSFP-echo. At long TR, little or no transverse magnetization survives through two TR intervals and the SSFP-echo is negligible. Thus, this technique is not used at long TR. However, as TR is reduced the SSFP-echo increases. The largest signal is generated using large flip angles and from tissues with the longest T2. At very short TR where S/N is highest, tissue contrast is primarily T2 weighted.

With the sufficient S/N and T2-weighted contrast being produced at very short TR, T2-enhanced GRE has been used in rapid 2D imaging for breathhold or perfusion studies (see 1.1214-17) and in 3D acquisitions.[2–4] Because the SSFP-echo signal is created by two RF pulses in adjacent TR intervals, this technique tends to be sensitive to motion and flow artifacts (see 1.1214-29 and 1.1214-31). With the absence of a 180° pulse, the technique is also subject to the same magnetic field errors as other GRE techniques (see 1.1214-6 and 1.1214-7). This includes chemical shift differences between fat and water that cause signal modulation with TE (see 1.1214-16), bulk susceptibility artifacts (see 1.1214-26), and accentuated artifacts from metal (see 1.1214-27).

Advantages

The T2-enhanced GRE technique provides good T2 weighting at very short TR when combined with larger flip angles, enabling rapid 2D and practical 3D imaging.

Disadvantages

The T2-enhanced GRE technique tends to have low S/N and is sensitive to flow and motion artifacts (see 1.1214-29 and 1.1214-31). Absence of the 180° RF pulse can accentuate magnetic field errors, such as signal modulation (see 1.1214-16), susceptibility artifact (see 1.1214-26), and increased metal artifact (see 1.1214-27).

Technical References

1. Tkach JA, Haacke EM. A comparison of fast spin echo and gradient field echo sequences. Magn Reson Imaging 1988; 6:373–389.
2. Gyngell ML. The application of steady-state free precession in rapid 2DFT NMR imaging: FAST and CE-FAST sequences. Magn Reson Imaging 1988;6:415–419.
3. Steinberg PM, Ross JS, Modic MT, et al. The value of fast gradient-echo MR sequences in the evaluation of brain disease. Am J Neuroradiol 1990;11:59–67.
4. Menick BJ, Bobman SA, Listerud J, Atlas SW. Thin-section, three-dimensional fourier transform, steady-state free precession MR imaging of the brain. Radiology 1992;183: 369–377.

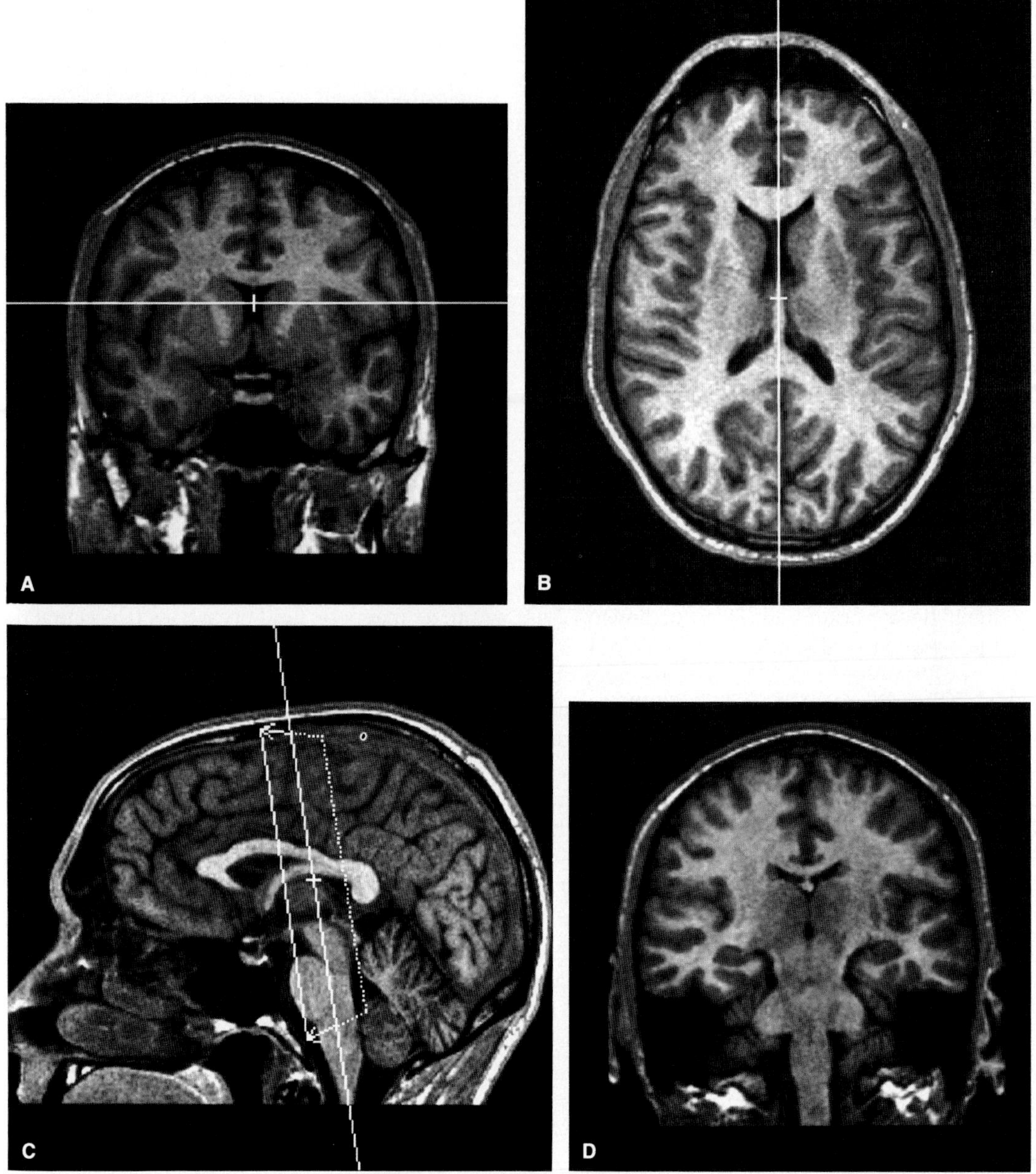

TECHNIQUE

Three-dimensional imaging and multiplanar reformatting

FINDINGS

(*A*) 3D spoiled GRE T1-weighted images were acquired in the coronal orientation (TR/TE/FA = 25/4/40°) with 0.9 × 0.9 × 0.9 mm isotropic resolution. MPR allows the display of axial (*B*), sagittal (*C*), or oblique sections (*D*) for better symmetry or visualization of structures. Isotropic acquisition maintains spatial resolution in all directions. Free curvilinear MPR is also demonstrated in the circular region drawn in (*E*) and displayed in the unraveling of the circuit of Papez (*F*). This allows projection of the complete spiral hippocampal formation and depiction of the amygdala (a), hippocampus (h), fimbria (f), body of the fornix (b), and mamillary bodies (m), not possible in normal planar acquisition or reformatting. MPR further enables partition stacking to display thicker sections for better S/N as shown at 0.9 mm (*G*) and at 5 mm (*H*). Spatial resolution losses are observed with MPR if anisotropic (*J*) instead of isotropic (*I*) acquisitions are displayed.

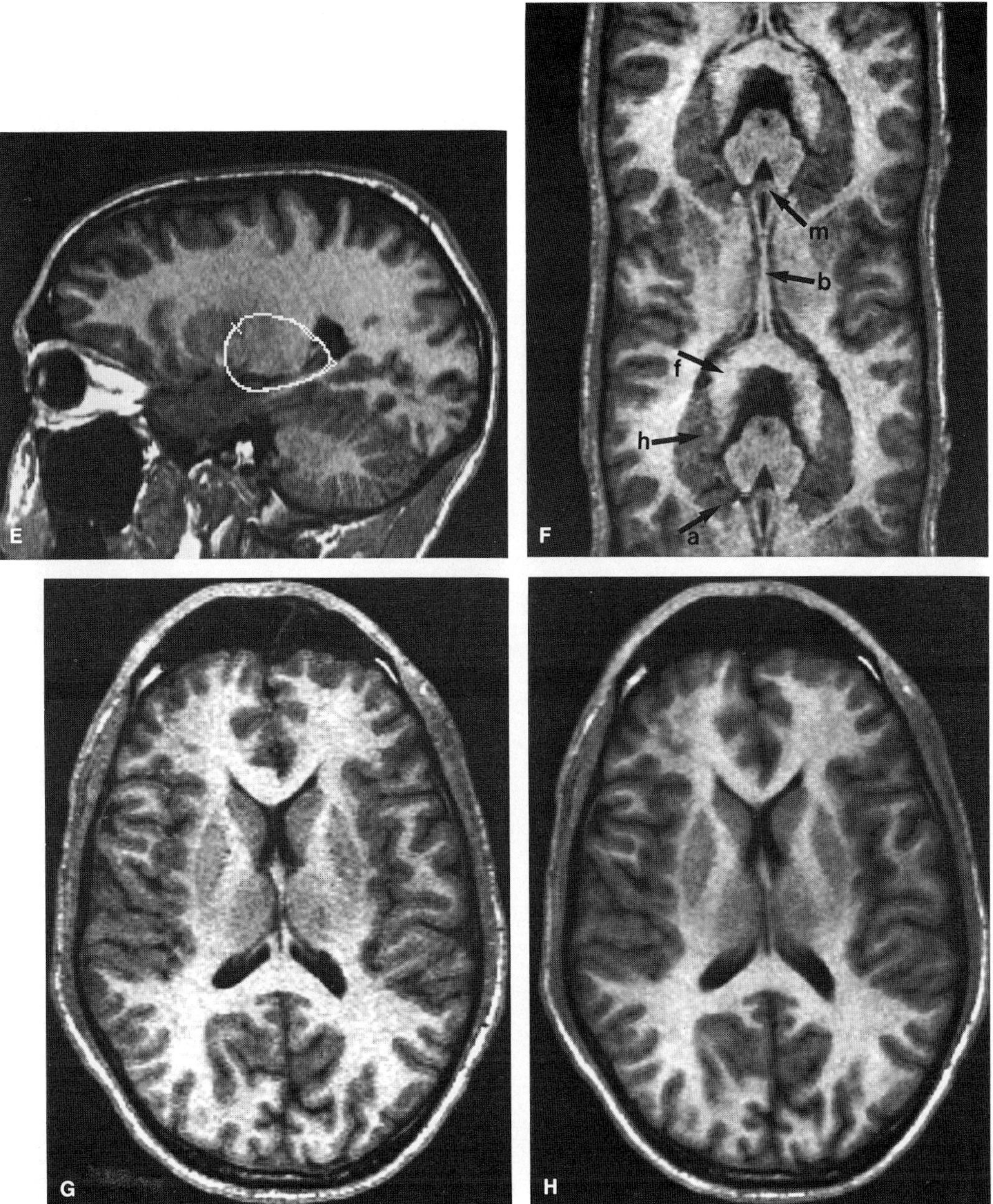

CONCLUSION

With 3D imaging, MPR in any plane is possible, including nonrectilinear formats. A loss in resolution occurs with anisotropic data.

DISCUSSION

The primary constraint on 3D MR is the necessity for rapid data acquisition. With the introduction of GRE techniques that allow rapid acquisition with a very short TR, 3D images can be obtained in reasonable scan times in a variety of ways with both T1- and T2-related contrast.[1–3] In conventional 2D MR, each slice is a separate and independent excitation volume with the pixels representing the projected sum of the signals through the entire section thickness. This leads to slice-to-slice interference that prevents obtaining contiguous cuts (see 1.1214-22), and limits thin-section capabilities resulting in partial voluming effects of small structures (see 1.1214-21).

In 3D MR, the third dimension becomes spatially phase encoded. When reconstructed, the sections or partitions uniquely represent true contiguity. Partition thicknesses can routinely be as thin as the in-plane dimensions of the pixels. Isotropic encoding yields voxels of

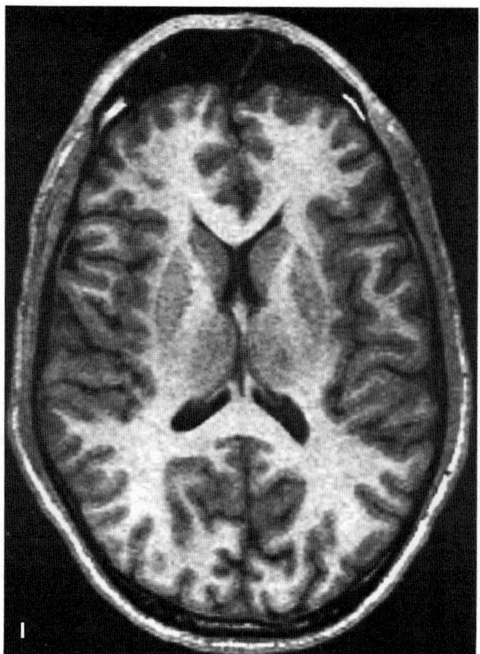

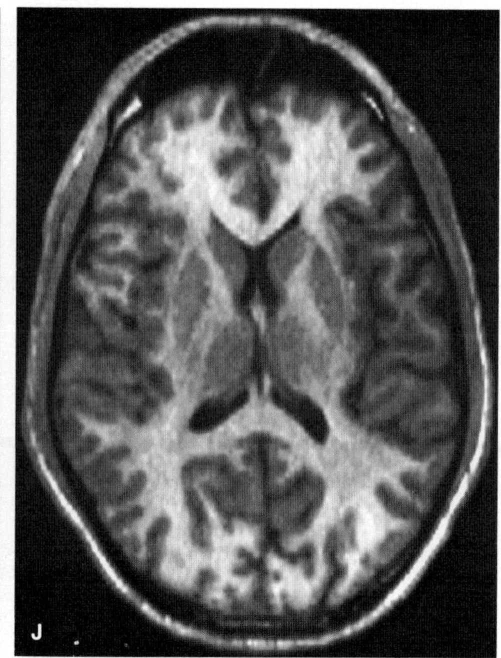

equal dimensions on all three sides and is primarily limited by S/N issues. To achieve reasonable imaging times, however, 3D MR requires a very short TR technique that generates good contrast and sufficient S/N. This restricts it to GRE methods using small RF flip angles (see 1.1214-6 to 1.1214-8), and therefore suffers the same potential artifacts as its 2D counterpart.

Because of its true contiguity and high resolution in the third dimension, 3D imaging allows MPR without a loss in spatial resolution from thick slices or poor image quality from information voids between sections. With the appropriate postprocessing capabilities, any plane through space can be visualized.[4–7] Free formatting of nonlinear planes can also be achieved with little difficulty. Partition averaging allows multiple sections to be combined which yields thicker slice representations for high S/N and superior image quality. Furthermore, volume and surface rendering of structures within the brain can be processed for 3D visualization.[5–7] These image processing capabilities may further aid in diagnosis as well as treatment and surgical planning.

Advantages

Three-dimensional imaging can provide true contiguous sections. Multiplanar reformatting in any plane and other postprocessing methods allow increased flexibility for visualization of structures at high resolution.

Disadvantages

Scan time requirements restrict 3D imaging techniques to short TR GRE methods (see 1.1214-6 to 1.1214-8), and may lead to artifacts not seen in 2D SE images.

Technical References

1. Frahm J, Haase A, Matthaei D. Rapid three-dimensional MR imaging using the FLASH technique. J Comput Assist Tomogr 1986;10:363–368.
2. Runge VM, Kirsch JE, Thomas GS, Mugler JP. Clinical comparison of three-dimensional MP-RAGE and FLASH techniques for MR imaging of the head. J Magn Reson Imaging 1991;1:493–500.
3. Menick BJ, Bobman SA, Listerud J, Atlas SW. Thin-section, three-dimensional fourier transform, steady-state free precession MR imaging of the brain. Radiology 1992;183:369–377.
4. Sherry CS, Harms SE, McCroskey WK. Spinal MR imaging: multiplanar representation from a single high resolution 3D acquisition. J Comput Assist Tomogr 1987;11:859–862.
5. Runge VM, Wood ML, Kaufman DM, et al. FLASH: clinical three-dimensional magnetic resonance imaging. Radiographics 1988;8:947–965.
6. Runge VM, Gelblum DY, Wood ML. 3-D imaging of the CNS. Neuroradiology 1990;32:356–366.
7. Bomans M, Hohne K-H, Laub G, et al. Improvement of 3D acquisition and visualization in MRI. Magn Reson Imaging 1991;9:597–609.

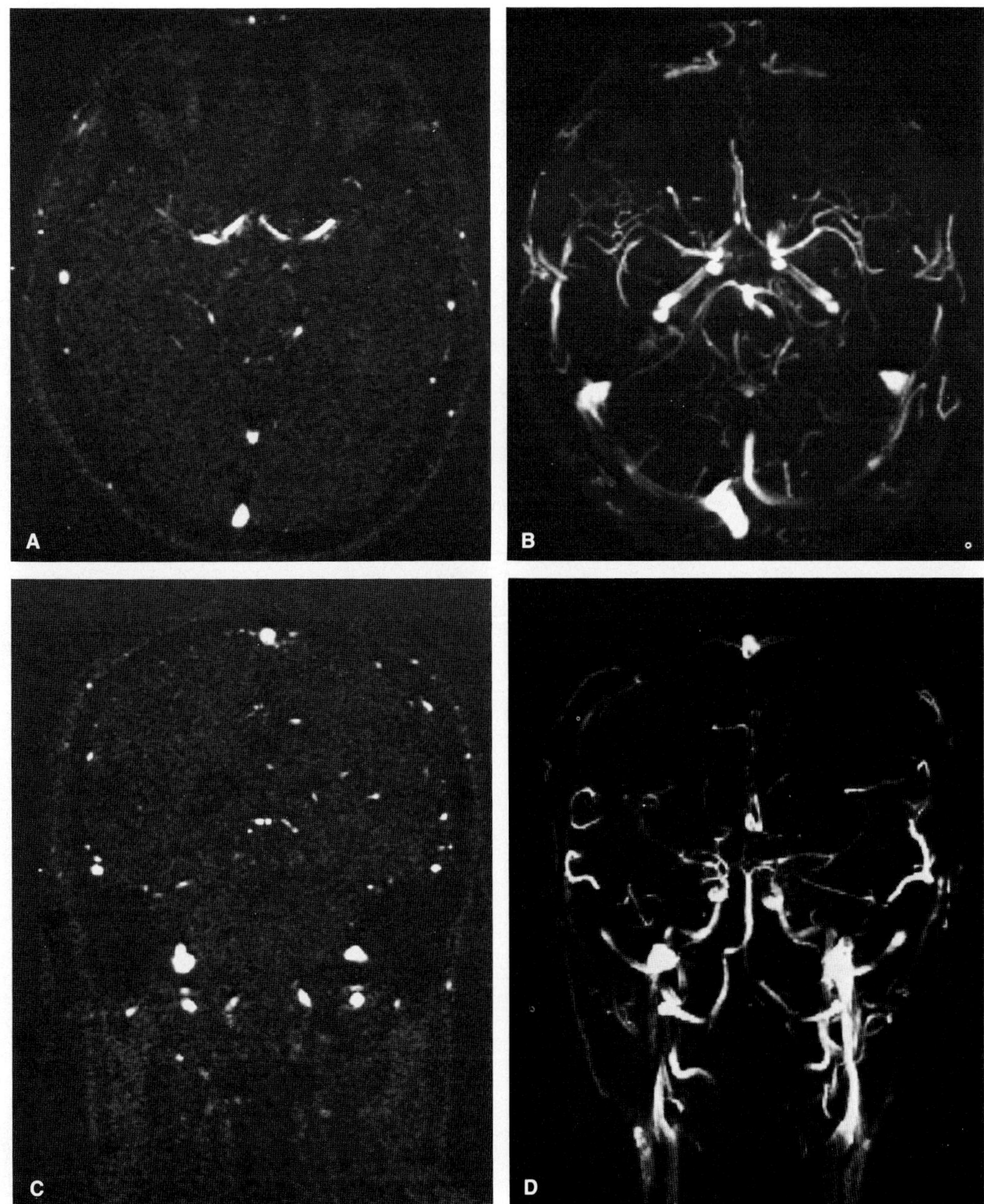

TECHNIQUE

Two-dimensional time-of-flight MR angiography, maximum intensity projection, and dependence on flow direction

FINDINGS

Fifty-five 2-mm 2D TOF MRA (TR/TE/FA=19/10/90°) slices of the circle of Willis were obtained with 1-mm overlap in the axial (*A*), coronal (*C*), and sagittal (*E*) orientations with corresponding MIPs (*B, D, and F,* respectively). Very high signal of through-plane vessels is observed with significant background tissue suppression yielding large contrast on the MIP displays. However, substantial loss of in-plane vessel structures is seen. Preferential flow and vessel depiction based on the direction of acquisition are shown on MIPs sagittally reformatted from coronal (*G*) and axial (*H*) acquisitions. Anterior/posterior vessel preference is seen in *G,* while inferior/superior preference is observed in *H.* By combining all three directions of acquisitions, no directionality is observed (*I*). However, this is only true in the volume that

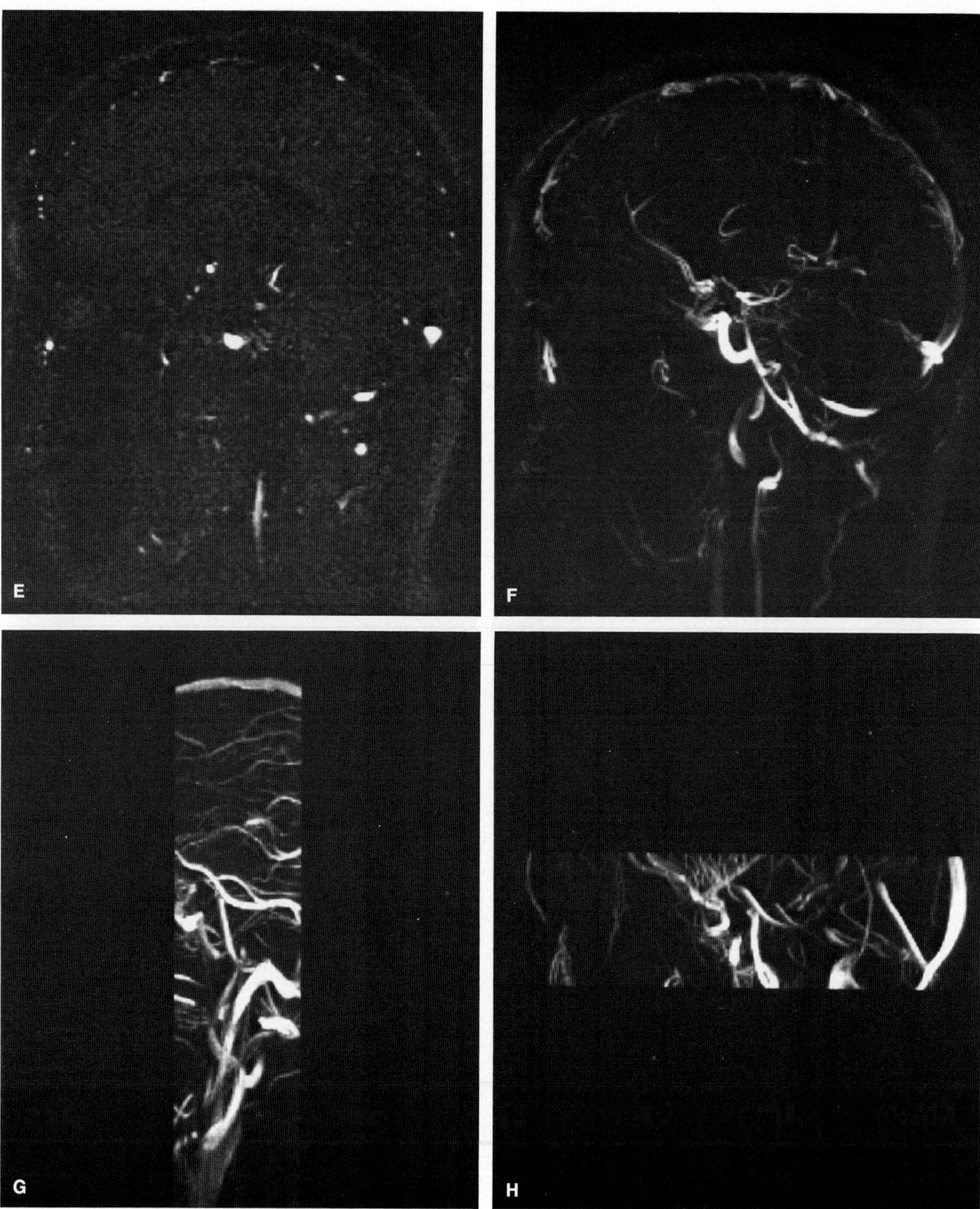

contains all three data sets as seen by the abrupt vessel voids (*arrows*) at acquisition boundaries (*J*).

CONCLUSION

Two-dimensional TOF MRA provides good visualization of vascular structures with MIP displays, but primarily of vessels perpendicular to the acquisition plane.

DISCUSSION

MRA is rapidly becoming a useful method for visualizing intracranial vasculature. Many MRA techniques exist but are all primarily variants of two distinct ways of detecting flow. Phase-contrast MRA (see 1.1214-12 and 1.1214-13) relies on the signal phase difference for vessel contrast between stationary and moving tissues. Contrast based on the signal amplitude difference between flowing blood and stationary tissue is the basis for TOF MRA.

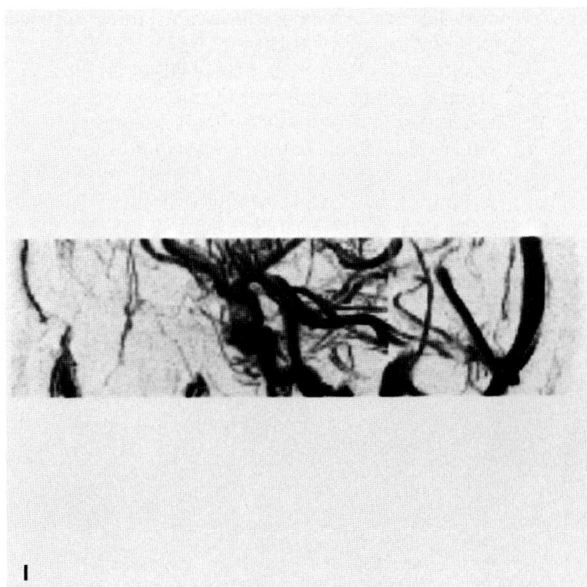

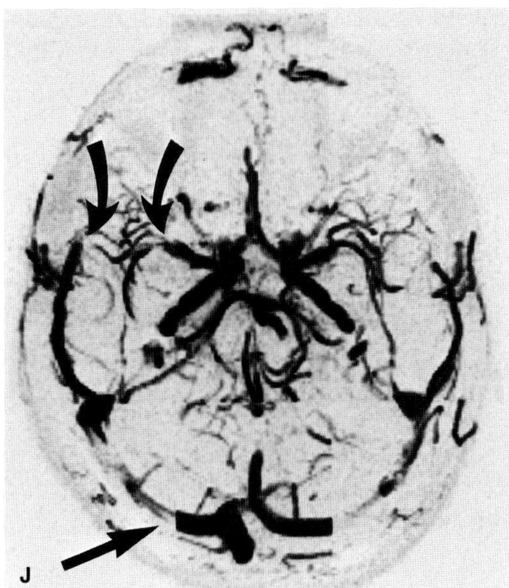

Contemporary TOF MRA relies on the inflow of blood into the imaging volume to enhance the signal in vessels relative to the background.[1] Conventional GRE techniques (see 1.1214-6 and 1.1214-7) are used with gradient moment nulling to minimize motion artifacts from flowing blood (see 1.1214-29). If a very short TR is used, stationary tissue signals become suppressed or saturated, experiencing a steady state of RF pulsing. "Fresh" unsaturated blood flowing into the 2D slice or 3D slab has not been exposed to the RF pulse and therefore generates signal as if it were based on an infinitely long TR.

Obtaining optimum vessel contrast in TOF MRA is not straightforward, ultimately depending on how long the blood resides in the imaging volume and how many times it becomes excited by RF. Factors that influence the contrast are physiologic parameters such as blood flow velocity, vessel directionality, and blood transit time in the imaging volume; measurement parameters such as technique, RF flip angle, slice or slab thickness, slice orientation, and TR; and relaxation parameters, T1 and T2, for blood and the background tissues.[1]

Two-dimensional TOF MRA has several advantages over 3D methodology (see 1.1214-11). It is typically faster, since individual slice selection allows the flexibility to target the region of study. Individual slices may also be preceded by presaturation pulses (see 1.1214-31) to selectively void the inflowing arterial or venous blood.[2,3] By using very thin slices, 2D methods can ensure that even slow-flowing blood has a relatively short transit time in the excitation volume providing high vessel contrast.[2–6]

With very short TR and a high RF flip angle, contrast is large and can exceed 3D capabilities. However, if vessels traverse laterally so that they remain within the slice, signal from blood becomes saturated and is quickly lost. This inherent directionality makes 2D TOF MRA less useful in the brain where vessels are tortuous and multidirectional, but valuable for carotid[4,5] and general body angiography.[6] Nevertheless, if 2D TOF MRA data sets are acquired in all three directions from a targeted region and subsequently combined, then most vessels can become well visualized regardless of their direction.

MIP is the most common way to postprocess MRA data for displaying complete vascular structures (see 1.1214-11). Although in-plane spatial resolution is high with 2D TOF MRA, it is limited in the slice direction. MIPs across a stack of slices typically show poor resolution since thicknesses of less than 1 mm are difficult to achieve. Furthermore, 2D slices are obtained sequentially in time, which leads to discrete breaks or shifts in vascular structures on an MIP display because of pulsatile or bulk motion.

Advantages

Thin-section 2D TOF MRA allows better vessel contrast, slow-flow visualization, and background suppression than 3D imaging (see 1.1214-11). Selective slice placement enables small-volume MRA in reduced scan times. MIP processing provides enhanced visualization of complete vascular structures.

Disadvantages

Two-dimensional TOF MRA provides mainly visualization of vessels perpendicular to the imaging plane with absence of lateral vascular branching. Spatial resolution in the slice direction is typically compromised on MIP displays.

Technical References

1. Ruggieri PM, Laub GA, Masaryk TJ, Modic MT. Intracranial circulation: pulse-sequence considerations in three-dimensional (volume) MR angiography. Radiology 1989;171:785–791.
2. Keller PJ, Drayer BP, Fram EK, et al. MR angiography with two-dimensional acquisition and three-dimensional display. Radiology 1989;173:527–532.
3. Edelman RR, Wentz KU, Mattle HP, et al. Intracerebral arteriovenous malformations: evaluation with selective MR angiography and venography. Radiology 1989;173:831–837.
4. Litt AW, Eidelman EM, Pinto RS, et al. Diagnosis of carotid artery stenosis: comparison of 2DFT time-of-flight MR angiography with contrast angiography in 50 patients. Am J Neuroradiol 1991;12:149–154.
5. Heiserman JE, Drayer BP, Fram EK, et al. Carotid artery stenosis: clinical efficacy of two-dimensional time-of-flight MR angiography. Radiology 1992;182:761–768.
6. Finn JP, Goldmann A, Edelman RR. Magnetic resonance angiography in the body. Magn Reson Q 1992;8:1–22.

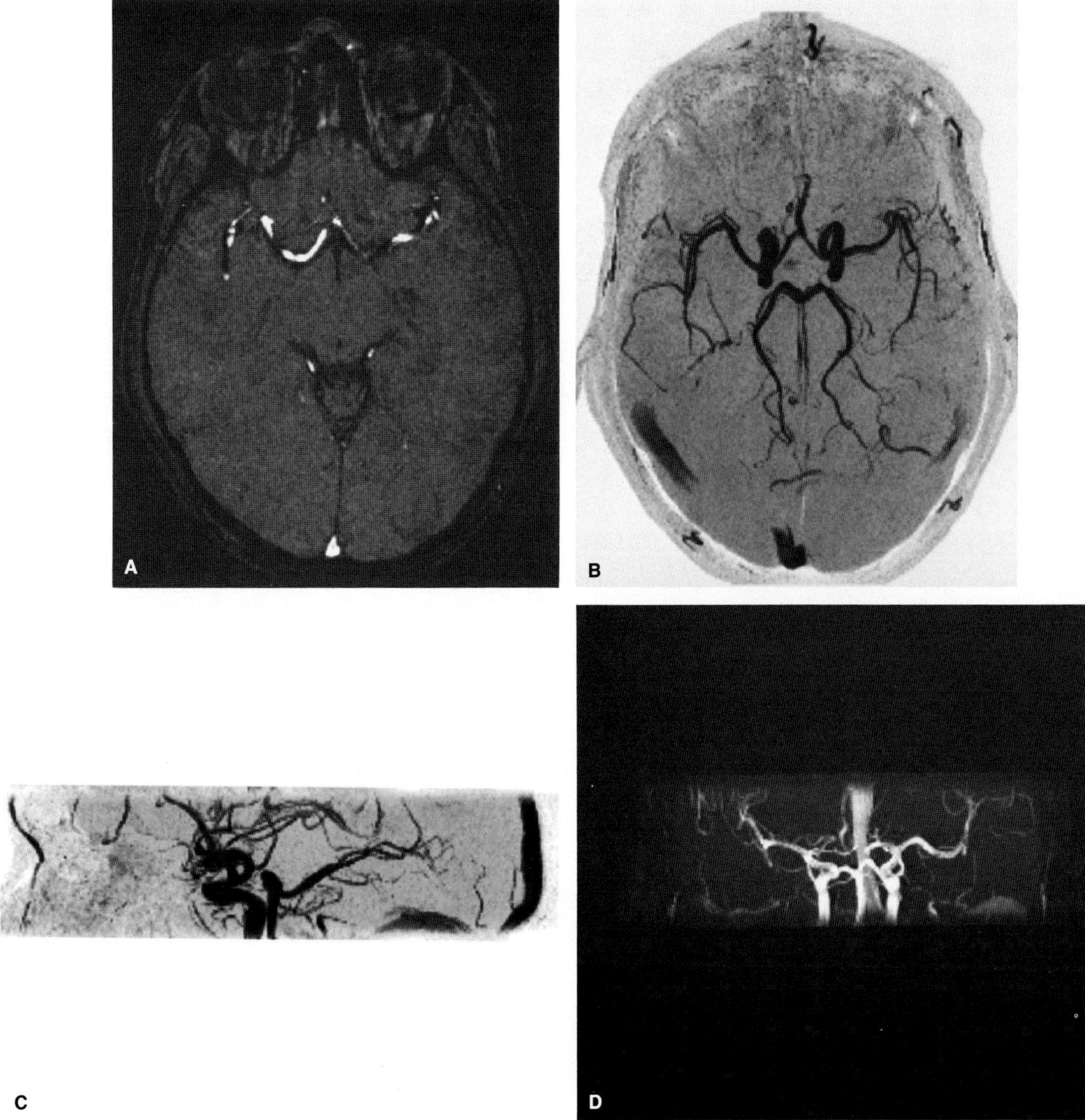

TECHNIQUE

Three-dimensional time-of-flight MR angiography, maximum intensity projection, and dependence on RF flip angle

FINDINGS

Sixty-four 3D TOF MRA partitions of the circle of Willis were acquired isotropically (0.8 × 0.8 × 0.8 mm) in the axial orientation with a rephased GRE technique (TR/TE/FA = 30/7/20°). (*A*) Individual partitions show moderate background tissue suppression with high vessel signal from inflow effects. MIPs of the axial (*B*) and sagittal (*C*) views show good delineation of primary and secondary vascular structures. (*D*) A complete coronal MIP demonstrates a large degree of vessel overlap that obscures details. Targeted MIPs of the carotid and middle cerebral arteries (*E*) eliminate overlap from the superior sagittal sinus (*F*). Structures such as the vertebral and basilar arteries (*G*) can also be isolated with targeted MIPs (*H*). Vessel contrast and depth penetration depend on RF flip angle as shown in sagittal MIPs acquired at 10° (*I*), 20° (*J*), 40° (*K*), and 80° (*L*). Higher contrast occurs at a larger flip angle, but depth penetration of inflow effects becomes less.

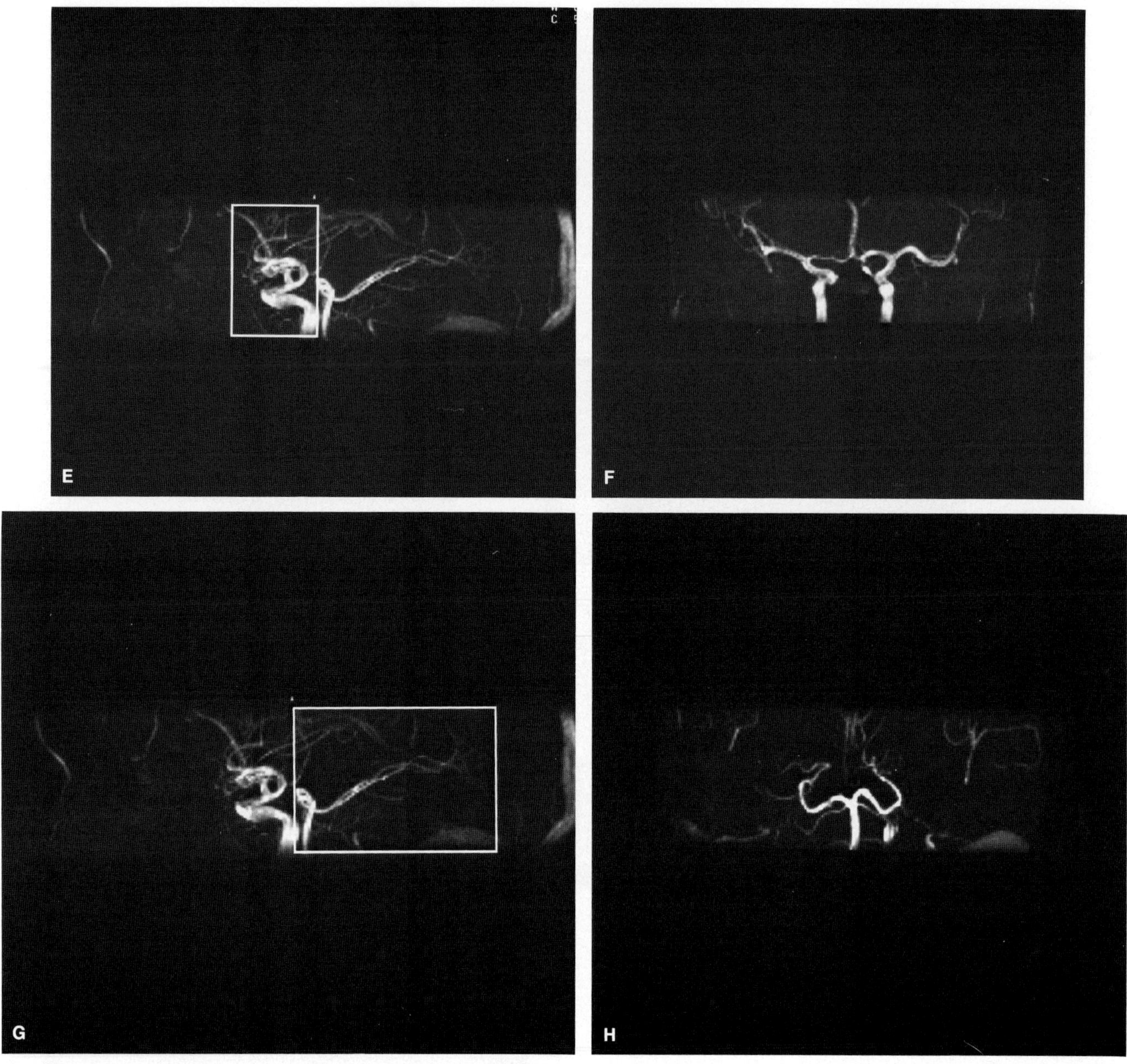

CONCLUSION

Three-dimensional TOF MRA provides good visualization of vascular structures in all directions using MIP and targeted MIP displays, using the optimal RF flip angle for greatest depth penetration and stationary signal suppression.

DISCUSSION

Three-dimensional TOF MRA is gaining acceptance as an MR method of choice to visualize intracranial vasculature.[1–3] In its contemporary form, it employs the principles of inflow and saturation effects to enhance the contrast between stationary tissues and moving blood. By combining conventional GRE techniques (see 1.1214-6 and 1.1214-7), 3D acquisition (see 1.1214-9), and gradient moment nulling (see 1.1214-29), tissue signal becomes suppressed with steady-state RF pulsing while inflowing "fresh" blood generates a high signal. These same TOF effects are used in 2D TOF MRA as well (see 1.1214-10).

The primary difference between 2D and 3D methods is the size of the excitation volume. Obtaining optimal vessel contrast in TOF MRA ultimately depends on how long the blood resides in the imaging volume and how many times it becomes excited by RF pulsing. Whereas in 2D the volume is a thin slice, 3D uses a comparatively

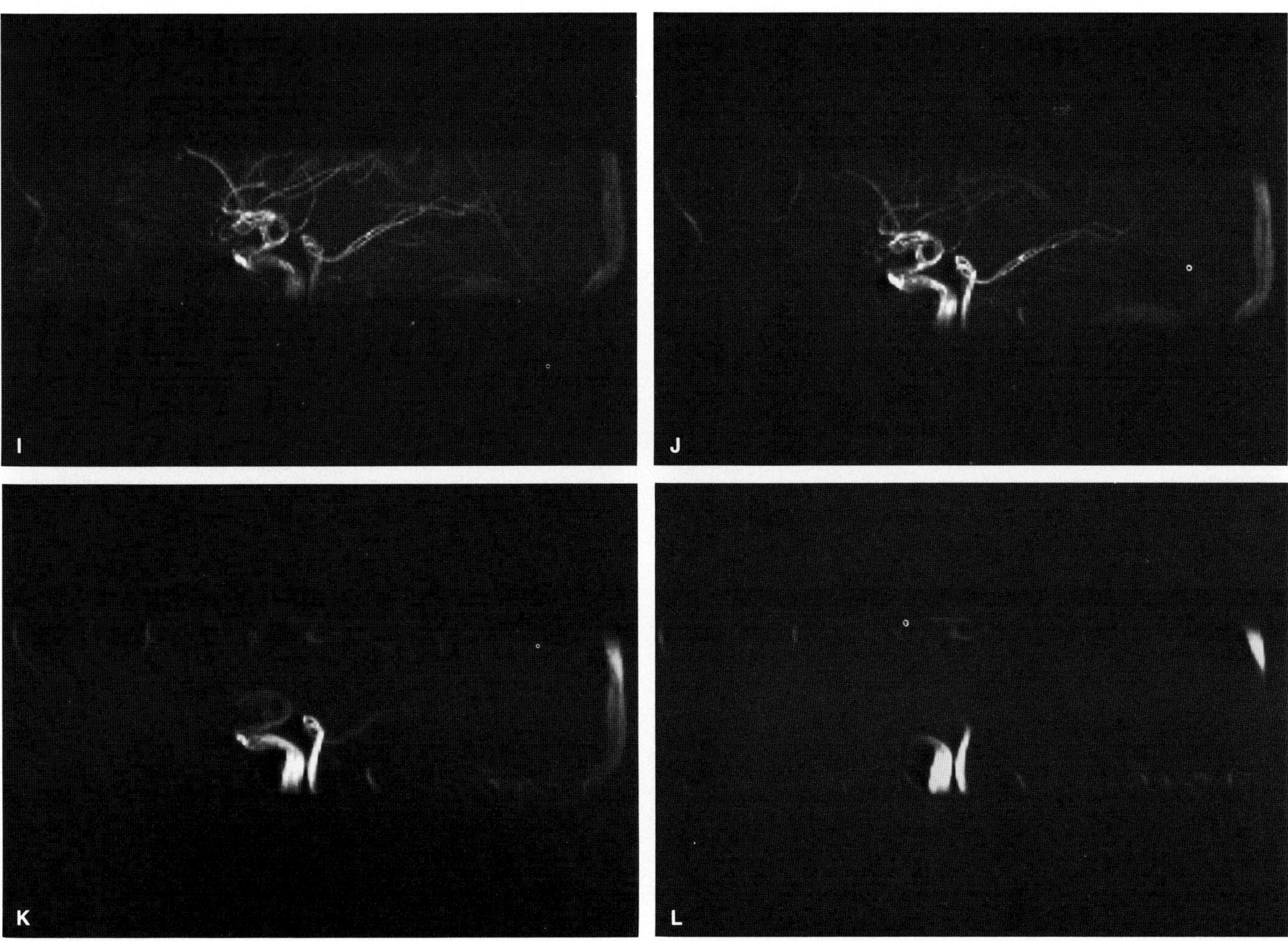

large slab that is spatially encoded in the third dimension, making vessel depth penetration a concern even with fast flow.

Large RF flip angles generate a large signal from blood at the immediate entry into the volume, which rapidly decreases as it penetrates the volume because of multiple RF excitations and approach to a suppressed steady state. As the flip angle is decreased, more RF excitations are required to reach a steady state resulting in better depth penetration. This yields better visualization of peripheral vessels, but the overall contrast is less than the entry signal at a large flip angle. If the flip angle is too small, the penetration may be greatest but the general contrast and S/N become insufficient. Therefore, for a given region of interest and slab thickness, good 3D TOF MRA requires careful selection of RF flip angle in conjunction with TR.[1,3]

The goal in angiography is to visualize vessels, and enhancing contrast in the acquisition between blood and stationary tissue is only part of the solution. A single partition image showing bright intensity in the vessel lumen makes it difficult to evaluate. MIP is a postprocessing method that creates projected 2D angiographic views through any rotation.[4]

MIP displays are created by "ray tracing" through a stacking of 2D slices or a 3D data set. This is done along a given direction through the data by projecting each ray as a pixel from the point of maximum intensity along the ray. The MIP image represents all the points of maximum intensity from the entire 3D data set at a given projected perspective. If blood yields the brightest signal in the acquisition, the MIP view displays primarily the vascular structures. *Targeted MIP* enables specific vessels within the acquisition volume to be depicted without overlap from surrounding vessels, and also reduces MIP-related artifacts such as vessel reduction caused by background variance.[5] Additionally, since the digital data represent a cube of information, oblique angle MIP displays may lose apparent spatial resolution.

TOF MR angiography has difficulty in certain situations. Regions of turbulence and higher order motion, such as at bifurcations, can result in regional vascular signal voids owing to insufficient moment nulling. Large velocity gradients at lumen walls typically result in overestimation of stenoses. Furthermore, very slow flow, in giant aneurysms, for example, is difficult to visualize with 3D TOF MRA since it closely resembles the static state of surrounding tissues and may be better seen with 2D TOF (see 1.1214-10) or phrase-contrast MRA (see 1.1214-12 and 1.1214-13).

Advantages

Three-dimensional TOF MRA provides greater vessel visualization in all directions and no vessel loss with lateral flow compared with 2D TOF MRA (see 1.1214-10). High isotropic spatial resolution is possible. MIP processing provides enhanced visualization of complete vascular structures.

Disadvantages

Three-dimensional TOF MRA produces less contrast and background suppression, and typically requires longer scan times than 2D TOF MRA. Slow flow is difficult to depict. Turbulent flow may cause vessel signal voids.

Technical References

1. Ruggieri PM, Laub GA, Masaryk TJ, Modic MT. Intracranial circulation: pulse-sequence considerations in three-dimensional (volume) MR angiography. Radiology 1989;171:785–791.
2. Masaryk TJ, Modic MT, Ross JS, et al. Intracranial circulation: preliminary clinical results with three-dimensional (volume) MR angiography. Radiology 1989;171:793–799.
3. Marchal G, Bosmans H, Van Fraeyenhoven L, et al. Intracranial vascular lesions: optimization and clinical evaluation of three-dimensional time-of-flight MR angiography. Radiology 1990;175:443–448.
4. Laub G. Dispays for MR angiography. Magn Reson Med 1990;14:222–229.
5. Anderson CM, Saloner D, Tsuruda JS, et al. Artifacts in maximum-intensity-projection display of MR angiograms. AJR 1990;154:623–629.

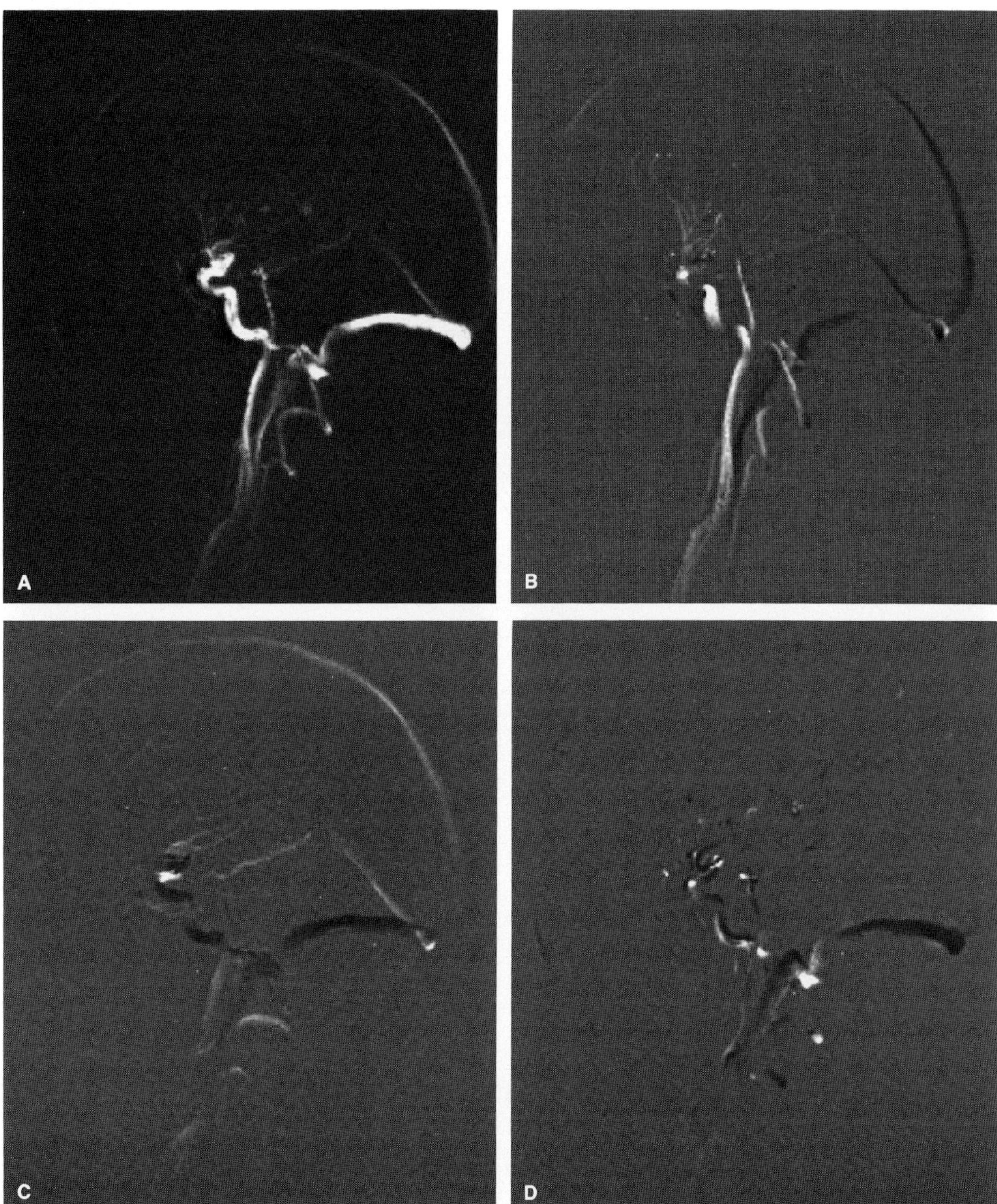

TECHNIQUE

Two-dimensional phase-contrast MR angiography, maximum intensity projection, and dependence on flow direction

FINDINGS

Sagittal (*A to D*) and coronal (*E to H*) 2D PC MRA (TR/TE/FA=30/12/20°) were acquired with a velocity encoding of 50 cm/s in all three directions. Magnitude MIPs (*A and E*) show near complete background tissue suppression and good visualization of major arterial and venous structures. Top/bottom (*B and F*), left/right (*C and G*), and in/out (*D and H*) flow is also depicted with directional "signed" MIP displays. Black vessels indicate one direction of flow, while white vessels indicate the opposite direction. The vessel pixel intensities are proportional to the average blood flow velocity.

CONCLUSION

Two-dimensional PC MRA provides good visualization of major vascular structures with velocity and direction information.

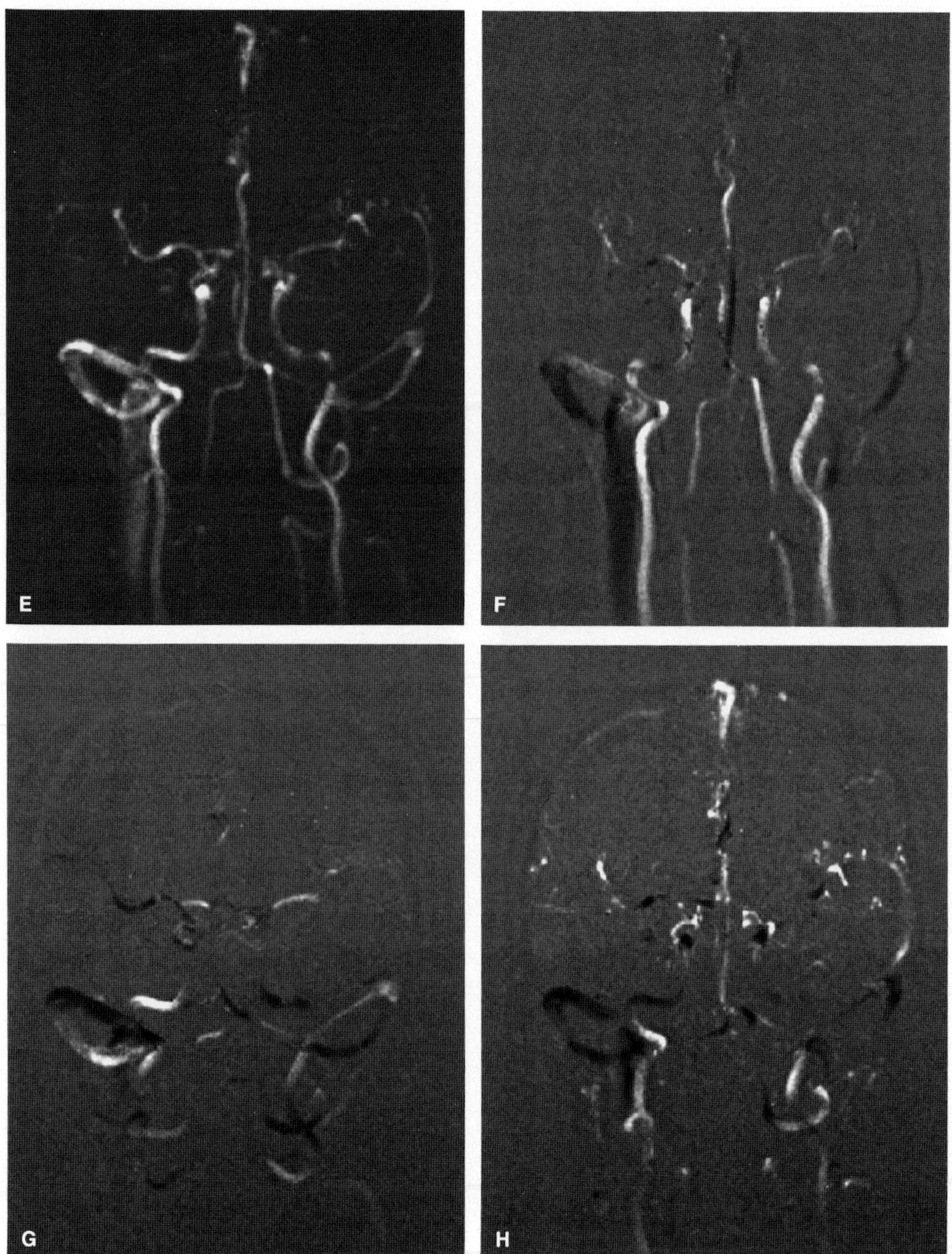

DISCUSSION

Many MRA techniques have been developed but all are primarily variants of two distinct ways of detecting flow. Contrast based on the signal amplitude difference between flowing blood and stationary tissue is the basis for TOF MRA (see 1.1214-10 and 1.1214-11). PC MRA relies on the signal phase difference for vessel contrast between stationary and moving tissues. Both methods have advantages and limitations in their ability to demonstrate vascular abnormalities.[1]

During the application of a field gradient, normally used to spatially encode the MR signal, spins from moving tissue such as blood undergo a signal phase deviation from stationary tissue. This phase difference becomes a signature of the velocity magnitude and direction. MR typically displays a magnitude or "modulus" image while discarding the mapping of the signal phase. If two phase images are subtracted, one that is a reference phase map and another that is "velocity encoded," the resulting phase-difference image corresponds only to the moving blood since no phase change has occurred in stationary tissue. Several methods are used to display a detected change; however, they all generate phase contrast in the image based on the phase deviations that exist from moving blood.[2]

Since velocity encoding occurs only when the motion is in the direction of the applied gradient, PC MRA must obtain at least four data sets to depict flow in all three directions, one for each direction that is velocity encoded and a fourth as a reference. Although this requires a significantly longer scan time than TOF MRA, it also contains unique quantitative information about the magnitude and direction of blood flow velocity. PC MRA can therefore display the vessels using MIP methods (see 1.1214-11), or it can selectively map the velocity and direction of the flow within the vasculature using "signed" MIPs. Unlike standard MIP displays, a "signed" MIP depicts a positive pixel intensity as velocity in one direction and negative pixel intensity as velocity in the other direction. The actual pixel value is directly proportional to the velocity itself.

Two-dimensional PC MRA has several advantages over 3D applications (see 1.1214-13). It is typically faster, since individual slice selection allows the flexibility to target the region of study or orient the projection of a thick section.[2–4] If flow is primarily unidirectional such as with the carotid arteries, scan time can be further reduced by velocity encoding only in the primary direction of the flow. Similar to 2D TOF techniques (see 1.1214-10), however, acquiring individual slices typically compromises the spatial resolution in the third dimension, and sequential slice acquisitions can yield discrete breaks or shifts in vascular structures on an MIP display owing to pulsatile or bulk motion. Time-resolved single-slice 2D PC analysis offers the capability of visualizing quantitative flow behavior and cine imaging, but its primary use has been in cardiac applications[4] or individual vessel evaluation.[5]

Advantages

PC MRA uniquely enables visualization of the velocity and direction of blood flow not possible in TOF MRA (see 1.1214-10 and 1.1214-11). Selective slice placement with 2D PC allows small-volume MRA in reduced scan times. MIP or "signed" MIP processing provides enhanced visualization of complete vascular structures and velocity information.

Disadvantages

Two-dimensional PC MRA provides primarily visualization of larger vessels. Spatial resolution in the slice direction is typically compromised on MIP displays. Artifacts of discrete vessel breaks or shifts due to pulsatile or bulk motion may occur.

Technical References

1. Huston J, Rufenacht DA, Ehman RL, Wiebers DO. Intracranial aneurysms and vascular malformations: comparison of time-of-flight and phase-contrast MR angiography. Radiology 1991;181:721–730.
2. Dumoulin CL, Hart HR. Magnetic resonance angiography. Radiology 1986;161:717–720.
3. Tsuruda JS, Shimakawa A, Pelc NJ, Saloner D. Dural sinus occlusion: evaluation with phase-sensitive gradient-echo MR imaging. Am J Neuroradiol 1991;12:481–488.
4. Pelc NJ, Herfkens RJ, Shimakawa A, Enzmann DR. Phase contrast cine magnetic resonance imaging. Magn Reson Q 1991;7:229–254.
5. Marks MP, Pelc NJ, Ross MR, Enzmann DR. Determination of cerebral blood flow with a phase-contrast cine MR imaging technique: evaluation of normal subjects and patients with arteriovenous malformations. Radiology 1992;182:467–476.

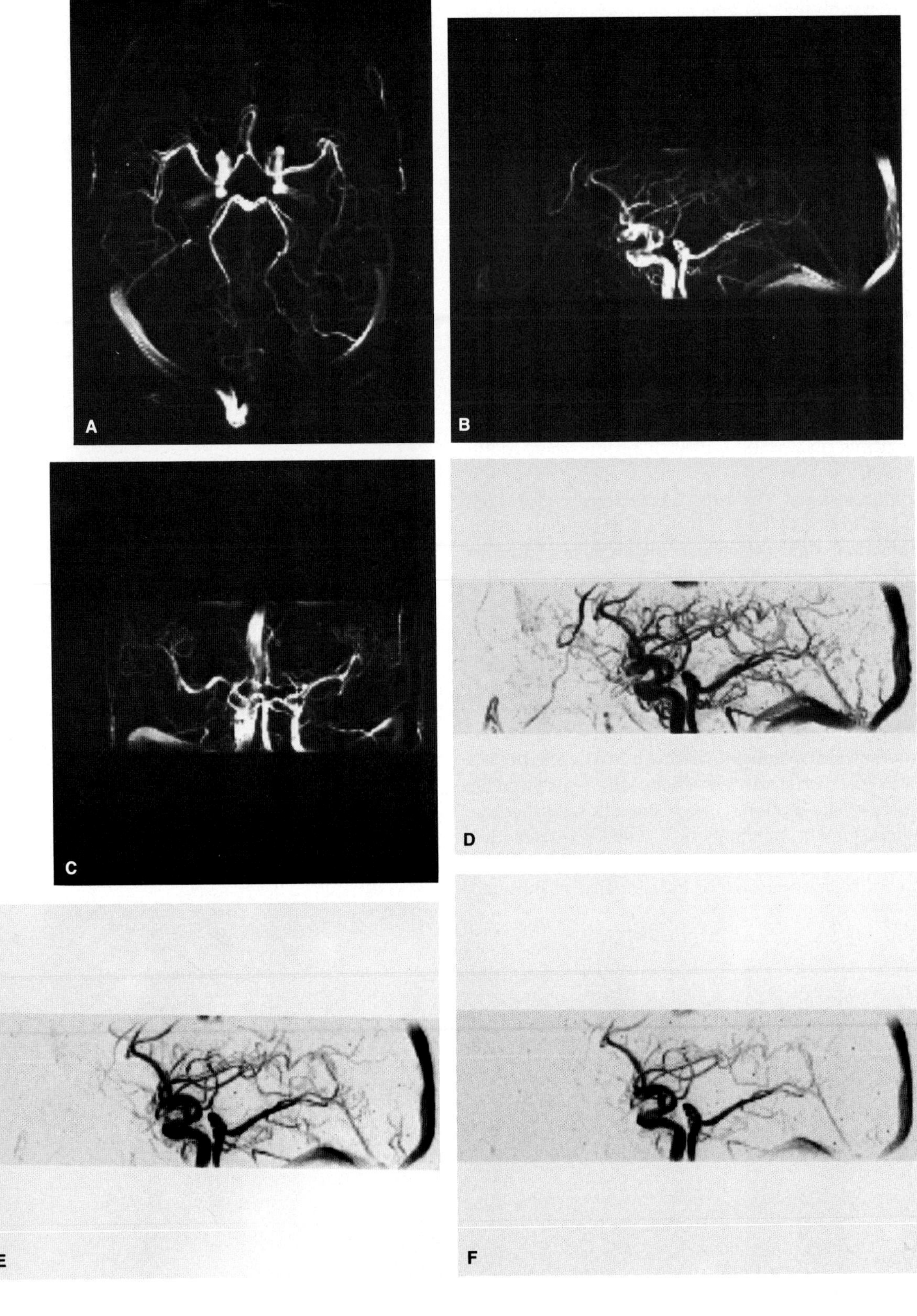
A
B
C
D
E
F

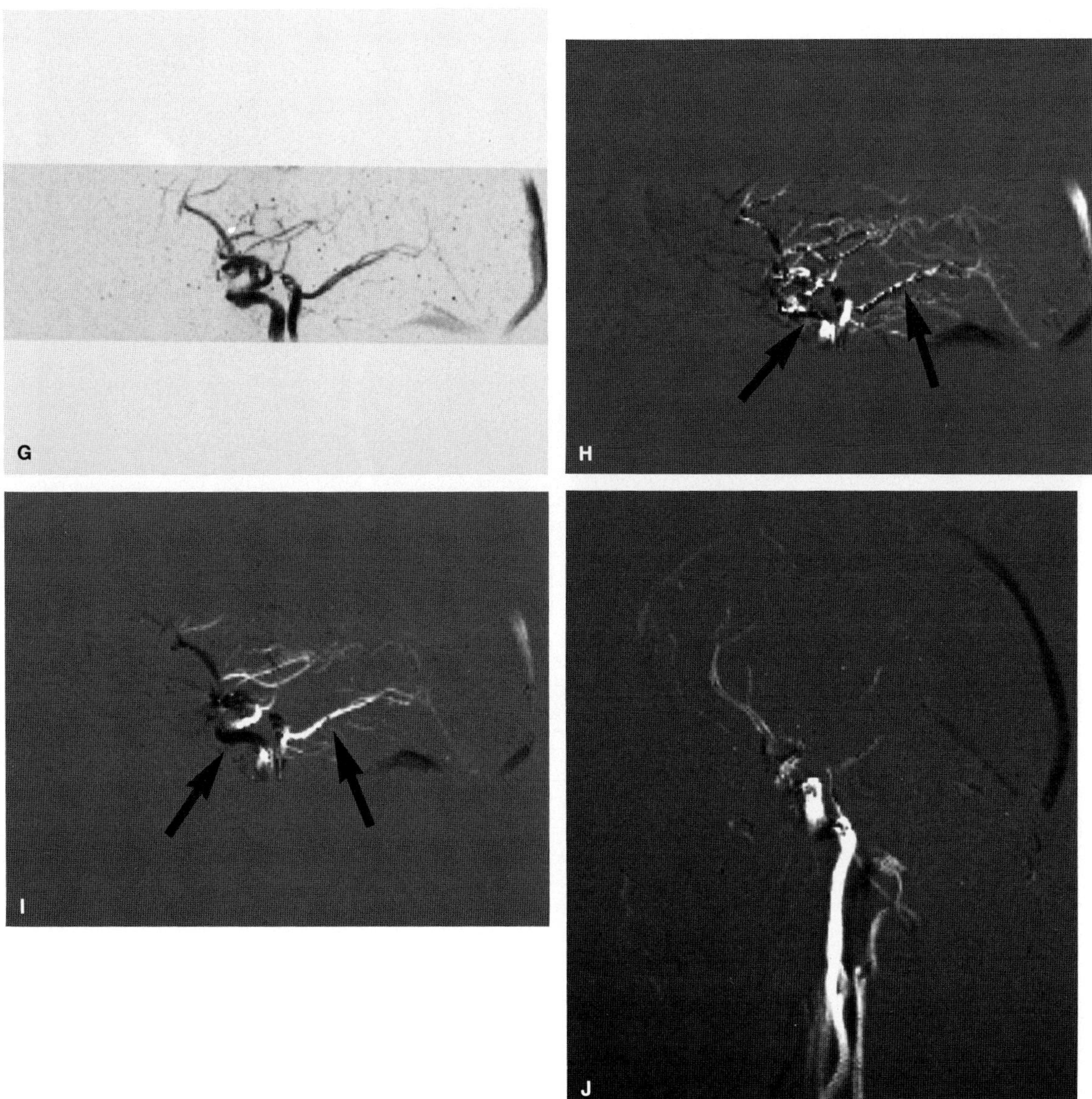

TECHNIQUE

Three-dimensional phase-contrast MR angiography, maximum intensity projection, and dependence on velocity encoding

FINDINGS

Sixty-four axial 3D PC MRA partitions (TR/TE/FA = 20/12/20°) were acquired with 15 cm/s velocity encoding in all three directions and 1 × 1 × 1 mm resolution. Axial (*A*), sagittal (*B*), and coronal (*C*) magnitude MIPs show near complete background tissue suppression and good visualization of primary and secondary arterial and venous structures. Vessel contrast and delineation decrease significantly with the degree of velocity encoding as demonstrated in sagittal MIPs at 15 (*D*), 30 (*E*), 50 (*F*), and 100 cm/s (*G*). However, directional "signed" MIP representations at 15 cm/s (*not shown*) and 30 cm/s (*H*) show severe phase aliasing of high velocity flow not seen at 50 cm/s (*I*) making interpretation difficult (*arrows*). "Signed" MIPs of sagittal (*J and K*) and coronal (*L and M*) 3D PC MRA partitions at 50 cm/s velocity encoding depict directional flow information. Inferior/superior arterial flow is shown as white pixels (*J and L*) with black pixels representing the reverse direction. Directionality is also demonstrated anterior/posterior (*K*), and left/right (*M*).

CONCLUSION

Improved vascular depiction with magnitude MIPs is obtained using slower-flow velocity encoding in 3D PC

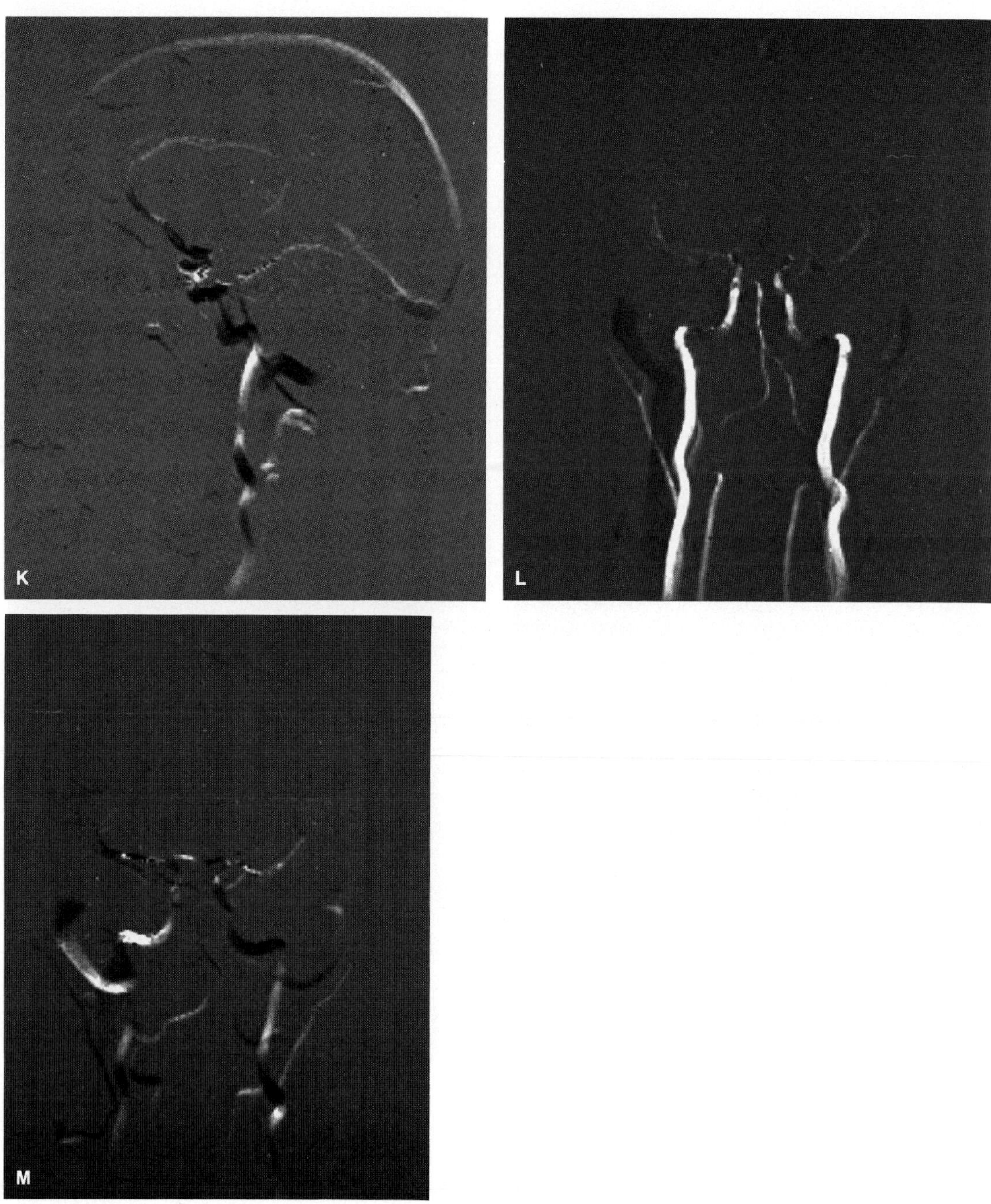

MRA. Directional velocity information without phase aliasing with "signed" MIPs is achieved using faster-flow velocity encoding.

DISCUSSION

Three-dimensional PC MRA[1] offers a unique wealth of vascular flow information not possible with TOF techniques (see 1.1214-10 and 1.1214-11) at high spatial resolution in all directions which is difficult to achieve with 2D PC MRA (see 1.1214-12). Phase-contrast imaging relies on the signal phase difference between stationary and moving tissues for vessel contrast. During an applied gradient field the signal phase from blood becomes "encoded" with information about its velocity. The phase differences are then mapped in the image between −180° and 180°, which are the limits associated with a particular velocity that is defined as the "velocity encoding" of the acquisition.

Since velocity encoding occurs only when the motion is in the direction of the applied gradient, it requires at least four data sets to depict flow in all three directions (see 1.1214-12). Although this leads to a significantly longer scan time than 3D TOF MRA (see 1.1214-11), it contains unique quantitative information about the magnitude and direction of blood flow velocity not attainable by TOF techniques.

Vascular structures are typically displayed using MIP methods (see 1.1214-11). However, phase-contrast methods can also selectively map the velocity and direction of the flow within the vasculature using "signed" MIPs, which depict positive pixel intensities as velocity in one direction and negative pixel intensities as velocity in the other direction (see 1.1214-12). The actual pixel value is directly proportional to the velocity. More sophisticated methods that determine flow streamlines within vessels, for example, have also been developed.[2]

The degree of velocity encoding is crucial to achieve high vascular contrast or to obtain useful velocity information.[3,4] Slow flow from secondary peripheral vessels or giant aneurysms is best visualized with PC techniques, but it requires a level of velocity encoding such that its resulting phase differences are significant. This, however, may accentuate pulsatile and bulk motion artifacts from faster flow unless electrocardiographic (ECG) gating is used. Furthermore, quantitative velocity information from fast flow becomes aliased and is lost if the measured phase difference exceeds the range of $-180°$ to $180°$.[5] Phase angles beyond this range from fast flow cannot be uniquely represented, and false aliased values become displayed in the signed MIP. Fast-flow velocity encoding retains unaliased velocity information but details in slow flow regions become lost as a result of insufficient phase contrast.

Three-dimensional PC MRA offers high vessel contrast, good visualization of slow flow, inherently little or no background, and the unique ability to quantitatively evaluate flow behavior if desired. However, such advantages may be overridden in favor of 3D TOF MRA (see 1.1214-11) because of lengthy scan times. Recent evaluations, nevertheless, indicate that both techniques may be useful in differing situations.[3]

Advantages

PC MRA uniquely enables visualization of the velocity and direction of blood flow not possible in TOF MRA (see 1.1214-10 and 1.1214-11). 3D PC MRA allows high spatial resolution in all directions and provides superior depiction of peripheral vessels with little or no background from stationary tissue. MIP or "signed" MIP processing provides enhanced visualization of complete vascular structures and velocity information.

Disadvantages

Three-dimensional PC MRA requires long scan times. Accentuated artifacts due to pulsatile or bulk motion may occur with high velocity encoding. PC MRA cannot selectively isolate venous or arterial flow.

Technical References

1. Dumoulin CL, Souza SP, Walker MF, Wagle W. Three-dimensional phase contrast angiography. Magn Reson Med 1989; 9:139–149.
2. Napel S, Lee DH, Frayne R, Rutt BK. Visualizing three-dimensional flow with simulated streamlines and three-dimensional phase-contrast MR imaging. J Magn Reson Imaging 1992;2:143–153.
3. Huston J, Rufenacht DA, Ehman RL, Wiebers DO. Intracranial aneurysms and vascular malformations: comparison of time-of-flight and phase-contrast MR angiography. Radiology 1991;181:721–730.
4. Pernicone JR, Siebert JE, Potchen EJ, et al. Three-dimensional phase-contrast MR angiography in the head and neck: preliminary report. Am J Neuroradiol 1990;11:457–466.
5. Axel L, Morton D. Correction of phase wrapping in magnetic resonance imaging. Med Phys 1989;16:284–287.

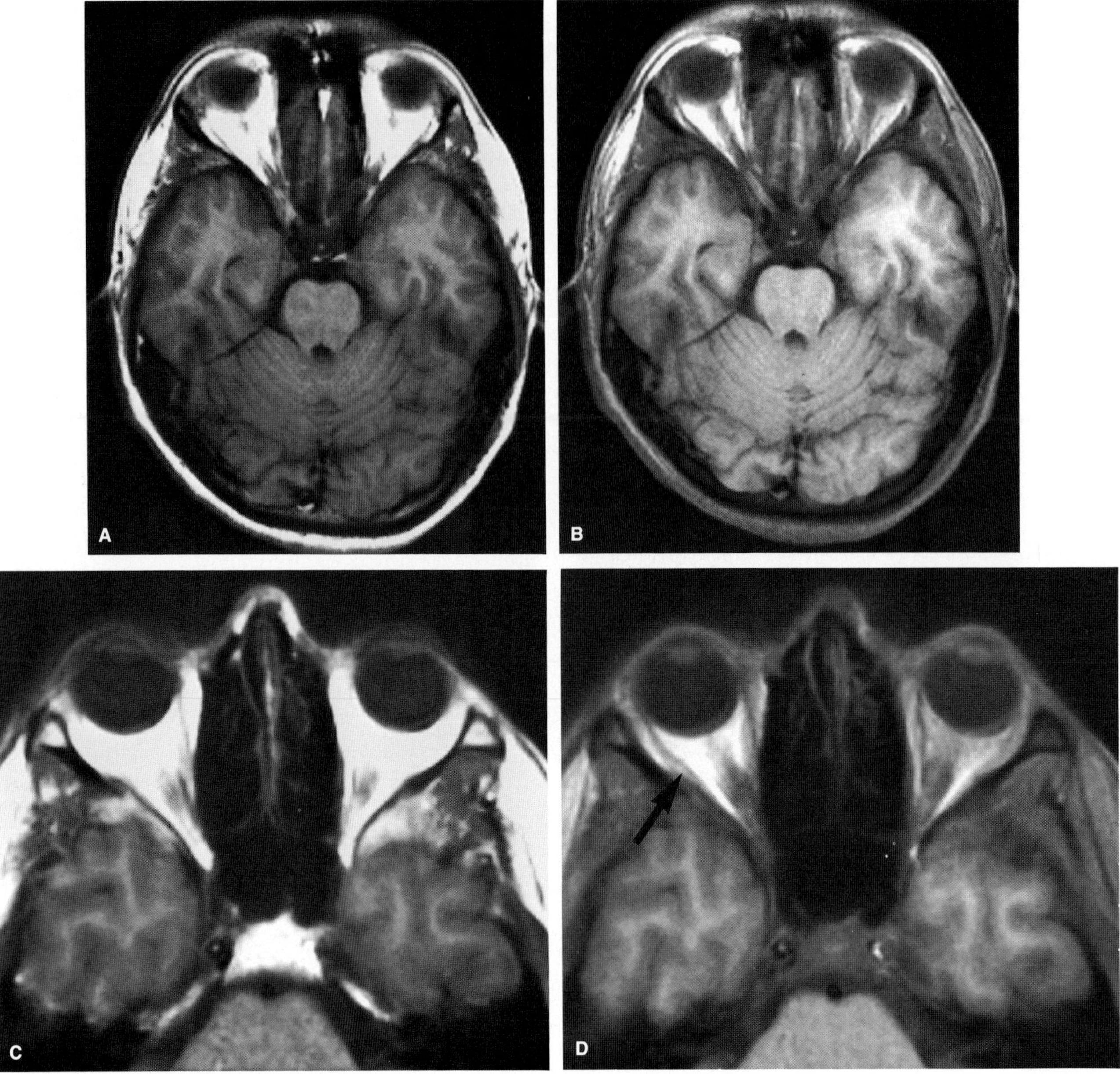

TECHNIQUE

Fat suppression by spectral saturation with the spin echo technique

FINDINGS

Similar contrast is demonstrated in regions devoid of fat on axial T1-weighted SE images (TR/TE = 500/15) without (*A and C*) and with (*B and D*) spectral fat suppression. Gray and white matter contrast remains similar with significant reduction in fat signal, particularly in the region of the optic nerve and pituitary gland. However, regional variations in the degree of suppression are clearly seen in *D* as a result of the sensitivity of the technique to magnetic field inhomogeneities (*arrow*).

CONCLUSION

Effective fat suppression by spectral saturation of fat signal is achieved; however, there are varying degrees of regional suppression.

DISCUSSION

MR possesses the ability to selectively isolate and image fatty tissues or water because of the fundamental differences between their NMR properties. Not only are their T1 and T2 values substantially different, but their inherent Larmor precessional frequencies are also different because of their chemical (spectral) shifts. Fat and water suppression techniques can offer enhanced diagnostic capabilities. Aside from providing fundamental information about the chemical nature of the tissue, they can allow increased visualization of structures otherwise obscured by fat, such as in the region of the orbits, and can aid in differentiating between fat and contrast-enhanced regions by suppressing the bright signal of fat.

Numerous techniques for suppressing fat or water have been developed.[1] All have met with varying degrees of success. Chemical shift selective (CHESS), frequency selective, or spectral saturation exploits the slight differences in the Larmor frequencies of fat and water and directly saturates the signal of either by applying a presaturation pulse prior to the imaging pulsing.[2–4] This can be incorporated into any technique and is similar to spatial presaturation (see 1.1214-30 and 1.1214-31), differing only in the fact that one is a spatial technique and the other is spectral.

This method of selective saturation, however, is difficult to achieve uniformly throughout the image. It is well known that free water (− OH) and lipids ($-CH_2$, for example) have sufficient differences in their chemical environments that the hydrogen protons associated with each complex have resonant frequencies that differ by approximately 3.5 ppm. At 1.5 T, this corresponds to a spectral frequency difference of only about 220 to 240 Hz. For spectral saturation to be effective, the presaturation pulse must only be applied to one chemical species and not the other. Therefore, it requires a very narrow bandwidth pulse. If the magnetic field changes slightly, the pulse will not be on resonance with the species and the desired suppression will not occur and could potentially simulate pathology.[5,6] This requires a high degree of field homogeneity throughout the imaging volume. Localized inhomogeneities such as those caused by susceptibility (see 1.1214-26) and metal (see 1.1214-27) compromise this technique further.

Advantages

Frequency selective saturation is a direct and effective method for suppressing fat or water without increased imaging time.

Disadvantages

Frequency selective saturation methods are highly sensitive to magnetic field inhomogeneities and can lead to regionally and highly localized ineffective suppression that can simulate pathology.

Technical References

1. Szumowski J, Simon JH. Proton chemical shift imaging. In: Stark DD, Bradley WG, eds. Magnetic resonance imaging, 2nd ed, vol 1. St Louis, Mosby–Year Book, 1992.
2. Rosen BR, Wedeen VJ, Brady TJ. Selective saturation NMR imaging. J Comput Assist Tomogr 1984;8:813–818.
3. Frahm J, Haase A, Hanicke W, et al. Chemical shift selective MR imaging using a whole-body magnet. Radiology 1985; 156:441–444.
4. Keller PJ, Hunter WW, Schmalbrock P. Multisection fat-water imaging with chemical shift selective presaturation. Radiology 1987;164:539–541.
5. Joseph PM, Shetty A. A comparison of selective saturation and selective echo chemical shift imaging techniques. Magn Reson Imaging 1988;6:421–430.
6. Anzai Y, Lufkin RB, Jabour BA, Hanafee WN. Fat-suppression failure artifacts simulating pathology on frequency-selective fat-suppression MR images of the head and neck. Am J Neuroradiol 1992;13:879–884.

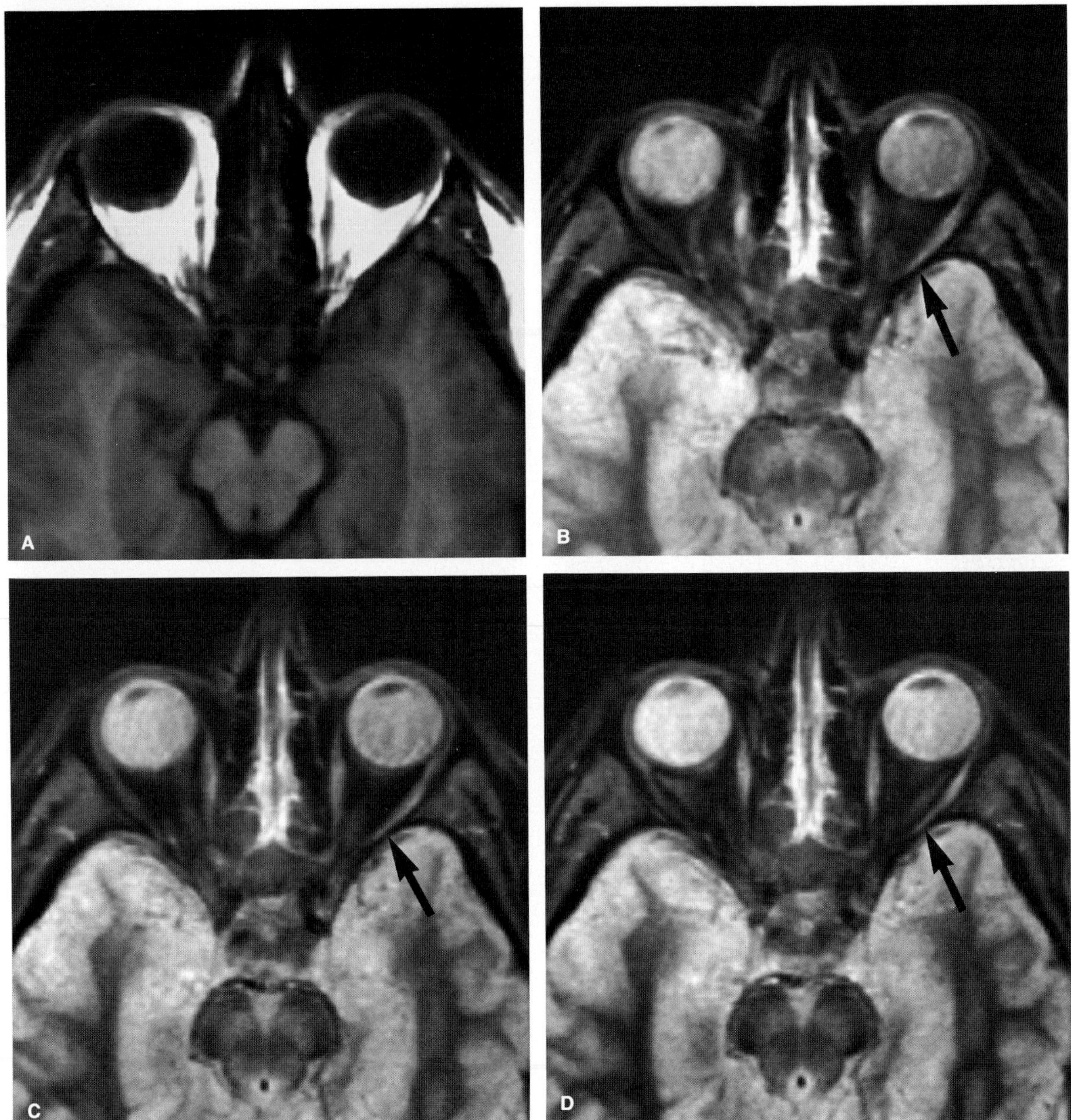

TECHNIQUE

Fat suppression using short tau inversion recovery (STIR)

FINDINGS

(*A*) An axial T1-weighted SE scan (TR/TE = 400/10) has hyperintense fat signal obscuring the optic nerve. Magnitude-reconstructed STIR images (TR/TE = 2000/20) at a TI of 140 (*B*), 190 (*C*), and 240 (*D*) show varying degrees of fat signal suppression (*arrows*) with the optimum obtained at 190 msec (*C*). In magnitude-reconstructed IR, T1-weighted contrast becomes inverted. At a different anatomic location (*E to H*), boundary artifacts are evident between fat and water (*arrow*), generated with magnitude reconstruction at a TI of 240 (*F*). Using phase-sensitive reconstruction, correct signal magnitude and T1 contrast is maintained (*G*), showing no boundary artifacts (*white arrow*). Suppression is better visualized by inverted display (*H*), and also allows better comparison with magnitude reconstruction under identical measurement conditions (*F*).

CONCLUSION

Good suppression of fat signal is obtained with STIR using the correct TI.

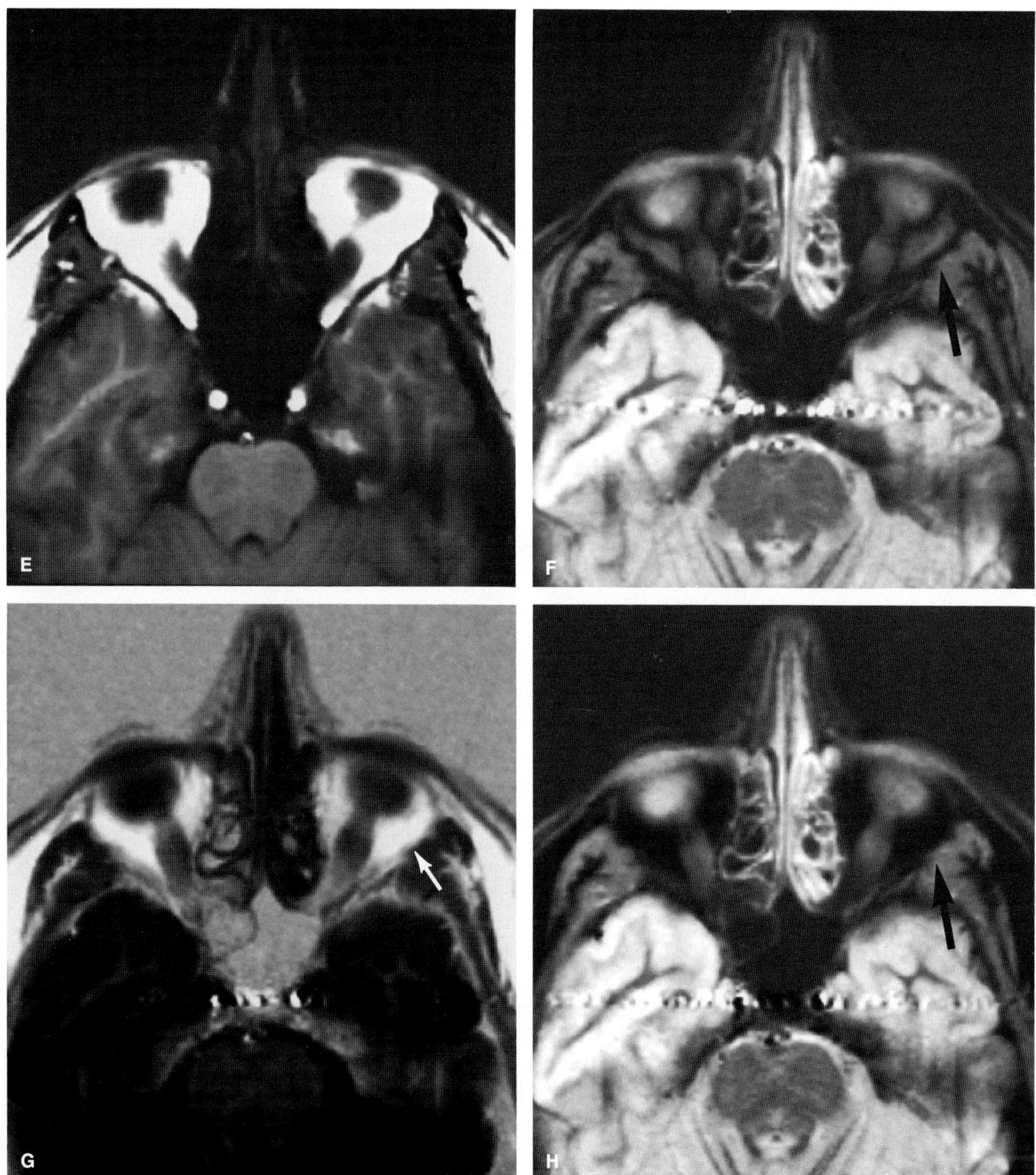

DISCUSSION

With the IR technique (see 1.1214-4 and 1.1214-5), strong T1 weighting and superb anatomic detail are obtained.[1] A unique aspect of IR is that the inverted magnetization must cross through a null point, or "bounce point," as it grows along the positive longitudinal direction. If the TI is chosen so that the signal is acquired precisely when a specific tissue of a given T1 value possesses zero longitudinal magnetization, the result is a minimal signal output and selective suppression of that tissue in the image. This phenomenon has been used to specifically suppress fat signal, and is called STIR.[1] Its use has been primarily for better visualization of the optic nerve[2] and hepatic lesions.[3,4]

Fat characteristically has the shortest T1 value and therefore is the first magnetization to pass through the null point. As a result, all neighboring tissues still possess negative magnetization and generate negative signals. An absolute or magnitude reconstruction of the STIR image inverts all the tissue signals that are negative to positive values. This produces reversed tissue contrast leading to a potentially confusing display (see 1.1214-4). Phase-sensitive reconstruction allows the sign of the tissue signals to be preserved thereby producing true T1 weighting (see 1.1214-5). When suppressing fat with the STIR technique, all tissues other than fat exhibit negative signal intensity, and background noise has the highest pixel intensity. Provided the correct TI is used, fat is suppressed in both magnitude and phase-sensitive reconstructed images.

A precise TI is necessary to null a given tissue signal and depends on both TR and T1. This is approximately equal to 70% of the T1 if a long TR is used. Because T1 is field strength dependent, the correct TI for good fat suppression also depends on field strength. If a larger TI is used, the fat signal becomes positive while all the other tissues are still negative. An absolute reconstruction and display of the STIR image then produces boundary artifacts at interfaces (see 1.1214-5). Even small deviations from the proper TI substantially compromise the suppression of the tissue.[5,6] On the other hand, this precise relation between T1 and TI makes it possible to selectively suppress not only fat but certain types of lesions as well, potentially increasing specificity.[6]

Advantages

Good fat suppression is obtained when the correct TI is used with the STIR technique (see 1.1214-4 and 1.1214-5). STIR yields good anatomic visualization of the optic nerve and orbit when fat is suppressed.

Disadvantages

Relatively long scan times are typical. Overall STIR contrast at the required TI for fat suppression may be difficult to interpret in comparison with the spin echo technique (see 1.1214-2) or other fat suppression methods (see 1.1214-14).

Technical References

1. Bydder GM, Young IR. MR imaging: clinical use of the inversion recovery sequence. J Comput Assist Tomogr 1985; 9:659–675.
2. Atlas SW, Grossman RI, Hackney DB, et al. STIR MR imaging of the orbit. J Radiol 1988;151:1025–1030.
3. Dwyer AJ, Frank JA, Sank VJ, et al. Short-TI inversion-recovery pulse sequence: analysis and initial experience in cancer imaging. Radiology 1988;168:827–836.
4. Dousset M, Weissleder R, Hendrick RE, et al. Short TI inversion-recovery imaging of the liver: pulse-sequence optimization and comparison with spin-echo imaging. Radiology 1989;171:327–333.
5. Shuman WP, Lambert DT, Patten RM, et al. Improved fat suppression in STIR MR imaging: selecting inversion time through spectral display. Radiology 1991;178:885–887.
6. Patrizio G, Pavone P, Testa A, et al. MR characterization of hepatic lesions by t-null inversion recovery sequence. J Comput Assist Tomogr 1990;14:96–101.

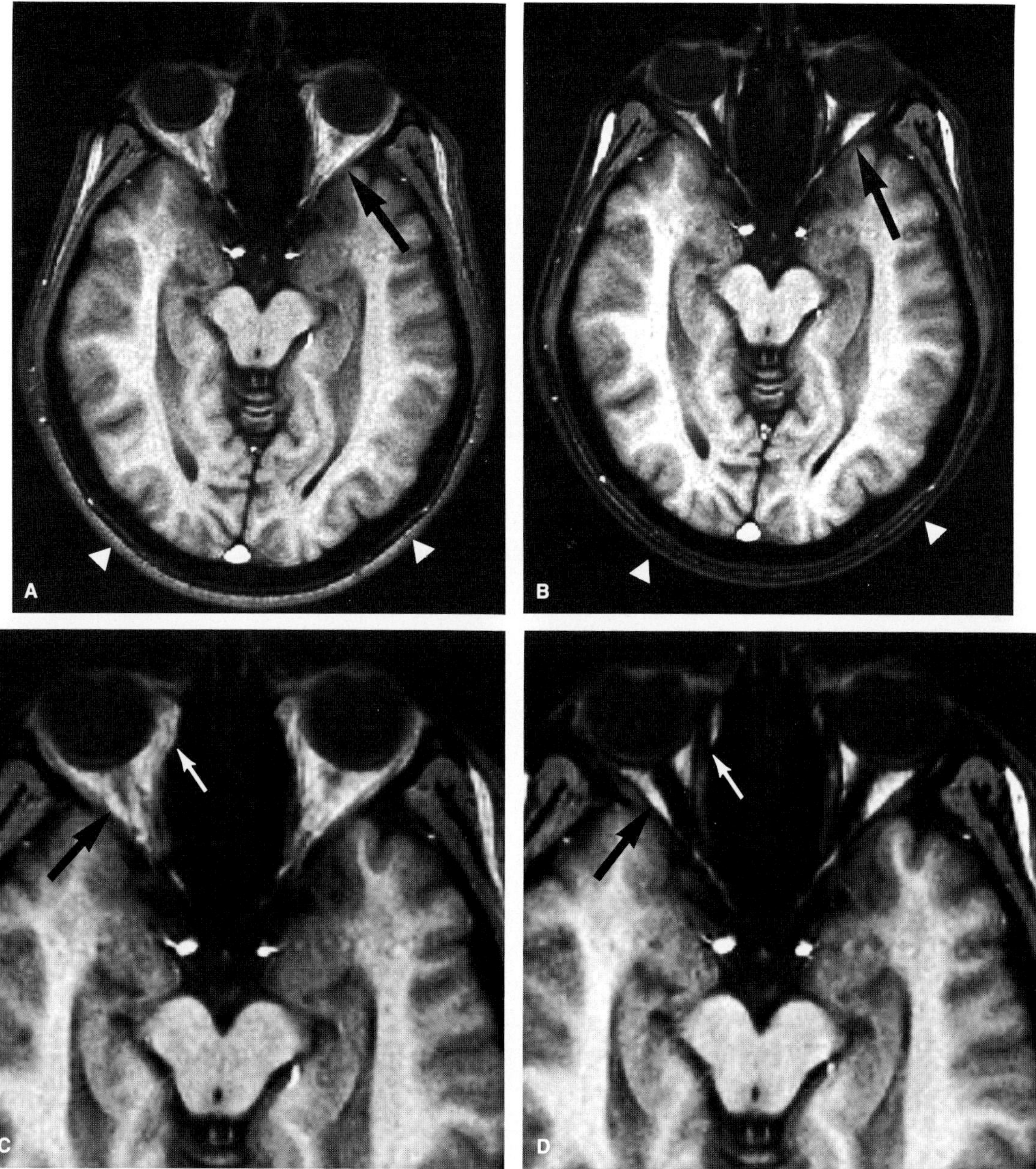

TECHNIQUE

Fat suppression by signal phase cycling with GRE techniques

FINDINGS

Spoiled GRE axial sections through the optic nerve were obtained under identical conditions (TR/FA = 150/60°) at TE = 9 (*A and C*) and TE = 7 (*B and D*). Contrast appears identical except in certain regions containing fat (*white arrowheads*) which in (*B*) show a marked decrease in its signal intensity. However, suppression occurs only in areas that contain water, and specifically is not seen in the fat surrounding the optic nerve (*black arrow*). Volume-averaged fat obscures the optic nerve in *C* but is substantially suppressed in *D,* as is the fat over the medial rectus muscle (*white arrow*). Fat immediately surrounding the optic nerve remains unsuppressed (*black arrow*).

CONCLUSION

Suppression of fat from signal phase cycling by varying TE in a GRE technique is possible when both fat and water are present.

DISCUSSION

In all SSFP techniques in which a gradient echo is formed to produce image data (see 1.1214-6 to 1.1214-8), the signal evolves as an FID. Although the characteristic time of decay for a given tissue is T2*, the FID may possess oscillatory behavior if both fat and water components are present in the signal. If the gradient echo is collected at a TE when the signal is a peak, fat in the image is hyperintense. On the other hand, if the echo is generated when the signal is a minimum, the fat has a certain degree of suppression.[1–3] All GRE techniques have this anomaly.

It is well known that a distinct chemical shift of the Larmor frequencies of fat (primarily the $-CH_2$ moiety) and water ($-OH$) exists that may cause a pixel misregistration in the frequency encoding direction of the image (see 1.1214-28). In addition, a cycling of the relative phase difference between the two signals occurs based on their relative frequency difference. Following an RF pulse, the fat and water signal begin in phase. Since one signal precesses at a faster rate than the other, the signals progress out of phase, and the FID oscillates in amplitude as it decays. Peaks occur when they are in phase, and minimums occur when they are 180° out of phase.

The chemical shift of fat and water is approximately 3.5 to 3.7 ppm, which corresponds to a 230-Hz frequency difference at 1.5 T. Thus, the FID oscillates about every 4.3 msec. Choosing the appropriate TE determines the intensity of the fat; it is relatively bright at TE = 4.3, 8.7, 13, n + 4.3 msec, and suppressed at TE = 6.5, 10.9, 15.2, n + 4.3 msec. The degree of suppression depends on the amount of water present. No suppression occurs if water is absent from the region, and complete suppression occurs if the signal is comprised of 50% fat and 50% water. Because most of the brain is water, this technique is more of an anomaly than a method for suppressing fat. It is of greater use in other areas of the body, especially in trabecular structures that possess tissues of both chemical species.[4,5]

Advantages

Simple minor adjustment of TE in a GRE scan (see 1.1214-6 to 1.1214-8) can produce fat suppression. The method is relatively insensitive to external magnetic field inhomogeneities.

Disadvantages

Signal phase cycling only suppresses fat in the presence of water and is primarily effective in body or spine imaging. In many cases, it is considered an artifact or an anomaly of GRE imaging.

Technical References

1. Wehrli FW, Perkins TG, Shimakawa A, Roberts F. Chemical shift-induced amplitude modulations in images obtained with gradient refocusing. Magn Reson Imaging 1987;5:157–158.
2. Wehrli FW. Fast-scan magnetic resonance: principles and applications. Magn Reson Q 1990;6:165–236.
3. Szumowski J, Simon JH. Proton chemical shift imaging. In: Stark DD, Bradley WG, eds. Magnetic resonance imaging, 2nd ed, vol 1. St Louis, Mosby–Year Book, 1992.
4. Wehrli FW, Ford JC, Attie M, et al. Trabecular structure: preliminary application of MR interferometry. Radiology 1991;179:615–621.
5. Sebag GH, Moore SG. Effect of trabecular bone on the appearance of marrow in gradient-echo imaging of the appendicular skeleton. Radiology 1990;174:855–859.

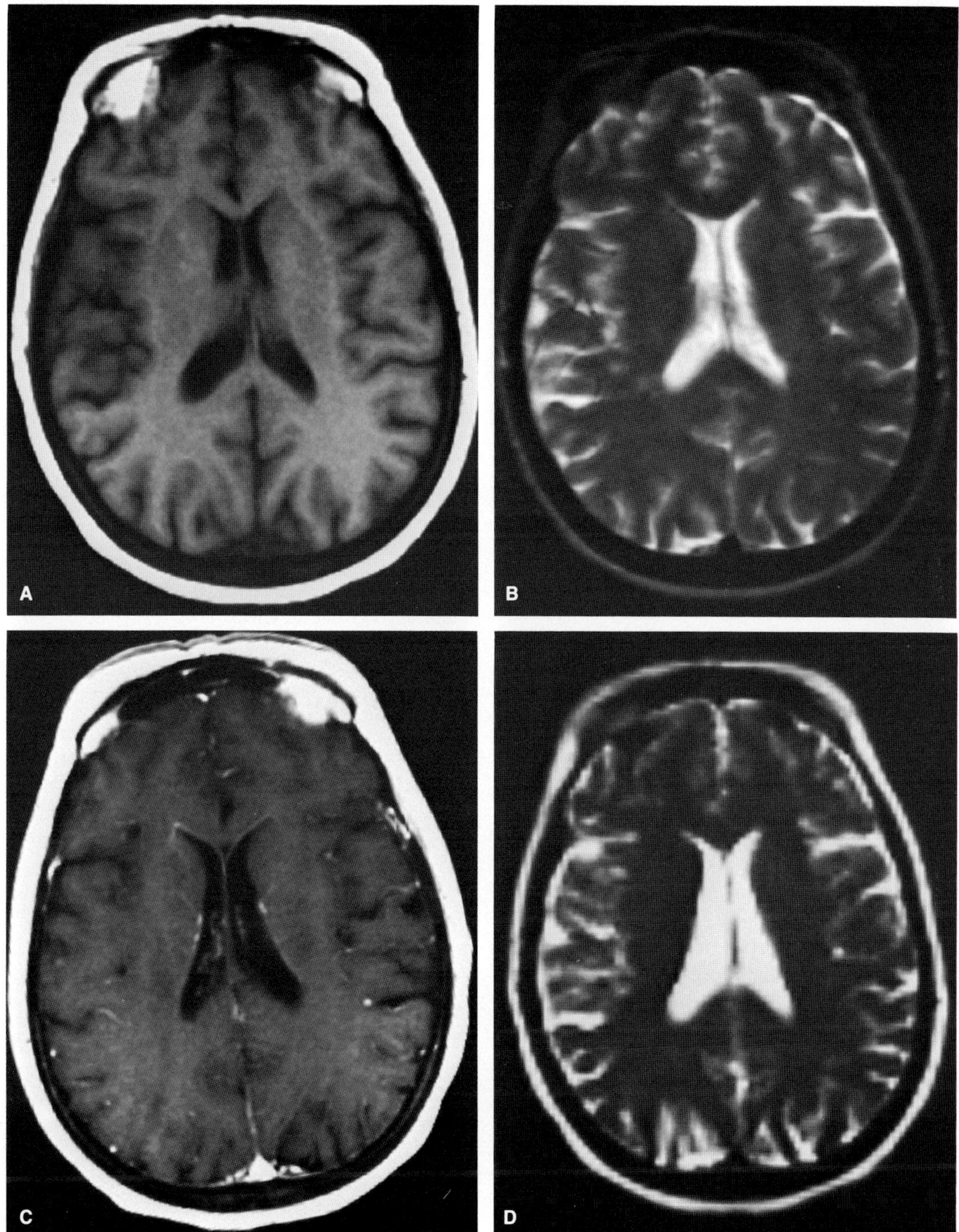

TECHNIQUE

Dynamic contrast-enhanced MR of microcirculatory perfusion

FINDINGS

Precontrast T1-weighted (TR/TE = 575/10) SE (*A*), T2-weighted (TR/TE = 3000/90) SE (*B*), and postcontrast T1-weighted (*C*) images are shown from a standard head protocol. During bolus contrast media administration, dynamic first-pass perfusion scans were obtained using a T2-enhanced GRE technique (TR/TE/FA = 12/18/90°) at 1-second intervals. Preinjection (*D*) and peak-of-bolus (*E*) images were divided on a pixel-by-pixel basis to obtain a relative indication of regional tissue blood volume (*F*). Gray matter shows a higher blood volume than white matter. Evaluating all time points during the first pass (*not shown*) allows a more accurate determination of regional blood volume.

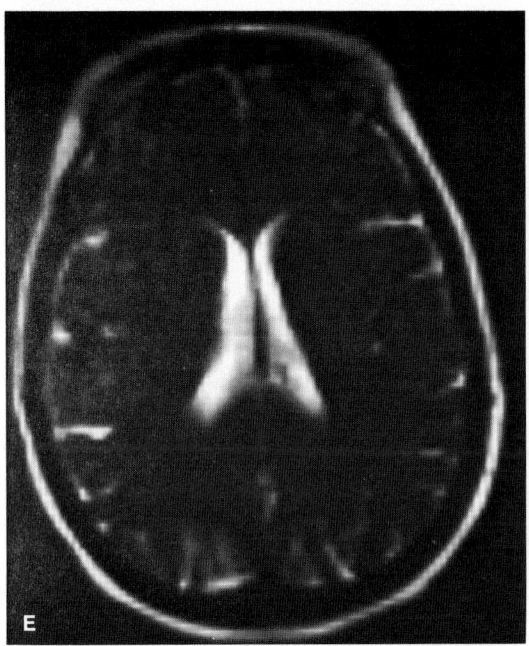

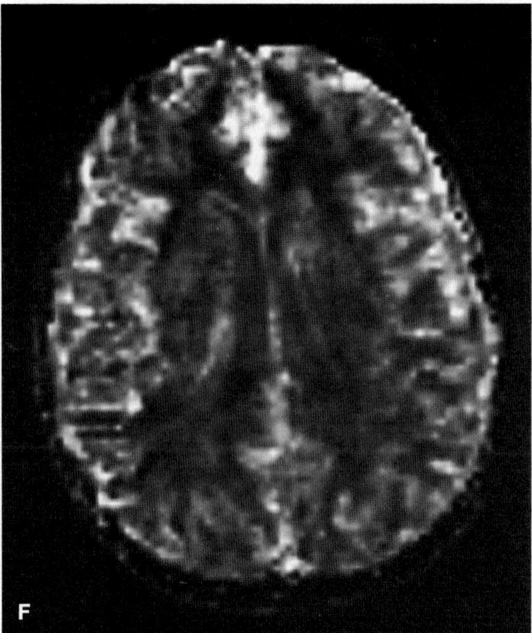

CONCLUSION

Dynamic MR allows the visualization of regional blood volume from signal changes in first-pass perfusion of a contrast agent bolus.

DISCUSSION

With the advent of fast imaging techniques in MR, observation of first-pass perfusion of a contrast agent bolus is possible. It is well known that in the presence of a paramagnetic, superparamagnetic, or ferromagnetic substance, NMR relaxation properties of T1, T2, and T2* become shortened thereby reducing or increasing the MR signal depending on the technique used.[1] After bolus injection of a contrast agent, first-pass transit of the bolus causes time-dependent regional signal changes that reflect the hemodynamic properties of the tissues.[2–6]

Measuring intensity variations over time in a given tissue allows a qualitative assessment of tissue perfusion. The accuracy of the technique depends on its time resolution, sensitivity to contrast agent concentration, and injection characteristics. Although numerous techniques have been investigated, they can be categorized as either negatively or positively enhancing. The former relies on T2 (relaxivity) or T2* (susceptibility) shortening and results in signal loss when the contrast agent is present.[2–5] The latter relies on T1 (relaxivity) shortening and results in signal gain.[6]

Quantitative evaluation of classic regional cerebral blood volume (rCBV) and regional cerebral blood flow (rCBF) requires evaluation of the concentration versus time behavior of the first-pass effect. This is difficult to achieve in MR because of the complex relation between MR signal intensity and contrast agent concentration.[4] Contrast agents other than pure susceptibility agents simultaneously alter all the relaxation properties, and no technique has the unique ability to isolate signal dependence due to T2 or T2* to allow a simple conversion of signal to concentration.

Advantages

The assessment of cerebral perfusion and hemodynamics in tissues may provide further diagnostic information. Initial studies indicate its ability to identify vascular abnormalities and stroke in its earliest stages.[7]

Disadvantages

The clinical relevance of imaging first-pass perfusion and cerebral hemodynamics is not yet proved. Accurate quantitative evaluation of rCBV and rCBF is difficult to achieve.

Technical References

1. Wolf GL, Joseph PM, Goldstein EJ. Optimal pulsing sequences for MR contrast agents. AJR 1986;147:367–371.
2. Majumdar S, Zoghbi SS, Gore JC. Regional differences in rat brain displayed by fast MRI with superparamagnetic contrast agents. Magn Reson Imaging 1988;6:611–615.
3. Villringer A, Rosen BR, Belliveau JW, et al. Dynamic imaging with lanthanide chelates in normal brain: contrast due to magnetic susceptibility effects. Magn Reson Med 1988;6:164–174.
4. Rosen BR, Belliveau JW, Chien D. Perfusion imaging by nuclear magnetic resonance. Magn Reson Q 1989;5:263–281.
5. Belliveau JW, Rosen BR, Kantor HL, et al. Functional cerebral imaging by susceptibility-contrast NMR. Magn Reson Med 1990;14:538–546.
6. Dean BL, Lee C, Kirsch JE, et al. Cerebral hemodynamics and cerebral blood volume: MR assessment using gadolinium contrast agents and T1-weighted turbo-FLASH imaging. Am J Neuroradiol 1992;13:39–48.
7. Warach S, Li W, Ronthal M, Edelman RR. Acute cerebral ischemia: evaluation with dynamic contrast-enhanced MR imaging and MR angiography. Radiology 1992;182:41–47.

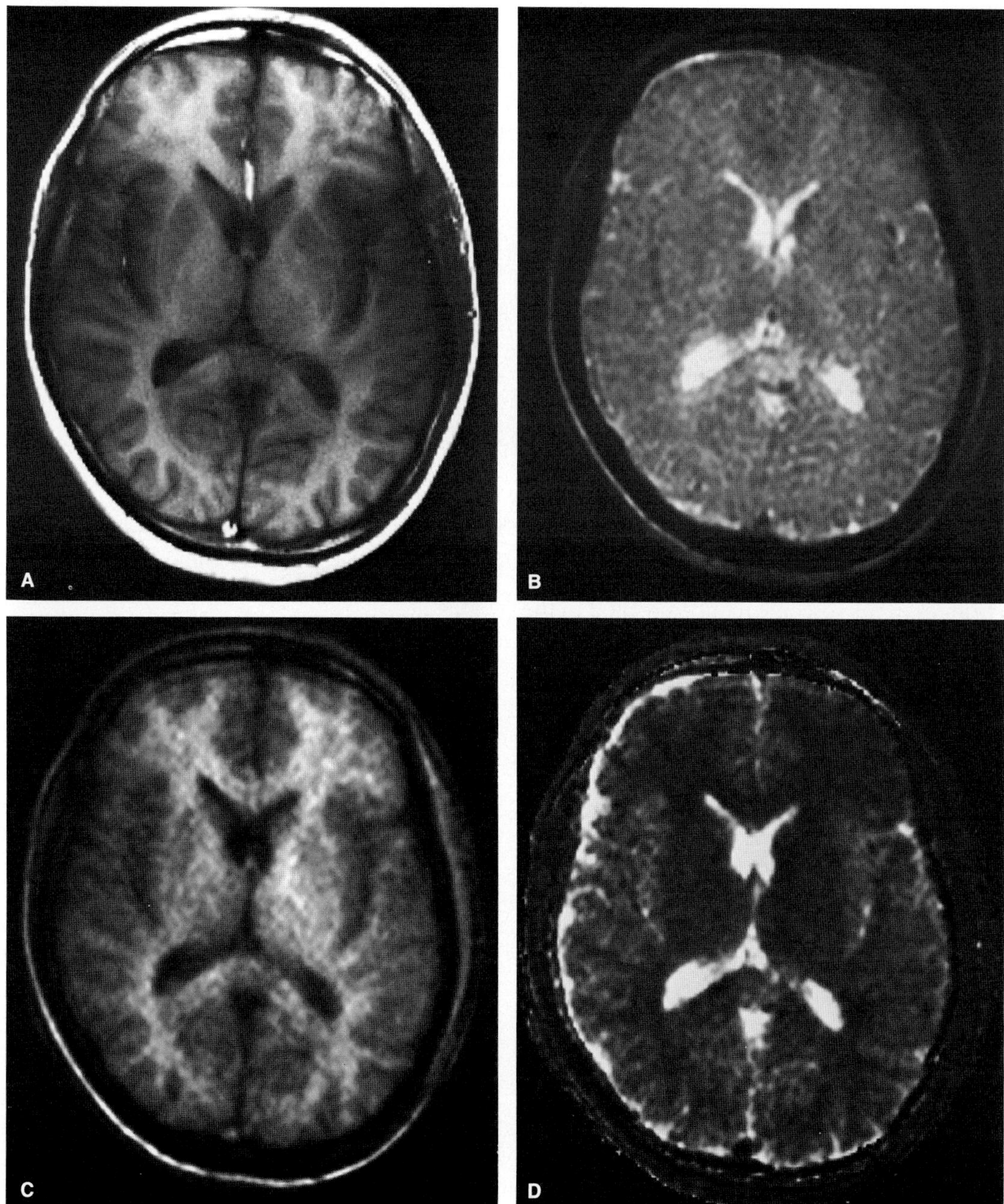

TECHNIQUE

Sensitivity of MR to molecular diffusion

FINDINGS

A conventional T1-weighted axial scan (*A*) is shown in comparison with a 1-second single-shot driven equilibrium scan (*B*) with strong T2 weighting. After sensitizing the latter to molecular diffusion and microscopic motion, the single shot technique demonstrates diffusion weighting (*C*) with substantial signal loss in regions of large diffusion such as the lateral ventricles and gray matter. Dividing *B* and *C* on a pixel-by-pixel basis produces an image (*D*) that gives a relative representation of apparent diffusion. Relative lack of microscopic motion is observed in fat and deep white matter.

CONCLUSION

Diffusional motion can produce large changes in signal allowing the evaluation of regional molecular diffusion in tissues.

DISCUSSION

It has been well known in NMR spectroscopy that molecular motions can affect the MR signal by causing a reduction in its amplitude. By altering the pulsing scheme, this phenomenon has been applied to determine the characteristic self-diffusion coefficient of a sample yielding information about the state of microscopic motion. This has been extended to imaging by incorporating features into existing MR techniques that sensitize the signal to diffusional motion, thereby obtaining additional unique information about the state of the tissues in vivo.[1,2]

In the process of applying magnetic gradient fields for the purposes of spatial encoding, any type of motion generates errors in the MR signal. This generally becomes reconstructed as motion-related artifacts throughout the image if it is not taken into account (see 1.1214-29). A number of different methods exist to minimize or eliminate this problem.[3,4] If extremely strong gradient fields are applied, it is possible to induce changes in the MR signal from even microscopic motions related to the diffusion of molecules. If the motion goes beyond an image pixel dimension, it becomes an artifact. If it remains within an image pixel, it simply reduces the signal intensity of that pixel. Therefore, the reduction in signal becomes a signature of the degree of molecular motion.

Diffusion-related contrast depends on the molecular motions of the tissue and the amount of "sensitizing" that is applied in the technique. To determine the degree of diffusion associated with a given tissue, it is necessary to determine the level of signal reduction. Therefore, an accurate assessment can only be made when comparing images from the same anatomic location before and after sensitization to diffusional motion. It has been suggested that cytoxic edema in the early stages of stroke is visualized on diffusion-weighted images as a result of the redistribution of water from extracellular to the more restrictive intracellular space.[5]

Directionality is also inherent in diffusion MR. Only those motions in the direction of the sensitizing gradient field yield a reduction in signal. In an isolated sample, most of the molecular motion is considered isotropic, or directionally independent. In human tissue, however, the movement of water can be anisotropic. Using the directionality of diffusion-weighted imaging may therefore provide not only useful information about the free mobility or restricted state of water in tissue but also unique insight into its directional dependence. Preliminary studies in diffusion-weighted imaging have shown that a strong anisotropy in water motion exists along the myelin tracts in white matter.[6]

Advantages

The state of molecular diffusion and the microscopic motion of water in tissues may provide further diagnostic information. Initial studies indicate its ability to identify stroke in its earliest stages.

Disadvantages

The clinical relevance of imaging diffusion and microscopic motion is not yet known. Sensitizing the signal to microscopic motion may also lead to accentuated bulk motion (see 1.1214-29) which compromises the image. Strong diffusion-weighted images have low S/N.

Technical References

1. Le Bihan D, Breton E, Lallemand D, et al. MR imaging of intravoxel incoherent motions: application to diffusion and perfusion in neurologic disorders. Radiology 1986;161: 401–407.
2. Le Bihan D, Turner R, Moonen CTW, Pekar J. Imaging of diffusion and microcirculation with gradient sensitization: design, strategy, and significance. J Magn Reson Imaging 1991;1:7–28.
3. Tsuruda JA, Chew WM, Moseley ME, Norman D. Diffusion-weighted MR imaging of the brain: value of differentiating between extraaxial cysts and epidermoid tumors. Am J Neuroradiol 1990;11:925–931.
4. Merboldt K-D, Hanicke W, Bruhn H, et al. Diffusion imaging of the human brain in vivo using high-speed STEAM MRI. Magn Reson Med 1992;23:179–192.
5. Moseley ME, Kucharczyk J, Mintorovitch J, et al. Diffusion-weighted MR imaging of acute stroke: correlation with T2-weighted and magnetic susceptibility-enhanced MR imaging in cats. Am J Neuroradiol 1990;11:423–429.
6. Hajnal JV, Doran M, Hall AS, et al. MR imaging of anisotropically restricted diffusion of water in the nervous system: technical, anatomic, and pathologic considerations. J Comput Assist Tomogr 1991;15:1–18.

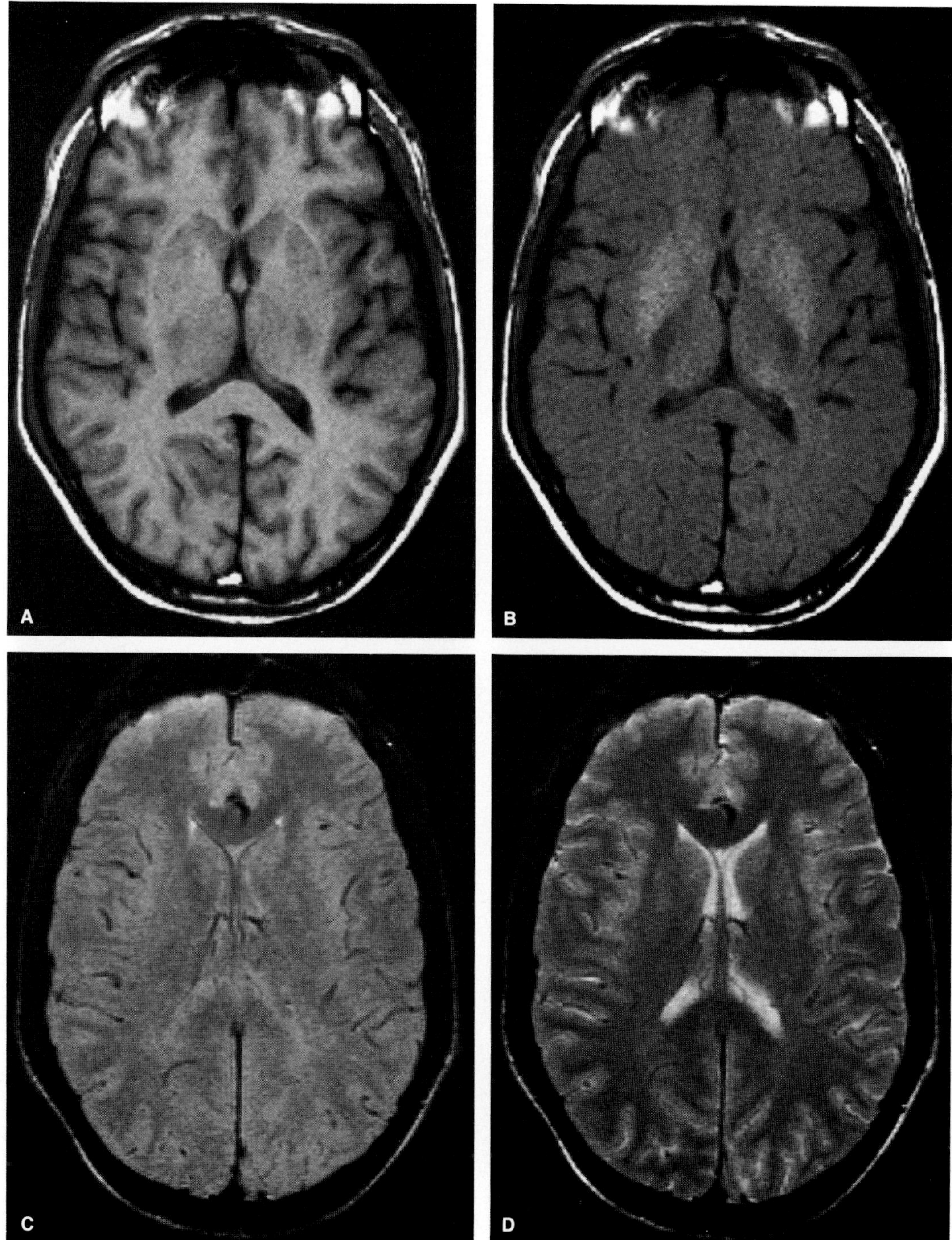

TECHNIQUE

Magnetization transfer spin echo as compared with conventional SE

FINDINGS

SE images without (*A*) and with (*B*) pulsed MT saturation are shown under otherwise identical measurement conditions (TR/TE = 400/15). Contrast changes appear similar to lengthening TR. However, the changes are associated with T1 shortening from the MT mechanism and are not readily observed in fat or CSF. Similar contrast changes are seen at TR/TE = 1400/60 without (*C*) and with (*D*) MT saturation, and at TR/TE = 2400/60 without (*E*) and with (*F*) MT saturation. The degree of signal change is a relative indication of the presence of a restricted hydrogen pool in the tissue. As expected, little change was seen in CSF since it primarily contains free water, although *B, D,*

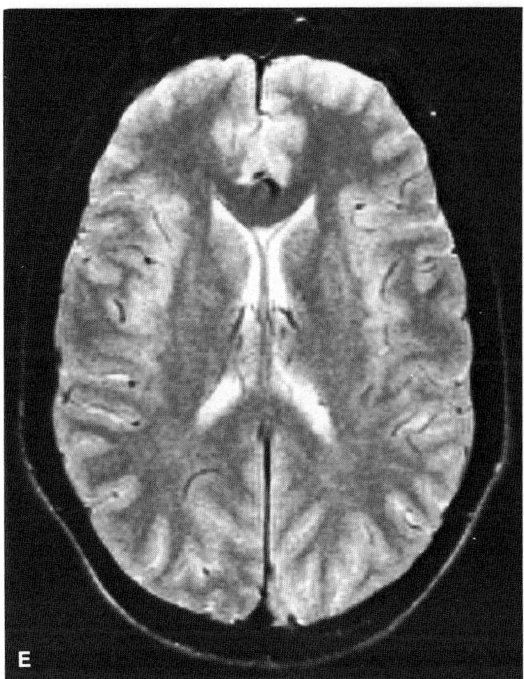

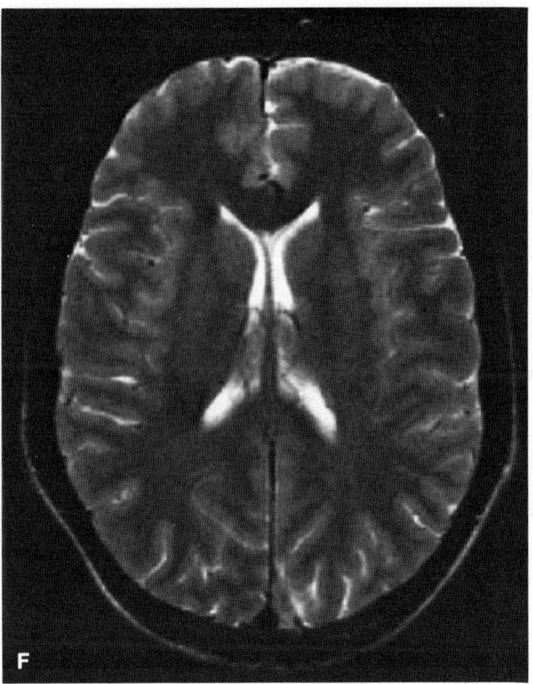

and *F* have been windowed differently for illustrative purposes.

CONCLUSION

Changes in tissue contrast are observed caused by MT from restricted hydrogen to free hydrogen.

DISCUSSION

MT is a mechanism well known in NMR spectroscopy. However, this intrinsic tissue characteristic has only recently been investigated regarding its clinical utility.[1–8] Normally, MR primarily demonstrates contrast among tissues based on spin density, T1, and T2 parameters of the tissues. The degree of their weighting in the image contrast depends on the imaging technique and the protocol (see 1.1214-2 through 1.1214-8). MT provides an additional contrast mechanism that may ultimately provide further diagnostic information.

In MR, the signal that eventually becomes encoded in the image is based primarily on a freely mobile hydrogen pool (Hf), which constitutes only a part of most tissues. A restricted hydrogen pool (Hr) also exists that is strongly bound to complex molecular structures within the tissue but that cannot be imaged by MR techniques because of its extremely short T2 values. In the application of MT, the Hr pool becomes saturated by RF excitation, and its magnetization is then transferred to the unexcited Hf pool. The primary effect is a shortening of the T1 value of the Hf pool. Less signal from the Hf pool also occurs since its available magnetization becomes saturated as well.[1–3]

Incorporating additional RF pulsing in a conventional MR technique, MT contrast is generated along with T1 and T2 contrast.[3–5] To observe the effects of MT, the Hr pool must become saturated by the RF without directly affecting the Hf pool. Two methods are used to apply MT. Off-resonance techniques[1–3] rely on saturating the Hr pool by applying RF away from the resonance of the Hf pool. On-resonance, or "pulsed" techniques,[4,5] apply RF pulses at the resonance of the Hf in a manner such that the effective flip angle experienced by the Hf pool is 0°.

MT contrast, manifested through the degree of T1 shortening and associated signal loss of the Hf pool, ultimately depends on the existence of an Hr pool. Assessment of the actual nature of Hr in tissues is possible only through comparison between images obtained with and without MT contrast.[6] Nevertheless, recent investigations using MT contrast for improved lesion conspicuity have been carried out in MRA,[7] early detection of stroke,[8] and tumor visualization.[9]

Advantages

MT offers an additional contrast mechanism in tissues that may lead to increased diagnostic information and better conventional contrast resolution, particularly in MR angiography.

Disadvantages

The diagnostic utility of MT is not yet known. In the presence of an Hr pool, the signal affected by MT is reduced leading to potentially poor image quality.

Technical References

1. Wolff SD, Balaban RS. Magnetization transfer contrast (MTC) and tissue water proton relaxation in vivo. Magn Reson Med 1989;10:135–144.
2. Balaban RS, Ceckler TL. Magnetization transfer contrast in magnetic resonance imaging. Magn Reson Q 1992;8:116–137.
3. Hajnal JV, Baudouin CJ, Oatridge A, et al. Design and implementation of magnetization transfer pulse sequences for clinical use. J Comput Assist Tomogr 1992;16:7–18.
4. Wolff SD, Eng J, Balaban RS. Magnetization transfer contrast: method for improving contrast in gradient-recalled-echo images. Radiology 1991;179:133–137.
5. Yeung HN, Aisen AM. Magnetization transfer contrast with periodic pulsed saturation. Radiology 1992;183:209–214.
6. Eng J, Ceckler TL, Balaban RS. Quantitative 1H magnetization transfer imaging in vivo. Magn Reson Med 1991; 17:304–314.
7. Pike GB, Hu BS, Glover GH, Enzmann DR. Magnetization transfer time-of-flight magnetic resonance angiography. Magn Reson Med 1992;25:372–379.
8. Ordidge RJ, Helpern JA, Knight RA, et al. Investigation of cerebral ischemia using magnetization transfer contrast (MTC) MR imaging. Magn Reson Imaging 1991;9:895–902.
9. Kurki TJI, Niemi PT, Lundbom N. Gadolinium-enhanced magnetization transfer contrast imaging of intracranial tumors. J Magn Reson Imaging 1992;2:401–406.

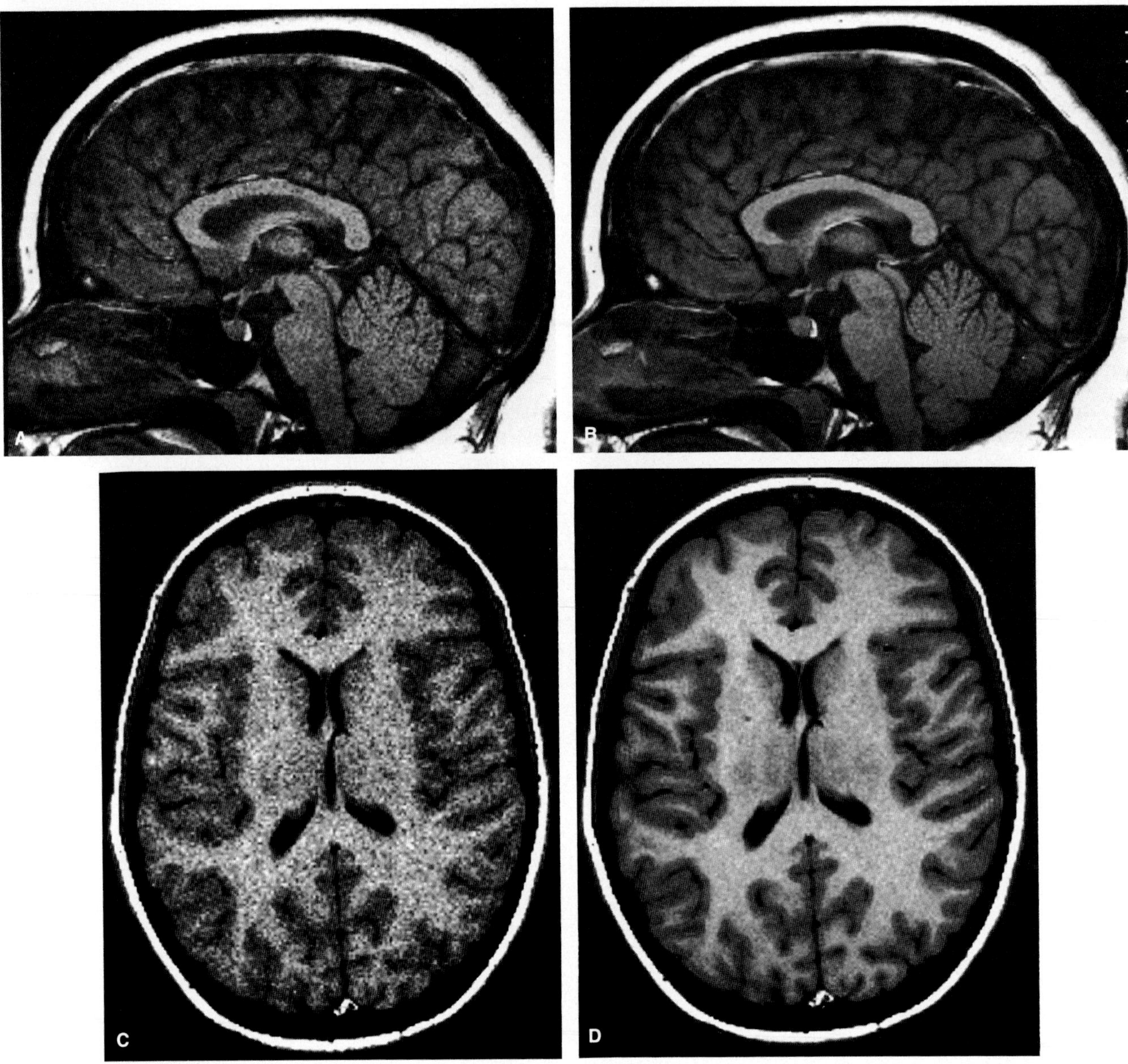

PARAMETER

Acquisitions, imaging time, and signal-to-noise ratio

FINDINGS

T1-weighted sagittal images (TR/TE = 400/15) were acquired with one acquisition (*A*) and four acquisitions (*B*) under otherwise identical conditions. Scan times were 1:47 and 6:54 minutes, respectively. T1-weighted axial images (TR/TE = 400/10) were also obtained with one acquisition (*C*) and eight acquisitions (*D*), and scan times of 1:44 and 13:41 minutes, respectively. S/N difference between *A* and *B* is 1:2. Sufficient differentiation between high contrast tissues is shown, but there is some loss in the delineation of small structures and low contrast regions in the image with lower S/N (*A*). Large differences in gray and white matter visualization are seen between *C* and *D*, where the S/N is 1:2.8. Substantial reduction in noise variation of the signal in *D* allows good depiction of low contrast structures such as the head of the caudate nucleus.

CONCLUSION

Increased acquisitions lead to higher S/N and better tissue differentiation.

DISCUSSION

S/N is an important consideration in maximizing C/N and improving tissue delineation (see 1.1214-1). Given the signal and contrast of an image based on the MR technique, protocol, and intrinsic MR parameters, the statistical noise can be reduced in order to further enhance image quality. This noise is uncorrelated and results in pixel-to-pixel signal variability in the image. Averaging of the signals by using multiple acquisitions, or number of excitations (NEX), reduces the image noise and increases the S/N and C/N.[1,2] Correlated or systematic noise from moving tissue structures or blood flow can obscure anatomic detail (see 1.1214-29 and 1.1214-31). Signal averaging also minimizes these image artifacts and further improves overall image quality.[3–5]

A compromise in scan time is made when increasing the number of acquisitions. Imaging time is linearly proportional to NEX. A factor of 4 increase in NEX doubles S/N, but total scan time also lengthens by a factor of 4. In many cases, increasing NEX can lead to prohibitively long scans. This is particularly true in T2-weighted studies where TR tends to be long. Its use is more frequent in T1-weighted scans with short TR, where an increase in NEX still allows reasonable imaging times.

Using multiple acquisitions can have diminishing returns. If the tissue signal is intrinsically large compared with the image noise or if the correlated noise is sufficiently large, signal averaging by increasing the NEX may not necessarily enhance S/N, C/N, or image quality.[5,6] Thus, it would result in lengthened scan time with little added benefit.

Advantages

Multiple acquisitions reduce image noise. Improved S/N leads to better tissue differentiation and structural detail (see 1.1214-1). Signal averaging also reduces motion and flow-related artifacts (see 1.1214-29 and 1.1214-31).

Disadvantages

An increase in acquisitions proportionally lengthens scan time.

Technical References

1. Edelstein WA, Bottomley PA, Hart HR, Smith LS. Signal, noise, and contrast in nuclear magnetic resonance imaging. J Comput Assist Tomogr 1983;7:391–401.
2. Hendrick RE, Raff U. Image contrast and noise. In: Stark DD, Bradley WG, eds. Magnetic resonance imaging, 2nd ed, vol 1. St Louis, Mosby–Year Book, 1992.
3. Wood ML, Henkelman RM. Suppression of respiratory motion artifacts in magnetic resonance imaging. Med Phys 1986;13:794–805.
4. Stark DD, Hendrick RE, Hahn PF, Ferrucci JT. Motion artifact reduction with fast spin-echo imaging. Radiology 1987;164:183–191.
5. Wood ML. Ineffectiveness of averaging for reducing motion artifacts in half-fourier MR imaging. J Magn Reson Imaging 1991;1:593–600.
6. Nalcioglu O, Cho ZH. Limits to signal-to-noise improvement by FID averaging in NMR imaging. Phys Med Biol 1984;29:969–978.

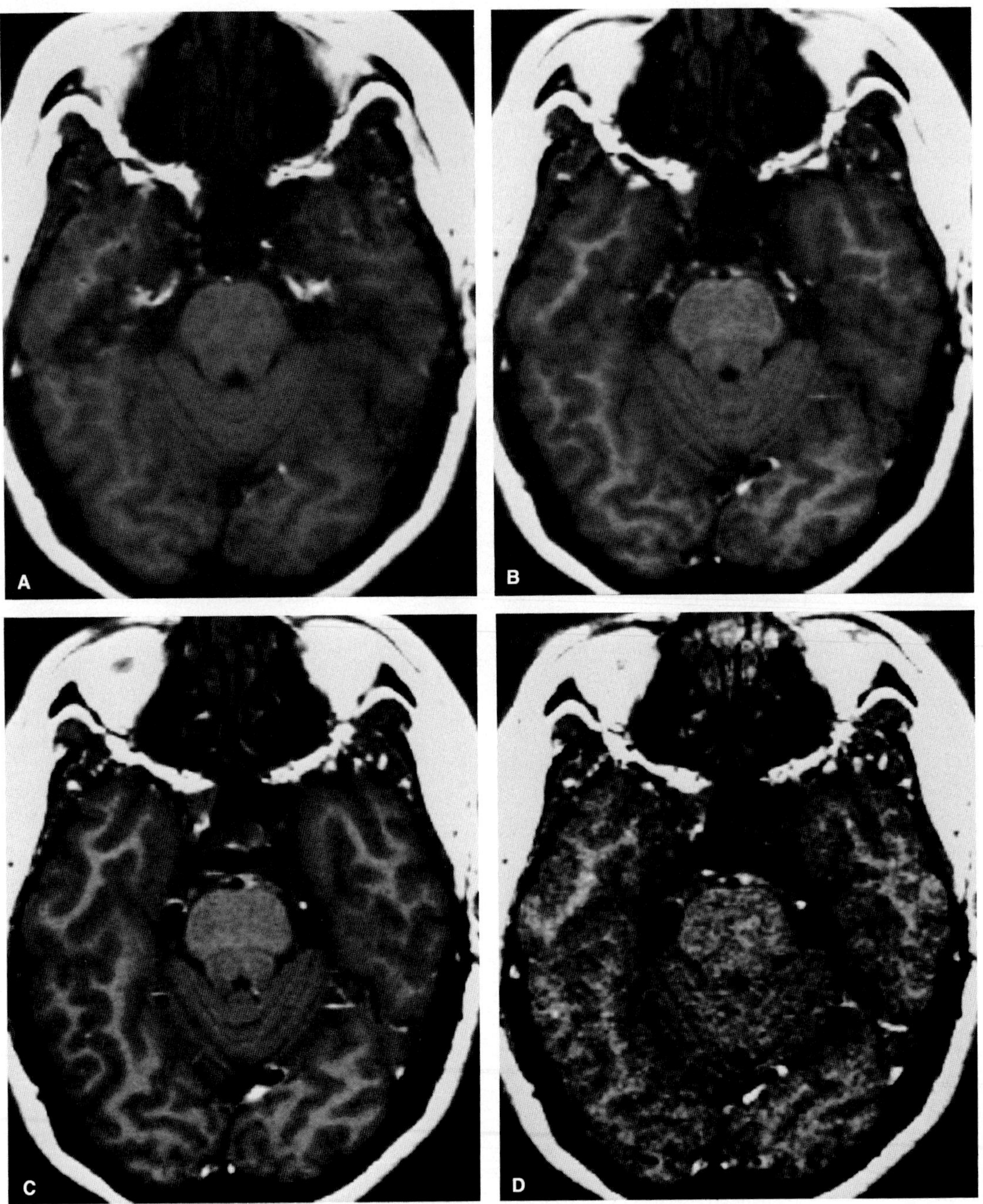

PARAMETER

Slice thickness, volume averaging, and signal-to-noise ratio

FINDINGS

Axial T1-weighted SE scans (TR/TE = 300/15) were acquired at section thicknesses of 8 mm (*A*), 4 mm (*B*), and 2 mm (*C*) under otherwise identical measurement conditions, including S/N. Substantial gray-to-white matter differentiation is lost with thick sections due to volume averaging, along with the near complete loss of the pituitary gland and fine details of the pons and cerebellum. However, thin sections require multiple acquisitions to regain S/N losses associated with reduced thicknesses. Scan time for *C* was 15:26 minutes compared with 1:02 minutes for *A*. (*D*) A 2-mm section was acquired in 1:02 minutes with an S/N reduction of 4:1 compared with an 8-mm section shown in *A*. Fine details and contrast are lost with thin sections as a result of the reduced S/N.

CONCLUSION

Partial voluming and loss of detail are observed using large slice thicknesses, and thin sections result in a substantial reduction in S/N.

DISCUSSION

Excitation of larger regions of tissue leads to an increase in signal. In general, S/N of the image is directly proportional to the slice thickness.[1] If the slice thickness is doubled, S/N is doubled. However, C/N and overall image quality may actually decrease with an increase in slice thickness due to volume averaging, or partial voluming. This is particularly true when the region of interest contains anatomic structures that are small compared with the slice thickness.[1–4]

Each pixel displayed in an image is a representation of the average signal produced by all the structures through the slice. The image, therefore, depicts a projection of all the anatomic detail contained within the section thickness. If structures are much smaller than the slice thickness, their delineation is compromised by averaging of all the neighboring tissues.[3,4] Furthermore, edges that traverse through the slice in a curved fashion such as at the boundary between gray and white matter tend to be blurred with large slice thicknesses. This results in a loss of boundary definition due to partial voluming.

Reduction in slice thickness may aid in differentiating small structures, enhancing tissue boundaries, and increasing contrast, but the resulting loss in S/N may negate these advantages. Increasing the number of acquisitions to regain the S/N may be sufficient (see 1.1214-20), but the longer imaging time may not always be an option as in the case of T2-weighted studies. Protocols are properly designed with thicknesses that minimize volume averaging effects while still maintaining S/N so that imaging time is not unreasonable. Small structures such as the pituitary require thin sections to be well visualized, and this inevitably leads to long scan times. In routine head screening, however, thicker slices can usually be afforded and may in fact be necessary for the purposes of sufficient coverage.

Advantages

Thick-section images have high S/N. Tissue delineation among large structures is improved. Thin slices have good small-structure visualization when obtained with sufficient S/N.

Disadvantages

Partial voluming effects associated with large slice thicknesses obscure small anatomic details and may decrease overall image quality. Thin slices have comparatively poor S/N.

Technical References

1. Crooks LE, Watts J, Hoenninger J, et al. Thin-section definition in magnetic resonance imaging. Radiology 1985;154:463–467.
2. Feinberg DA, Crooks LE, Hoenninger JC, et al. Contiguous thin multisection MR imaging by two-dimensional fourier transform techniques. Radiology 1986;158:811–817.
3. Bradley WG, Glenn BJ. The effect of variation in slice thickness and interslice gap on MR lesion detection. Am J Neuroradiol 1987;8:1057–1062.
4. Webb WR, Moore EH. Differentiation of volume averaging and mass on magnetic resonance images of the mediastinum. Radiology 1985;155:413–416.

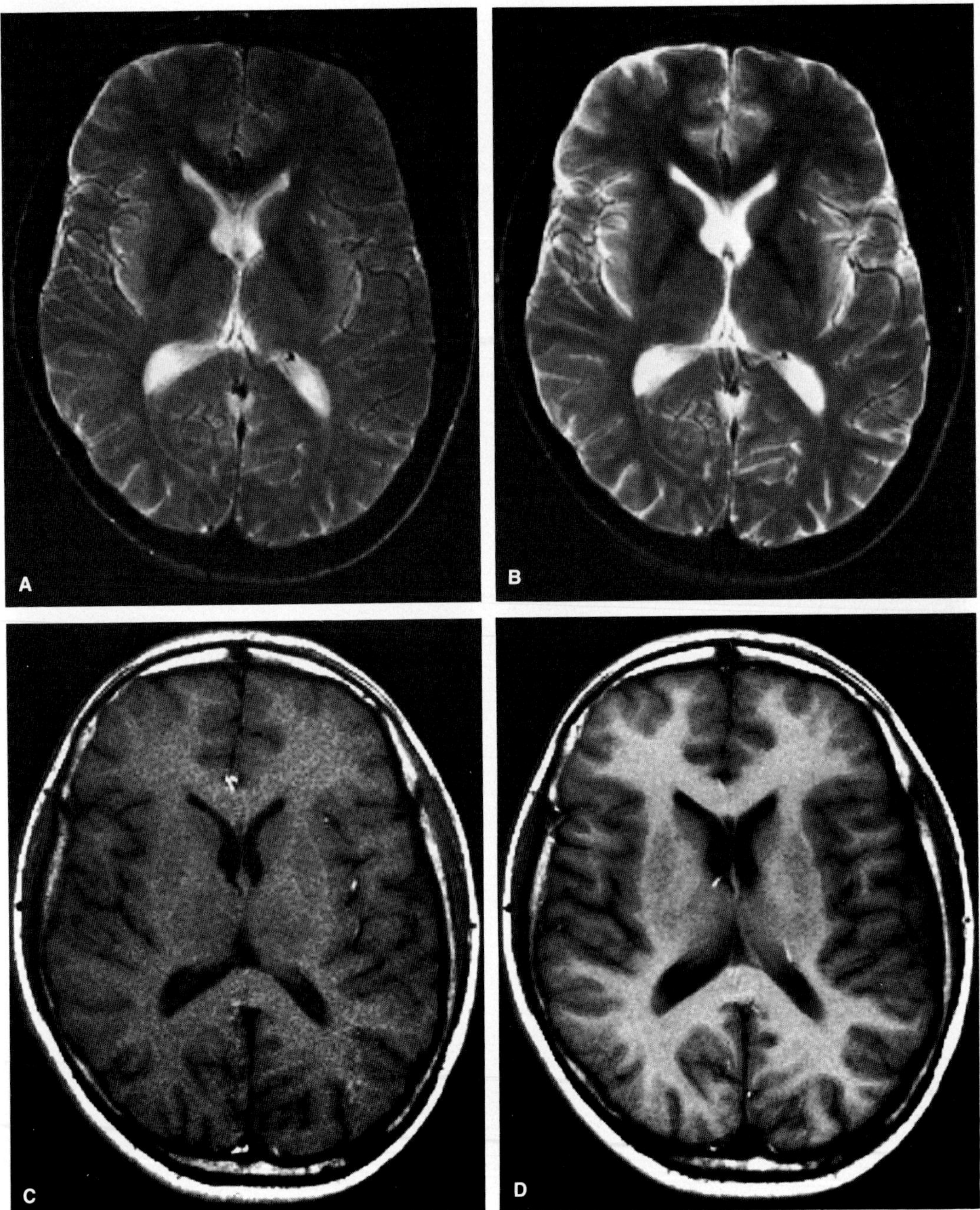

PARAMETER

Slice gap, slice-to-slice interference, and image quality

FINDINGS

(*A*) Contiguous-slice acquisitions yield reduced S/N and a loss of contrast as seen in a T2-weighted (TR/TE = 2500/90) SE scan. (*B*) With a 100% gap under otherwise identical conditions, contrast and S/N are maintained. The effect of slice interference is more severe on a T1-weighted examination (TR/TE = 300/20) as demonstrated in slices obtained at 0% gap (*C*) and 100% gap (*D*). Significant loss of gray-to-white matter differentiation is seen in *C* along with a large reduction in S/N.

CONCLUSION

Loss in S/N and decreased tissue contrast result from a reduced slice gap.

DISCUSSION

Ideally, a slice in MR should experience a uniform RF excitation throughout its thickness. Sharp, distinct edges should exist with no excitation extending beyond slice boundaries. In practice, however, the spatial excitation of spins is invariably a distribution ranging from the correct RF flip angle of excitation at the center of the slice to largely reduced flip angles at the ill-defined edges that excite regions well beyond the desired thickness.

In multislice imaging, a slice of interest may suffer interference, or "crosstalk," from neighboring slices caused by RF excitation that extends beyond their slice boundaries. S/N loss and contrast changes within each slice may result[1–4] along with potential artifacts.[5] When the gap between slices is reduced, slice-to-slice interference becomes more probable. True contiguity is theoretically not possible in 2D multislice MR, and the worst effects are seen at 0% slice gaps, where interference among slices is the greatest. Conversely, the best results occur when the gap is large enough so that neighboring slice excitations do not interfere with each other.

For a given slice gap, it is possible to minimize the effect of slice-to-slice interference. Its extent depends on the relative time between excitation of two adjacent slices. If a slice is given sufficient time for T1 and T2 relaxation to occur within it, its effect on neighboring slices is negligible regardless of the gap.[6] This depends on TR and how many slices are excited within the TR. For coverage purposes, acquiring the maximum number tends to produce the largest interference effects. Interleaving the acquisition by chronologically altering the order in which slices are excited reduces the influence.[1] Efforts have also been made to craft RF profiles so that a more uniform slice with sharper boundaries is excited, thereby minimizing interference between the slices.[7,8]

Although increasing the gap reduces crosstalk, information from the skipped regions is lost and small lesions can potentially be missed. On the other hand, slice interference with small gaps or in a contiguous mode voids the signal in the outerlying boundaries of the slice, effectively reducing slice thickness and leads to information loss as well.

Advantages

Small slice gaps may provide more complete coverage. Large gaps yield better S/N, tissue contrast, and overall image quality within each slice.

Disadvantages

A small interslice gap results in loss of S/N, tissue differentiation, and overall image quality. Large gaps may miss small lesions between slices.

Technical References

1. Kneeland JB, Shimakawa A, Wehrli FW. Effect of intersection spacing on MR image contrast and study time. Radiology 1986;158:819–822.
2. Bradley WG, Glenn BJ. The effect of variation in slice thickness and interslice gap on MR lesion detection. Am J Neuroradiol 1987;8:1057–1062.
3. Kucharczyk W, Crawley AP, Kelly WM, Henkelman RM. Effect of multislice interference on image contrast in T2- and T1-weighted MR images. Am J Neuroradiol 1988;9:443–451.
4. Schwaighofer BW, Yu KK, Mattrey RF. Diagnostic significance of interslice gap and imaging volume in body MR imaging. AJR 1989;153:629–632.
5. Crawley AP, Henkelman RM. A stimulated echo artifact from slice interference in magnetic resonance imaging. Med Phys 1987;14:842–848.
6. Feinberg DA, Crooks LE, Hoenninger JC, et al. Contiguous thin multisection MR imaging by two-dimensional fourier transform techniques. Radiology 1986;158:811–817.
7. Loaiza F, Lim KT, Warren WS, et al. Crafted pulses and pulse sequences for MR imaging. Health Care Instrum 1986;1:188–194.
8. Runge VM, Wood ML, Kaufman DM, Silver MS. MR imaging section profile optimization: improved contrast and detection of lesions. Radiology 1988;167:831–834.

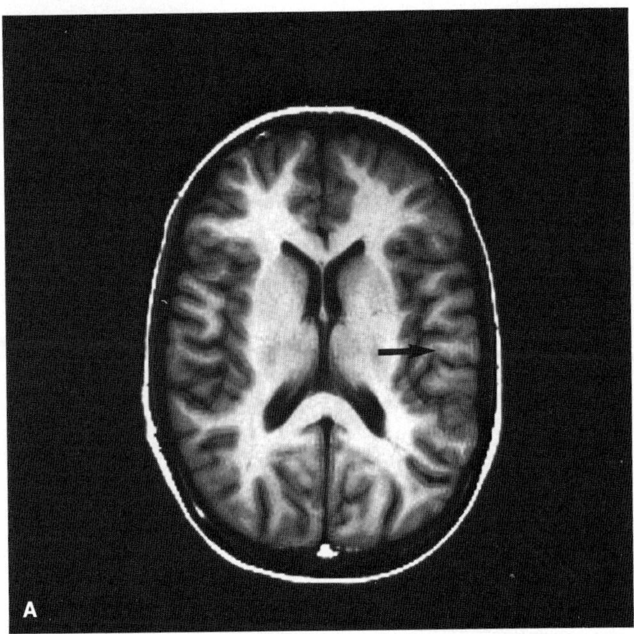

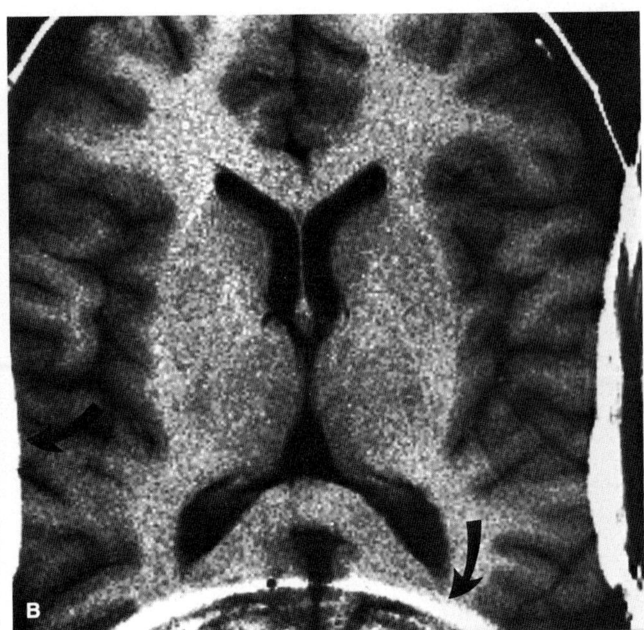

PARAMETER

Field-of-view, spatial resolution, and image quality

FINDINGS

(*A*) Acquired with an FOV of 256 mm, this T1-weighted scan (TR/TE = 500/15) possesses high S/N and good contrast with a relatively low spatial resolution of 1 mm. Some truncation artifacts are apparent (*arrow*). (*B*) T1-weighted scan taken under the same measurement conditions but with an FOV of 128 mm and a comparatively high pixel resolution of 0.5 mm. S/N is significantly reduced in conjunction with a loss in the detectability of low contrast structures. Aliasing artifact is seen at boundaries in both dimensions (*curved arrow*).

CONCLUSION

Higher spatial resolution is achieved with a smaller FOV at the expense of reduced S/N.

DISCUSSION

In MR, the FOV can be easily prescribed to achieve any degree of spatial resolution within the constraints of the system hardware. The pixel dimensions in the image are determined by the FOV divided by the acquisition matrix in each direction (see 1.1214-24). If the matrix size is held constant, the spatial resolution is increased with a smaller FOV allowing for better visualization of small structures. However, determining the appropriate FOV for a clinical study is not easy. The detectability of a lesion is associated not only with the spatial resolution but also with the contrast resolution, which is dependent on S/N (see 1.1214-1). The influence of FOV on these more diagnostically relevant parameters is complex and ultimately depends on the individual case being investigated.[1–3]

The most severe compromise with a reduced FOV is in the S/N.[1,3–5] If the FOV is halved, the S/N is reduced by a factor of 4. As the pixel size gets smaller, the amount of signal representing the pixel reduces in two dimensions. Simple geometry dictates that the area of a square reduces as the product of its sides. Background noise, however, remains the same since the amount of noise is associated with the number of pixels and not their size (see 1.1214-24). As a result, S/N reduces as the square of the FOV for a given matrix size. This large compromise may outweigh the benefits of increased resolution.

If the FOV is reduced to the extent that its boundaries lie within the region of excitation and spatial encoding, then aliasing artifacts occur. Any signal that lies beyond the FOV folds back into the image and can potentially obscure regions of interest (see 1.1214-32). On the other hand, reducing the FOV can minimize truncation artifacts (see 1.1214-34). With a large FOV, high spatial frequency signal can be "truncated" from the received signal, which can lead to an image with significant ringing artifacts. A smaller FOV reduces the degree of ringing.

High-resolution MR is difficult to accomplish without necessarily lengthening scan times. Because of the substantial loss in S/N with reduced FOVs, good image quality may be attainable only by increasing the number of acquisitions which inevitably increases the imaging time (see 1.1214-20). At a short TR, T1-weighted scans with multiple acquisitions to regain the loss in S/N may still be obtained in a reasonable amount of time. On the other hand, T2-weighted studies that have inherently long scan times may not benefit from higher resolution at the expense of prohibitively long examinations.

Advantages

A smaller FOV provides higher spatial resolution and better delineation of smaller tissue structures. A larger FOV has better S/N.

Disadvantages

A small FOV has poor S/N and may produce aliasing artifacts (see 1.1214-32). A large FOV has poorer spatial resolution with loss of structural detail, and may possess accentuated truncation artifacts (see 1.1214-34).

Technical References

1. Bradley WG, Kortman KE, Crues JV. Central nervous system high-resolution magnetic resonance imaging: effect of increasing spatial resolution on resolving power. Radiology 1985;156:93–98.
2. Runge VM, Wood ML, Kaufman DM, et al. The straight and narrow path to good head and spine MRI. Radiographics 1988;8:507–531.
3. Owen RS, Wehrli FW. Predictability of SNR and reader preference in clinical MR imaging. Magn Reson Imaging 1990; 8:737–745.
4. Crooks LE, Hoenninger J, Arakawa M, et al. High-resolution magnetic resonance imaging: technical concepts and their implementation. Radiology 1984;150:163–171.
5. Constable RT, Henkelman RM. Contrast, resolution, and detectability in MR imaging. J Comput Assist Tomogr 1991; 15:297–303.

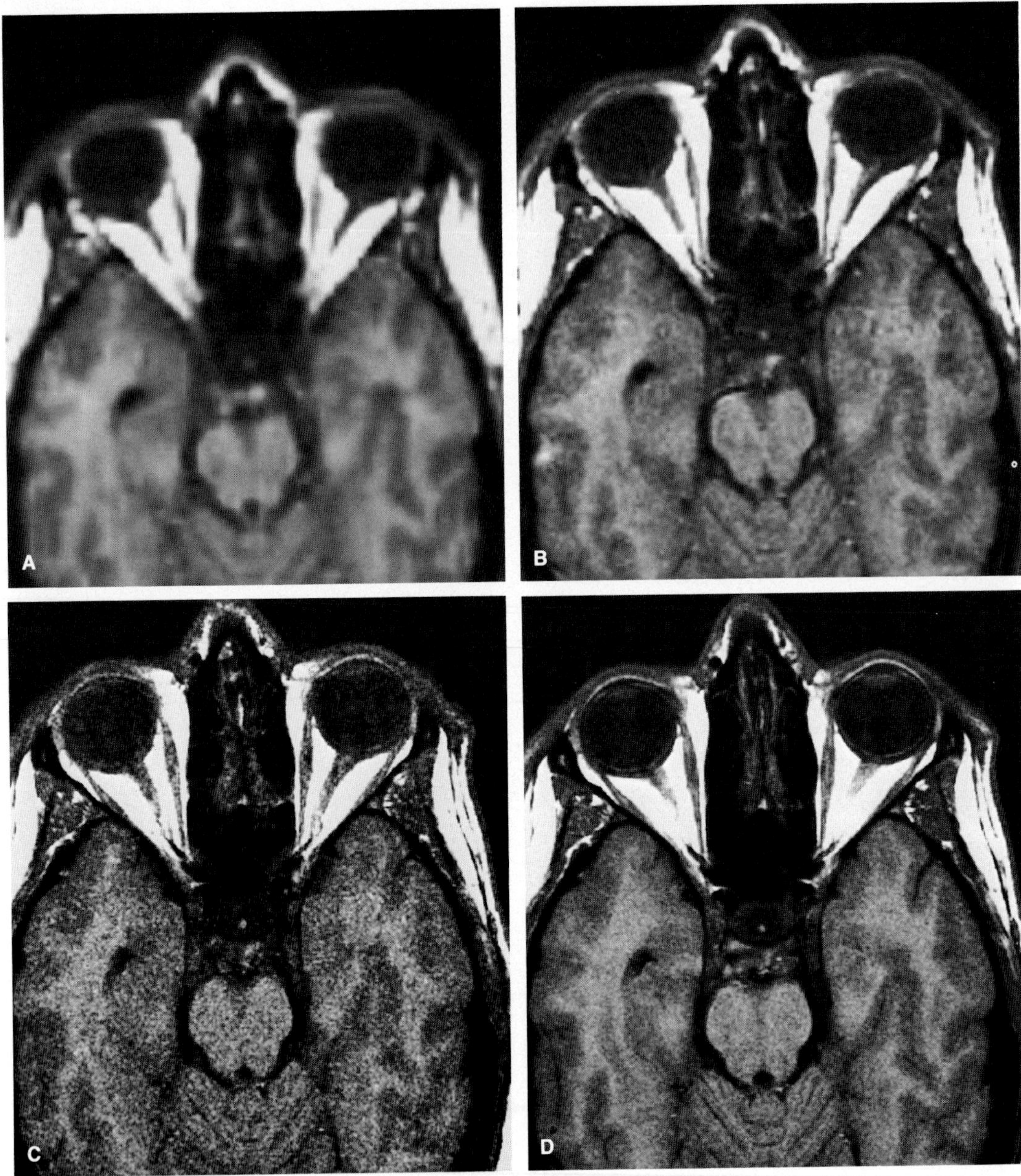

PARAMETER

Matrix size, spatial resolution, image quality, and scan time

FINDINGS

T1-weighted axial SE (TR/TE = 350/15) images were obtained at 128 (*A*), 256 (*B*), and 512 matrix size (*C*) associated with 2, 1, and 0.5 mm pixels, and acquisition times of 0:50, 1:34, and 3:04 minutes, respectively. High S/N but poor spatial resolution is observed in *A*. Increased matrix size reduces S/N, contrast, and detectability, despite the corresponding increase in spatial resolution (*C*). (*D*) Improving S/N with multiple acquisitions enhances image quality substantially at high resolution at the expense of imaging time (12:01 minutes). The cerebellum is well delineated, and the pons, pituitary gland, and orbit show small structures not observed in *A* or *B*.

CONCLUSION

Higher spatial resolution is achieved with a larger matrix at the expense of reduced S/N and longer scan times.

DISCUSSION

The effect of matrix size on the S/N and the imaging time is straightforward. Determining the appropriate matrix size for a clinical study is not as easy. The detectability of a lesion is associated with contrast resolution, which is dependent on S/N, and with the true spatial resolving power, which is not necessarily equal to the size of a pixel or voxel (see 1.1214-1). The influence of matrix size on these more diagnostically relevant parameters is complex and ultimately depends on the individual case being investigated.[1–3]

The pixel dimensions of an MR image are determined by the FOV divided by the matrix size in each direction (see 1.1214-23). If the FOV along with other user-selectable parameters is held constant, then the S/N increases with reduced matrix size.[1,4,5] Although background noise increases with a reduced matrix, the signal increases more for a given FOV because of the increase in pixel size. Therefore, the overall S/N improves.

Higher S/N may improve detection because of better contrast resolution, but a larger pixel size may counter this because of the loss in spatial resolution, particularly with small structures. Additionally, truncation artifacts may become evident at a smaller matrix (see 1.1214-34). It has been shown that with larger matrices there is also less sensitivity to field inhomogeneities caused, for example, by metal (see 1.1214-27).[6]

The total scan time also depends on the matrix size. A 2D MR image is acquired by encoding one dimension in frequency and the other in phase. In 3D MR an additional third dimension of phase encoding is incorporated (see 1.1214-9). The number of phase encoding steps equals the number of pixels in the phase encoding direction of the image, provided partial data methods are not employed (see 1.1214-25). The total imaging time is directly proportional to the total number of phase-encoded signals that are acquired. Therefore, although some advantages can be gained by using large matrix sizes, the drawback of increased imaging time limits their routine use.

Advantages

Large matrices provide higher spatial resolution and better delineation of smaller tissue structures. Smaller matrices have better S/N and shorter scan times.

Disadvantages

A larger matrix requires longer scan times. Small matrices have poorer spatial resolution with loss of structural detail, and may possibly possess truncation artifacts (see 1.1214-34).

Technical References

1. Bradley WG, Kortman KE, Crues JV. Central nervous system high-resolution magnetic resonance imaging: effect of increasing spatial resolution on resolving power. Radiology 1985;156:93–98.
2. Runge VM, Wood ML, Kaufman DM, et al. The straight and narrow path to good head and spine MRI. Radiographics 1988;8:507–531.
3. Owen RS, Wehrli FW. Predictability of SNR and reader preference in clinical MR imaging. Magn Reson Imaging 1990;8:737–745.
4. Crooks LE, Hoenninger J, Arakawa M, et al. High-resolution magnetic resonance imaging: technical concepts and their implementation. Radiology 1984;150:163–171.
5. Constable RT, Henkelman RM. Contrast, resolution, and detectability in MR imaging. J Comput Assist Tomogr 1991; 15:297–303.
6. Young IR, Cox IJ, Bryant DJ, Bydder GM. The benefits of increasing spatial resolution as a means of reducing artifacts due to field inhomogeneities. Magn Reson Imaging 1988;6:585–590.

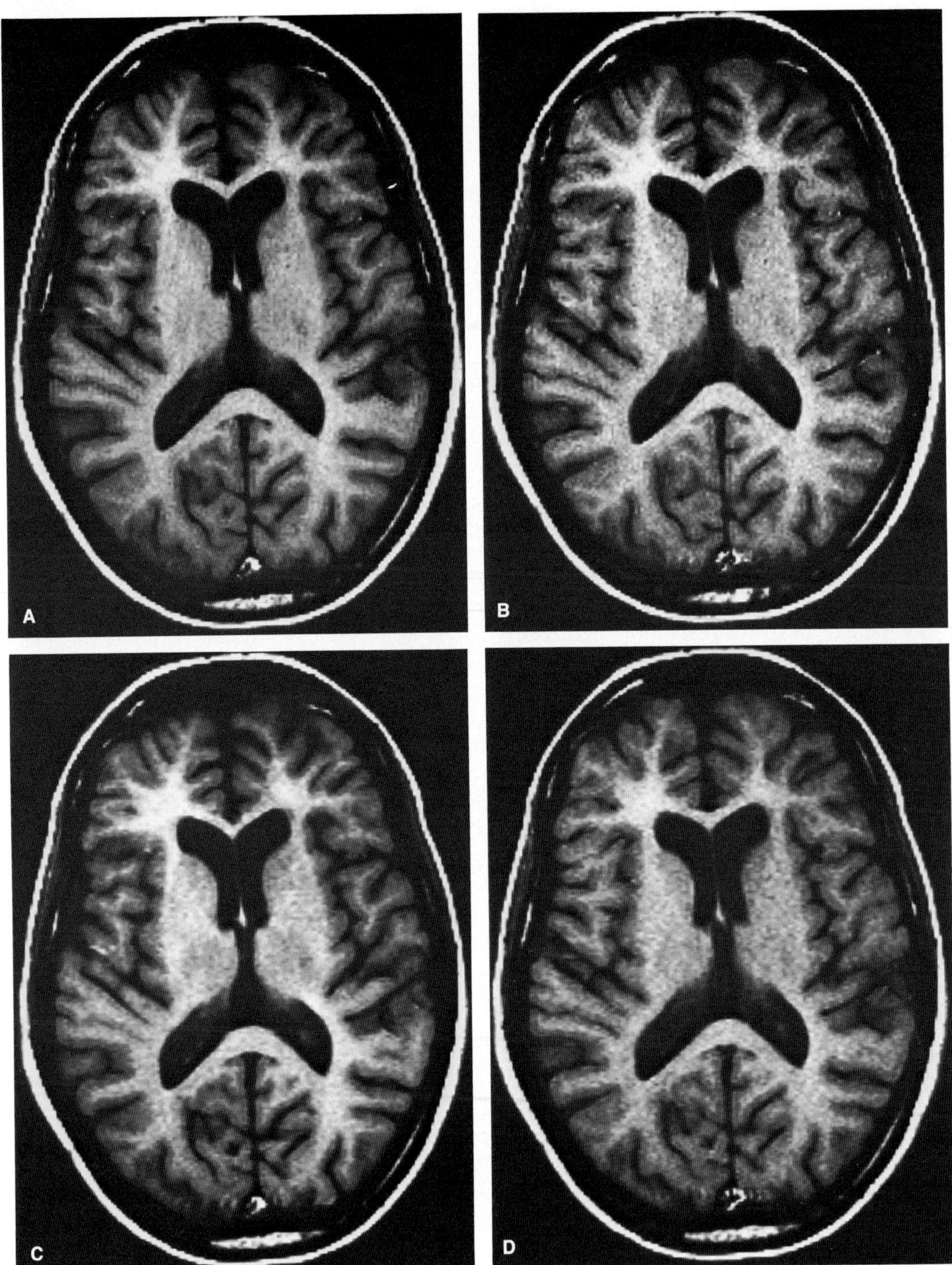

PARAMETER

Partial data methods with reduced scan time

FINDINGS

(*A*) A full 256 × 256 matrix acquisition of a T1-weighted (TR/TE = 400/15) SE scan obtained in 6:54 minutes. Contrast between gray and white matter is high, and spatial resolution is 0.9 × 0.9 mm. (*B*) A half-fourier acquisition acquired in 3:55 minutes under otherwise identical conditions. S/N is reduced from approximately 1.4:1, but spatial resolution is maintained. (*C*) A rectangular FOV acquisition acquired in 4:21 minutes with no loss in spatial resolution and only a slight reduction in S/N. (*D*) SE scan obtained with a partial data acquisition that combines both half-fourier and rectangular FOV methods. S/N re-

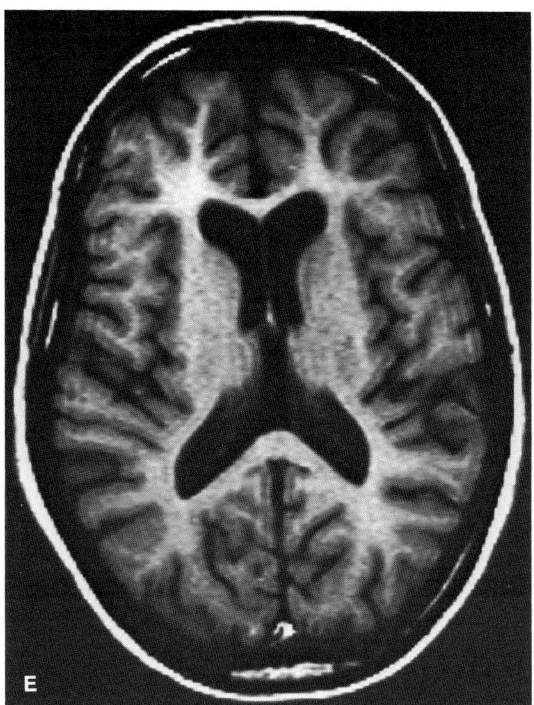

duction is noticeable; however, spatial resolution is still maintained and the total imaging time was only 2:38 minutes. (*E*) This scan demonstrates a rectangular pixel acquisition that improves S/N while reducing scan time (4:21 minutes); however, left/right spatial resolution is reduced and truncation artifacts are seen.

CONCLUSION

Scan time is reduced using partial data schemes, with compromises in either S/N or spatial resolution.

DISCUSSION

Moderate- to high-resolution examinations with large matrix sizes may require long scan times (see 1.1214-24). This is particularly true if a long TR is used to acquire proton density or T2-weighted data (see 1.1214-2). Additionally, breathhold imaging and ultrafast techniques for dynamic perfusion studies (see 1.1214-17) require total scan times of very short duration, the latter requiring less than a second per image for accurate evaluation. Therefore, many incentives exist to reduce total scan time. Collecting only part of the total data is one way that this can be accomplished.

Normally, a complete 2D data set is composed of a repeated acquisition of phase encoding steps, or "views," that equals the number of pixels in the direction of phase encoding in the image. Total imaging time, therefore, is proportional to the TR times the number of phase encoding steps. The exception is hybrid (see 1.1214-3) and echo planar techniques. In half-fourier or "half-scan" imaging, collecting only half the data and synthesizing the remainder halves the imaging time without substantial losses in the inherent detail of the image.[1–4] This method, however, comes at the expense of a reduction in the S/N.

Other partial data schemes are possible with different compromises. A rectangular FOV along with a proportionate reduction in phase encoding steps, also known as "strip scanning," maintains spatial resolution but reduces the S/N.[5] Aliasing artifact (see 1.1214-32) may also occur in this direction if the image boundaries are reduced too severely. If the FOV is maintained, decreased matrix in the phase encoding direction yields rectangular pixels with poorer resolution, but with a gain in S/N. This may also be accompanied by truncation artifact (see 1.1214-34).

Partial data schemes can be combined for fast scan applications.[6] For example, reducing the resolution of the pixel in conjunction with half-fourier reconstruction would result in no S/N change and one fourth the imaging time. Such a dramatic decrease in time may override deleterious effects of the loss in spatial resolution. On the other hand, a significant decrease in S/N from using only part of the data may reduce contrast resolution to a point that may render the image of little diagnostic utility (see 1.1214-1).

Advantages

Scan time is reduced with partial data schemes. Half-fourier and rectangular FOV methods maintain spatial resolution. Rectangular pixel methods increase S/N.

Disadvantages

Half-fourier and rectangular FOV methods suffer S/N loss. Aliasing (see 1.1214-32) can occur with severely asymmetric views. Rectangular pixel methods lose spatial resolution (see 1.1214-24) and may demonstrate truncation artifact (see 1.1214-34).

Technical References

1. Margosian P, Schmitt F, Purdy D. Faster MR imaging: imaging with half the data. Health Care Instrum 1986;1:195–197.
2. Feinberg DA, Hale JD, Watts JC, et al. Halving MR imaging time by conjugation: demonstration at 3.5 kG. Radiology 1986;161:527–531.
3. Runge VM, Wood ML. Half-fourier MR imaging of CNS disease. Am J Neuroradiol 1990;11:77–82.
4. Terk MR, Simon HE, Udkoff RC, Colletti PM. Halfscan: clinical applications in MR imaging. Magn Reson Imaging 1991;9:477–483.
5. Feinberg DA, Hoenninger JC, Crooks LE, et al. Inner volume MR imaging: technical concepts and their application. Radiology 1985;156:743–747.
6. Martin JF, Edelman RR. Fast MR imaging. In: Edelman RR, Hesselink JR, eds. Clinical magnetic resonance imaging. Philadelphia, WB Saunders. 1990.

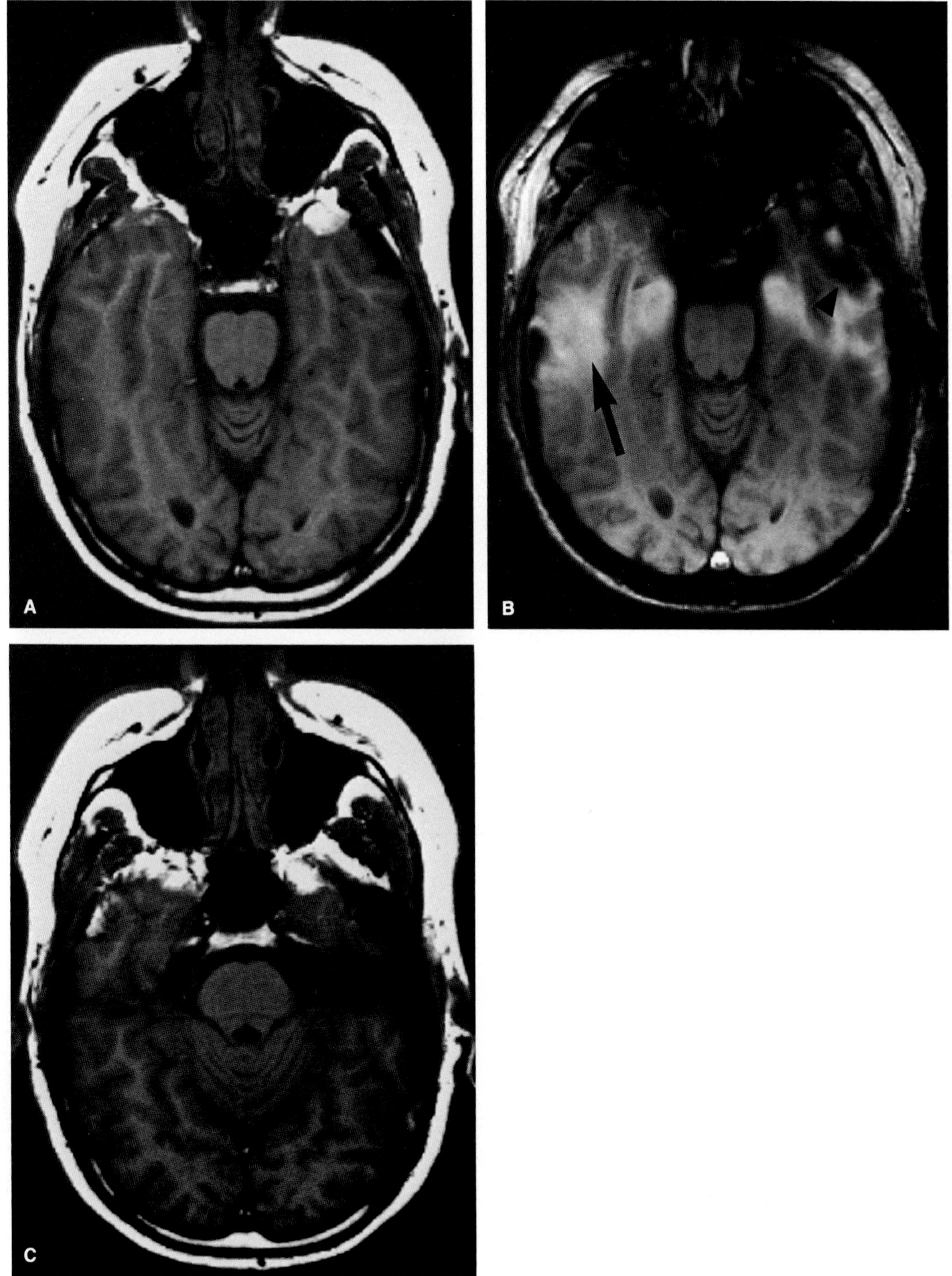
A
B
C

ARTIFACT

Magnetic susceptibility artifact in gradient echo imaging

FINDINGS

In comparison with a T1-weighted (TR/TE = 450/15) SE scan (*A*), a spoiled GRE acquisition (TR/TE/FA = 450/15/90°) obtained under identical measurement conditions demonstrates large susceptibility artifacts (*B*). Hyperintense regions (*arrow*) and signal voids (*arrowhead*) are characteristic (*B*) and can usually be attributed to the presence of air/tissue interfaces in neighboring slices, as illustrated on the adjacent SE scan (*C*).

CONCLUSION

Regional signal voids and loss in contrast caused by magnetic susceptibility differences are accentuated with GRE techniques.

DISCUSSION

Magnetic susceptibility (χ) is a property of tissues that defines the degree to which a material becomes magnetized. Not all tissues or substances experience the same magnetic field internally, even though they exist in the presence of the same external field. Differences in χ result in field gradients across boundaries, no matter how slight or small. These localized regions of field inhomogeneity can lead to T2* shortening, spin dephasing, and potential losses in MR signal.[1]

The influence of χ depends on the type of MR technique that is employed. In the SE technique (see 1.1214-2), the 180° RF pulse reverses the effect of χ field errors and little signal loss occurs in regions of even large differences in χ. However, in GRE techniques (see 1.1214-6 to 1.1214-8) that are missing a 180° pulse, χ effects do not cancel. The degree of signal loss depends on the degree of difference in susceptibility between two regions. Air, for example, has a value of χ significantly different from most tissues. Thus, air–tissue interfaces show large susceptibility effects. This would include such regions as the sinuses, the pituitary, and the internal auditory canal. The frontal lobe of the brain also commonly shows susceptibility artifacts because of its proximity to the ethmoid sinuses.[2,3]

Susceptibility artifacts can become accentuated in several ways. If TE is increased, signal errors accumulate and susceptibility artifacts become more prominent. Also, if the sampling bandwidth (see 1.1214-28) is lowered, thereby increasing the overall magnetic field sensitivity, regions with errors induced by susceptibility are mapped to a larger degree. Conversely, these artifacts can be minimized by using a short TE, higher bandwidth, or other means of correction currently being investigated.[4,5]

Most tissues have similar intrinsic χ values. There are some instances, however, when tissues may be introduced with substances that change their susceptibility. The presence of ferromagnetic or paramagnetic material either biochemically (eg, hemosiderin) or artificially (eg, contrast agents) can generate microscopic susceptibility-induced field inhomogeneities on a molecular level that can lead to enhanced contrast rather than image artifact (see 1.1214-17).[6]

Advantages

Differences in susceptibility of tissues may enhance contrast under certain conditions (see 1.1214-17 and 1.1214-19).

Disadvantages

Large-bulk magnetic susceptibility differences cause regional signal voids and contrast loss, obscuring structural detail, particularly with GRE techniques (see 1.1214-6 to 1.1214-8).

Technical References

1. Ludeke KM, Roschmann P, Tischler R. Susceptibility artifacts in NMR imaging. Mag Reson Imaging 1985;3:329–343.
2. Schick RM, Wismer GL, Davis KR. Magnetic susceptibility effects secondary to out-of-plane air in fast MR scanning. Am J Neuroradiol 1988;9:439–442.
3. Czervionke LF, Daniels DL, Wehrli FW, et al. Magnetic susceptibility artifacts in gradient-recalled echo MR imaging. Am J Neuroradiol 1988;9:1149–1155.
4. Haacke EM, Tkach JA, Parrish TB. Reduction of T2* dephasing in gradient field-echo imaging. Radiology 1989;170:457–462.
5. Cho ZH, Ro YM. Reduction of susceptibility artifact in gradient-echo imaging. Magn Reson Med 1992;23:193–200.
6. Young IR, Bydder GM, Khenia S, Collins AG. Assessment of phase and amplitude effects due to susceptibility variations in MR imaging of the brain. J Comput Assist Tomogr 1989;13:490–494.

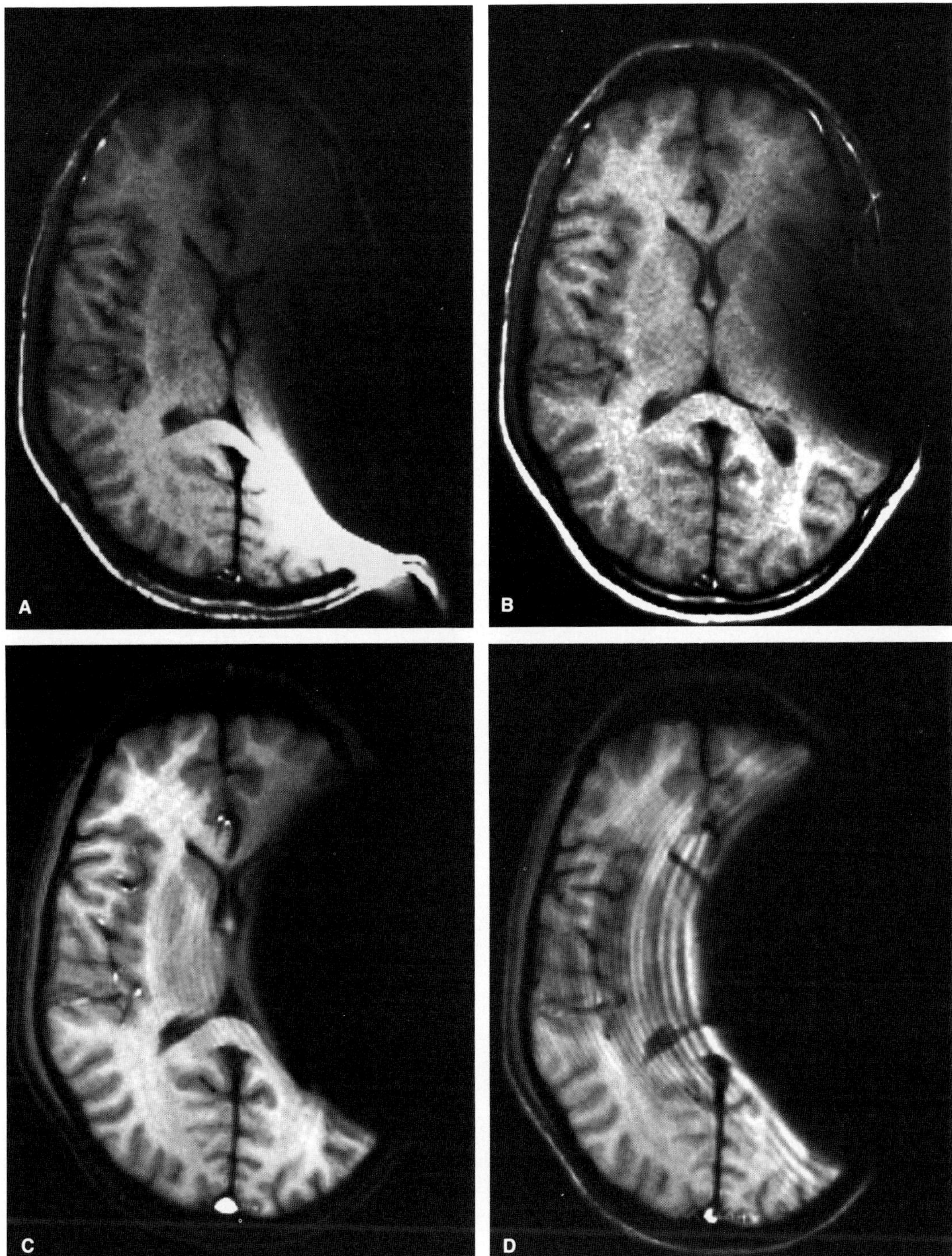

ARTIFACT

Metal artifact in spin echo and gradient echo imaging at low and high sampling bandwidths

FINDINGS

(*A*) On an axial T1-weighted (TR/TE = 350/24) SE scan acquired with low sampling bandwidth (56 Hz/pixel), there is a large region of signal void with a rim of hyperintensity and peripheral image distortion due to the presence of metal. (*B*) At a high sampling bandwidth (325 Hz/pixel) under otherwise identical measurement conditions, the metal artifacts are substantially reduced. (*C*) In comparison with *B*, a spoiled GRE (TR/TE = 350/7/90°) scan at the same high bandwidth shows an expanded region of signal void, despite a reduced echo time. (*D*) An increase in echo time (TE = 14) accentuates the metal artifact substantially and produces a rippling that emanates through the entire section.

CONCLUSION

Signal loss and local image distortions caused by magnetic field errors are generated by the presence of metal and are accentuated using a low sampling bandwidth or GRE techniques with longer TE.

DISCUSSION

Ferromagnetic and nonferromagnetic metals are well known to locally distort the main external magnetic field.[1–4] As a result, the MR signal frequency, phase, and amplitude in their vicinity are altered. In general, the main field is made as homogeneous as possible so that the errors in the signal are minimized to yield high image quality and accurate anatomic representation. Deviations in the signal frequency and phase can lead to spatially mismapped pixels and image distortions. Errors in the magnetic field can also lead to local T2* shortening, reduced signal amplitude, and regional intensity voids in the image.

Artifacts caused by the presence of metal can become accentuated when low sampling frequency bandwidths are used as a result of the increased sensitivity to magnetic field errors (see 1.1214-28). This is seen primarily in the frequency encoding direction of the image and is independent of the type of MR technique that is used.

The severity of metal artifact, however, can also depend on technique. In SE imaging (see 1.1214-2), the 180° RF pulse tends to cancel minor magnetic field inhomogeneities thereby minimizing the artifacts caused by metal. Higher spatial resolution (see 1.1214-23 and 1.1214-24) can also reduce the extent of artifacts.[5] On the other hand, the absence of a 180° pulse in GRE techniques (see 1.1214-6 to 1.1214-8) allows errors to accumulate, which leads to larger artifacts. Longer echo times further increase the propagation of error, accentuating signal loss and distortion in the image.

If the influence of the metal extends beyond the dimension of the image pixel, the result is an artifact. Dental materials,[1,6,7] mascara,[8] hairpins, surgical clips,[1,4] and prosthetic devices[1–4] are typical sources. However, microscopic field inhomogeneities can be generated by the presence of paramagnetic, superparamagnetic, or ferromagnetic substances introduced either biochemically (eg, hemosiderin) or injected as a negatively enhancing contrast agent (eg, iron particulates). The primary effect is T2* shortening and signal reduction of the tissue in its presence (see 1.1214-17 and 1.1214-26).

Advantages

Metal substances used as negatively enhancing contrast agents can improve lesion conspicuity (see 1.1214-17). Intrinsic changes in the iron content of tissue may provide additional diagnostic information.

Disadvantages

Metallic objects lead to large regions of signal loss and spatial distortion that can be accentuated by the technique used.

Technical References

1. New PFJ, Rosen BR, Brady TJ, et al. Potential hazards and artifacts of ferromagnetic and nonferromagnetic surgical and dental materials and devices in nuclear magnetic resonance imaging. Radiology 1983;147:139–148.
2. Laakman RW, Kaufman B, Han JS, et al. MR imaging in patients with metallic implants. Radiology 1985;157:711–714.
3. Augustiny N, von Schulthess GK, Meier D, Bosiger P. MR imaging of large nonferromagnetic metallic implants at 1.5T. J Comput Assist Tomogr 1987;11:678–683.
4. Teitelbaum GP, Bradley WG, Klein BD. MR imaging artifacts, ferromagnetism, and magnetic torque of intravascular filters, stents, and coils. Radiology 1988;166:657–664.
5. Young IR, Cox IJ, Bryant DJ, Bydder GM. The benefits of increasing spatial resolution as a means of reducing artifacts due to field inhomogeneities. Magn Reson Imaging 1988;6:585–590.
6. Fache JS, Price C, Hawbolt EB, Li DK. MR imaging artifacts produced by dental materials. Am J Neuroradiol 1987;8: 837–840.
7. Hinshaw DB, Holshouser BA, Engstrom HIM, et al. Dental material artifacts on MR images. Radiology 1988;166:777–779.
8. Smith FW, Crosher GA. Mascara—an unsuspected cause of magnetic resonance imaging artifact. Magn Reson Imaging 1985;3:287–289.

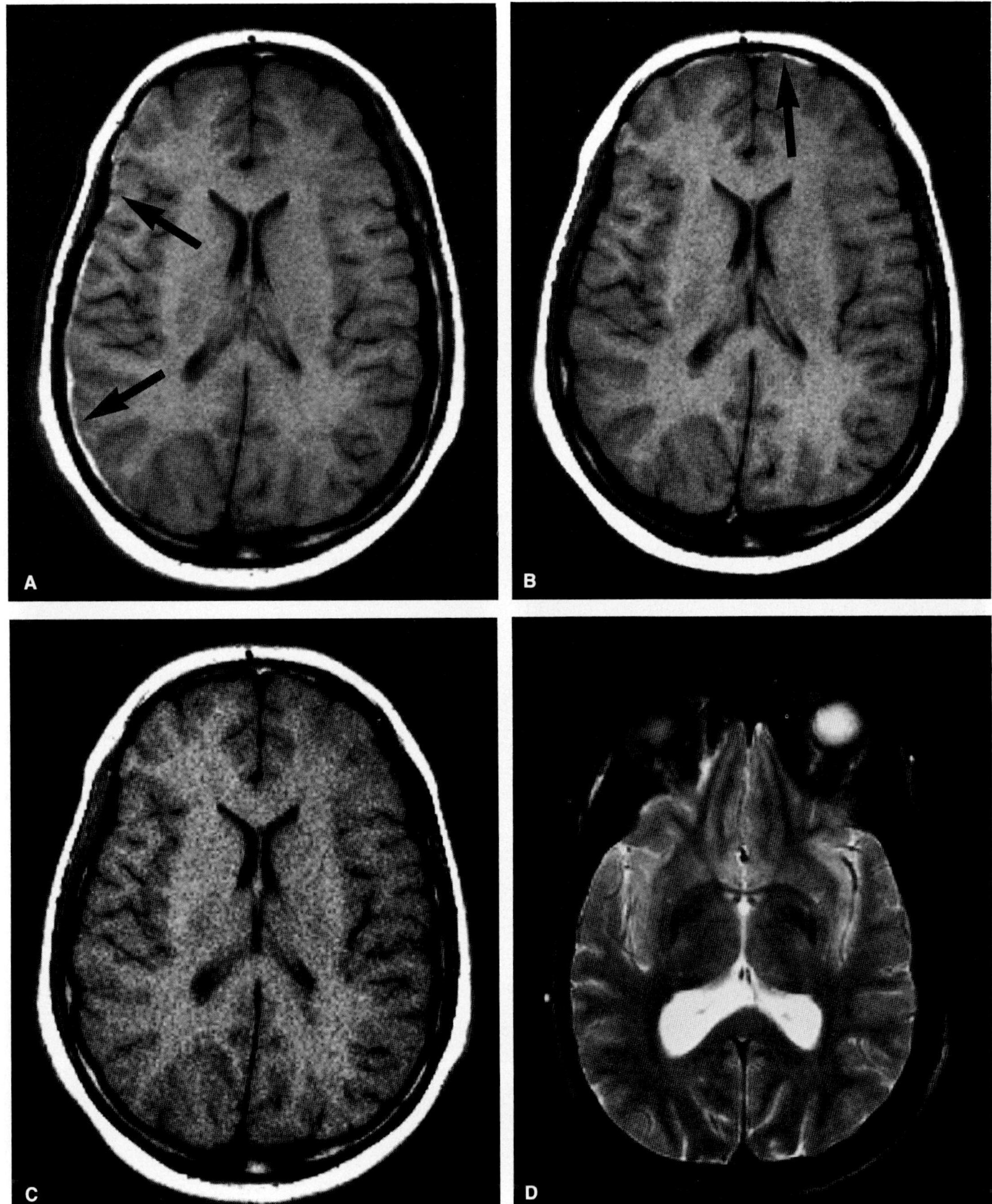

ARTIFACT

Chemical shift artifact and sampling bandwidth

FINDINGS

On a low sampling bandwidth (56 Hz/pixel) axial T1-weighted (TR/TE = 300/24) scan, frequency encoding was left to right (*A*), and anterior to posterior (*B*). In *A*, there is a rim of hyperintensity mimicking abnormality on one side (*arrows*) and increased subdural space on the other indicating a wholesale left/right shift of the brain relative to fat. A similar hyperintense periphery is evident in *B*, although anteriorly (*arrow*), suggesting an anterior/posterior shift of the brain relative to fat. (*C*) At a high sampling bandwidth (230 Hz/pixel), no artificial hyperintensities or regional shifts are seen. However, a substantial decrease in S/N and image quality is apparent. (*D*) On a T2-weighted (TR/TE = 2500/90) scan with low bandwidth (56 Hz/pixel), contrast and S/N are high with no visible pixel shift artifacts owing to the absence of signal from fat.

CONCLUSION

An artifactual pixel shift between tissues containing fat and water is observed, which is increased using reduced sampling bandwidths.

DISCUSSION

A common artifact in MR is chemical shift pixel misregistration. Early investigations showed wholesale shifts in regions of images between tissues containing fat and water.[1–3] This pixel misregistration is caused by a spectroscopic chemical shift phenomenon.

All MR signals carry spectroscopic information about the chemical nature of the tissue. At imaging magnetic field strengths, primarily fat and water manifest themselves in the hydrogen MR signal. The spectral, or frequency, difference between the two is about 3.5 ppm or roughly 230 Hz at 1.5 T (see 1.1214-14). Since one of the two directions of an MR image is spatially mapped according to frequency, this difference causes the fat and the water signal to be mapped in two different pixel positions of the frequency-encoded direction in the image. No pixel shift occurs in the other image direction of phase encoding.

Depending on the chemical makeup and anatomic structure of the tissues, chemical shift artifacts can have varying appearances, producing edge artifacts[4] or misleading subdural enhancement.[5] Errors are most prominent in regions containing fat that surrounds soft tissue structures such as the pituitary[6] and the optic nerve.[7]

The extent to which fat and water become misregistered depends on the range of frequencies that are encoded in the image. This is determined by the sampling frequency bandwidth which is independent of the type of MR technique, and is defined by the rate at which the signal is digitally collected. If this sampling rate is slow, the frequency bandwidth is small and the image becomes encoded at small-frequency increments from pixel to pixel. For a 230-Hz difference, fat and water become separated by a large number of pixels with low-frequency-bandwidth encoding, but may accurately reside within the same pixel if the signal was collected at a high sampling bandwidth. Thus, low bandwidth imaging results in a large degree of chemical shift artifact.

Several other effects are associated with the sampling rate and frequency bandwidth. An advantage of low sampling bandwidth is that it substantially reduces the statistical noise of the image. This increases the S/N and C/N, and may improve overall image quality.[8] Because it encodes a small range of frequencies over a large number of pixels, however, magnetic field errors resulting in signal frequency errors become accentuated. Extrinsic factors such as field inhomogeneity and metal objects warp the magnetic field causing large distortions and signal loss in the image when low bandwidth sampling is used (see 1.1214-27).

Reduced bandwidth imaging is frequently implemented on the later echoes of a T2-weighted study in which S/N is inherently low and fat signal has effectively decayed away.[5,9] At short TE and long TR in spin density weighting, overall S/N is large enough and fat signal is high so that low sampling bandwidths tend not to be used. Although the S/N is relatively low on T1-weighted studies, these have a substantial amount of fat signal that may cause a large chemical shift artifact and are thus typically acquired at high bandwidths.

Advantages

High sampling bandwidth minimizes chemical shift misregistration between fat and water tissues. Low sampling bandwidth reduces statistical noise, while improving S/N and image quality.

Disadvantages

Low sampling bandwidth increases chemical shift misregistration between fat and water. High sampling bandwidth increases statistical image noise, while reducing S/N and image quality.

Technical References

1. Soila KP, Viamonte M, Starewicz PM. Chemical misregistration effects in MRI. Radiology 1984;153:819–820.
2. Dwyer AJ, Knop RH, Hoult DI. Frequency shift artifacts in MR imaging. J Comput Assist Tomogr 1985;9:16–18.
3. Weinreb JC, Brateman L, Babcock EE, et al. Chemical shift artifact in clinical magnetic resonance images at 0.35T. AJR 1985;145:183–185.
4. Babcock EE, Brateman L, Weinreb JC, et al. Edge artifacts in MR images: chemical shift effect. J Comput Assist Tomogr 1985;9:252–257.
5. Smith AS, Weinstein MA, Hurst GC, et al. Intracranial chemical-shift artifacts on MR images of the brain: observations and relation to sampling bandwidth. AJR 1990;154:1275–1283.
6. Haughton VM, Prost R. Pituitary fossa: chemical shift effect in MR imaging. Radiology 1986;158:461–462.
7. Daniels DL, Kneeland JB, Shimakawa A, et al. MR imaging of the optic nerve and sheath: correcting the chemical shift misregistration effect. Am J Neuroradiol 1986;7:249–253.
8. Hendrick RE. Sampling time effects on signal-to-noise and contrast-to-noise ratios in spin-echo MRI. Magn Reson Imaging 1987;5:31–37.
9. Simon JH, Foster TH, Ketonen L, et al. Reduced-bandwidth MR imaging of the head at 1.5T. Radiology 1989;172:771–775.

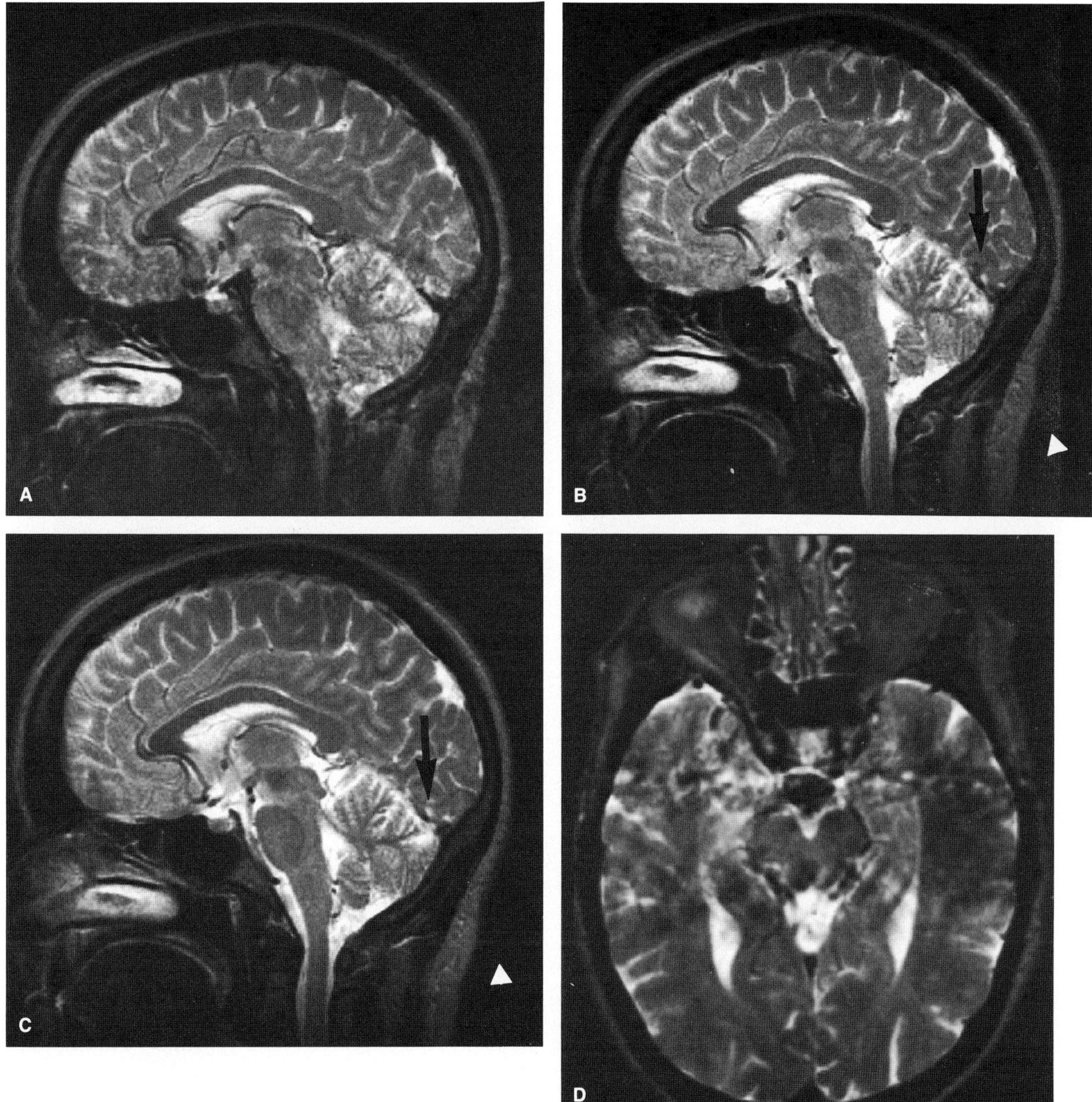

ARTIFACT

Motion-related artifacts and gradient moment nulling compensation

FINDINGS

Sagittal T2-weighted (TR/TE = 2500/90) SE scans of the midline are shown with static (zeroth-order) (*A*), velocity (first-order) (*B*), and acceleration (second-order) (*C*) gradient moment nulling motion compensation. A strong CSF signal on T2 weighting demonstrates significant motion/flow related artifacts left to right in the phase encoding direction (*A*). Velocity correction in *B* substantially improves image quality by reducing CSF flow artifacts; however, slight pulsation artifacts persist in the straight sinus (*arrow*) and pons. Pulsation artifacts are absent in *C* with acceleration compensation. Axial T2-weighted (TR/TE = 2800/90) SE scans are shown with static (*D*), velocity (*E*), and acceleration compensation (*F*). Although most artifacts are absent in *E*, regional signal voids from pulsation (*curved arrows*) can mimic abnormalities not present with acceleration compensation (*F*).

CONCLUSION

Motion artifacts, particularly from CSF flow and bulk motion on T2-weighted studies, are reduced with gradient

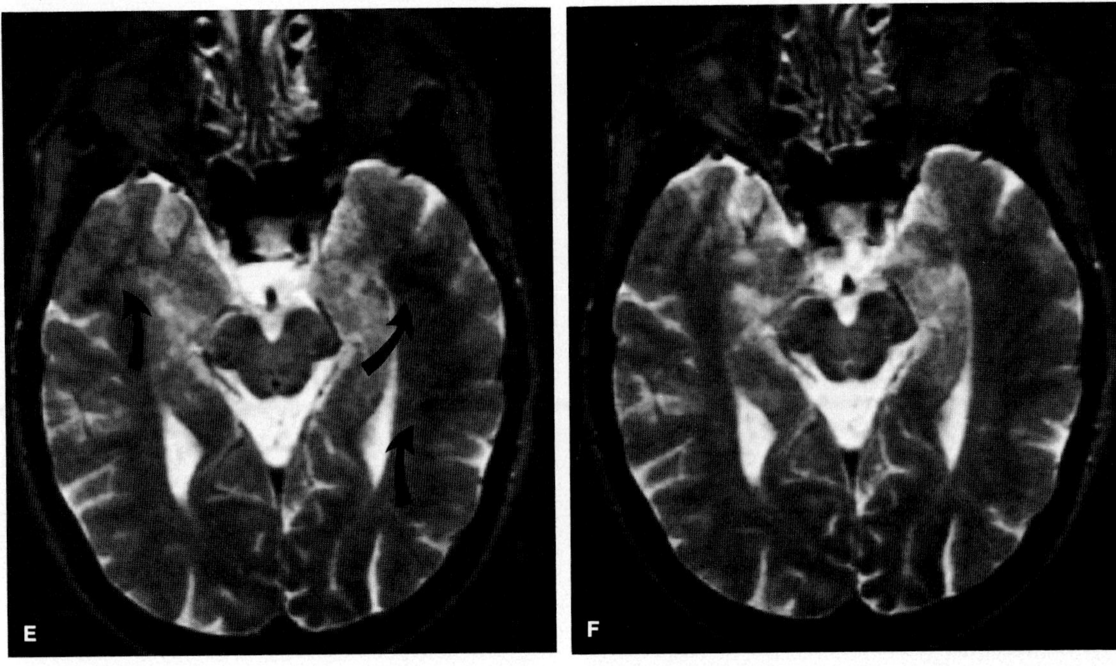

moment nulling compensation, improving overall image quality.

DISCUSSION

The MR signal from moving tissues such as blood, CSF, or the body, deviates from stationary tissues and becomes mismapped as ghost artifacts in an image. Motion generated in any direction manifests itself as an artifact in the reconstructed phase encoding direction if it remains uncorrected. In the display, these errors may constructively add to the static tissues to yield higher intensity, or destructively cancel to create regions of signal void. In both situations, motion-related artifacts give the image an overall splotchy appearance.

There are many ways to compensate for motion error in MR, one of which is gradient moment nulling. It has also been described as flow compensation, gradient motion rephasing, motion artifact suppression technique (MAST), or gradient motion refocusing.[1–4] By incorporating additional gradient pulses into an MR technique, the phase error induced in moving spins can be eliminated without compromising the spatial encoding of static spins. As a result, signal caused by motion is mapped in the correct position of the image along with the signal from stationary tissue, improving overall image quality.[5–7] Most MR techniques can be implemented with gradient moment nulling.

Motion has numerous components associated with it. First-order motion pertains to velocity. Second-order motion refers to acceleration. Higher orders of motion also exist, particularly in areas of random, pulsatile, or turbulent flow. In most imaging techniques, only the first-order, or moment, is nulled. Tissues moving with constant velocity become properly encoded in the image. In many situations this may be sufficient. If acceleration components exist, however, ghosts still become generated and more complete compensation of the higher orders may be required, as in MRA.

Motion also tends to be multidirectional. To compensate the error, gradient pulses must be added in each direction to gain the full advantage of artifact removal.[8] Difficulty arises in accomplishing motion reduction in T1 studies where TE is kept as short as possible, but motion reduction lends itself well to T2 studies where TE tends to be long. Nevertheless, T1-weighted scans that generate a large signal from fat or regions of contrast agent uptake may benefit from gradient moment nulling if a small compromise in TE is tolerable.[9]

Advantages

Compensation of bulk motion and flow by gradient moment nulling reduces artifacts and improves image quality. Compensation of motion from acceleration further increases image quality.

Disadvantages

This compensation technique requires additional gradient pulsing in the imaging technique and may restrict the choice of TE, particularly for T1-weighted scans.

Technical References

1. Constantinesco A, Mallet JJ, Bonmartin A, et al. Spatial or flow velocity phase encoding gradients in NMR imaging. Magn Reson Imaging 1984;2:335–340.
2. Waluch V, Bradley WG. NMR even echo rephasing in slow laminar flow. J Comput Assist Tomogr 1984;8:594–598.
3. Pattany PM, Phillips JJ, Chiu LC, et al. Motion artifact suppression technique (MAST) for MR imaging. J Comput Assist Tomogr 1987;11:369–377.
4. Haacke EM, Lenz GW. Improving MR image quality in the presence of motion by using rephasing gradients. AJR 1987;148:1251–1258.
5. Elster AD. Motion artifact suppression technique (MAST) for cranial MR imaging: superiority over cardiac gating for reducing phase-shift artifacts. Am J Neuroradiol 1988;9:671–674.
6. Colletti PM, Raval JK, Benson RC, et al. The motion artifact suppression technique (MAST) in magnetic resonance imaging: clinical results. Magn Reson Imaging 1988;6:293–299.
7. Quencer RM, Hinks RS, Pattany PM, et al. Improved MR imaging of the brain by using compensating gradients to suppress motion-induced artifacts. Am J Neuroradiol 1988;9:431–438.
8. Duerk JL, Pattany PM. Analysis of imaging axes significance in motion artifact suppression technique (MAST): MRI of turbulent flow and motion. Magn Reson Imaging 1989;7:251–263.
9. Richardson DN, Elster AD, Williams DW. Gd-DTPA-enhanced MR images: accentuation of vascular pulsation artifacts and correction by using gradient-moment nulling (MAST). Am J Neuroradiol 1990;11:209–210.

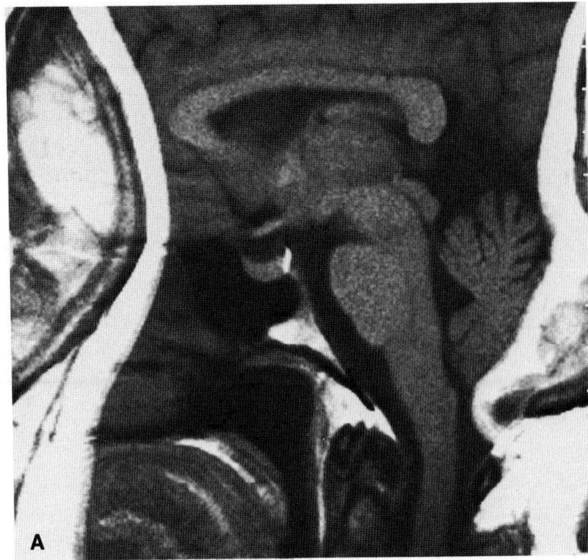

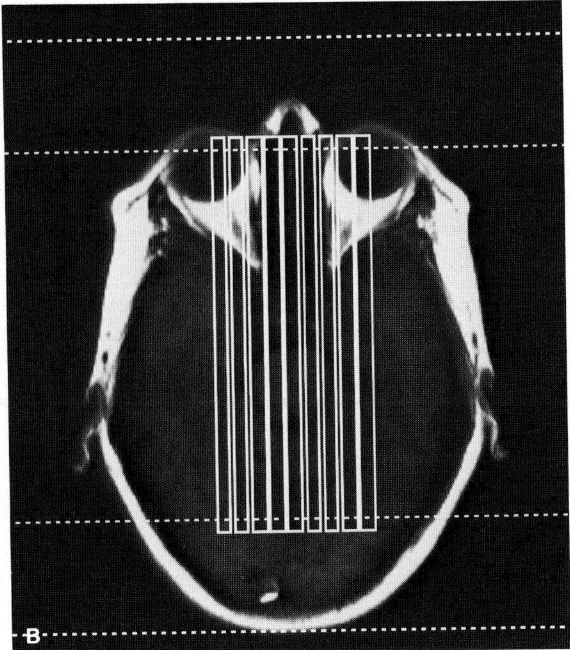

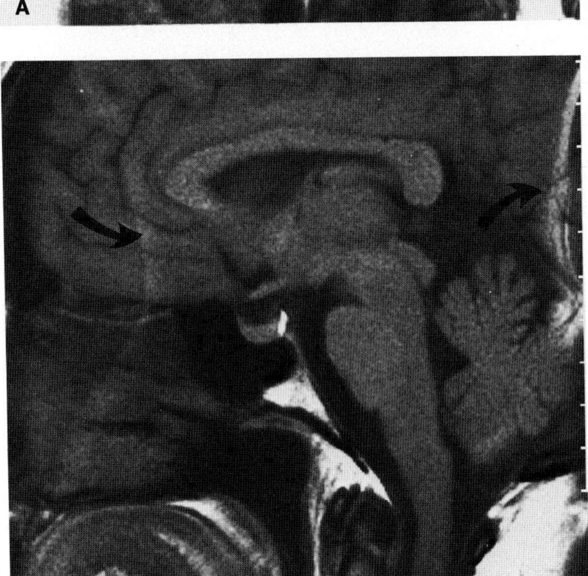

ARTIFACT

Through-plane spatial presaturation for suppression of undesirable signal

FINDINGS

(*A*) A high resolution, small FOV T1-weighted (TR/TE = 400/10) sagittal scan shows a large degree of aliasing artifact on the left and right boundaries in the phase encoding direction. Placement of large through-plane presaturation regions (*dotted lines*) at the borders of the sagittal slices (*solid lines*) substantially reduces aliasing artifacts anteriorly (*B*) and posteriorly (*C*).

CONCLUSION

Signal artifacts such as aliasing can be effectively removed by using through-plane spatial presaturation to suppress the signal.

DISCUSSION

Spatial presaturation[1–3] is an effective method for minimizing motion (see 1.1214-29) or aliasing (see 1.1214-32) artifacts resulting from a signal that would otherwise obscure image details. If a signal is suppressed by through-plane spatial presaturation, then the artifact associated with it also becomes minimized. Spatial presaturation is also used to minimize blood flow artifacts by placing presaturation slabs parallel to the slice to void the blood signal moving through the slice (see 1.1214-31).

Presaturation prevents the growth of longitudinal magnetization of the tissue being suppressed by saturating the spins in the region just before executing the imaging technique.[4] This is accomplished by applying an additional spatially selective RF pulse to the presaturation region. The effectiveness of presaturation depends in a complex manner on the imaging technique parameters, the T1 relaxation time of the tissue being saturated, and the delay time between the presaturation and the imaging pulses. The technique can be incorporated into any imaging application and has also been used to selectively void venous or arterial blood in TOF MRA (see 1.1214-11).[5]

Several disadvantages exist with the introduction of a presaturation pulse into an MR technique. Each presaturation pulse that is applied to suppress a region requires additional time. The use of many pulses reduces the total slice capability of the technique. Presaturation pulsing also increases the specific absorption rate (SAR) and may significantly increase the RF exposure to the patient. Nevertheless, spatial presaturation can effectively reduce artifacts from unwanted tissues by suppressing their signal and may greatly enhance the diagnostic image quality.

Advantages

Through-plane spatial presaturation substantially reduces unwanted signal in the image from aliasing (see 1.1214-32) or in-plane motion (see 1.1214-29).

Disadvantages

Additional RF pulsing required for presaturation decreases the time available for multislice imaging and increases the SAR to the patient.

Technical References

1. Felmlee JP, Ehman RL. Spatial presaturation: a method for suppressing flow artifacts and improving depiction of vascular anatomy in MR imaging. Radiology 1987;164:559–564.
2. Edelman RR, Atkinson DJ, Silver MS, et al. FRODO pulse sequences: a new means of eliminating motion, flow, and wraparound artifacts. Radiology 1988;166:231–236.
3. Ehman RL, Felmlee JP. Flow artifact reduction in MRI: a review of the roles of gradient moment nulling and spatial presaturation. Magn Reson Med 1990;14:293–307.
4. Mugler JP, Brookeman JR. The design of pulse sequences employing spatial presaturation for the suppression of flow artifacts. Magn Reson Med 1992;23:201–214.
5. Edelman RR, Wentz KU, Mattle HP, et al. Intracerebral arteriovenous malformations: evaluation with selective MR angiography and venography. Radiology 1989;173:831–837.

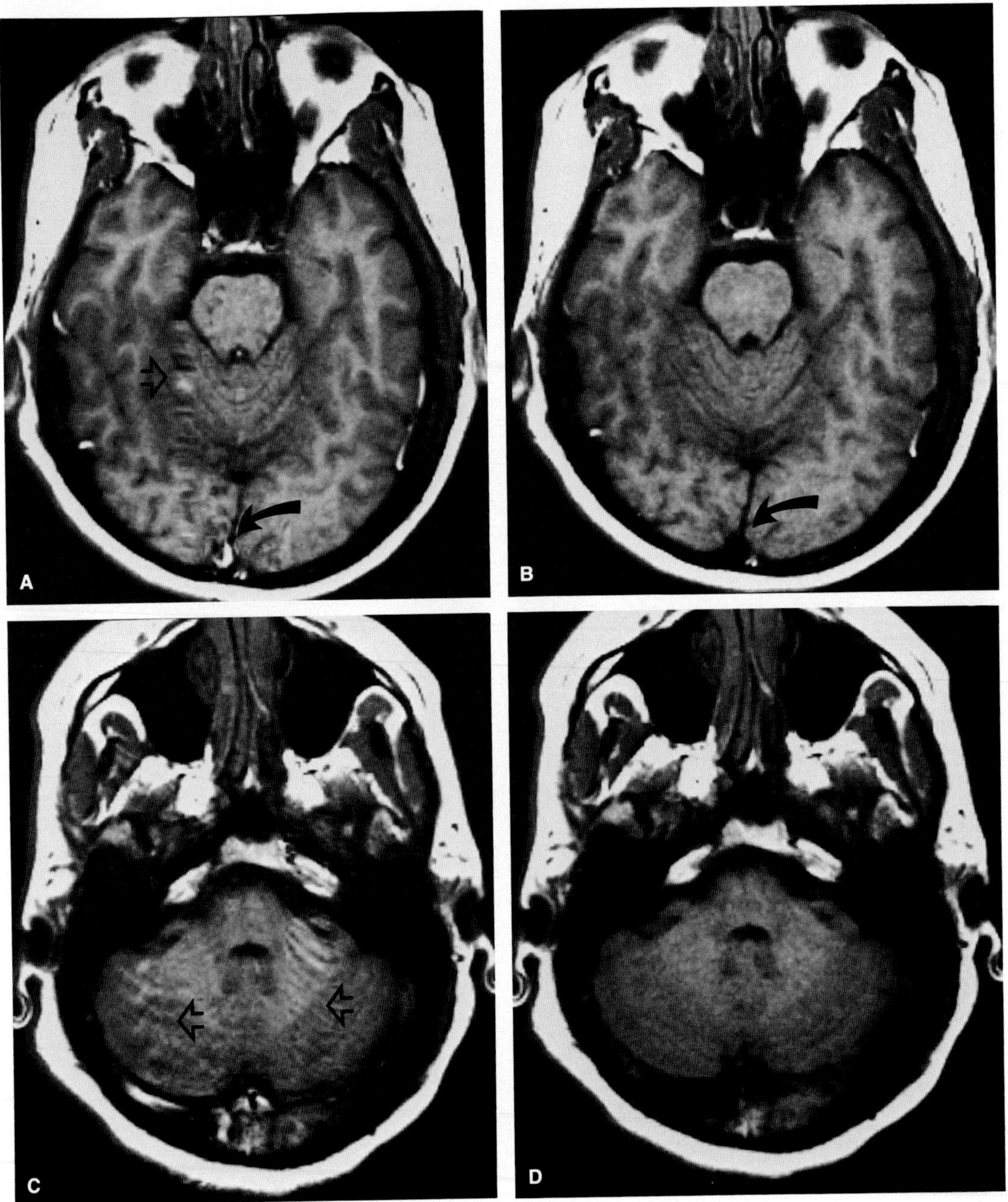

ARTIFACT

Parallel spatial presaturation for suppression of flow-related artifacts

FINDINGS

(*A*) A T1-weighted (TR/TE = 400/15) axial scan shows a significant degree of vertical pulsation artifact throughout the image (*open arrow*) from vessels with large signal (*curved arrow*). (*B*) Placement of presaturation regions parallel to the slices substantially reduces flow artifacts from vessels by voiding the signal from flow (*curved arrow*). (*C*) A more inferior section shows flow-related artifacts from both venous and arterial structures (*open arrows*), obscuring details in nearly the entire cerebellum. (*D*) With parallel presaturation, flow signal is voided and associated artifacts are absent.

CONCLUSION

Effective removal of flow-related artifacts is achieved using parallel spatial presaturation.

DISCUSSION

Parallel spatial presaturation is an effective way to minimize flow-related artifacts resulting from vessels that traverse through the slice.[1–3] If signal originating from inflowing blood is suppressed, the motion artifact associated with it is suppressed in the image. This can be accomplished parallel to the plane of imaging by saturating the spins from the blood flowing through the slice, and is sometimes referred to as "flow voiding." Spatial presaturation is also used to minimize in-plane motion or aliasing artifacts (see 1.1214-30).

The concept of presaturation is to suppress the growth of longitudinal magnetization by saturating the unwanted spins through the application of an additional spatially selective RF pulse to the region just prior to the imaging technique. Its effectiveness depends in a complex manner on the imaging technique parameters, the T1 relaxation time and velocity of the blood being saturated, the distance between the saturation plane and the imaging plane, and the delay time between the presaturation and the imaging pulses.[4] These determinants are similar issues addressed in TOF MRA techniques (see 1.1214-10 and 1.1214-11).

Several disadvantages exist with the introduction of a presaturation pulse into an MR technique. Each presaturation pulse that is applied to suppress a region requires additional time. The use of two pulses on either side of the imaging volume to saturate inflowing spins reduces the total slice capability of the technique. Presaturation pulsing also increases the SAR when it is applied and may significantly increase the RF exposure to the patient. Nevertheless, parallel spatial presaturation can effectively reduce flow-related artifacts and may greatly enhance the diagnostic image quality.

Advantages

Parallel spatial presaturation substantially reduces unwanted signal in the image from flow.

Disadvantages

Additional RF pulsing required for presaturation decreases the time available for multislice imaging and increases the SAR to the patient.

Technical References

1. Felmlee JP, Ehman RL. Spatial presaturation: a method for suppressing flow artifacts and improving depiction of vascular anatomy in MR imaging. Radiology 1987;164:559–564.
2. Edelman RR, Atkinson DJ, Silver MS, et al. FRODO pulse sequences: a new means of eliminating motion, flow, and wraparound artifacts. Radiology 1988;166:231–236.
3. Ehman RL, Felmlee JP. Flow artifact reduction in MRI: a review of the roles of gradient moment nulling and spatial presaturation. Magn Reson Med 1990;14:293–307.
4. Mugler JP, Brookeman JR. The design of pulse sequences employing spatial presaturation for the suppression of flow artifacts. Magn Reson Med 1992;23:201–214.

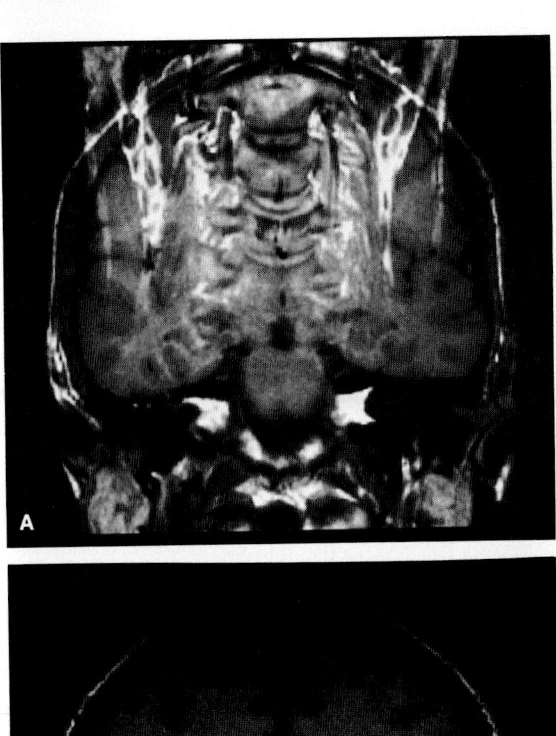

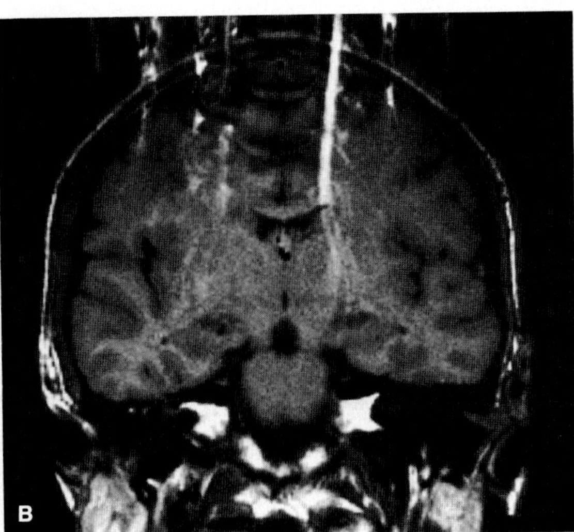

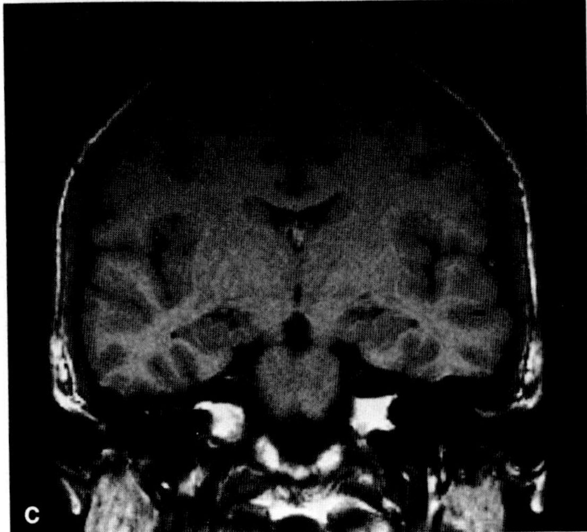

ARTIFACT

Aliasing artifact and oversampling in 2D MR

FINDINGS

Severe (*A*) and moderate (*B*) aliasing artifacts are shown in coronal T1-weighted SE (TR/TE = 400/15) images. Signal from the neck becomes superimposed on the top of the head, making interpretation difficult or impossible in the aliased region. (*C*) Oversampling in the vertical direction completely eliminates the artifact.

CONCLUSION

Image wraparound occurs from signal extending beyond the boundaries of the FOV obscuring the details of underlying structures; it is eliminated by oversampling.

DISCUSSION

Aliasing, sometimes referred to as "foldover" or "wraparound," is strictly a digital phenomenon and is a well-known artifact in MR.[1–4] The MR signal is typically encoded with many frequencies and phases and carries with it information about its spatial origin within the body. At times, however, the digital sampling of the signal is not fast enough to accurately represent the highest frequencies and largest phases that come from regions far from the center of the image. As a result, signal from outside one boundary of the FOV becomes wrapped to the opposite boundary, overlaying itself on the image and obscuring details.

The FOV of the image relative to the size of the tissue in the region governs the extent of the aliasing. Therefore, there is more danger of aliasing with a small FOV than a large one. In routine examinations in which high spatial resolution is not required, the FOVs are comparatively large and aliasing is unlikely to occur since the tissue signal typically lies well within the FOV. However, a high-resolution study that necessitates a small FOV runs the risk of large degrees of aliasing (see 1.1214-23). One way of eliminating this artifact is to simply expand the FOV so that the signal from all sides lies within the boundaries. The matrix size is increased accordingly in order to maintain spatial resolution. This, however, leads to longer scan times.

A number of other methods exist for minimizing or eliminating aliasing. The most direct way is to increase the amount of sampling, or to "oversample" the signal. In MR, elimination of aliasing in the frequency encoding direction of the image is accomplished by sampling the signal faster. This can be achieved with no compromise in S/N or imaging time. Oversampling in the phase encoding direction, whether in 2D or 3D (see 1.1214-33), may also be done. However, this comes at the expense of imaging time since more phase encoding steps in the acquisition are required to accomplish this task.

Another strategy to minimize aliasing artifacts is to ensure that signals from beyond the boundaries are suppressed and do not obscure the underlying structures when they become aliased. This can be accomplished by using spatial presaturation to reduce the signal outside of the boundaries (see 1.1214-30).[5] Use of surface coils also may offer an effective way of minimizing aliasing by only receiving signal from a small region near the coil. Finally, minimization of signal beyond the FOV can be accomplished by using filters before image reconstruction that reduce those signals that lie beyond the boundary limits. This, however, can be done only in the frequency encoding direction.

Advantages

Oversampling of the MR data minimizes aliasing artifact.

Disadvantages

Aliasing artifacts obscure details of underlying structures in the image. Oversampling in the phase encoding direction increases imaging time.

Technical References

1. Henkelman RM, Bronskill MJ. Artifacts in magnetic resonance imaging. Rev. Magn Reson Med 1987;2:1–126.
2. Pusey E, Lufkin RB, Brown RKJ, et al. Magnetic resonance imaging artifacts: mechanism and clinical significance. Radiographics 1986;6:891–911.
3. Porter BA, Hastrup W, Richardson ML, et al. Classification and investigation of artifacts in magnetic resonance imaging. Radiographics 1987;7:271–287.
4. Bellon EM, Haacke EM, Coleman PE, et al. MR artifacts: a review. AJR 1986;147:1271–1281.
5. Edelman RR, Atkinson DJ, Silver MS, et al. FRODO pulse sequences: a new means of eliminating motion, flow, and wraparound artifacts. Radiology 1988;166:231–236.

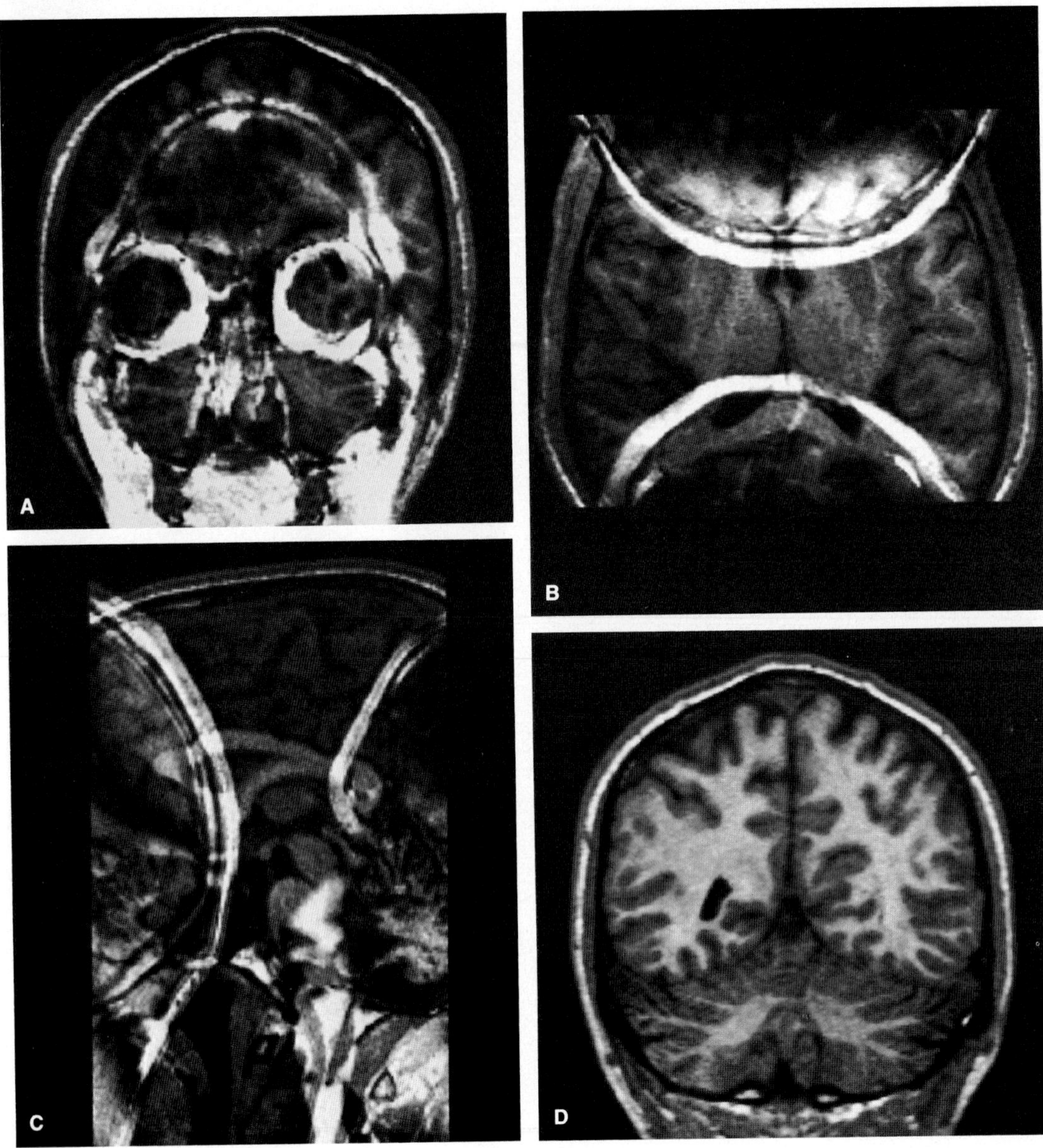

ARTIFACT

Aliasing artifact in 3D MR

FINDINGS

(*A*) A posterior coronal partition of a coronally acquired T1-weighted spoiled GRE 3D acquisition (TR/TE/FA = 25/4/40°) shows aliasing in the third dimension from an anterior partition obscuring the entire image. Multiplanar reformatting in the axial (*B*) and sagittal (*C*) planes demonstrates the degree of aliasing, indicating that only the middle coronal partitions are unaliased. (*D*) The same anatomic coronal partition as in *A* is depicted but with no 3D aliasing.

CONCLUSION

Double-exposed images occur from signal that extends beyond the boundaries of the 3D slab thickness obscuring details of the underlying structures.

DISCUSSION

Aliasing artifacts, or wraparound, occurs whenever the MR signal extends beyond the boundaries of the FOV. In 2D imaging, a signal from outside one boundary of the FOV becomes wrapped to the opposite boundary, overlaying itself on the image and obscuring details (see 1.1214-32). This occurs in both the frequency and phase encoding directions if a signal exists beyond the boundary in their respective dimension. In 3D imaging (see

1.1214-9), a large slab is selectively excited which then becomes spatially phase encoded. If the signal extends further than the encoded portion of the slab, aliasing also occurs.

In the third dimension, a signal beyond one side of the 3D-encoded slab is wrapped to the opposite side of the slab. Therefore, 3D aliasing is uniquely observed as a double-exposed image consisting of the correctly encoded 3D partition image and the aliased partition from the other side of the slab.[1–3] This primarily arises regardless of slab thickness because the boundaries of the excited slab region are not sharp and extend beyond the encoding of the third dimension.

Several methods exist for minimizing or eliminating 3D aliasing. The most direct way is to spatially encode the third dimension farther than the limits of the slab excitation thickness. This can be accomplished by increasing the number of 3D partitions concomitant with an increase in the 3D boundary, but it correspondingly increases imaging time. Extending the encoded boundaries without increasing the number of partitions results in larger partition thicknesses. Alternatively, slab thickness can be reduced for the same extent of encoding. With any strategy, there is a certain degree of compromise.

Advantages

Encoding the third dimension beyond the boundaries of the slab minimizes aliasing artifact.

Disadvantages

Aliasing artifacts obscure details of underlying structures in the image. Encoding beyond the slab may lead to either increased imaging time or increased partition thickness.

Technical References

1. Wehrli FW. Fast-scan magnetic resonance: principles and applications. Magn Reson Q 1990;6:165–236.
2. Kirsch JE. Fundamentals of magnetic resonance imaging. In: Runge VM, ed. Magnetic resonance imaging: clinical principles. Philadelphia, JB Lippincott, 1992.
3. Wood ML. Fourier imaging. In: Stark DD, Bradley WG, eds. Magnetic resonance imaging, 2nd ed, vol 1. St Louis, Mosby–Year Book, 1992.

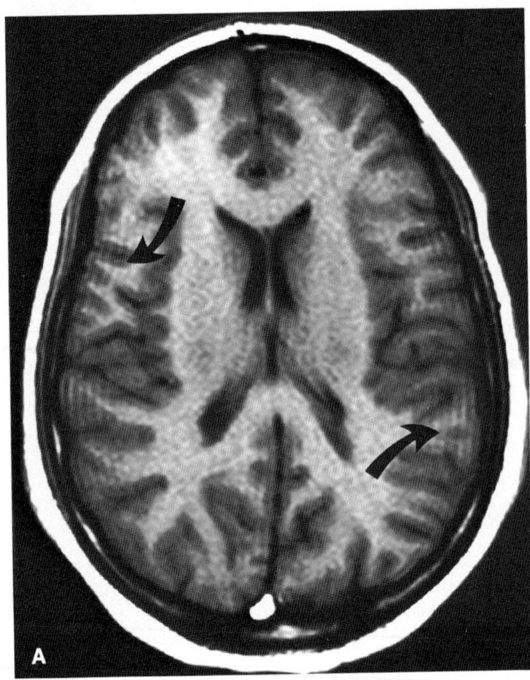

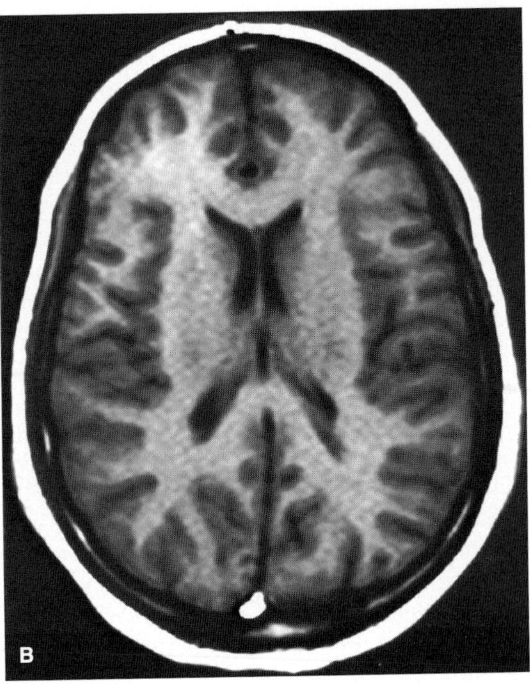

ARTIFACT

Truncation and filtering

FINDINGS

(*A*) An axial T1-weighted (TR/TE = 400/10) SE scan acquired with a reduced horizontal matrix (192 × 256) shows ringing artifacts (*curved arrows*). The left/right ringing emanates into the brain from the high contrast boundary of the fat, and replicates the anatomic contour. (*B*) With appropriate filtering, the artifacts are substantially reduced without significant loss in edge detail or spatial resolution.

CONCLUSION

Data truncation results in loss of edge definition and ringing artifacts emanating from high contrast interfaces that can be minimized by filtering.

DISCUSSION

Truncation artifact is a frequently observed phenomenon in MR.[1-3] It is also referred to as "ringing" or "Gibbs artifact" and can be recognized by a characteristic rippling of signal intensity in the vicinity of and parallel to high contrast tissue boundaries such as in the region of the internal auditory canal[4] or spinal cord.[5]

Since the MR signal is not infinitely sampled, a certain degree of this artifact is introduced on fourier transform image reconstruction. By necessarily starting and stopping the sampling, some of the signal is never collected. This missing information is usually associated with the fine detail of edges and small structures throughout the image. In addition to potentially losing edge definition, truncation of the data sampling results in an approximation error of the edges during image reconstruction. This is seen as a rippling effect that emanates away from the edge and eventually dies away at a certain distance. The ringing or rippling of edges is larger if the truncation of the sampled data is greater, and occurs if large tissue contrast exists at sharp boundaries. The artifact is less severe if only smooth boundaries exist. Ringing can exist in either the frequency or phase encoding direction of an MR image provided there is a tissue boundary that possesses sharp edge definition and large contrast in that direction.

Various types of data filters can be applied before reconstruction to smooth the severity of abrupt truncation of the sampled signal information.[3] This minimizes the rippling effect in the image caused by data truncation, but it does not improve the actual edge detail and may actually even increase blurring. Other more sophisticated methods of data processing have been investigated that do not compromise the inherent detail in the image.[6]

Acquiring the data with a smaller FOV (see 1.1214-23), larger matrix (see 1.1214-24), or at higher spatial resolution are alternative ways to minimize truncation artifact. However, there is an inherent loss in S/N associated with the reduction in FOV and longer imaging times with larger matrices that may compromise the image quality at the expense of removing the ringing.

Advantages

Data filtering can minimize truncation artifact ringing and may reduce image noise.

Disadvantages

Truncation artifacts can mimic or obscure anatomic structures or abnormalities. Data filtering to remove the artifact leads to reduced spatial resolution and edge blurring.

Technical References

1. Wood ML, Henkelman RM. Truncation artifacts in magnetic resonance imaging. Magn Reson Med 1985;2:517–526.
2. Lufkin RB, Pusey E, Stark DD, et al. Boundary artifact due to truncation errors in MR imaging. AJR 1986;147:1283–1287.
3. Czervionke LF, Czervionke JM, Daniels DL, Haughton VM. Characteristic features of MR truncation artifacts. Am J Neuroradiol 1988;9:815–824.
4. Daniels DL, Czervionke LF, Breger RK, et al. "Truncation" artifact in MR images of the internal auditory canal. Am J Neuroradiol 1987;8:793–794.
5. Levy LM, DiChiro G, Brooks RA, et al. Spinal cord artifacts from truncation errors during MR imaging. Radiology 1988;166:479–483.
6. Constable RT, Henkelman RM. Data extrapolation for truncation artifact removal. Magn Reson Med 1991;17:108–118.

CHAPTER
TWO

Magnetic Resonance Imaging of the Brain,
edited by Val M. Runge.
J. B. Lippincott Company, Philadelphia © 1994.

Skull and Its Contents

Val M. Runge
Mitchell A. Brack
Robert A. Garneau

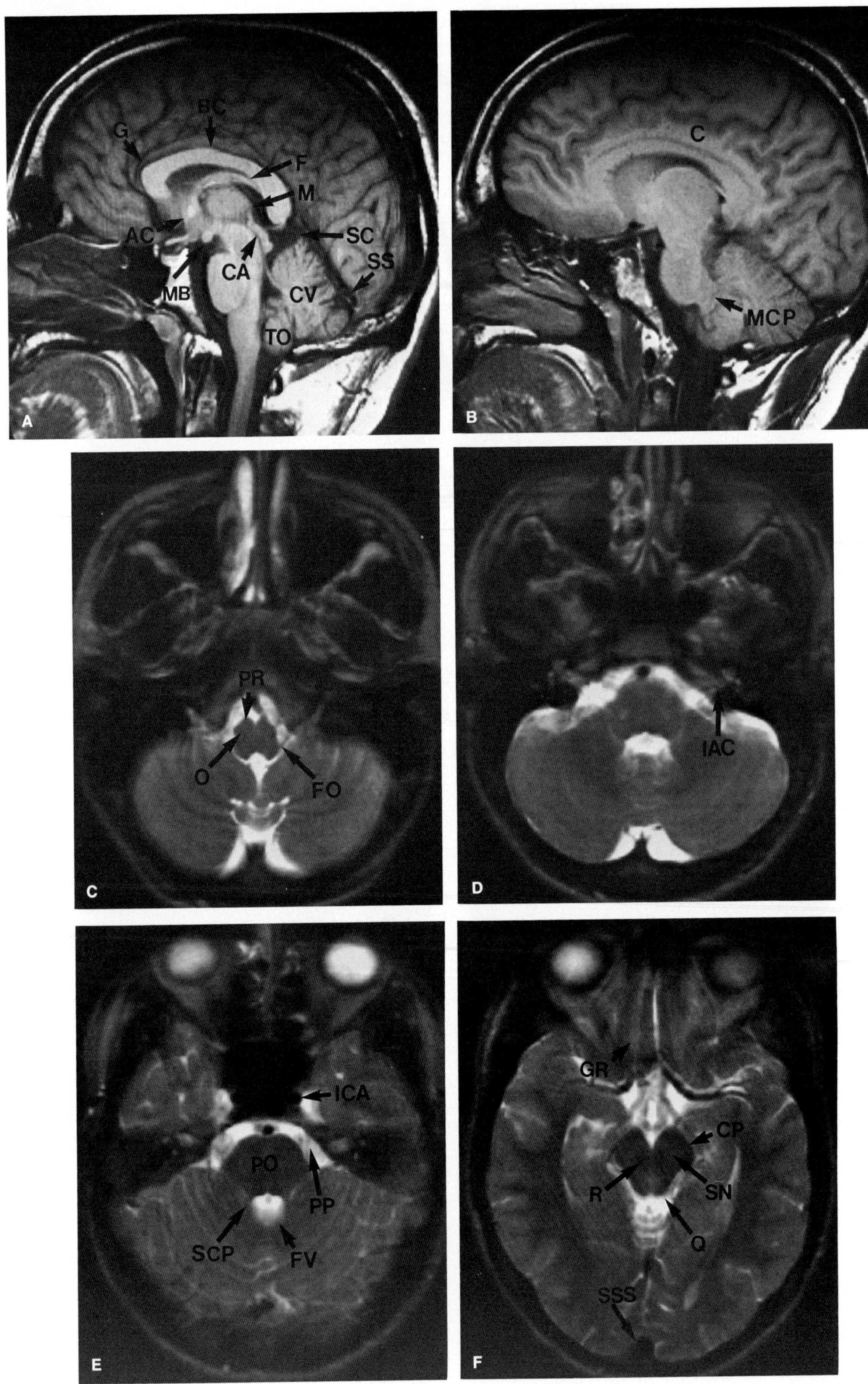
BC
G
F
M
AC
SC
SS
CA
MB
CV
TO
A
C
MCP
B
PR
O
FO
C
IAC
D
ICA
PO
PP
SCP
FV
E
GR
CP
R
SN
Q
SSS
F

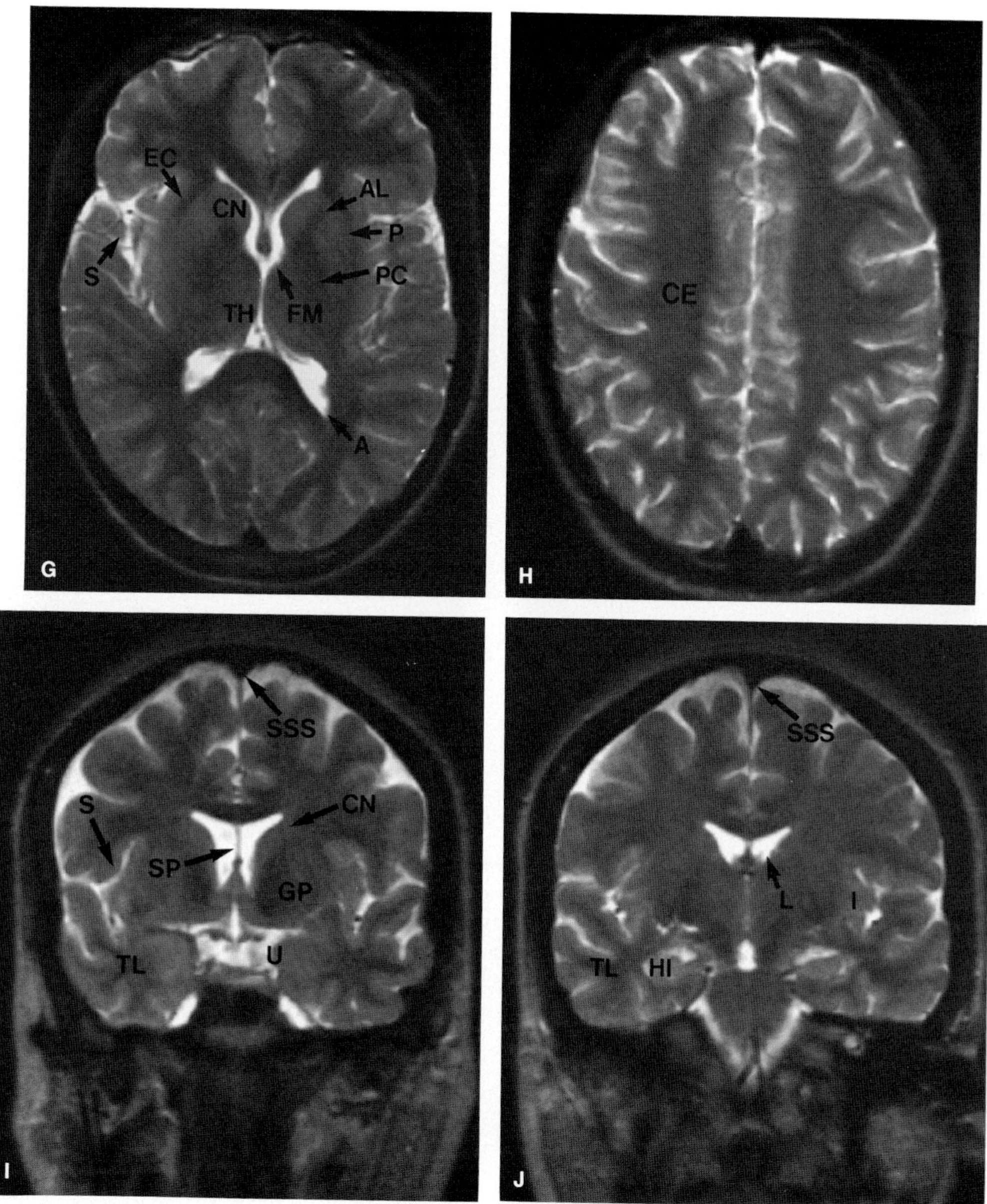

HISTORY

Noncontributory

FINDINGS

Sagittal (*A and B*), axial (*C to H*), and coronal (*I to K*) T2-weighted images are presented for interpretation.

A, atrium of the lateral ventricle
AC, anterior commissure
AL, anterior limb of the internal capsule
BC, body of the corpus callosum
C, cingulate gyrus
CA, cerebral aqueduct
CE, centrum semiovale
CN, caudate nucleus
CP, cerebral peduncle
CV, cerebellar vermis
EC, external capsule
F, fornix
FV, fourth ventricle
FM, foramen of Monroe
FO, foramen of Magendie
G, genu of the corpus callosum
GP, globus pallidus
GR, gyrus rectus
H, hypothalamus
HI, hippocampus
I, insular cortex
IAC, internal auditory canal
ICA, internal carotid artery
L, lateral ventricle
M, mass intermedia
MB, mamillary body
MCP, middle cerebellar peduncle
O, olive
P, putamen
PC, posterior limb of the internal capsule
PO, pons
PP, prepontine cistern
PR, pyramid
Q, quadrigeminal plate (tectum)
R, red nucleus
S, sylvian fissure
SC, superior cerebellar cistern
SCP, superior cerebellar peduncle
SN, substantia nigra
SP, septum pellucidum
SS, straight sinus

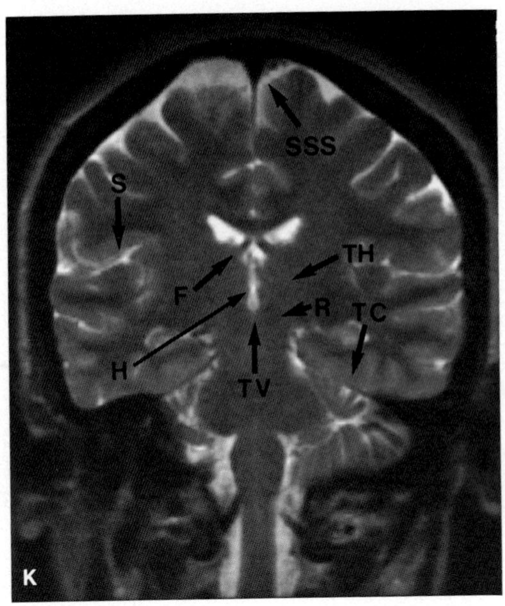

SSS, superior sagittal sinus
TC, tentorium cerebelli
TH, thalamus
TL, temporal lobe
TO, tonsil
TV, third ventricle
U, uncus

DIAGNOSIS

Normal intracranial anatomy

DISCUSSION

The frontal lobe is demarcated posteriorly from the parietal lobe by the central sulcus, and inferiorly from the temporal lobe by the lateral sulcus (fissure of Sylvius). The primary motor area (Brodmann area 4) occupies the precentral gyrus. The primary somesthetic area (Brodmann areas 1, 2, and 3) occupies the postcentral gyrus.

The parietal lobe is separated from the occipital lobe by the parietooccipital sulcus. On the surface of the brain the parietal lobe is separated inferiorly from the temporal lobe by the lateral sulcus and its continuation posteriorly as an imaginary line.

Clinical References

1. Fisher HW, Ketonen L. Radiographic neuroanatomy: a working atlas. New York, McGraw-Hill, 1991.
2. Stark DD, Bradley WG. Magnetic resonance imaging. St Louis, Mosby–Year Book, 1992;557–634.
3. Iwasaki S, Nakagawa H, Fukusumi A, et al. Identification of pre- and postcentral gyri on CT and MR images on the basis of the medullary pattern of cerebral white matter. Radiology 1991;179:207–213.

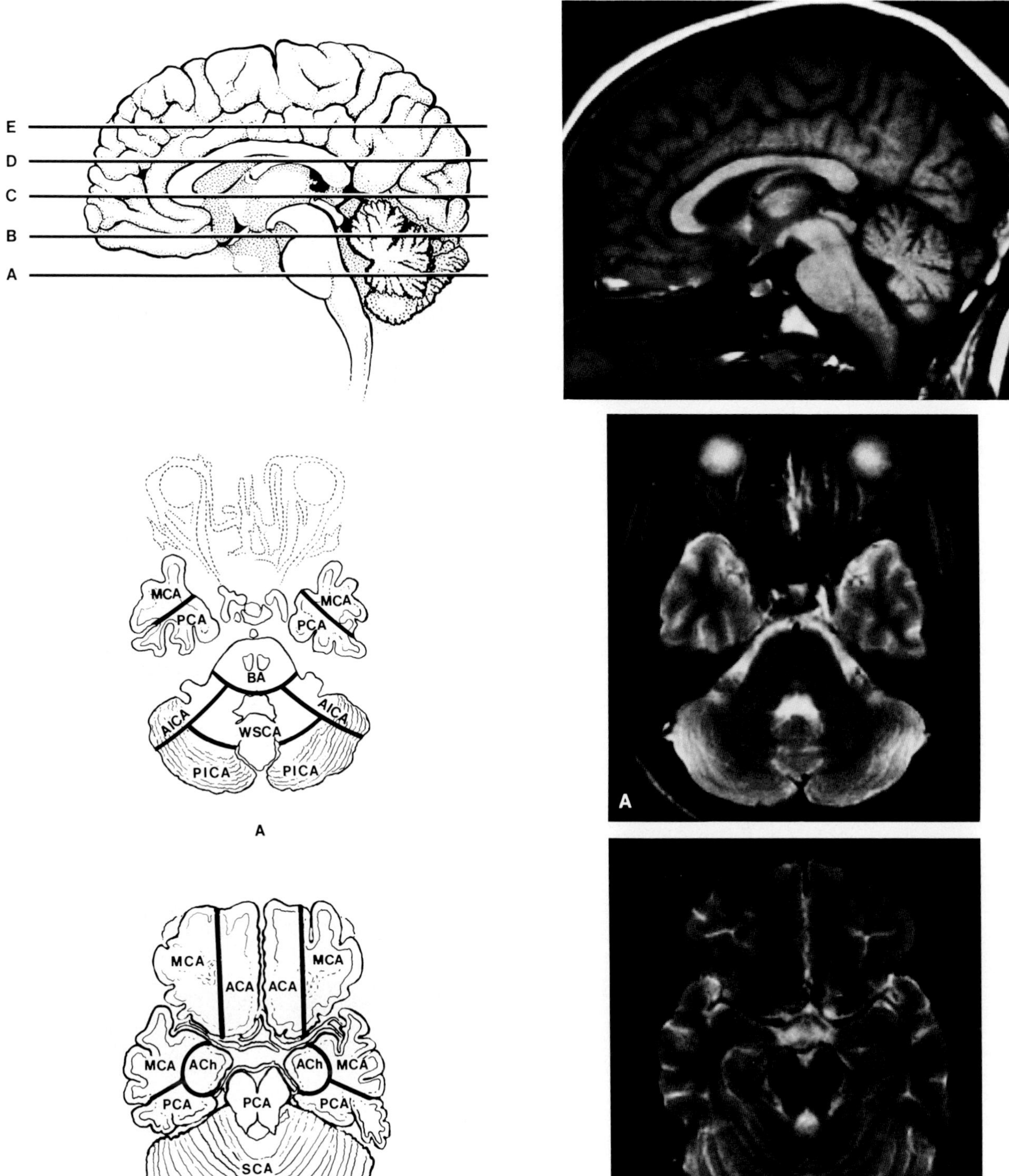
E
D
C
B
A
MCA
PCA
MCA
PCA
BA
AICA
AICA
WSCA
PICA
PICA
A
MCA
ACA
ACA
MCA
MCA
ACh
ACh
MCA
PCA
PCA
PCA
SCA
B
A
B

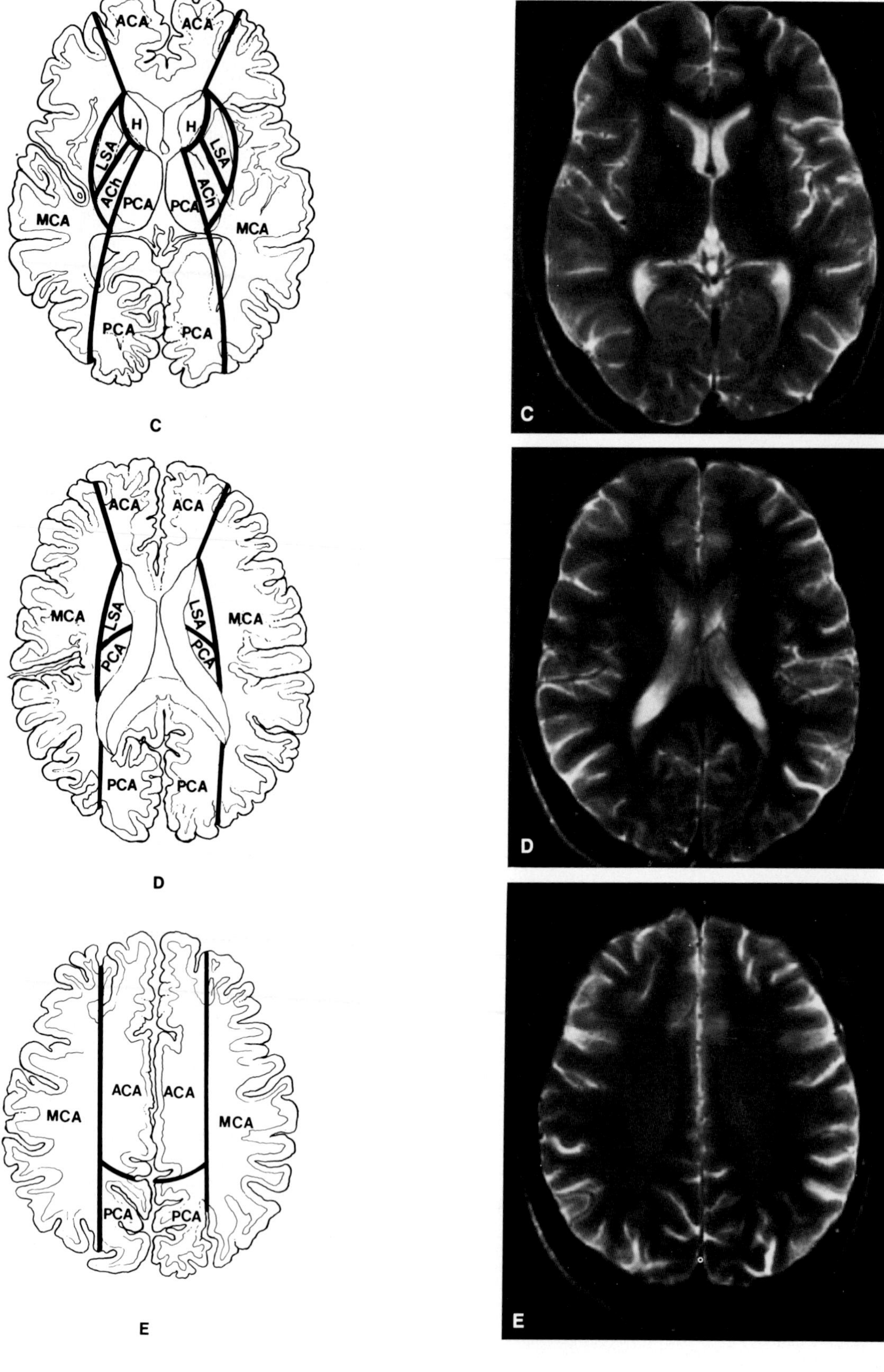
ACA
ACA
H
H
LSA
LSA
ACh
ACh
PCA
PCA
MCA
MCA
PCA
PCA
C
C
ACA
ACA
MCA
MCA
LSA
LSA
PCA
PCA
PCA
PCA
D
D
ACA
ACA
MCA
MCA
PCA
PCA
E
E

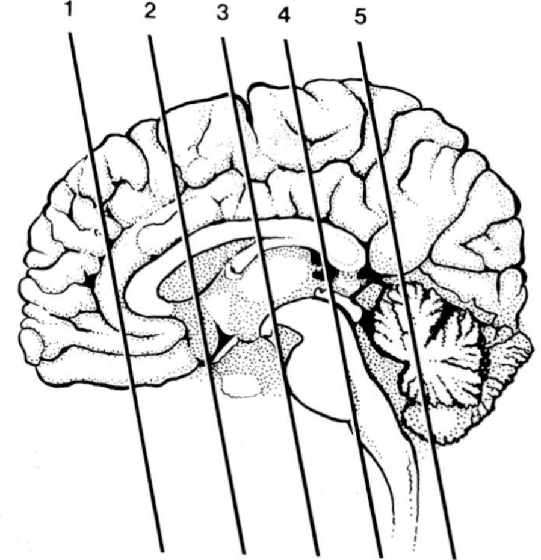
1
2
3
4
5

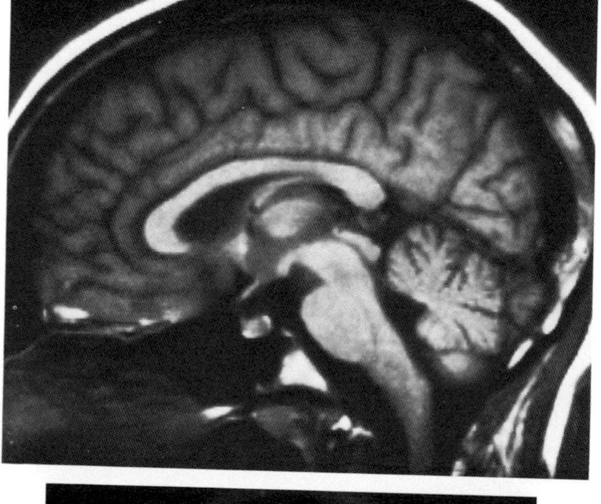

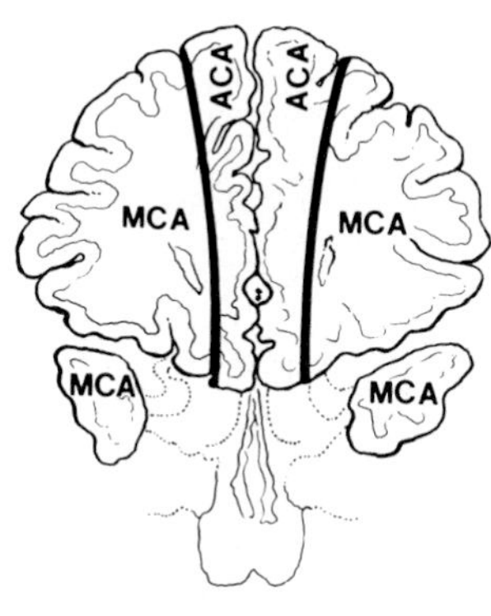
ACA
ACA
MCA
MCA
MCA
MCA

1

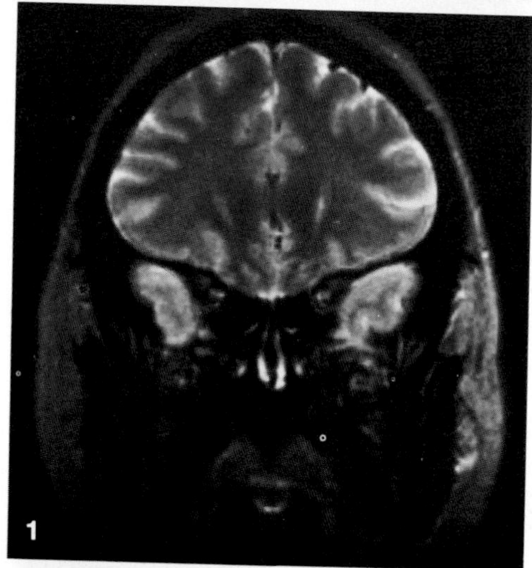
1

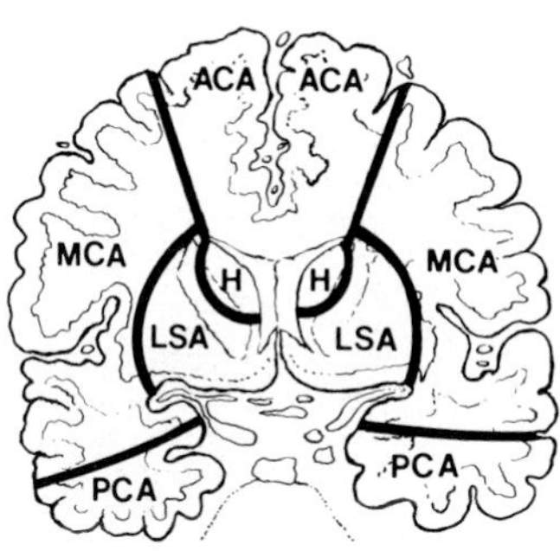
ACA
ACA
MCA
MCA
H
H
LSA
LSA
PCA
PCA

2

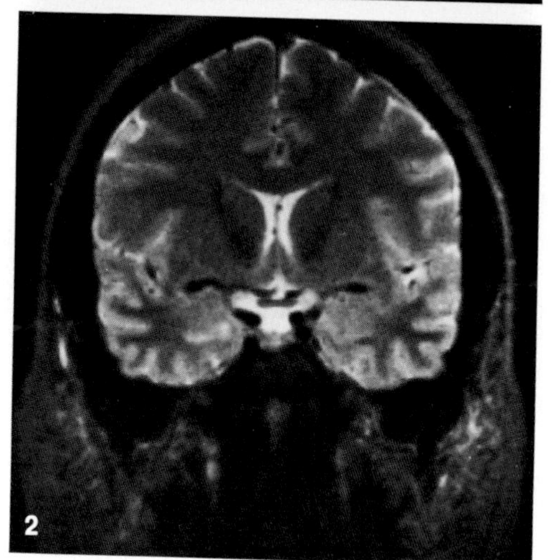
2

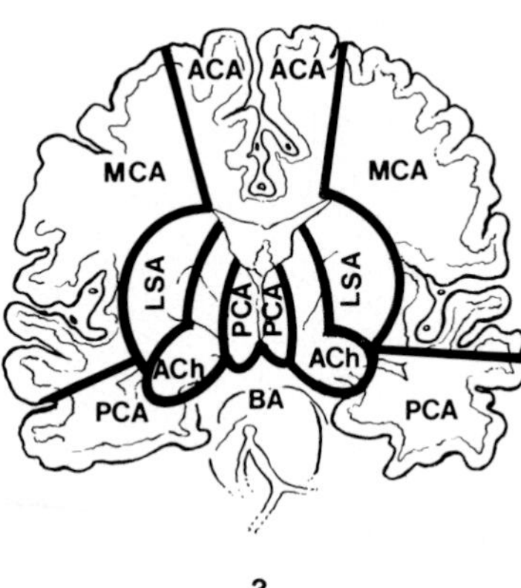
ACA
ACA
MCA
MCA
LSA
LSA
PCA
PCA
ACh
ACh
PCA
BA
PCA

3

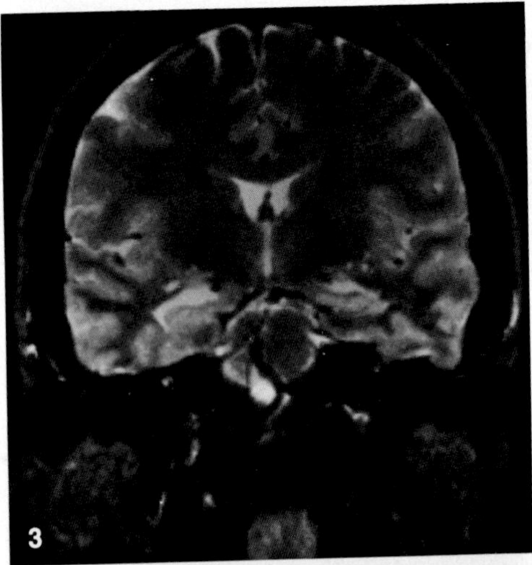
3

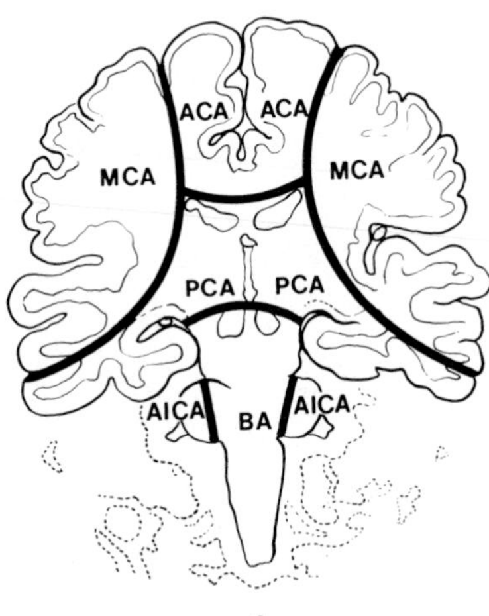
ACA
ACA
MCA
MCA
PCA
PCA
AICA
BA
AICA

4

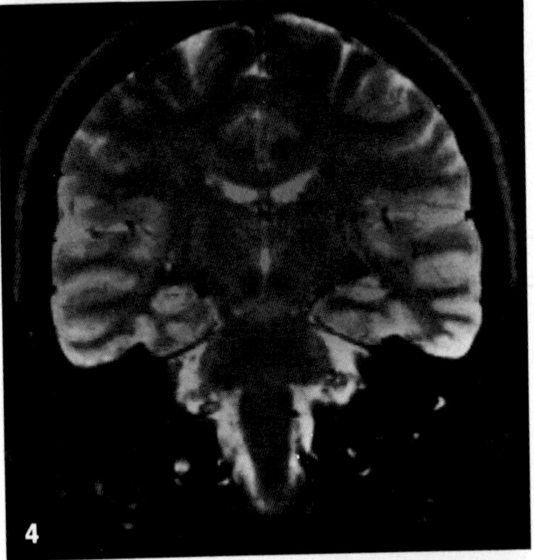
4

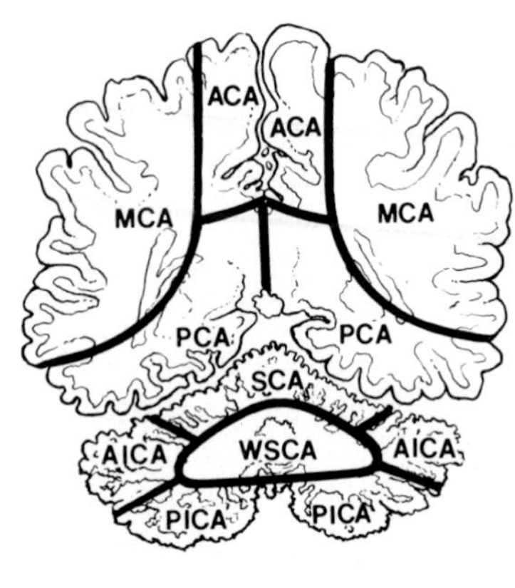
ACA
ACA
MCA
MCA
PCA
PCA
SCA
AICA
WSCA
AICA
PICA
PICA

5

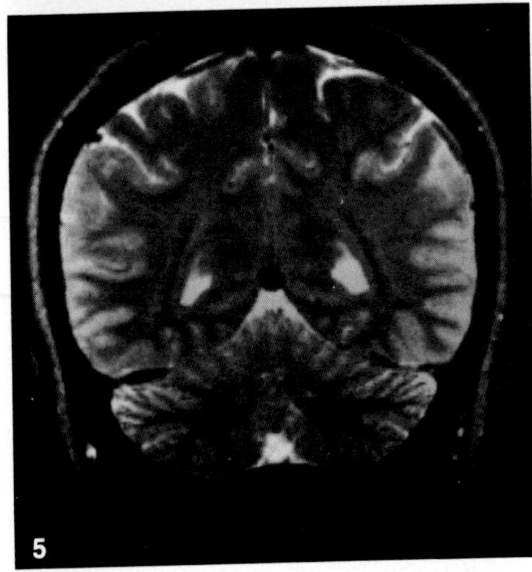
5

HISTORY

Noncontributory

FINDINGS

A sagittal T1-weighted localizer, axial T2-weighted images (*A to E*), and a second sagittal T1-weighted localizer with corresponding coronal T2-weighted images (*1 to 5*) are presented for interpretation.

ACA, anterior cerebral artery
ACh, anterior choroidal artery
AICA, anterior inferior cerebellar artery
BA, perforating branches of the basilar artery
H, recurrent artery of Heubner
LSA, lenticulostriate arteries
MCA, middle cerebral artery
PCA, posterior cerebral artery
PICA, posterior inferior cerebellar artery
SCA, superior cerebellar artery
WSCA, watershed region supplied predominantly by the SCA

DIAGNOSIS

Arterial vascular territories

DISCUSSION

The anterior cerebral artery supplies the anterior two thirds of the medial cerebral surface and approximately 1 cm of superomedial tissue over the convexity. The recurrent artery of Heubner arises from the A1 or A2 segment of the anterior cerebral artery and supplies the head of the caudate nucleus, anterior limb of the internal capsule and the rostral putamen.[1] The anterior choroidal artery arises from the posterior aspect of the supraclinoid internal carotid artery and supplies the posterior limb of the internal capsule, choroid plexus and portions of the thalamus, hypothalamus, caudate nucleus, globus pallidus, and cerebral peduncle.

The middle cerebral artery supplies most of the lateral surface of the cerebrum, as well as the insular cortex and the anterior and lateral aspects of the temporal lobe. The lenticulostriate branches arise from the M1 segment of the middle cerebral artery and supply portions of the basal ganglia and anterior limb of the internal capsule.[2]

The posterior cerebral artery supplies the occipital lobe and medial portion of the temporal lobe. The thalamoperforating arteries arise from the posterior communicating artery and the P1 segment of the posterior cerebral artery and supply the medial ventral thalamus and a portion of the posterior limb of the internal capsule.[3]

The posterior inferior cerebellar artery supplies the inferior vermis, tonsil, inferior surface of the cerebellum, and choroid plexus of the fourth ventricle. The anterior inferior cerebellar artery supplies the anterior portion of the cerebellar hemisphere.

The superior cerebellar artery supplies the superior surface of the cerebellar hemisphere.[4]

Clinical References

1. Berman SA, Hayman LA, Hinck VC. Correlation of CT cerebral vascular territories with function. I. Anterior cerebral artery. AJNR 1980;1:259–263.
2. Berman SA, Hayman LA, Hinck VC. Correlation of CT cerebral vascular territories with function. III. Middle cerebral artery. AJR 1984;142:1035–1040.
3. Berman SA, Hayman LA, Hinck VC. Correlation of CT cerebral vascular territories with function. II. Posterior cerebral artery. AJR 1981;137:13–19.
4. Osborn AG. Introduction to cerebral angiography. Philadelphia, JB Lippincott, 1980:167–326.

(From Runge VM. Clinical magnetic resonance imaging. Philadelphia, JB Lippincott, 1990.)

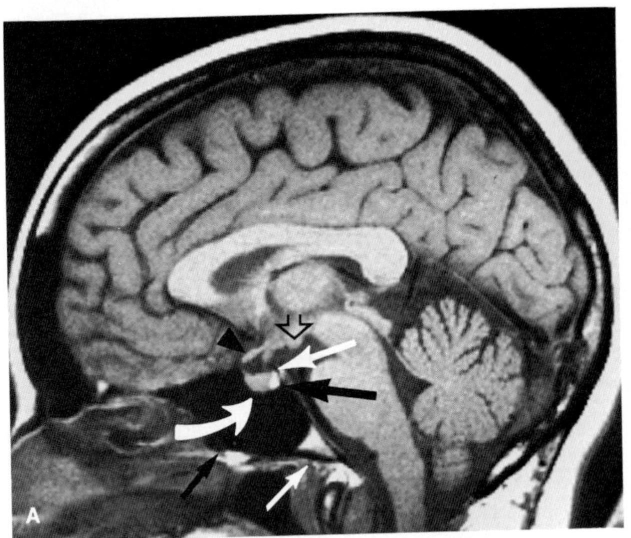

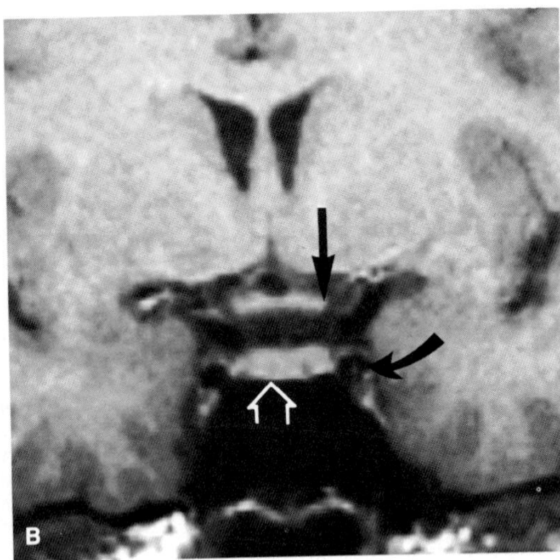

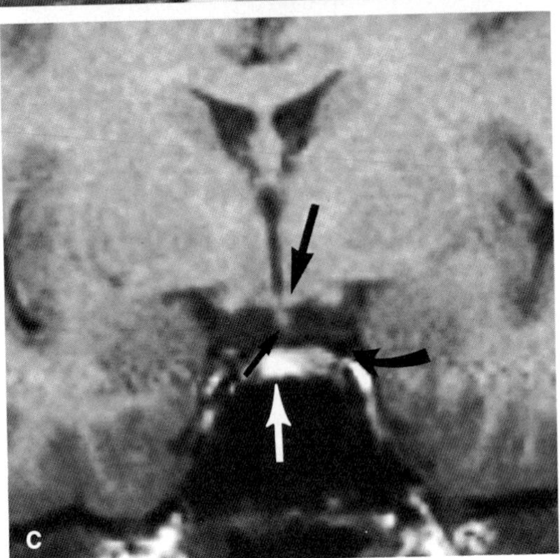

HISTORY

Noncontributory

FINDINGS

Precontrast sagittal (*A*) and coronal (*B and C*) T1-weighted images are presented for interpretation.

A: Curved arrow indicates adenohypophysis (anterior pituitary); large black arrow, neurohypophysis (posterior pituitary); large white arrow, infundibulum; arrowhead, optic chiasm; open arrow, mamillary bodies; small black arrow, sphenoid sinus; small white arrow, clivus.

B: Curved arrow indicates cavernous carotid artery; black arrow, optic chiasm; open white arrow, adenohypophysis.

C: Curved arrow indicates cavernous carotic artery; black arrow, optic tract; white arrow, neurohypophysis; small black arrow, infundibulum.

DIAGNOSIS

Pituitary gland, normal anatomy

DISCUSSION

An upward convexity of the pituitary gland measuring less than 10 mm in height is a normal finding in young women.[1] The normal pituitary gland should measure no more than 7 mm high in patients under 12 years of age.[2,3] The posterior pituitary is of hyperintensity on T1-weighted images in 50% to 90% of subjects; the absence of this hyperintensity does not necessarily indicate pathology. Small low-signal-intensity foci are seen within the pituitary gland in about 15% of contrast-enhanced studies in asymptomatic patients; these may represent colloid cysts, pars intermedia cysts, or asymptomatic microadenomas.

The blood–brain barrier is not present in the pituitary gland (or in the choroid plexus, tuber cinereum, area postrema, and pineal gland); thus, the gland enhances intensely after administration of a gadolinium chelate.

Clinical References

1. Johnsen DE, Woodruff WW, Allen AS, et al. MR imaging of the sellar and juxta sellar regions. Radiographics 1991; 11:727–758.
2. Swartz JD, Russel KB, Basile BA, et al. High-resolution computed tomographic appearance of the intrasellar contents in woman of childbearing age. Radiology 1983;147:115–117.
3. Elster AD, Chen MYM, Williams DW, et al. Pituitary gland: MR imaging of physiologic hypertrophy in adolescence. Radiology 1990;174:681–685.

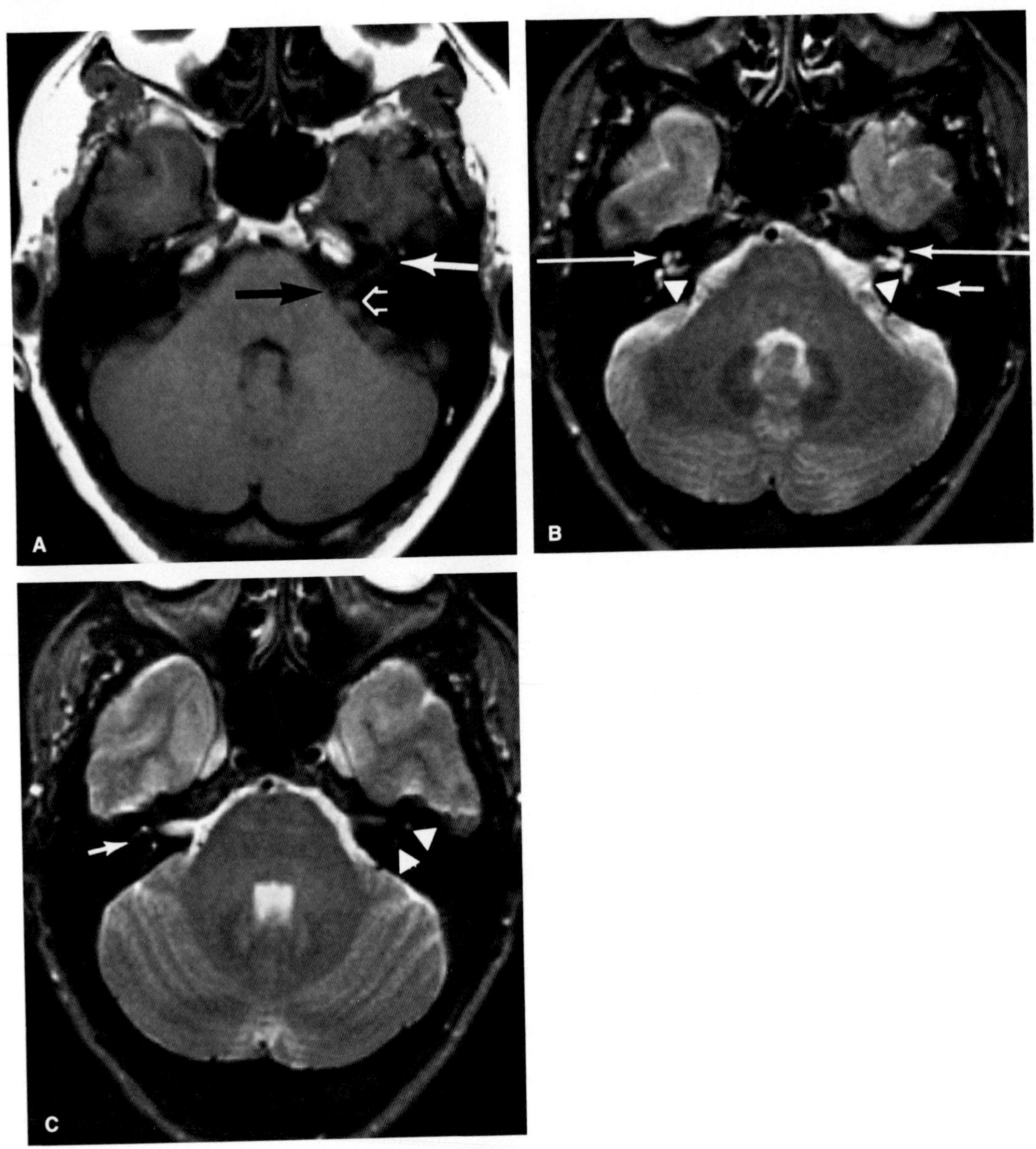

HISTORY

Noncontributory

FINDINGS

(*A*) T1-weighted axial image demonstrates the normal seventh and eighth nerve complex (*black arrow*) exiting the lateral aspect of the brain stem bilaterally, and traveling in the internal auditory canal (IAC). The seventh nerve (*white arrow*) beyond the IAC is also seen on the same image, running obliquely, adjacent to the inner ear. The flocculus (*open white arrow*), a normal small lobe of the cerebellum, is located just posterolateral to the origin of the seventh and eighth nerve complex. (*B and C*) Cerebrospinal fluid (CSF)–filled internal auditory canal is well seen on T2-weighted axial images. The cochlea (*thin white arrows in B*) lies anterior to the IAC, within the inner ear. The vestibule (*white arrowheads in B*) is located posterior to the cochlea. The horizontally oriented lateral semicircular canal (*small white arrows in B and C*) is seen in its entirety. The superior semicircular canal (*white arrowheads in C*) is seen in cross section.

DIAGNOSIS

Internal auditory canal, normal anatomy

DISCUSSION

The IAC is a bony foramen within the petrous portion of the temporal bone that contains structures traveling from the brain stem to the inner ear. The seventh (facial) and eighth (vestibulocochlear) nerves exit the lateral aspect of the pontomedullary groove and together enter the IAC. The IAC is divided into two compartments by a horizontal bony septum, the crista falciformis.[1] The facial nerve occupies the anterosuperior aspect of the IAC and courses laterally to join the geniculate ganglion, which gives rise to several branches, portions of which are well seen with MR.[2] The cochlear division of the eighth nerve occupies the anteroinferior compartment of the IAC, and innervates the cochlea, which lies anteriorly in the inner ear.[3] The superior and inferior vestibular nerves occupy the entire posterior compartment of the IAC, and provide equilibrium information to the brain from the vestibule and semicircular canals. The labyrinthine artery, a branch of either the basilar or anterior inferior cerebellar artery, also travels in the IAC.

The facial and vestibulocochlear nerves are isointense to brain on all pulse sequences and are best seen on T1-weighted images. The cochlea, vestibule, semicircular canals, and IAC all contain fluid and are well seen on T2-weighted images as high-signal-intensity structures.

MR Technique

Thin cuts (3 mm or less) should be used for evaluation of the IAC. This can be accomplished with routine 2D SE, or 3D GRE techniques. In addition, postcontrast T1-weighted images are necessary to rule out small intracanalicular lesions.

Clinical References

1. Valvassori G, Morales F, Palacios E, et al. MR of the normal and abnormal internal auditory canal. AJNR 1988;9:115–119.
2. Brogan M, Chakeres D, Schmalbrock P. High-resolution 3DFT MR imaging of the endolymphatic duct and soft tissues of the otic capsule. AJNR 1991;12:1–11.
3. Armington W, Harnsberger H, Smoker W, et al. Normal and diseased acoustic pathway: evaluation with MR imaging. Radiology 1988;167:509–515.

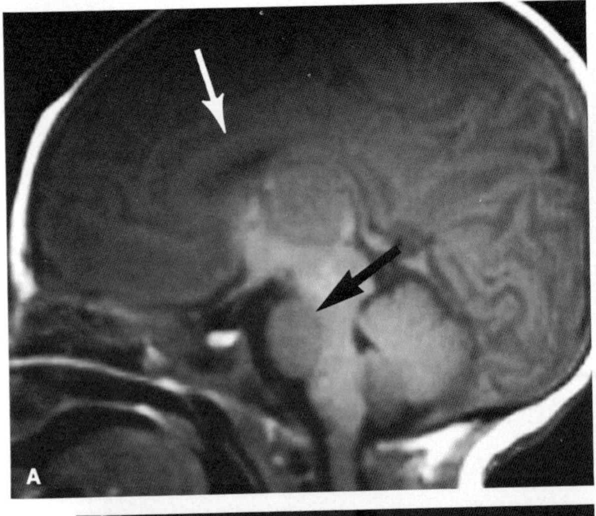

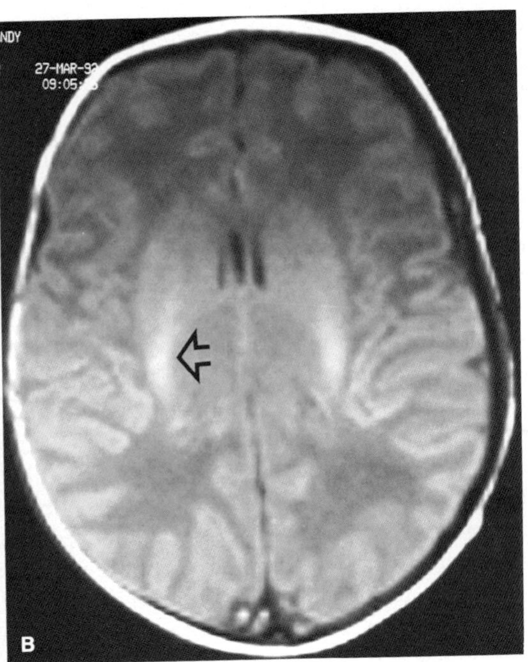

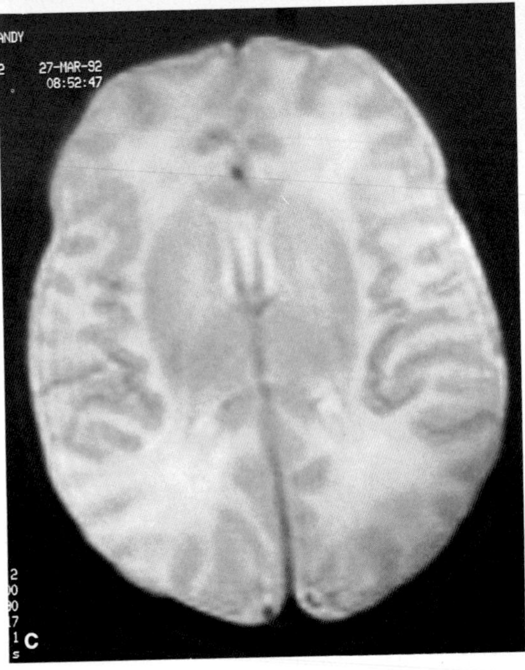

HISTORY

A 1-week-old full-term infant

FINDINGS

(*A*) On the sagittal T1-weighted image the ventral pons (*black arrow*) is of lower signal intensity than the dorsal pons, indicating that it is not yet myelinated. The corpus callosum is also not myelinated (*white arrow*). (*B*) Axial T1-weighted image reveals the posterior portion of the posterior limb of the internal capsule (*open arrow*) to be of slight hyperintensity, indicating some myelination. (*C*) The subcortical white matter is of diffusely increased signal intensity on the axial T2-weighted image, indicating that it is not myelinated.

DIAGNOSIS

Normal myelination in a newborn

DISCUSSION

Myelination of the brain begins during the fifth fetal month. At birth, the dorsal pons, portions of the inferior and superior cerebellar peduncles, the decussation of the superior cerebellar peduncles, the posterior limb of the internal capsule, and the ventral lateral thalamus are partially myelinated.[1] These sites are of decreased signal intensity on T2-weighted images in newborns; unmyelinated white matter is hyperintense and partially myelinated structures are isointense relative to gray matter on T2-weighted images. Unmyelinated white matter is hypointense on T1-weighted images. Myelinated structures appear hyperintense on T1-weighted images.[2]

Brain maturation is an orderly process that begins first in the brain stem and progresses to the cerebellum and the cerebrum. During the first month after birth, myelination advances in the corona radiata in the direction of the sensory cortex and thereafter in the direction of the motor cortex. After 3 or 4 months, myelination proceeds in a frontal direction.

By 3 months of age, the cerebellum has an adult appearance. Myelination of the optic tracts begins at 1 month of age. By 4 months, the calcarine fissure demonstrates some myelination. The internal capsule myelinates in a posterior to anterior direction.

Myelin is composed of a bilayer of lipids with several large proteins. The outer layer of the membrane is close to 50% cholesterol, the remainder being predominantly composed of glycolipid. It is known that cholesterol causes shortening of the T1 relaxation rate of water; proteins also cause T1 shortening of water. As myelin matures it becomes increasingly hydrophobic secondary to an inner layer of phospholipids. This hydrophobic layer results in fewer aqueous protons and a decrease in signal intensity on T2-weighted images.

T1-weighted sequences are most useful in monitoring brain development during the first 6 to 8 months of life; T2-weighted images are more useful after 6 months of age.

MR Technique

Neonatal brain tissue has very long T1 and T2 relaxation rates, and it is necessary to use a longer TR (3500 to 4000) with T2-weighted sequences than is typically employed in adults in order to obtain sufficient tissue contrast for diagnostic purposes.

Clinical References

1. Barkovich AJ, Kjos BO, Jackson DE, et al. Normal maturation of the neonatal and infant brain: MR imaging at 1.5 T. Radiology 1988;166:173–180.
2. van der Knaap MS, Valk J. MR imaging of the various stages of normal myelination during the first year of life. Neuroradiology 1990;31:459–470.

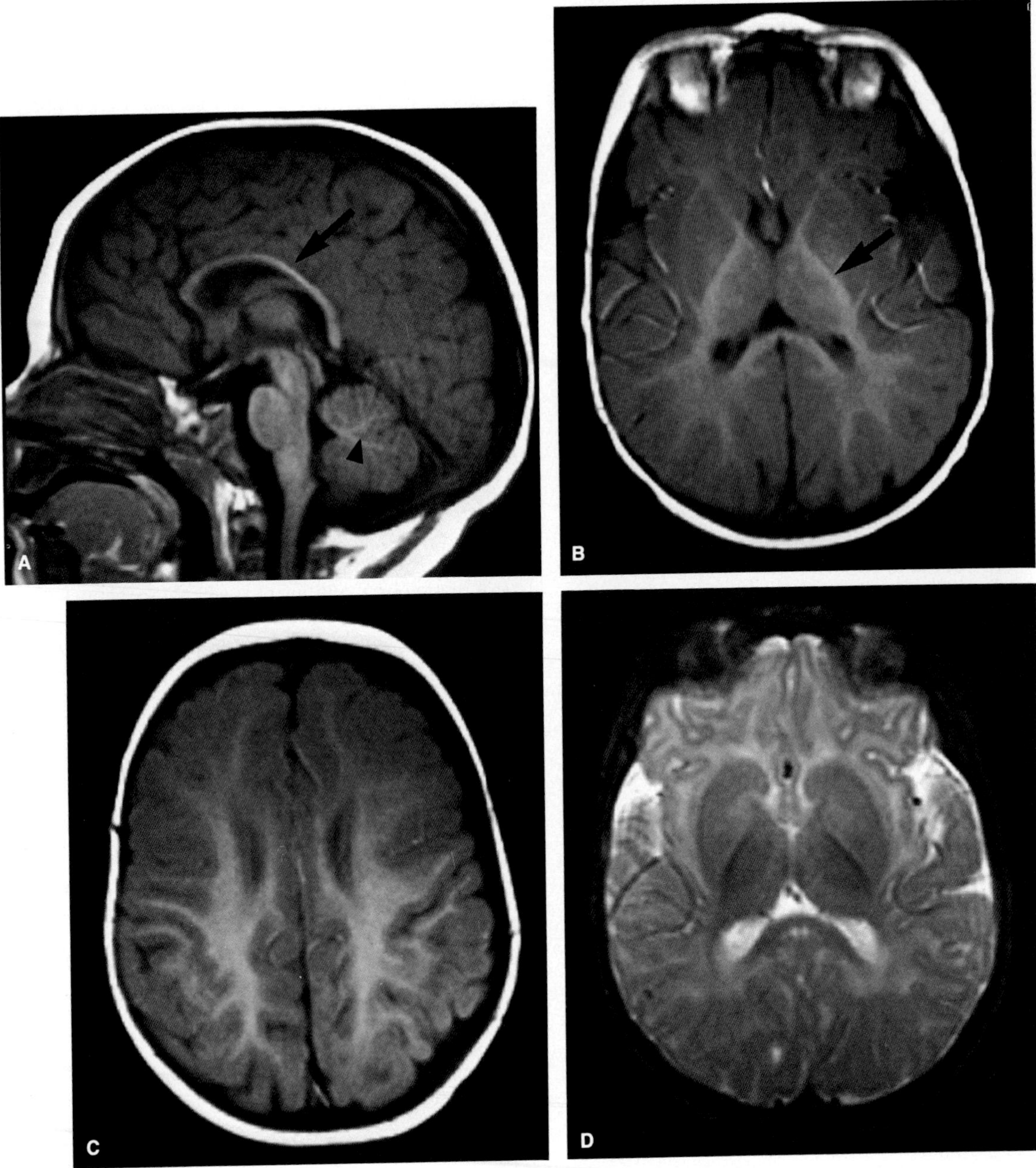

HISTORY

A 6-month-old infant

FINDINGS

(*A*) Although the corpus callosum (*arrow*) is thin, it is of relative increased signal intensity (indicating that it is myelinated) on the sagittal T1-weighted image. The cerebellar white matter (*arrowhead*) also demonstrates myelination. (*B*) The posterior limb and genu of the internal capsule (*arrow*) demonstrate increased signal intensity when compared to gray matter (indicating myelination) on the axial T1-weighted image. The occipital lobe white matter demonstrates myelin signal intensity on the axial T1-weighted image. The white matter in the frontal lobes cannot as of yet be well differentiated from gray matter. (*C*) On an axial T1-weighted image through the centrum semiovale, it is evident that myelination has progressed further in the posterior portion of the centrum semiovale than the anterior portion. (*D*) The posterior limb of the internal capsule demonstrates low signal intensity consistent with myelination on the axial T2-weighted image. The periatrial, parietal, and occipital white matter still have immature signal intensity on T2-weighted images.

DIAGNOSIS

Normal myelination at 6 months

DISCUSSION

Myelination of the white matter causes a decrease in T1 and T2 relaxation rates. At 2 months of age, unmyelinated white matter is slightly hyperintense on T2-weighted sequences. The short T2 relaxation time (which leads to low signal intensity) seen in adult white matter pathways is secondary to heavy myelination.

Most deep white matter tracts myelinate between 6 and 12 months of age. The posterior limb of the internal capsule myelinates at 4 to 7 months, but the anterior limb of the internal capsule is rarely myelinated by 6 months. The splenium of the corpus callosum usually develops high signal intensity on T1-weighted images by 4 months, and the genu by 6 months.[1]

The optic radiations typically progress to maturity, as assessed on T1-weighted images, by 6 months of age.[2] Deep white matter myelinates in a dorsal to rostral direction, with the deep occipital white matter maturing first and the frontal white matter last. Peripheral extension and increasing complexity of arborization of the subcortical white matter continues until 7 months in the occipital white matter and 8 to 11 months in the frontal white matter. An adult pattern of myelination is seen on T1-weighted images at 9 to 12 months.

Clinical References

1. Barkovich AJ, Kjos BO, Jackson DE, et al. Normal maturation of the neonatal and infant brain: MR imaging at 1.5 T. Radiology 1988;166:173–180.
2. Bird RC, Hedberg M, Drayer BP, et al. MR assessment of myelination in infants and children: usefulness of marker sites. AJNR 1989;10:731–740.

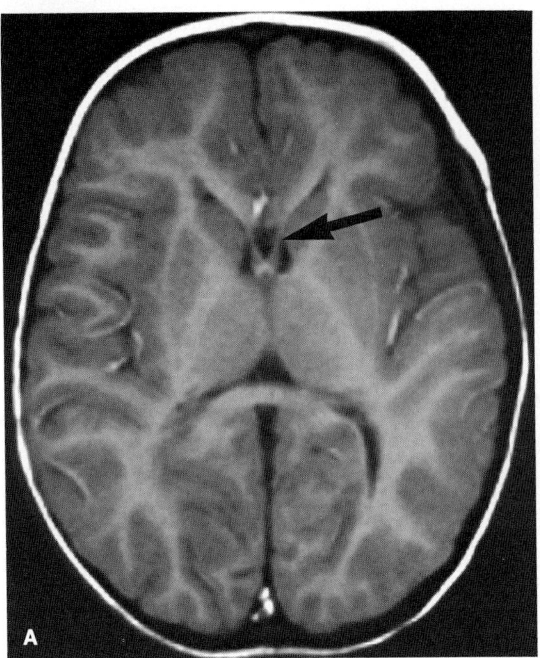

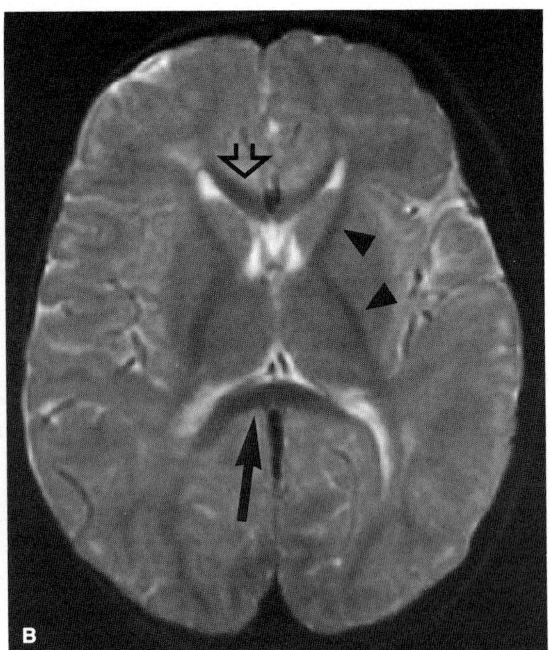

HISTORY

A 1-year-old child

FINDINGS

(*A*) The brain appears normal on the T1-weighted axial image. The degree of myelination is normal, with an adult pattern of signal intensity in both the deep and peripheral white matter. Incidentally noted is a cavum septum pellucidum (*arrow*). (*B*) T2-weighted axial image at the same level also shows that the brain is normal for age. The deep white matter is mature, and has low signal intensity on T2-weighted images. This is seen in the anterior and posterior limbs of the internal capsule (*arrowheads*), and the splenium (*arrow*) and genu (*open arrow*) of the corpus callosum. The peripheral subcortical white matter is not yet mature, and its signal intensity is isointense to gray matter.

DIAGNOSIS

Normal myelination at 1 year

DISCUSSION

Myelination of the brain begins in the fifth month of fetal life and continues in infancy and childhood in an organized, predictable pattern, starting in the brain stem and progressing to the cerebellum and cerebrum.[1] The degree of myelination is therefore a reliable marker for determining the degree of brain maturity.[2] The pattern of myelination in the brain on T1-weighted images should have a normal, mature adult appearance by the age of 9 months. Only minimal changes in peripheral arborization in the frontal white matter may be seen after this age.[1] Therefore, assessment of myelination in a 1-year-old child requires inspection of T2-weighted images, which are of lesser utility in younger children.

Normally myelinated structures have low signal intensity on T2-weighted images, primarily because of low water content.[2] In general, white matter maturation proceeds from central to peripheral, from inferior to superior, and from posterior to anterior.[1] At the age of 1 year, there is mature myelin in the anterior limb of the internal capsule and the genu of the corpus callosum, in addition to the other deep, compact white matter structures that mature earlier (ie, the posterior limb of the internal capsule, corona radiata, splenium of the corpus callosum, optic radiations, cerebellar white matter and cerebellar peduncles, and brain stem). At this age, however, the deep and superficial white matter of the frontal, temporal, parietal, and occipital lobes is only partially myelinated and has signal intensity isointense to gray matter on T2-weighted images.[2]

Clinical References

1. Barkovich A, Kjos B, Jackson D, et al. Normal maturation of the neonatal and infant brain: MR imaging at 1.5 T. Radiology 1988;166:173–180.
2. Bird C, Hedberg M, Drayer B, et al. MR assessment of myelination in infants and children: usefulness of marker sites. AJNR 1989;10:731–740.

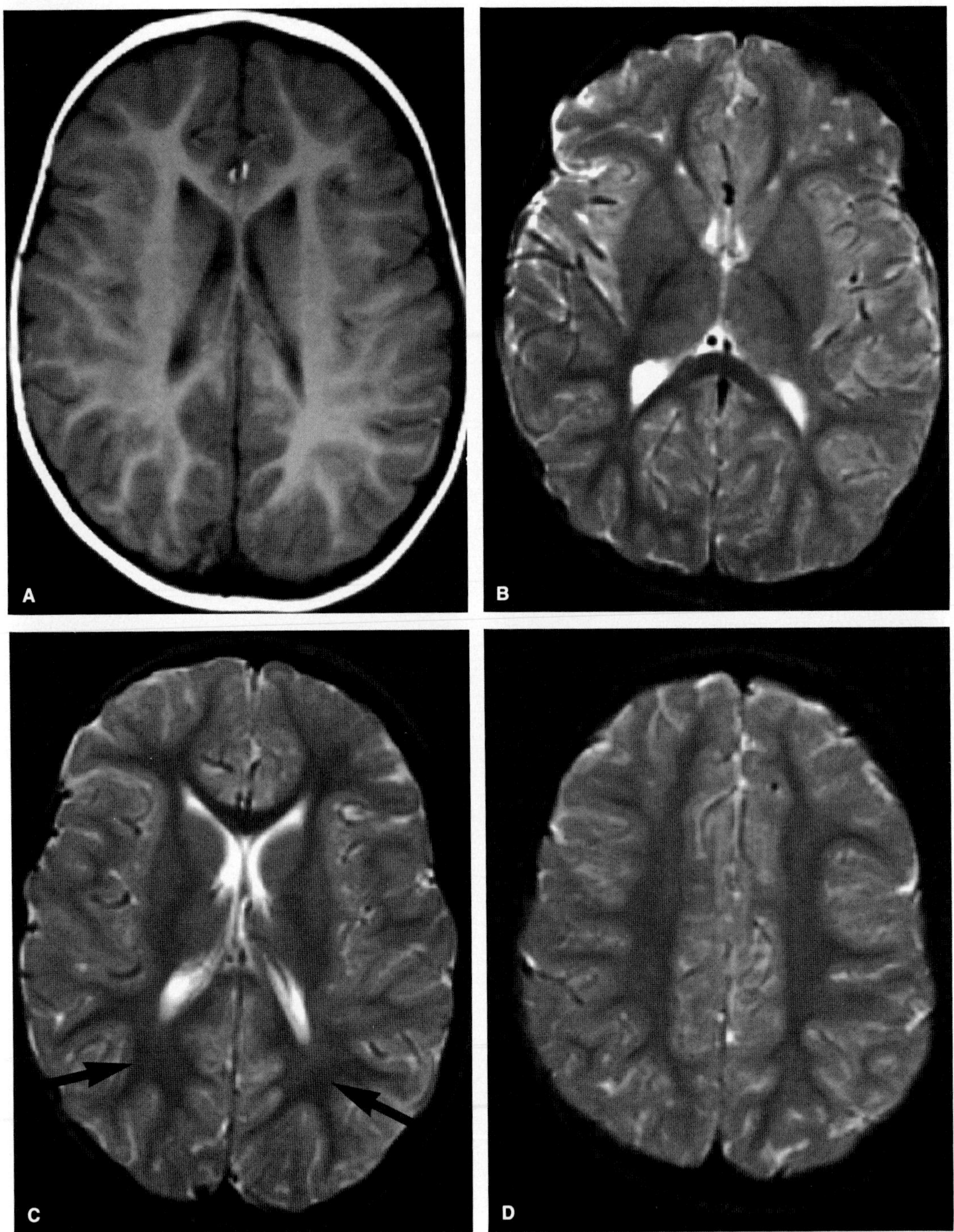

HISTORY

A 2-year-old child

FINDINGS

(*A*) The brain is unremarkable on the T1-weighted axial image. (*B through D*) T2-weighted axial images are also normal. The signal intensity of the peripheral subcortical white matter is much lower than the adjacent gray matter on the T2-weighted images. The peripheral branching, or "arborization," of the white matter between the gyri is normal. The deep white matter of the parietal lobes (*arrows in C*) has a slightly higher signal intensity than the frontal white matter.

DIAGNOSIS

Normal myelination at 2 years

DISCUSSION

The degree of myelination within white matter structures in the brain is a reliable indicator of brain maturity.[1] By the age of 9 months, the pattern of myelination in the brain on T1-weighted images should have a normal, mature adult appearance. Therefore, T2-weighted images are most useful for evaluation of myelination beyond the age of 6 to 9 months.

At 2 years of age, the deep and superficial white matter of the frontal, temporal, parietal, and occipital lobes should be homogeneously hypointense relative to the adjacent gray matter, approaching an adult pattern on T2-weighted images. However, the signal intensity may not yet be as low as the internal capsule, which is often used as an internal standard for mature myelination.[1] The signal intensity within peripheral white matter usually becomes isointense to the posterior limb of the internal capsule sometime in the third year of life.[1]

The deep white matter of the parietal lobes, dorsal and superior to the ventricular trigones, shows the slowest progression of myelination in the brain.[1] Indistinctly marginated, homogeneous mild hyperintensity on T2-weighted images persists in these regions beyond the age of 2 years. This is caused by the slow myelination of fiber tracts originating in the posterior inferior parietal and posterior temporal cortex. This mild hyperintensity usually disappears by the age of 10 years.[2]

Pitfalls in Image Interpretation

The normal persistence of high signal intensity dorsal and superior to the ventricular trigones should not be mistaken for periventricular leukomalacia (PVL). PVL is associated with loss of white matter volume, has abnormal high signal intensity on intermediate T2-weighted images, and always involves the white matter directly adjacent to the ventricles.[3]

Clinical References

1. Bird C, Hedberg M, Drayer B, et al. MR assessment of myelination in infants and children: usefulness of marker sites. AJNR 1989;10:731–740.
2. Barkovich A, Kjos B, Jackson D, et al. Normal maturation of the neonatal and infant brain: MR imaging at 1.5 T. Radiology 1988;166:173–180.
3. Baker L, Stevenson K, Enzmann D. End-stage periventricular leukomalacia: MR evaluation. Radiology 1988;168:809–815.

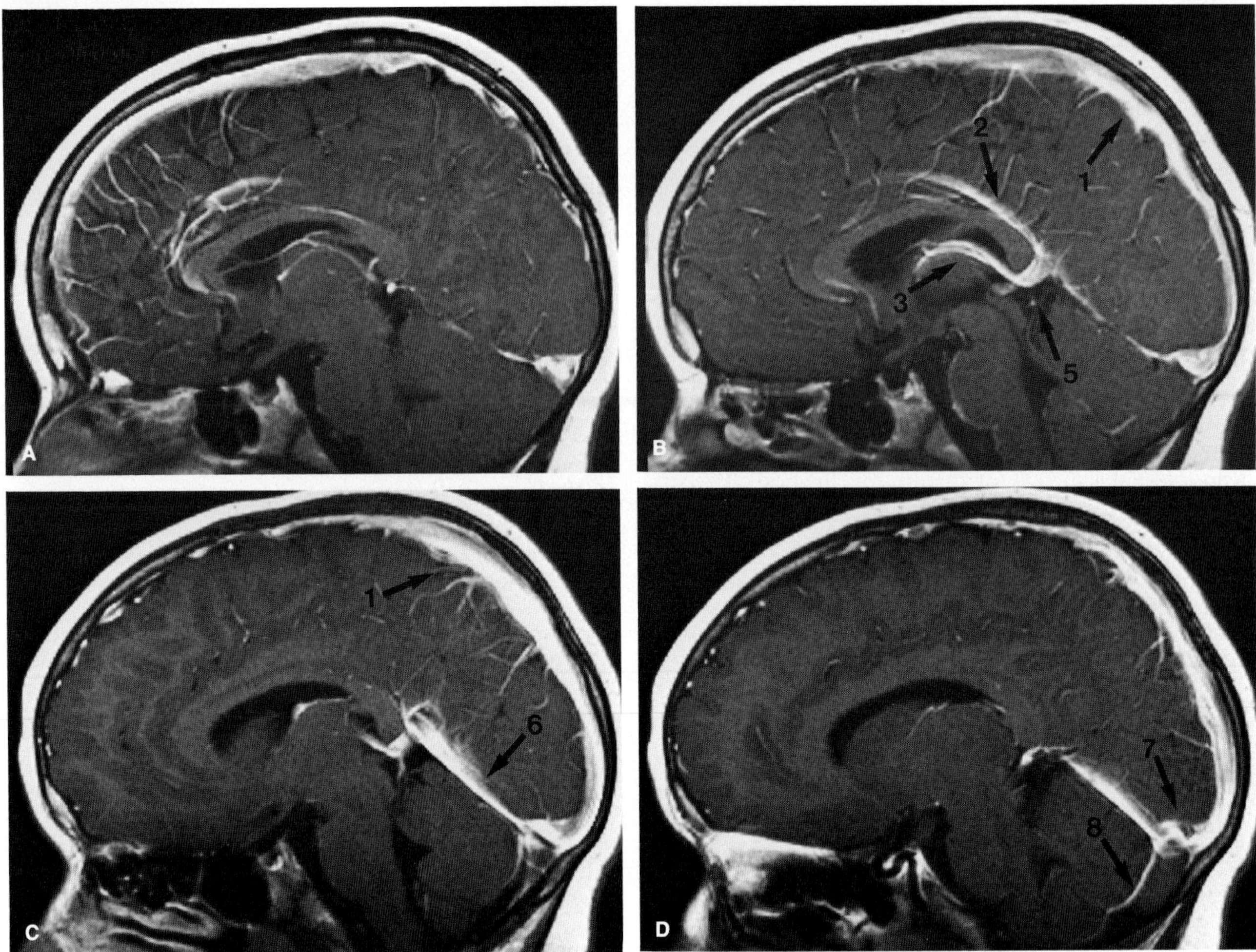

HISTORY

Noncontributory

FINDINGS

(*A to D*) The central venous anatomy of the brain is depicted on adjacent sagittal postcontrast T1-weighted images. Venous congestion, secondary to transverse sinus thrombosis (*not shown*), leads to excellent visualization of the venous system in this patient. The superior sagittal sinus (1), inferior sagittal sinus (2), internal cerebral veins (3), vein of Galen (5), straight sinus (6), torcular Herophili (7), and occipital sinus (8) are illustrated.

(*E to G*) MR venography acquired with 2D TOF technique in a normal volunteer: lateral projection (*E*), high-resolution targeted lateral projection of the deep cerebral veins (*F*), and AP projection (*G*). The superior sagittal sinus (1), internal cerebral veins (3), basal vein of Rosenthal (4), vein of Galen (5), straight sinus (6), and torcular Herophili (7) are well identified. Additional veins depicted on the lateral and AP projections include superficial cerebral veins (8), transverse sinus (9), sigmoid sinus (10), jugular bulb (11), and internal jugular vein (12). Depiction of the smaller deep veins—including the thalamostriate veins (13), internal cerebral veins, vein of Galen, basal vein of Rosenthal, and straight sinus—is improved on the high-resolution targeted lateral projection.

DIAGNOSIS

Normal venous anatomy

DISCUSSION

The superficial cerebral veins lie along the cortical surface of the brain and drain into the dural sinuses. There are three large, named superficial veins: the superficial middle cerebral vein, which lies along the sylvian fissure

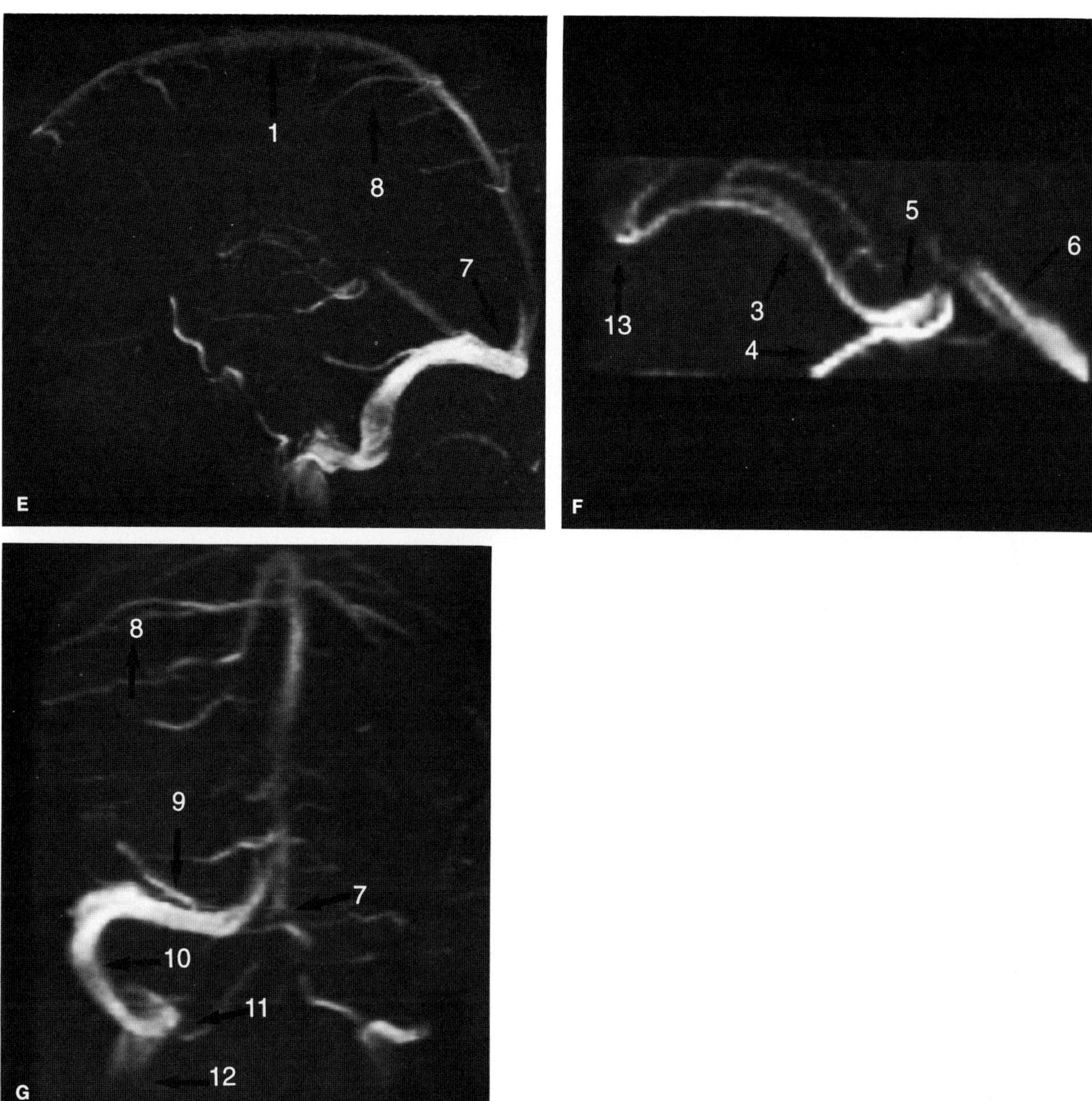

and drains into the cavernous or sphenoparietal sinuses; the vein of Trolard, which joins the superficial middle cerebral vein posteriorly with the superior sagittal sinus; and the vein of Labbé, which joins the superficial middle cerebral vein and the transverse sinus. The deep white matter and basal ganglia are drained centrally by the deep cerebral veins. The paired internal cerebral veins run posteriorly in the velum interpositum, uniting just behind the splenium of the corpus callosum with the basal vein of Rosenthal to form the vein of Galen. The vein of Galen joins the inferior sagittal sinus at the tentorial incisura to form the straight sinus, which extends toward the internal occipital protuberance to the torcular Herophili. The superior sagittal sinus lies midline along the inner table of the skull, often originating near the crista galli and increasing in size as it drains posteriorly to the torcular Herophili. Within the free edge of the falx lies the inferior sagittal sinus. The occipital sinus, which is only occasionally identified, drains superiorly and posteriorly to join the torcular Herophili. From this point, flow continues in the transverse sinuses, which are often asymmetric, the right usually appearing dominant. The transverse sinuses turn downward and medially at the petrous bone to become the sigmoid sinuses, which exit through the jugular foramen to become the internal jugular veins. The jugular bulb represents a prominent consistent enlargement of the internal jugular vein near its origin.[1]

MR Technique

Visualization of the venous system is improved on conventional planar SE MR images following intravenous (IV) gadolinium chelate administration. 2D TOF and 3D PC MRA techniques are also sensitive to slow flow and can be used for depiction of venous anatomy. With these techniques, contrast administration is not typically employed. On 3D TOF MRA (which is typically used to depict arterial anatomy), IV contrast administration markedly improves the visualization of venous structures.[2]

Clinical References

1. Veins of the head and neck. In: Osborn AG, ed. Introduction to cerebral angiography. Philadelphia, Harper & Row, 1980.
2. Chakeres DW, Schmalbrock P, Brogan M, et al. Normal venous anatomy of the brain: demonstration with gadopentetate dimeglumine in enhanced 3-D MR angiography. AJR 1991;156:161–172.

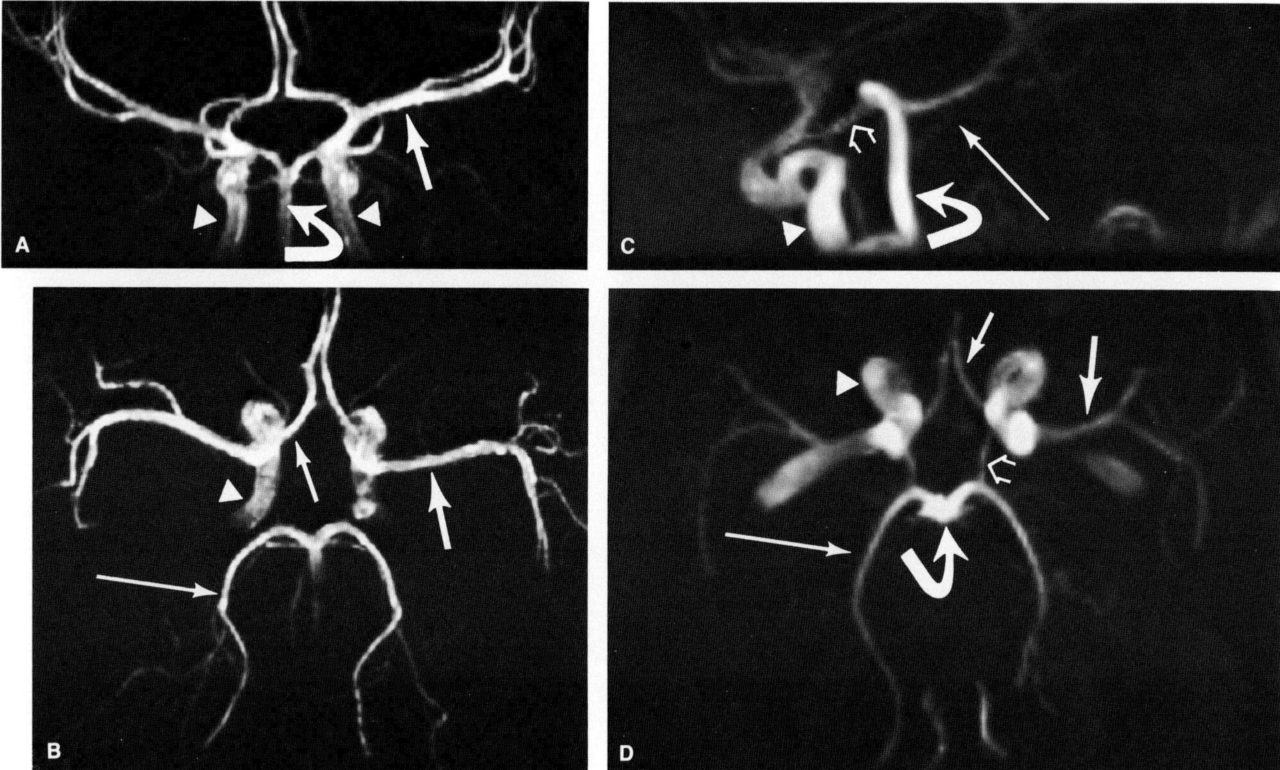

HISTORY

Noncontributory

FINDINGS

Anteroposterior (AP) (*A*) and craniocaudal (*B*) projections from a 3D TOF MRA study in one patient, and lateral (*C*) and craniocaudal (*D*) projections from a similar study in a second patient are presented for interpretation. Magnetization transfer (MT) was used for improved background suppression in *A* and *B,* but not in *C* and *D.*

A: Arrowheads indicate internal carotid arteries; large arrow, middle cerebral artery; small arrow, A1 segment of the anterior cerebral artery; curved arrow, basilar artery; large open arrow, P1 segment of the posterior cerebral artery.

B: Arrowhead indicates internal carotid artery; large arrow, middle cerebral artery; small arrow, A1 segment of the right anterior cerebral ártery; long arrow, posterior cerebral artery.

C: Arrowhead indicates internal carotid artery; long arrow, posterior cerebral artery; curved arrow, basilar artery; small open arrow, posterior communicating artery.

D: Arrowhead indicates internal carotid artery; large arrow, middle cerebral artery; small arrow, A1 segment of the anterior cerebral artery; long arrow, posterior cerebral artery; curved arrow, basilar artery; small open arrow, posterior communicating artery. No anterior communicating artery is identified.

DIAGNOSIS

Normal arterial anatomy

DISCUSSION

Approximately 25% of the population have a complete circle of Willis. Fetal origin of the posterior cerebral artery is a common anatomic arterial variant and is present in 22% of the population; the P1 segment is usually hypoplastic in this variant. The posterior communicating artery is hypoplastic in 34%; the anterior communicating artery is hypoplastic in 15%; the A1 segment is hypoplastic in 10% of the population.[1]

Pitfalls in Image Interpretation

Small-caliber intracranial vessels may not be as well visualized on MRA as on conventional angiography. Thus, differentiation is not possible at present between a very small diameter communicating artery (which is not visualized on MRA) and an incomplete circle of Willis.

Clinical References

1. Osborn AG. Handbook of neuroradiology. St Louis, Mosby–Year Book, 1991:28.

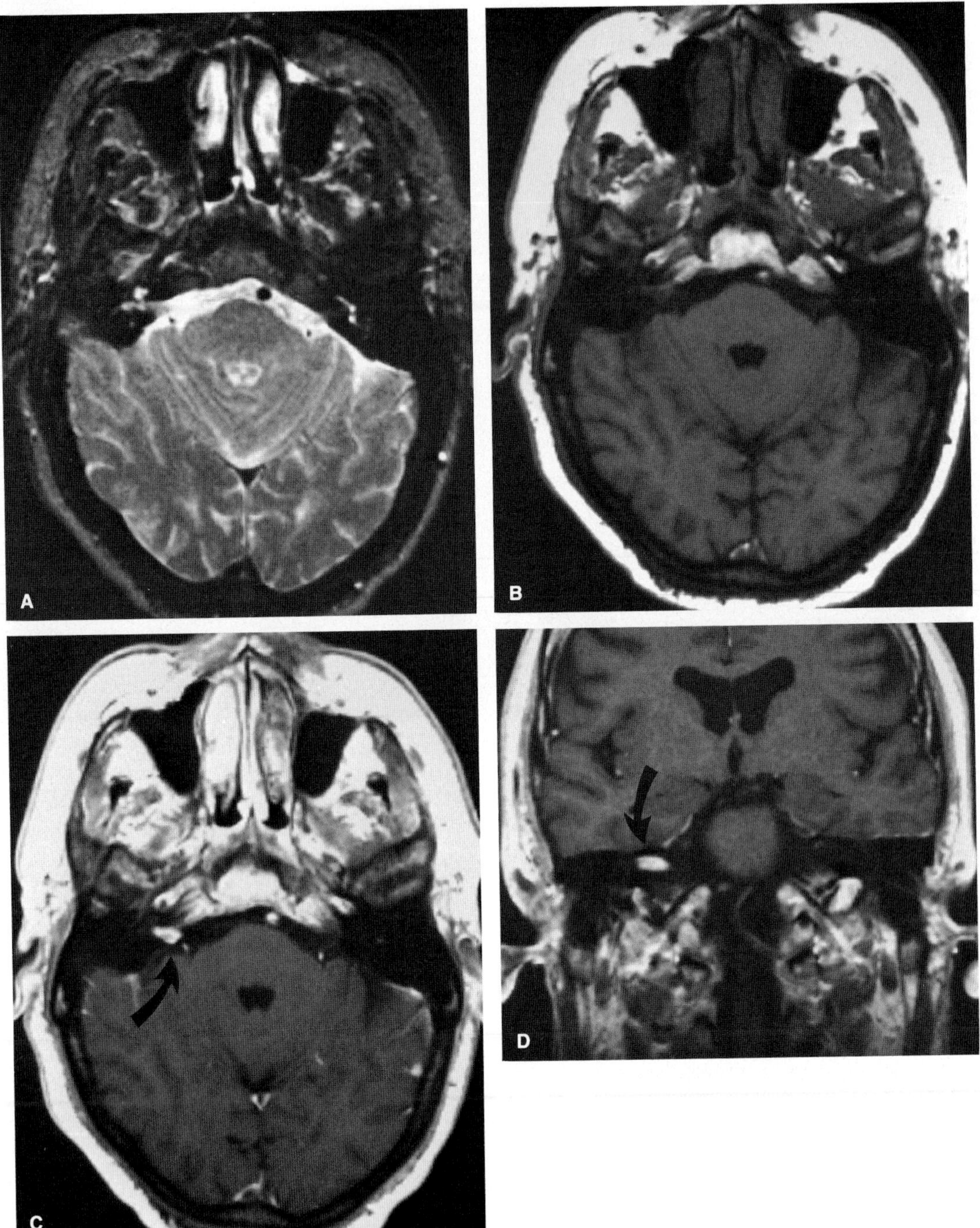

HISTORY

PATIENT 1: Right-sided hearing loss for many years

PATIENT 2: Lung carcinoma with known metastatic disease to the liver and bone. There are no symptoms attributable to central nervous system (CNS) involvement.

PATIENT 3: Resolving expressive aphasia of 3½ weeks' duration

FINDINGS

PATIENT 1: Inspection of T2-weighted (*A*) (TE = 90 msec) and T1-weighted (*B*) axial sections obtained before the administration of IV contrast raises the question of a soft tissue abnormality within the right internal auditory canal. There is, however, only subtle asymmetry between the presumed normal left side and the right side. On axial

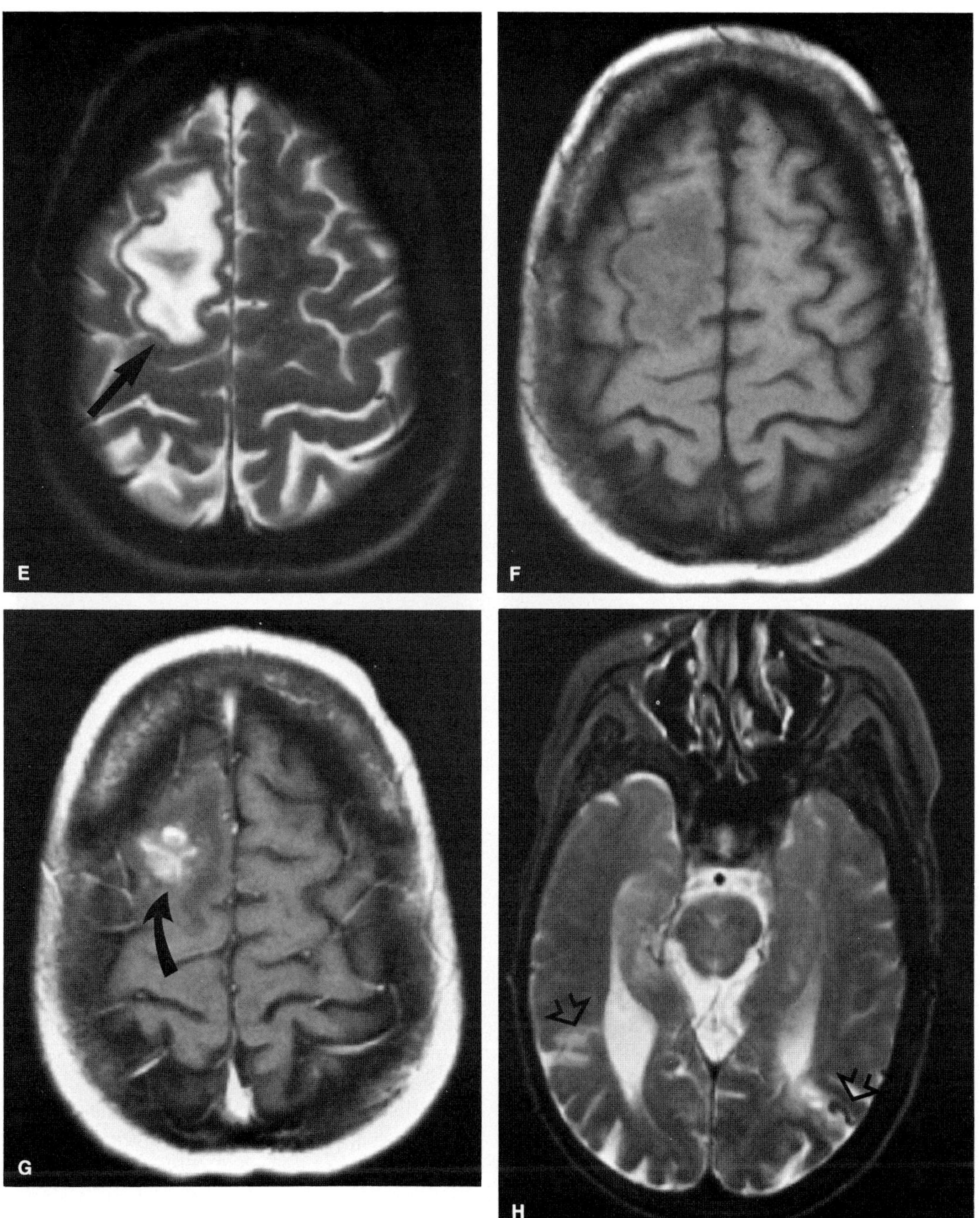

(*C*) and coronal (*D*) postcontrast T1-weighted images, a soft tissue lesion with prominent contrast enhancement (*curved arrows*) is readily identified. The enhancement in this case is due to intrinsic lesion vascularity. The contrast agent used was gadopentetate dimeglumine at a dose of 0.1 mmol/kg IV.

PATIENT 2: Axial precontrast T2-weighted (*E*) (TE = 90 msec) and T1-weighted (*F*) images reveal edema (*arrow* in *E*) in the right frontal lobe near the convexity. No underlying lesion could be visualized on precontrast images. (*G*) The postcontrast T1-weighted axial image demonstrates abnormal enhancement (*curved arrow*) owing to blood–brain barrier disruption, which permits identification of the underlying metastatic focus. The contrast agent used was gadoteridol at a dose of 0.1 mmol/kg IV.

PATIENT 3: (*H*) T2-weighted (TE = 90 msec) axial image raises the question of abnormalities bilaterally (*open arrows*) in the watershed territory between the middle cerebral artery (MCA) and posterior cerebral artery (PCA) distributions. (*I*) Precontrast T1-weighted image reveals abnormal hyperintensity (*arrow*) outlining a gyrus on the left. This appearance is due to the presence of petechial

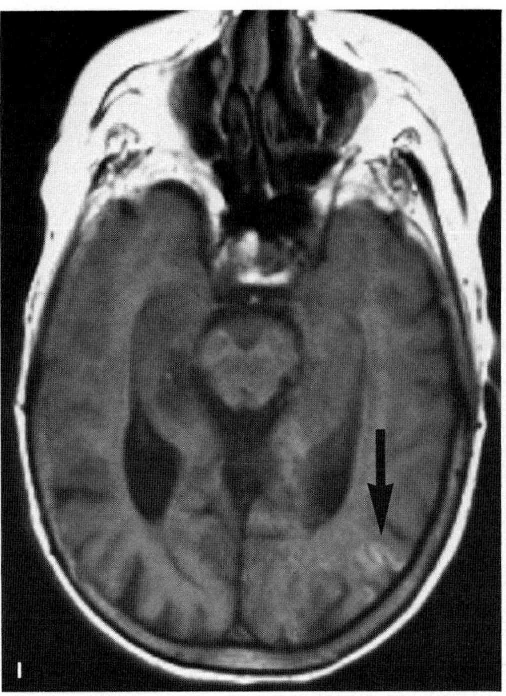

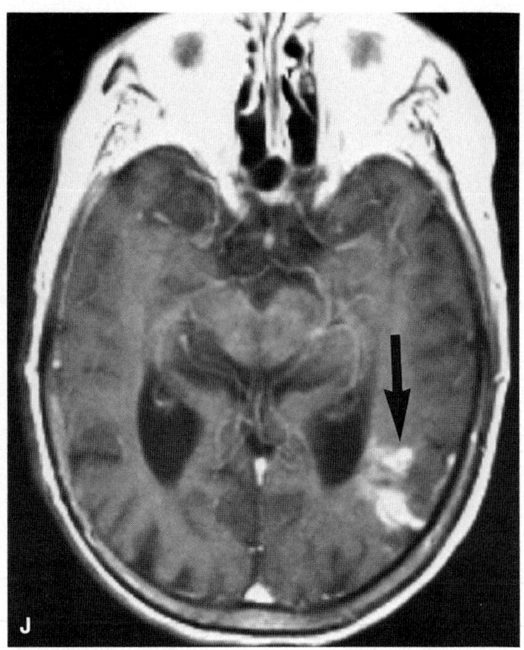

hemorrhage, specifically in the form of methemoglobin. Focal atrophy is noted in the right watershed territory, indicating that this lesion is chronic in nature. (*J*) Abnormal enhancement (*arrow*) on the postcontrast T1-weighted image identifies more completely the full extent of tissue involvement on the left. Contrast enhancement, which in this case is due to disruption of the blood–brain barrier, also permits improved dating of the lesion. The contrast agent used was gadoteridol at a dose of 0.1 mmol/kg IV.

DIAGNOSIS

Examples of use of IV contrast media:

PATIENT 1: Intracanalicular acoustic neuroma

PATIENT 2: Metastatic lung carcinoma

PATIENT 3: Subacute watershed infarction (with petechial hemorrhage)

DISCUSSION

MR is unique among diagnostic imaging modalities because tissue contrast is determined by a multitude of parameters and because the specific measurement technique employed greatly influences the observed contrast.[1] With respect to current clinical use of MR in head imaging, the different contrast agents available act principally by the alteration of tissue relaxation, specifically T1. All paramagnetic agents, however, affect both T1 and T2. Paramagnetic agents enhance tissue relaxation, resulting in a reduction of both T1 and T2, the effect on T1 leading to increased signal intensity and that on T2 to decreased signal intensity. Thus, the relation between concentration of a contrast agent and the resultant change in signal intensity on MR is complex and specifically not linear (unlike computed tomography [CT]). Fortunately, at the concentrations typically achieved in brain tissue, positive enhancement is encountered. Negative enhancement, which could occur on the basis of T2 shortening, has not been reported in the brain with standard imaging techniques. In the bladder, a reduction in signal intensity can be routinely demonstrated after administration of a gadolinium chelate as a result of hyperconcentration of the agent in the urine.

There are four metal chelates in current clinical use as IV contrast agents for MR.[2] All share similar T1 relaxivity and enhancement characteristics. Gadopentetate dimeglumine (Magnevist) was approved for clinical use in the United States in 1988. Gadoteridol (ProHance) completed clinical trials in the United States in 1990. The latter agent is nonionic, unlike gadopentetate dimeglumine, which must be formulated as a salt. Furthermore, the ligand or chelate in gadoteridol is a rigid macrocycle, which improves the stability of the complex relative to metal ion exchange. Clinical trials have been pursued using doses of gadoteridol up to 0.3 mmol/kg, with no laboratory abnormalities attributable to contrast injection noted. Gadodiamide (Omniscan) has also been evaluated in recent clinical trials in the United States, although questions have been raised concerning possible demetalation and metabolism of this complex in vivo. Gadoterate meglumine (Dotarem), the last of the four agents, is approved in several European and South American countries for clinical use.

In the United States, gadolinium chelates are employed intravenously in about half of all head MR examinations, with use continuing to expand.[3] Indications for application are broad, with some studies recommending their use in all patients except potentially children and young adults with a low clinical suspicion of disease. Normal structures that demonstrate enhancement include the choroid plexus, pituitary (anterior lobe and infundibulum), and nasal mucosa. Enhancement of venous and arterial structures is common, although influenced markedly by flow rate, turbulence, choice of pulse sequence, and other factors.

For detection of small extraaxial neoplastic lesions, contrast use is mandatory (see patient 1). The full extent of large extraaxial lesions is also better determined postcontrast. Enhancement of these lesions is seen on the basis of intrinsic vascularity. In sharp distinction, intraaxial lesions display contrast enhancement principally as a result of blood–brain barrier disruption. With many primary and secondary intraaxial lesions, tumor bulk, necrosis, and tumor grade are best assessed postcontrast (see patient 2). Contrast use is mandatory in screening for metastatic disease. As noted in later cases, the detection of metastatic disease can be improved even further by the use of doses greater than 0.1 mmol/kg IV. Identification of tumor recurrence after surgery is also an important indication for contrast use. In the study of sella and parasellar abnormalities, contrast enhancement has proved useful for both small and large lesions. In certain instances, a microadenoma can be identified only postcontrast. With respect to large lesions in this anatomic area, contrast enhancement can improve the delineation of tumor extent and identify cavernous sinus invasion. In infection, contrast enhancement permits both delineation of the lesion and assessment of disease activity. With demyelinating diseases and specifically multiple sclerosis (MS), IV contrast is used to assess lesion activity. In a small number of MS patients, lesions can be identified postcontrast that are not visible on unenhanced MR. In cerebral infarction, vascular enhancement is seen 1 to 3 days postictus, presumably as a result of vascular engorgement and slow flow. Slightly later, abnormal enhancement of adjacent meninges can be visualized. In the subacute time frame, parenchymal enhancement due to blood–brain barrier disruption is noted (see patient 3). Some subacute infarcts appear isointense on both T1- and T2-weighted images, with identification possible only following contrast administration. Detection of recent cerebral infarction is particularly difficult in the elderly population with significant underlying chronic white matter ischemia, with contrast agent use also having a major impact here. Contrast enhancement can improve the visualization of arteriovenous abnormalities, in particular abnormal venous structures. In this instance, it is the presence of the contrast agent at high levels within the blood that leads to improved vessel visualization.

For brevity and clarity, in the cases that follow, reference will not be made to the specific contrast agent used unless pertinent to the case or illustration. One major exception is in the discussion of cases in which a dose greater than 0.1 mmol/kg has been used, since in this instance clinical experience is predominantly limited to gadoteridol (with the safety of this agent also clearly established at high doses). Other than dose, and possible differences with regard to clinical safety, the four gadolinium chelates mentioned should be considered interchangeable with respect to enhancement properties. Thus, reference in the patient cases is commonly limited to "enhancement with a gadolinium chelate" or "postcontrast," with all such statements implying IV administration and a dose of 0.1 mmol/kg. Unless otherwise stated, postcontrast images depicted were obtained within the first 5 to 10 minutes of contrast injection.

MR Technique

In clinical practice, T1-weighted SE images are typically employed for detection of enhancement following IV administration of a gadolinium chelate. Excellent contrast detectability can be achieved with TRs of 400 to 600 msec and TEs of 10 to 25 msec.

Pitfalls in Image Interpretation

It is strongly recommended that T1-weighted SE scans be obtained both before and after IV contrast administration in all patients. In this manner, abnormal contrast enhancement can be identified with certainty. On postcontrast examinations alone, fat (such as that in a lipoma), blood (specifically methemoglobin), fluid with elevated protein content, and Pantopaque can be confused with abnormal contrast enhancement.

Clinical References

1. Runge VM, ed. Contrast media in magnetic resonance imaging: a clinical approach. Philadelphia, JB Lippincott, 1992.
2. Runge VM. Magnetic resonance contrast agents. In: Katzberg RW, ed. The contrast media manual. Baltimore, Williams & Wilkins, 1992.
3. Runge VM. MR imaging contrast agents. Curr Opin Radiol 1992;4:3–12.

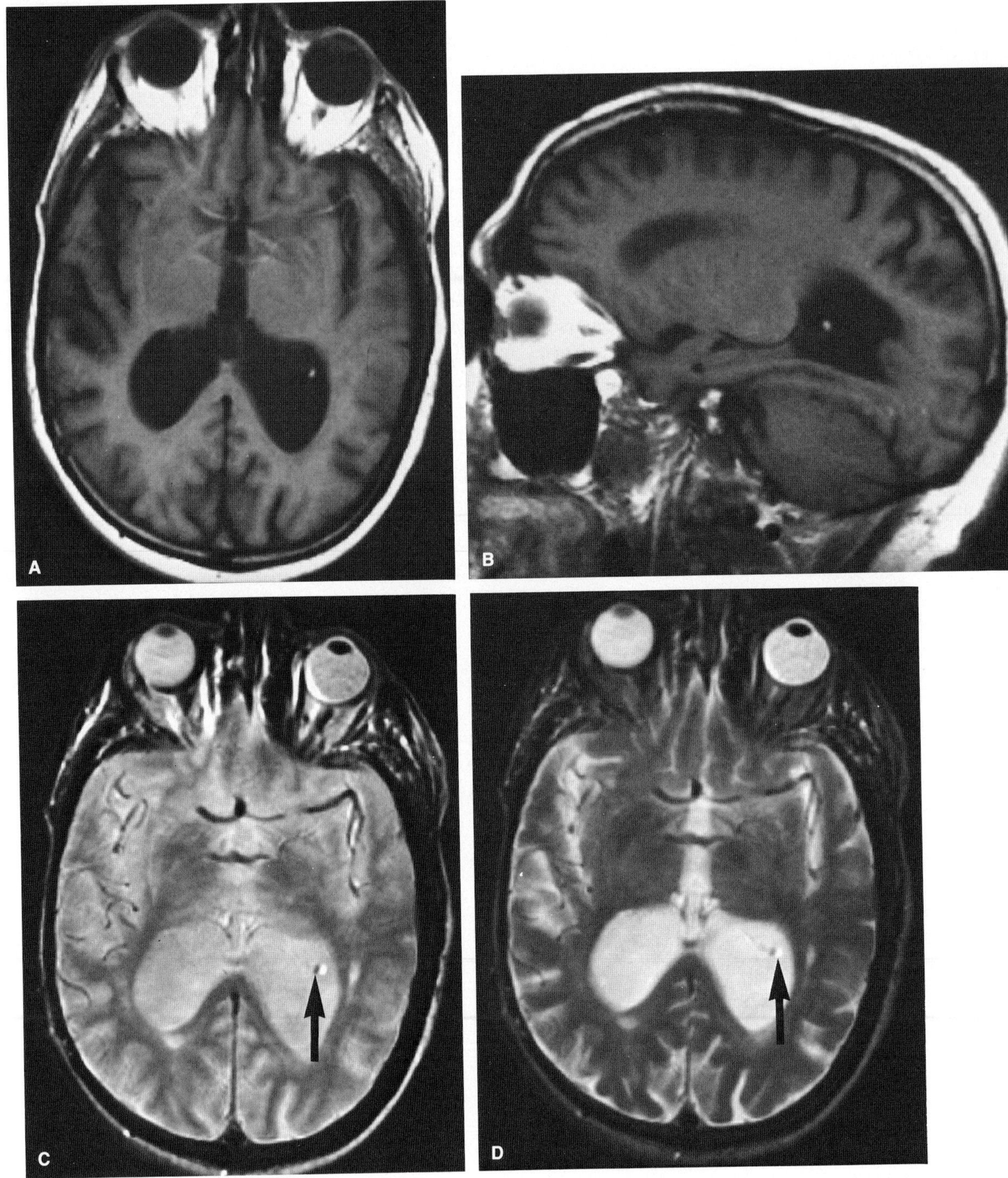

HISTORY

Noncontributory

FINDINGS

Axial (*A*) and sagittal (*B*) T1-weighted images identify a small round mass of increased signal intensity in the trigone of the left lateral ventricle. First (*C*) and second (*D*) echoes of axial T2-weighted sequences show chemical shift artifact (*black arrows*) in the frequency encoding direction at the interface of this mass with CSF.

DIAGNOSIS

Calcified choroid plexus

DISCUSSION

The glomus portion of the choroid plexus is contained in the atria of the lateral ventricles and is the most frequent portion of the choroid plexus to calcify. Glomus calcification can occur as early as 3 years of age but is uncommon under 9 years. The size and shape of calcifications vary, but they are usually globular and bilateral. Calcification of the choroid plexus in the third or fourth ventricles is rare.[1]

Intracranial calcification can have a variety of signal intensities on MR. It can be of low, intermediate, or increased signal intensity on T1-weighted images (as well as imperceptible). On T2-weighted images, intracranial calcification is manifested by decreased signal intensity.[2,3] There are several possible explanations for the cause of the increased signal intensity of calcifications on T1-weighted images. Certain calcifications contain a fatty matrix (as in this case); other calcifications have a large microscopic crystal surface area of particulate calcium. The latter has been shown to result in T1 shortening.

Chemical shift artifact is produced by spatial misregistration of signal intensity that occurs in the frequency encoding direction. Chemical shift artifacts appear as bright or dark rims at the boundary between fatty and watery tissues. The width of these rims correlates with the degree of spatial misregistration. In fat, the most common chemical component containing hydrogen (protons) is the CH group. The resonant frequency of the CH group differs from that of water by approximately 3.5 ppm. The hydrogen molecules in fat precess at a slower rate than the hydrogen molecules in water. When the gradient coil is turned on, fat protons are shifted to a lower frequency with respect to water protons; therefore, the fat signal appears to originate from an incorrect location.[4]

The effect of chemical shift is always in the direction of frequency encoding. At 1.5 T, the fat–water chemical shift is 220 Hz. The distance of the chemical shift artifact is directly proportional to the strength of the magnetic field and the field-of-view (FOV); it is inversely proportional to the sampling bandwidth. Low-bandwidth pulse sequences are desirable for head MR imaging in most instances because they result in increased S/N. The amount of noise is proportional to the square root of the bandwidth. However, low-bandwidth sequences have more prominent chemical shift artifact.

Clinical References

1. Osborn AG. Handbook of neuroradiology. St Louis, Mosby–Year Book, 1991:157.
2. Dell LA, Brown MS, Orrison WW, et al. Physiologic intracranial calcification with hyperintensity on MR imaging: case report and experimental model. AJNR 1988;9:1145–1148.
3. Henkelman RM, Watts JF, Kucharczyk W. High signal intensity in MR images of calcified brain tissue. Radiology 1991;179:199–206.
4. Smith AS, Weinstein MA, Hurst GC, et al. Intracranial chemical-shift artifacts on MR images of the brain: observations and relation to sampling bandwidth. AJR 1990;154:1275–1283.

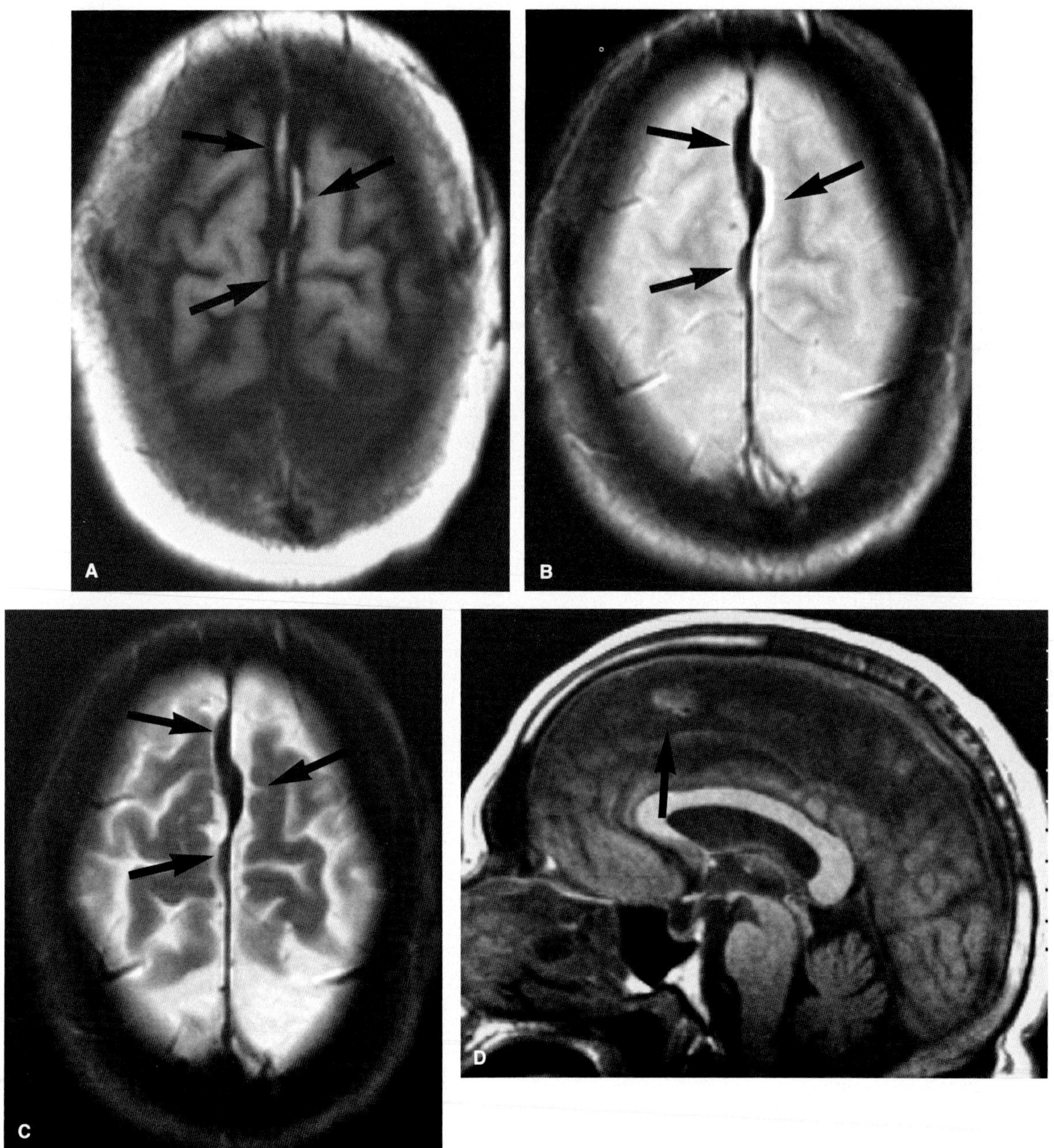

HISTORY

A 65-year-old with headaches

FINDINGS

(*A*) High signal intensity is seen in the falx cerebri (*arrows*) on this precontrast T1-weighted axial image. On intermediate weighted (*B*) and heavily T2-weighted (*C*) axial images, there is very low signal intensity in the corresponding portions of the falx (*arrows*). In addition, there is a subtle high-signal-intensity band along the left lateral aspect of the low-signal-intensity falx in *B,* which represents a chemical shift artifact. A chemical shift artifact occurs along the frequency encoding axis at fat–water interfaces and is explained in detail in 1.1341. (*D*) Midline T1-weighted sagittal image demonstrates high signal intensity within the falx (*arrow*).

DIAGNOSIS

Falx ossification

DISCUSSION

The term *falx calcification* is often used to refer to either calcium deposition or ossification of the falx cerebri.[1] Both calcification and ossification of the falx exist, and there is probably a spectrum containing both elements.[1] Increased density of the falx, representing either calcification or ossification, is seen in up to 42% of adult patients on CT. Calcification of the falx is usually an incidental finding on CT or MR of the brain and is probably degenerative in etiology, although the exact cause is not known. A higher incidence of falx calcification is reported in hyperparathyroidism and hypoparathyroidism, hypervitaminosis A and D, basal cell nevus syndrome, and pseudoxanthoma elasticum.[2]

The normal falx is composed of fibrous connective tissue and has low signal intensity on both T1- and T2-weighted images. Therefore, calcification within a falx of normal thickness is not usually detected by MR. Falx ossification, on the other hand, has a characteristic appearance on MR. The fat within the marrow of an ossified falx has high signal intensity on T1-weighted images. As with all fat, the signal intensity of falx ossification decreases on T2-weighted images. The cortical bone surrounding the marrow has low signal intensity on both T1- and T2-weighted images, and dominates the appearance on T2-weighted images. The ossification is usually located on one side or the other of midline, corresponding to the leaves of the falx. The affected leaf of the falx usually demonstrates focal enlargement.

Pitfalls in Image Interpretation

Pathologic entities that may occur in the region of the falx include meningioma, myeloid metaplasia, primary falx osteosarcoma, metastases, and leukemic infiltration of the falx.[2] High signal intensity on T1-weighted images does not occur in any of these entities. Meningiomas are commonly isointense to gray matter on both T1- and T2-weighted images, and show intense homogeneous enhancement after contrast infusion.

Clinical References

1. Lee D, Larson T, Norman D. Falx ossification: MR visualization. Can Assoc Radiol J 1988;39:260–262.
2. Sands S, Farmer P, Alvarez O, et al. Fat within the falx: MR demonstration of falcine bony metaplasia with marrow formation. J Comput Assist Tomogr 1987;11:602–605.

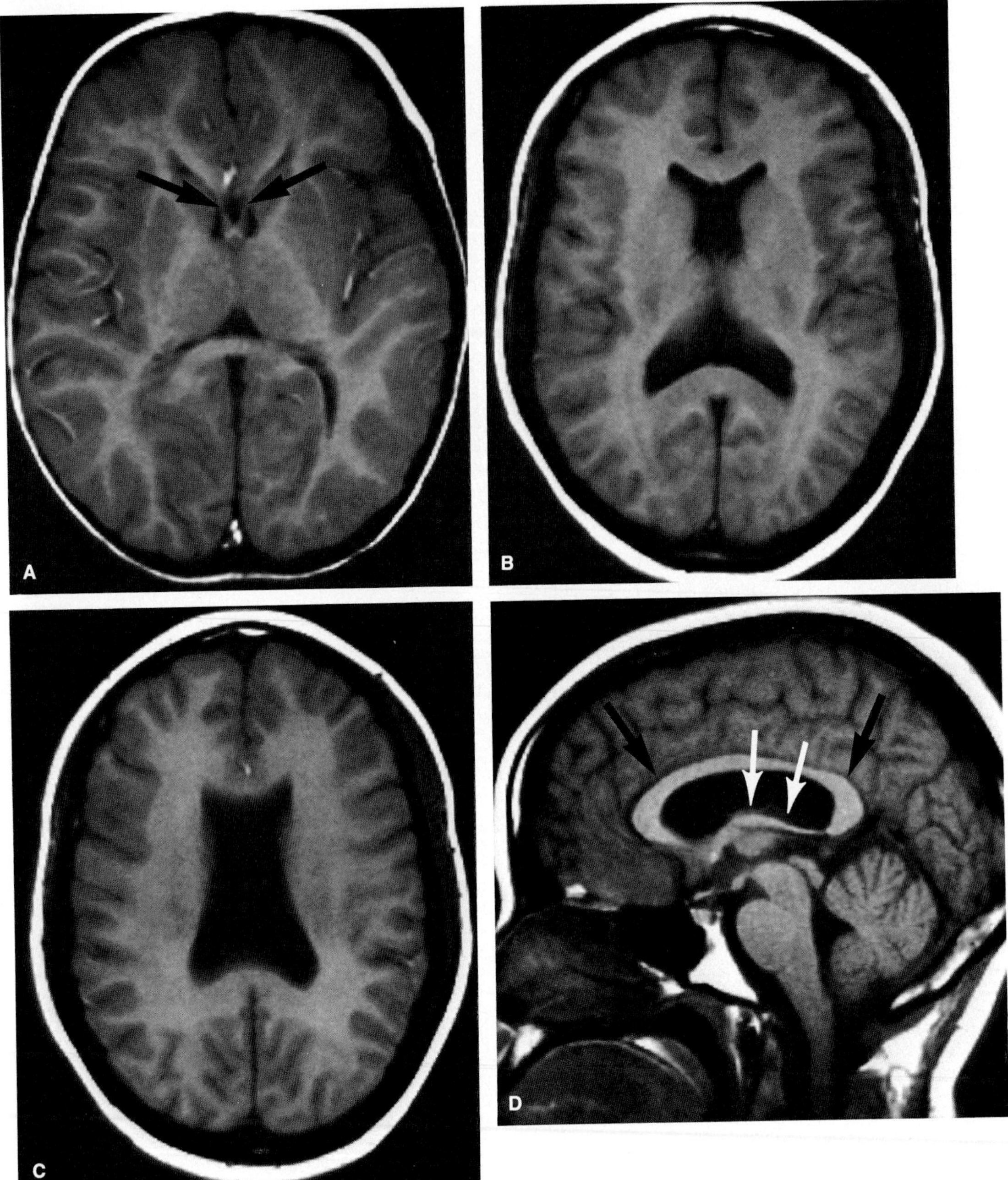

HISTORY

PATIENT 1: 1-year-old with behavioral changes

PATIENT 2: 28-year-old with headaches but no visual changes or other neurologic signs or symptoms

FINDINGS

PATIENT 1: (*A*) The leaves of the septum pellucidum (*black arrows*) are separated on the T1-weighted axial image, and there is CSF intensity between them. This fluid was of CSF intensity on intermediate- and T2-weighted images as well (*not shown*).

PATIENT 2: (*B and C*) The frontal horns and bodies of the lateral ventricles are not separated by a midline septum on the T1-weighted axial images (*D*). The fornix (*white arrows*) lies in an abnormally low position and has a horizontal orientation on the T1-weighted sagittal image, because of the lack of superior tethering by a septum pellucidum. The corpus callosum (*black arrows*) is normal, and there is no evidence of hydrocephalus.

DIAGNOSIS

PATIENT 1: Cavum septum pellucidum

PATIENT 2: Absence of the septum pellucidum

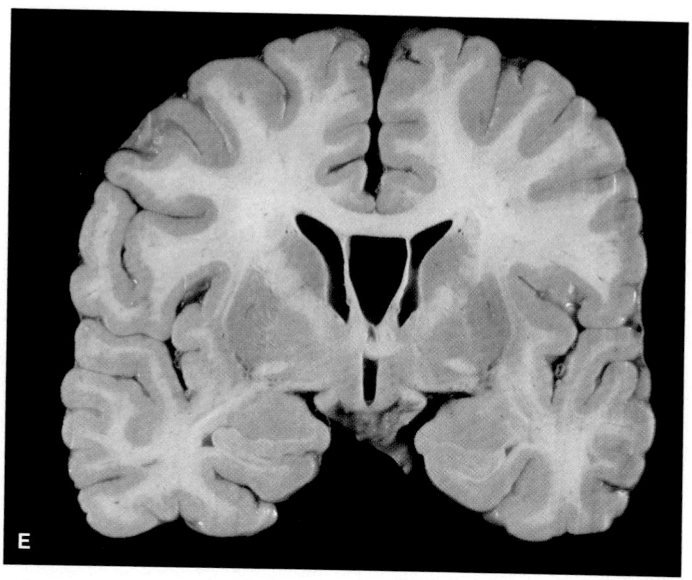

DISCUSSION

The septum pellucidum is a thin translucent (*pellucidum* is Latin for "transparent") plate of two laminae that lies in the midline between the frontal horns of the lateral ventricles. Contrary to widely held belief, the septum pellucidum is not functionless; it is an important relay station in the limbic system, linking the hippocampus and the hypothalamus.[1] Therefore, abnormalities of the septum pellucidum may be associated with subtle neuropsychiatric symptoms.

A cavum septum pellucidum (CSP) is a normal embryologic space between the two leaves of the septum pellucidum that is seen in 100% of fetuses and premature infants.[1] Subsequent growth of the brain and fusion of the leaves causes the prevalence of CSP to decrease to 15% by the age of 3 to 6 months. CSP can persist into adulthood and is simply a normal variant. Very wide separation of the leaves of the septum pellucidum, greater than 1 cm with outward bowing, is termed a cyst of the septum pellucidum and may rarely cause symptoms because of obstruction of CSF flow at the foramina of Monro.[1]

Absence of the septum pellucidum is a rare anomaly, present in 2 to 3 per 100,000 population.[2] It almost always signifies substantial neurologic disease[1,2] and is associated with several congenital anomalies of the brain: holoprosencephaly, septooptic dysplasia, agenesis of the corpus callosum, anterior basilar encephaloceles, hydranencephaly, and the Chiari II malformation. Therefore, absence of the septum pellucidum should provoke a search for further abnormalities of the brain. Absence of the septum pellucidum may also be acquired, usually a sequela of severe long-standing hydrocephalus, which actually causes rupture and disintegration of the leaves of the septum.[1]

MR Technique

Coronal images are helpful in evaluating the interhemispheric fissure and the optic chiasm. There is fusion across the midline, usually of the frontal lobes, in patients with holoprosencephaly, which manifests as incomplete formation of the interhemispheric fissure. The optic nerves and chiasm are small on MR in about half the patients with septooptic dysplasia.

Pathologic Correlate

(*E*) Coronal gross section demonstrates wide separation of the leaves of the septum pellucidum. This CSP was asymptomatic and was an incidental finding at autopsy.

Clinical References

1. Sarwar M. The septum pellucidum: normal and abnormal. AJNR 1989;10:989–1005.
2. Barkovich A, Norman D. Absence of the septum pellucidum: a useful sign in the diagnosis of congenital brain malformations. AJR 1989;152:353–360.

(*E courtesy of Daron G. Davis, MD.*)

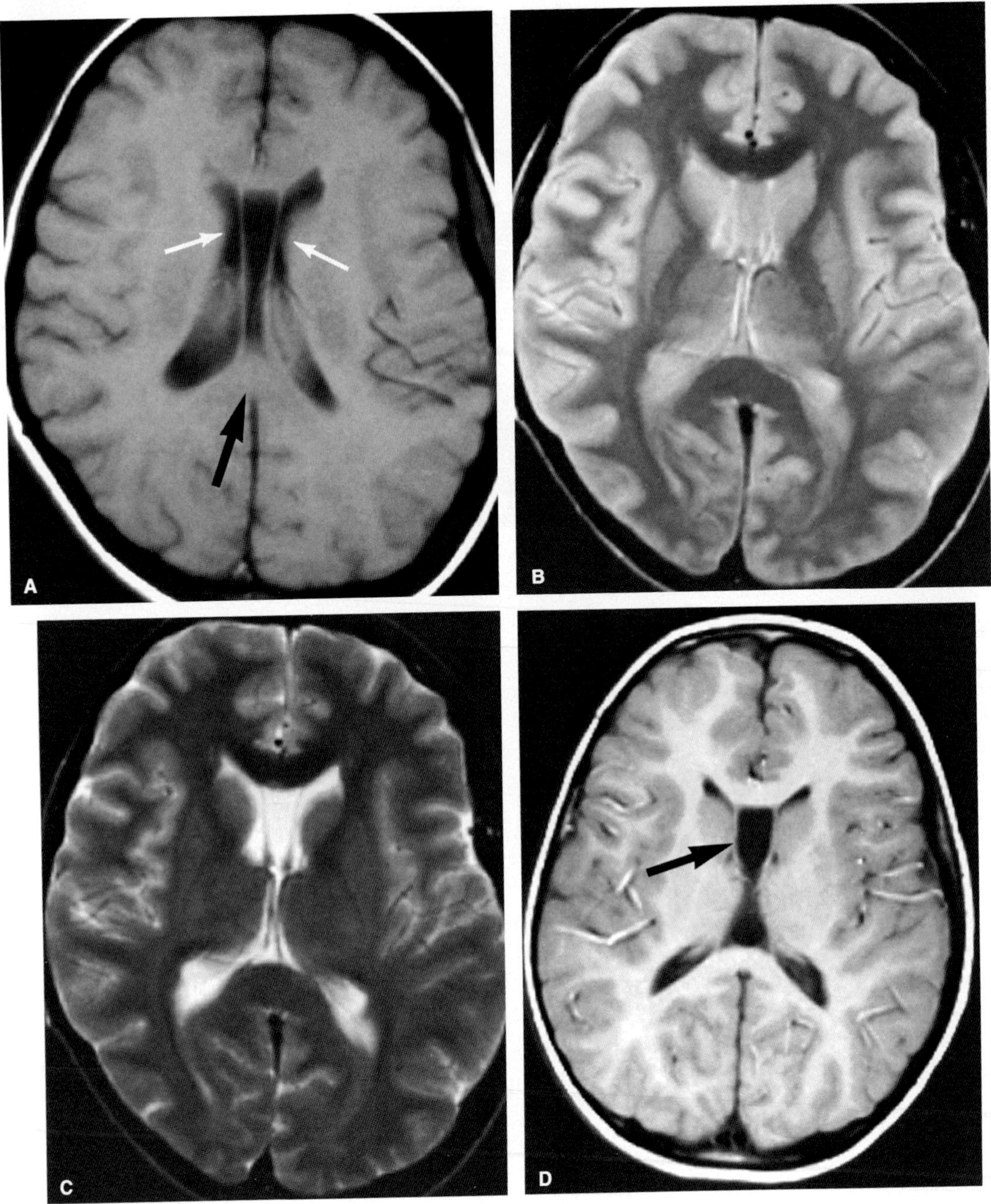

HISTORY

A 26-year-old with nosebleeds and headaches

FINDINGS

(*A*) T1-weighted axial image at the level of the lateral ventricles demonstrates separation of the two leaves of the septum pellucidum (*small white arrows*), with formation of a cavity between the frontal horns. The posterior extent of the cavity is demarcated by the splenium of the corpus callosum (*black arrow*). The fluid within the cavity has the signal intensity of CSF on T1-weighted (*A*), intermediate-weighted (*B*), and heavily T2-weighted (*C*) axial images. The size of the lateral ventricles is within normal limits.

(*D*) T1-weighted axial image from a different patient shows similar findings, with the posterior extension of the midline cavity (*arrow*) having a more flask-shaped appearance.

DIAGNOSIS

Cavum septum pellucidum (CSP) and cavum vergae

DISCUSSION

CSP and cavum vergae are normal embryologic cavities found in the midline of all fetal brains.[1] Cavum vergae is located directly behind the CSP, and is essentially a posterior extension of the same structure. Cavum vergae is defined as the portion of the midline cavity that is located posterior to an arbitrary vertical plane formed by the columns of the fornix.[2] The midline of the posterior wall of cavum vergae ends at the splenium of the corpus callosum. Cava vergae usually begin to disappear at about 6 months of gestation, are present in about 30% of full-term infants, and are seen in only approximately 1% of children over the age of 10 years.[3]

Small CSPs and cava vergae in children and adults are asymptomatic and are considered normal anatomic variants. There have been reports of associated structural and neurologic abnormalities when these cavities are wider than 1 cm.[1,4] However, there is no definite evidence that a large CSP or cavum vergae is clinically significant, unless it is large enough to cause obstruction of CSF flow. Obstruction, when present, usually occurs at the foramina of Monro.[2]

On MR, cavum vergae appears as a midline CSF-filled cavity that is flask-shaped on axial images and is positioned directly posterior to the CSP.[1]

Pitfalls in Image Interpretation

Cavum velum interpositum (CVI) is a CSF-containing space that develops from a separation of the crura of the fornix between the thalami and above the third ventricle,[1] and is seen in the posterior midline of the brain. Cavum vergae can be differentiated from CVI easily by MR, particularly with coronal images: cavum vergae lies superior to the internal cerebral veins, while these two vessels lie within a CVI.[1]

Clinical References

1. Miller M, Kido D, Horner F. Cavum vergae: association with neurologic abnormality and diagnosis by magnetic resonance imaging. Arch Neurol 1986;43:821–823.
2. Shaw C, Alvord E. Cava septi pellucidi et vergae: their normal and pathological states. Brain 1969;92:213–224.
3. Nakanno S, Hojo H, Kataoka K, et al. Age-related incidence of cavum septum pellucidum and cavum vergae on CT scans of pediatric patients. J Comput Assist Tomogr 1981; 5:348–349.
4. Schaefer G, Bodensteiner J. Wide cavum septum pellucidum: a marker of disturbed brain development. Pediatr Neurol 1990;6:391–394.

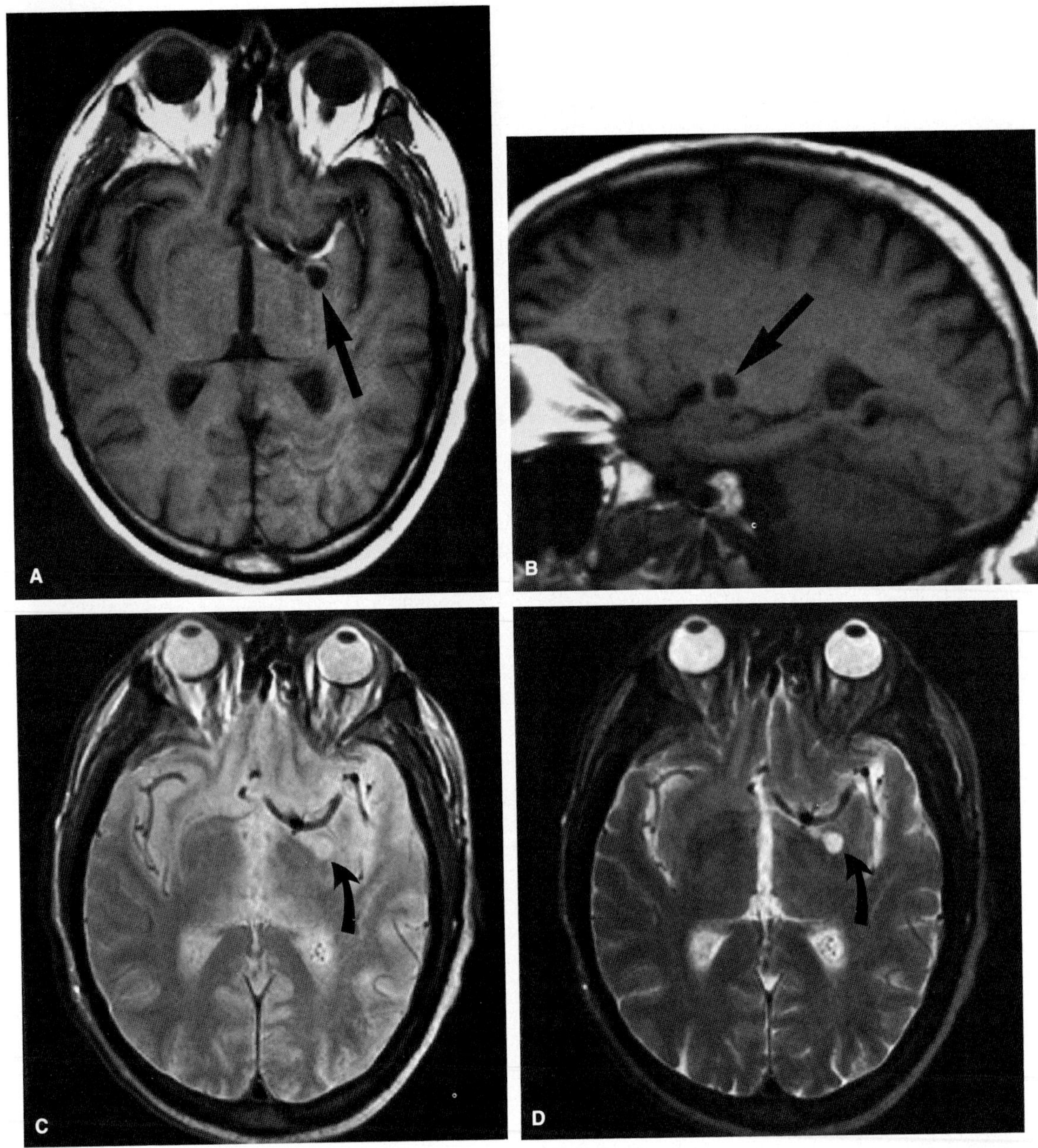

HISTORY

Noncontributory

FINDINGS

PATIENT 1: A small, round low-signal-intensity lesion (*arrow*) is noted in the inferior one third of the left basal ganglia adjacent to the anterior commissure on axial (*A*) and sagittal (*B*) T1-weighted images. First (*C*) and second (*D*) echoes of T2-weighted scan show that the lesion (*curved arrow*) is of CSF signal intensity. No abnormal contrast enhancement was noted (*images not shown*).

PATIENT 2: Small bilateral foci of CSF signal intensity are identified in the cerebral peduncles on the first (*E*) and second (*F*) echoes of the T2-weighted scan. (*G*) On the axial T1-weighted image these foci are barely discernible, being only slightly hypointense to brain.

DIAGNOSIS

Dilated perivascular spaces (DPVSs)

DISCUSSION

The perivascular space, also known as the Virchow-Robin space, normally surrounds perforating arteries that enter the brain and represents an invagination of the subarach-

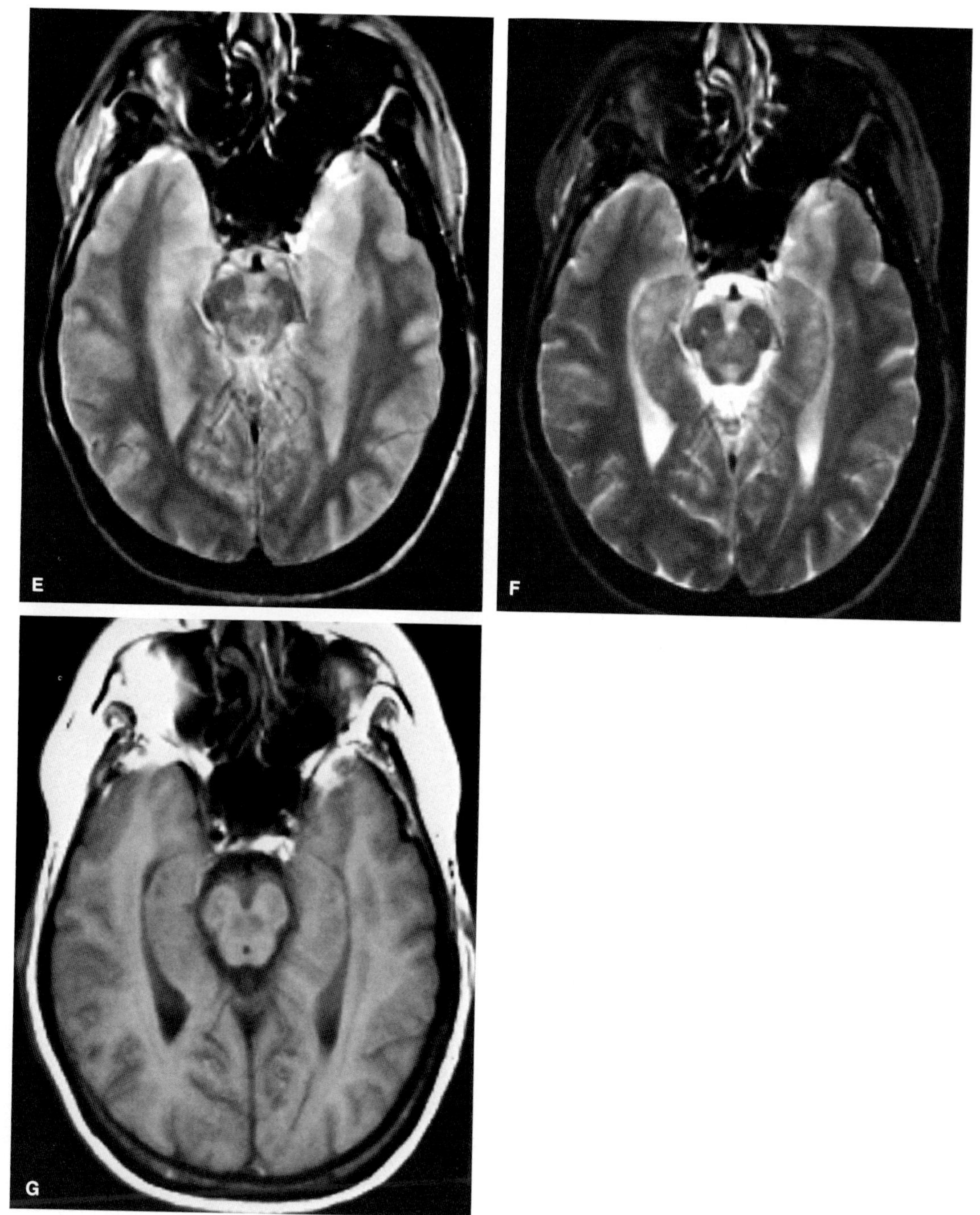

noid space surrounding these vessels as they course from the subarachnoid space into the brain parenchyma. The term *état criblé* indicates a dilated Virchow-Robin space, with or without associated changes of gliosis or demyelination in the surrounding brain parenchyma.[1]

DPVSs are most commonly seen in the inferior third of the basal ganglia adjacent to the anterior commissure where they follow the course of the lenticulostriate arteries as they enter the basal ganglia. DPVSs are also commonly identified in the high-convexity white matter of the centrum semiovale, where they follow the course of penetrating nutrient arteries. The latter are usually no more than 1 or 2 mm in diameter.[2,3] DPVSs are also occasionally identified on MR in the midbrain. These appear as punctate or linear foci typically located near the junction of the substantia nigra and cerebral peduncle in the lower mesencephalon. In the midbrain, DPVSs are typically 1 to 1.5 mm in greatest diameter and correspond to branches of the collicular or accessory collicular arteries, which are branches of the posterior cerebral artery.[4]

MR demonstrates perivascular spaces as small foci of CSF intensity on all pulse sequences. The artery within the perivascular space is not typically delineated by MR since the associated perivascular space is much larger than the size of the vessel. Although perivascular spaces are usually less than 5 mm in diameter, they can be larger.

Lacunar infarcts can be confused with dilated perivascular spaces. Lacunae are small infarcts caused by penetrating branch artery occlusion. On MR lacunar infarcts are usually ovoid or slitlike in configuration, occur in the upper two thirds of the basal ganglia, and are usually not of CSF intensity on all pulse sequences. They are typically less than 1 cm in greatest diameter, and hyperintense to brain parenchyma on T2-weighted sequences.

MR Technique

The first echo of the T2-weighted sequence is helpful in differentiating a dilated perivascular space from a subacute lacunar infarct. On scans with mild to moderate T2 weighting, a dilated perivascular space is isointense to CSF, whereas a subacute lacunar infarct is of increased signal intensity.

Pitfalls in Image Interpretation

Large perivascular spaces can be difficult to distinguish from chronic cavitated lacunar infarcts on MR.

Clinical References

1. Braffman BH, Zimmerman RA, Trojanowski JQ, et al. Brain MR: pathologic correlation with gross and histopathology: 1. Lacunar infarction and Virchow-Robin spaces. AJR 1988; 151:551–558.
2. Jungreis CA, Kanal E, Hirsch WL, et al. Normal perivascular spaces mimicking lacunar infarction: MR imaging. Radiology 1988;169:101–104.
3. Heier LA, Bauer CJ, Schwartz RD, et al. Large Virchow-Robin spaces: MR-clinical correlation. AJNR 1989;10:929–936.
4. Elster AD, Richardson DN. Focal high signal on MR scans of the midbrain caused by enlarged perivascular spaces: MR pathologic correlation. AJR 1991;156:157–160.

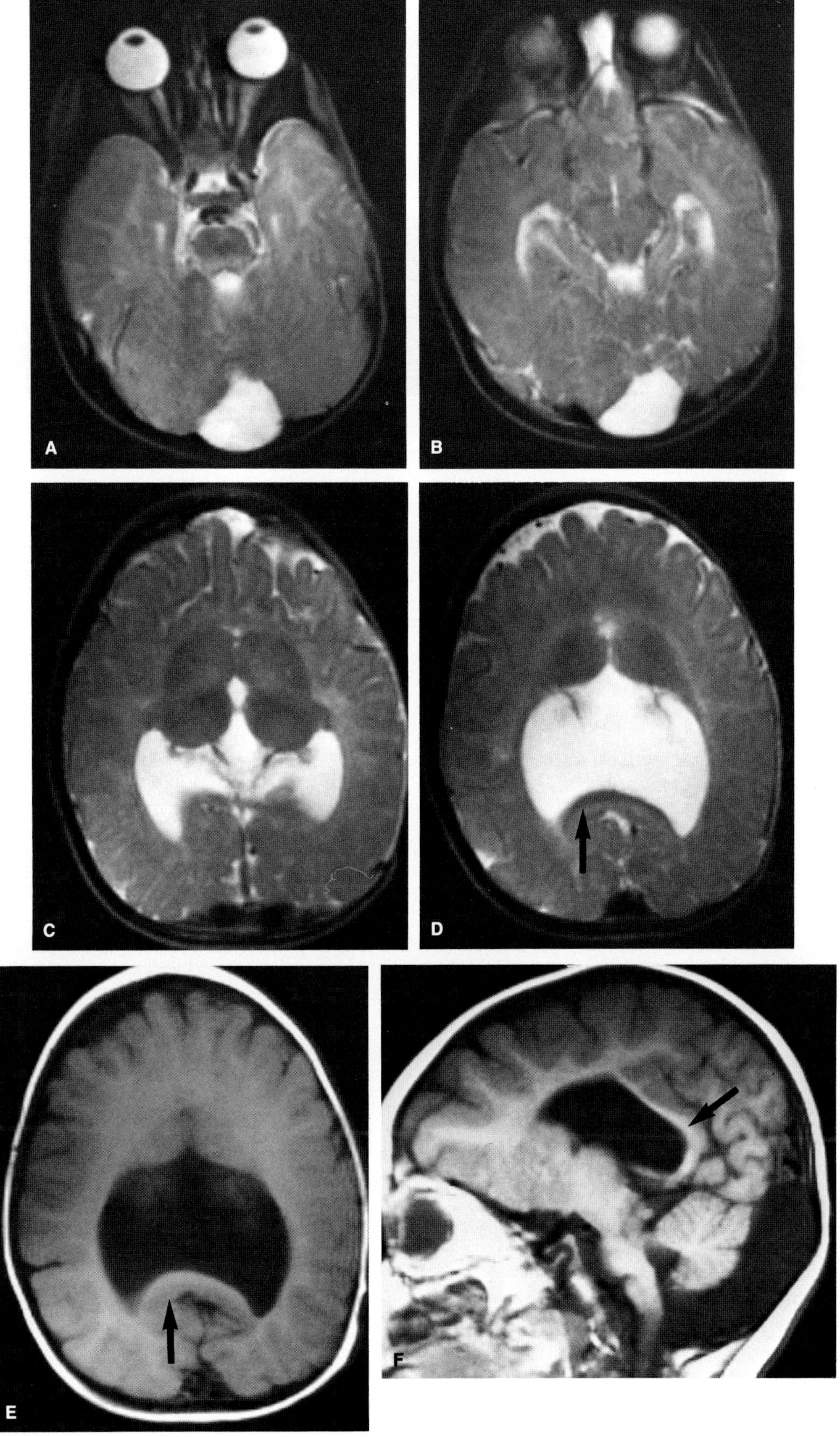
A
B
C
D
E
F

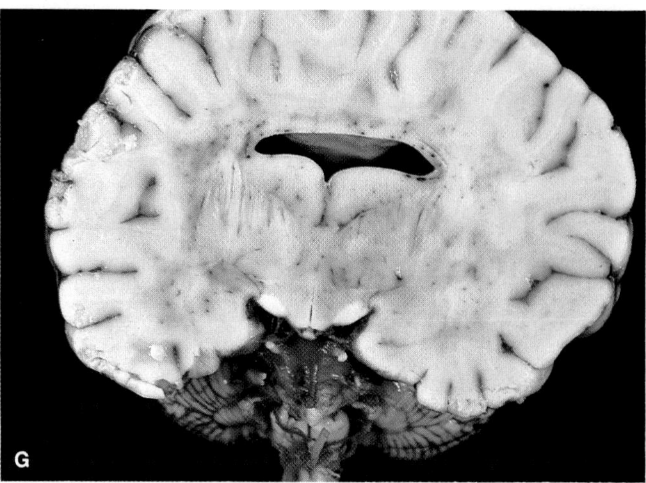

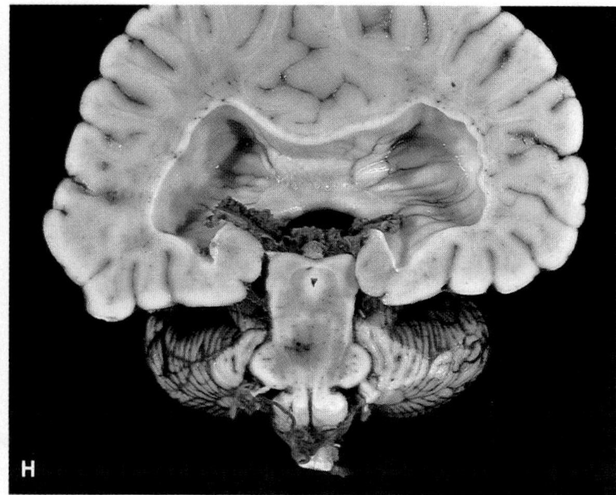

HISTORY

A 9-month-old infant with microcephaly and developmental delay

FINDINGS

(*A to D*) Axial T2-weighted, and axial (*E*), and sagittal (*F*) T1-weighted images are presented. There is hypotelorism (*A*), rudimentary formation of the temporal horns (*B*), a small third ventricle with fusion of more anterior structures (*C*), and preservation of the splenium of the corpus callosum (*arrow in D*). No frontal horns can be identified. The fusion of anterior structures (with absence of the falx anteriorly), as well as the presence of the corpus callosum posteriorly (*arrows in E and F*), is confirmed on the axial and sagittal T1-weighted images. Incidentally noted on *F* is a large retrocerebellar cyst.

DIAGNOSIS

Semilobar holoprosencephaly

DISCUSSION

The term *holoprosencephaly*[1] is used for a subgroup of congenital malformations of the brain, characterized by failure of cleavage and differentiation in the forebrain (prosencephalon) during embryogenesis. In this disorder, there is a failure of both lateral cleavage (which in the normal embryo results in distinct cerebral hemispheres) and transverse cleavage (which results in separation of the diencephalon–thalamus, hypothalamus, and globus pallidus from the telencephalon–caudate, putamen, and cerebral hemispheres). Clinical presentation due to microcephaly, seizures, or developmental delay is common. In the more severe forms of holoprosencephaly, facial dysmorphism is frequent, in particular hypotelorism and midline facial clefts.

Holoprosencephaly has been divided into three subcategories: alobar, semilobar, and lobar, listed in order of decreasing severity.[2] This separation is artificial, however, with the different subcategories simply part of the disease spectrum. In alobar holoprosencephaly, the most severe form, the thalami are fused, the third ventricle is absent, and the falx cerebri is absent (with no interhemispheric fissure). A single crescent-shaped ventricle joins a large dorsal cyst, the latter dominating the intracranial contents. The alobar form of disease is rarely imaged radiologically, with most infants either stillborn or of short life span. In semilobar holoprosencephaly, the disease subcategory of intermediate severity, the interhemispheric fissure and falx cerebri may be present posteriorly, with partial separation of the thalami by a small third ventricle. There is rudimentary temporal horn formation. The splenium of the corpus callosum may be present. Facial anomalies can be mild or absent. In lobar holoprosencephaly, the least severe form of disease, the falx and interhemispheric fissure extend into the frontal region, with the anterior falx commonly dysplastic. The frontal horns demonstrate an abnormal configuration and the frontal lobes may be hypoplastic. In all forms of holoprosencephaly, the septum pellucidum is absent.

MR Technique

Coronal T1-weighted images are recommended, in addition to axial and sagittal images, for improved diagnostic interpretation in complex congenital brain anomalies. For example, apparent atypical callosal dysgenesis (presence of the splenium with absence of the genu)

can be seen in two entities, agenesis of the corpus callosum and semilobar holoprosencephaly. Coronal imaging permits differentiation, with demonstration of an enlarged hippocampal commissure in the first entity and a dorsal interhemispheric commissure (resembling a true splenium) in the second.[3]

Pitfalls in Image Interpretation

Although the presence of a major brain anomaly is obvious in the current case, in other patients abnormalities may be subtle. Absence of the septum pellucidum, which has not been reported as an isolated finding, can be a clue to diagnosis.[4] Absence of the septum pellucidum can be seen in holoprosencephaly, agenesis of the corpus callosum, septooptic dysplasia, hydrocephalus (chronic, severe), basilar encephaloceles, schizencephaly, and porencephaly or hydranencephaly.

Pathologic Correlates

Coronal gross sections at the level of the thalami (which are fused) (*G*) and through the cerebral aqueduct (*H*) in a case of lobar holoprosencephaly are presented for correlation. Note the absence of dorsal midline structures, including the interhemispheric fissure, septum pellucidum, and fornices.

Clinical References

1. Byrd SE, Osborn RE, Radkowski MA, et al. Disorders of midline structures: holoprosencephaly, absence of corpus callosum, and chiari malformations. Semin Ultrasound CT MR 1988;9:201–215.
2. Barkovich AJ. Congenital malformations of the brain. In: Barkovich AJ, ed. Pediatric neuroimaging. New York, Raven Press, 1990.
3. Barkovich AJ. Apparent atypical callosal dysgenesis: analysis of MR findings in six cases and their relationship to holoprosencephaly. AJNR 1990;11:333–339.
4. Barkovich AJ, Norman D. Absence of the septum pellucidum: a useful sign in the diagnosis of congenital brain malformations. AJR 1989;152:353–360.

(G and H from Okazaki H, Scheithauer B. Slide atlas of neuropathology. New York, Gower Medical Publishing, 1988. By permission of Mayo Foundation.)

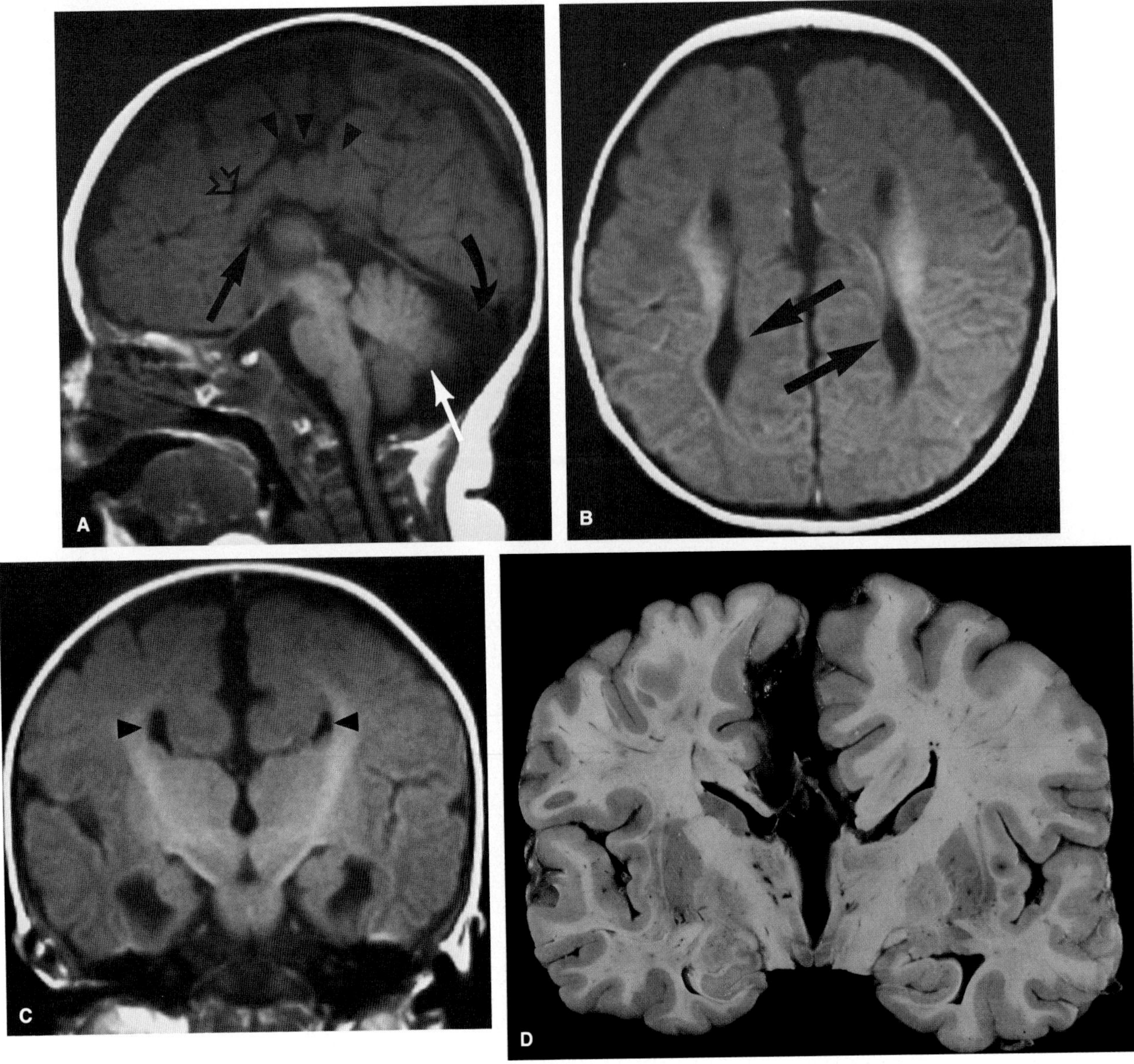

HISTORY

A 4-month-old infant with new onset of seizures

FINDINGS

(*A*) The midline sagittal T1-weighted image shows a small, dysplastic genu of the corpus callosum (*arrow*). The remainder of the corpus callosum is absent. There is a moderate-sized CSF collection (*curved arrow*) posterior to the cerebellum, although the cerebellar vermis (*white arrow*) is normal. Adjacent to the intact genu of the corpus callosum the cingulate gyrus (*open arrow*) has a normal orientation. However, the cerebral gyri (*arrowheads*) have an abnormal radiating appearance where the corpus callosum is absent. (*B*) The lateral ventricles (*arrows*) are widely separated and oriented parallel to each other on the T1-weighted axial image. (*C*) On the T1-weighted coronal image, the bodies of the lateral ventricles (*black arrowheads*) have an abnormal crescentic appearance, with medial indentation. The temporal horns of the lateral ventricles are abnormally enlarged, secondary to malformed hippocampi.

DIAGNOSIS

Agenesis of the corpus callosum

DISCUSSION

The corpus callosum is the largest interhemispheric commissure in the brain and is the major pathway of association fibers between the two cerebral hemispheres.[1,2] The corpus callosum develops between the 8th and 20th weeks of fetal life, forming in an orderly fashion. Development proceeds from anterior to posterior, with the genu forming first, followed by the body, and then the splenium. The exception to this anterior-to-posterior rule is the rostrum, which forms last, despite its anterior position.[1] Primary dysgenesis of the corpus callosum is caused by an insult (eg, vascular, toxic, infectious) during its development. The degree of dysgenesis ranges from total agenesis, caused by an insult early in development, to partial agenesis with an intact genu and body, caused by a later insult.

While the corpus callosum is forming, the entire brain is also developing at the same time, and agenesis of the corpus callosum is associated with other anomalies of the brain in 80% of cases.[2] The most commonly associated congenital brain anomalies are the Chiari II malformation, Dandy-Walker cysts and variants, interhemispheric cysts, neuronal migration anomalies, and basilar encephaloceles. These associated anomalies are commonly the cause of symptoms such as seizures since isolated agenesis of the corpus callosum is usually clinically silent.

Agenesis of the corpus callosum causes characteristic anatomic brain abnormalities that are easily seen with MR. Axons from the cerebral hemispheres that normally cross the midline by way of the corpus callosum continue along the medial borders of the lateral ventricles parallel to the interhemispheric fissure, forming Probst bundles. This causes wide separation and parallel orientation of the lateral ventricles. Probst bundles also invaginate the superomedial borders of the lateral ventricles, giving them a characteristic crescentic shape on coronal images.[1] The lack of a corpus callosum also allows superior extension of the third ventricle between the lateral ventricles, and abnormal dilatation of the trigones and occipital horns of the lateral ventricles, termed *colpocephaly*. Eversion of the cingulate gyrus with uninterrupted radial arrangement of the mesial hemispheric gyri and sulci to the roof of the third ventricle is also pathognomonic.

MR Technique

The corpus callosum itself, or lack thereof, is best seen on midline sagittal images.

Pathologic Correlate

(*D*) Coronal gross specimen from a patient with agenesis of the corpus callosum is presented. The third ventricle is "high riding," extending between the bodies of the lateral ventricles. Because of the absence of a corpus callosum the interhemispheric fissure extends all the way down to the roof of the third ventricle.

Clinical References

1. Barkovich A, Norman D. Anomalies of the corpus callosum: correlation with further anomalies of the brain. AJNR 1988;9:493–501.
2. Atlas S, Zimmerman R, Bilaniuk L, et al. Corpus callosum and limbic system: neuroanatomic MR evaluation of developmental anomalies. Radiology 1986;160:355–362.

(D *courtesy of Daron G. Davis, MD.*)

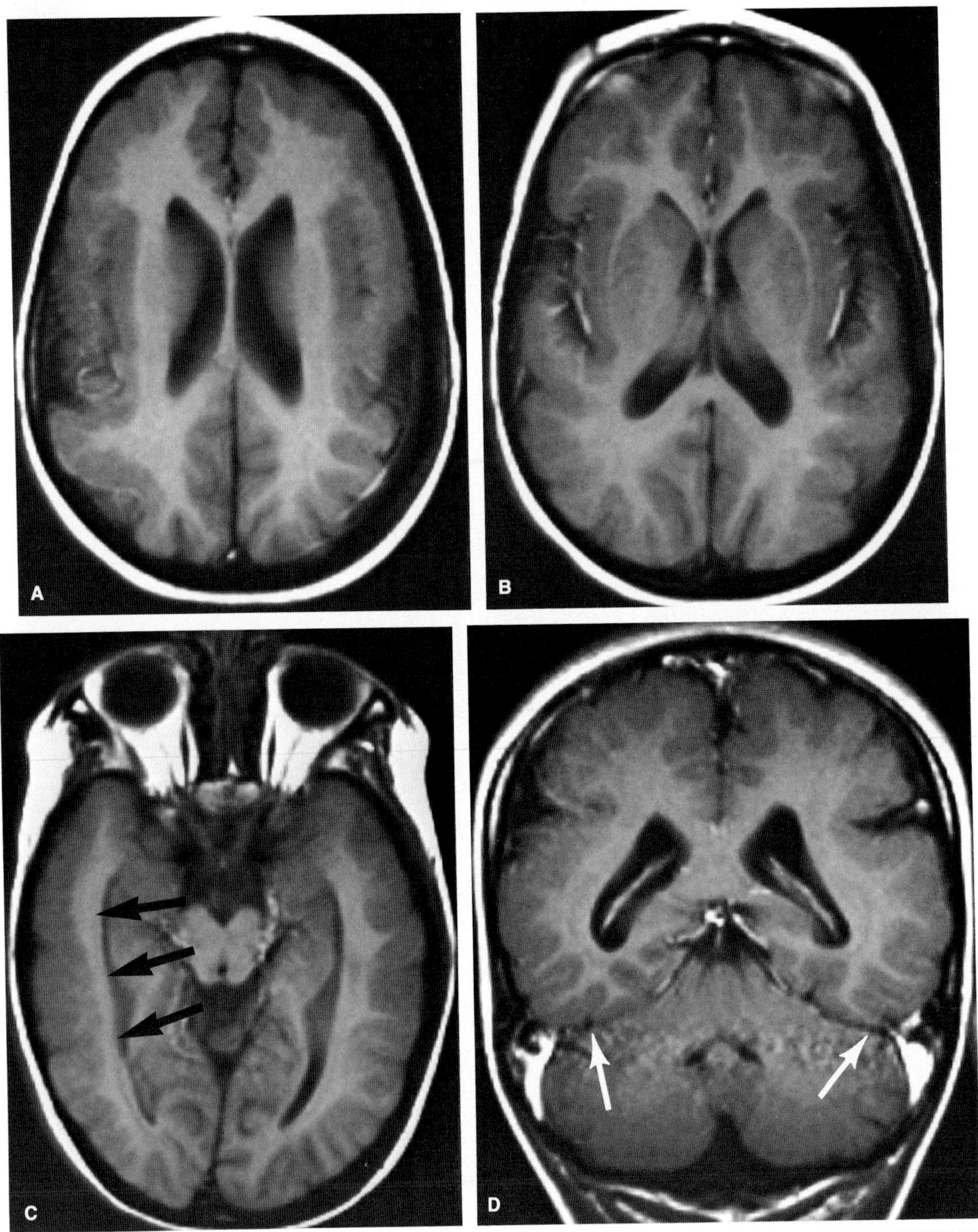

HISTORY

A 5-year-old child with seizures

FINDINGS

(*A and B*) T1-weighted axial images at two levels through the bodies of the lateral ventricles demonstrate a decreased number of abnormally broad cortical gyri. The gyri are abnormal bilaterally and involve most of the visualized brain. The gray matter is also abnormally thick. (*C*) A T1-weighted axial image at a more inferior position shows a smooth contour of the inner aspect of the gray matter (*arrows*) of the right temporal lobe. (*D*) The broad gyri of the parietal and superior temporal lobes are also well seen on the T1-weighted coronal image. However, the inferior gyri of the temporal lobes (*white arrows*) are normal.

DIAGNOSIS

Pachygyria

DISCUSSION

Pachygyria, agyria, and *lissencephaly* are terms used to describe a continuum of the most severe form of neuronal migrational abnormality. These congenital developmental anomalies are characterized by a simplified gyral pattern. The gyri are broad, and there are fewer gyri than normal. *Agyria* and *lissencephaly* are synonyms that refer to the most severe form of the continuum, in which the brain resembles that of an immature fetus with few rudimentary gyri separated by primary sulci and fissures.[1] Pachygyria is the least severe degree of the continuum, with abnormal but more completely developed gyri and sulci. Pachygyria may be focal and unilateral but is most commonly a diffuse, bilateral abnormality with relative sparing of the temporal lobes.

Neuronal migrational abnormalities are probably caused by a complex combination of genetic susceptibility and an in utero insult, the latter during brain development.[1] The result is an abnormally thickened cortex that contains a cell-sparse zone representing an area of laminar necrosis. Neuronal migration through this region is impaired.[1] The cell-sparse zone can sometimes be seen on T2-weighted images as a rim of high signal intensity within the outer cortex, a sign that is useful in distinguishing pachygyria from polymicrogyria. However, pachygyria can be proved only histologically.

Pachygyria can be associated with agenesis of the corpus callosum, and with other focal masses of heterotopic gray matter. The brain stem is usually small because of the lack of development of the corticospinal tracts. Patients often are microcephalic and have seizures, mental retardation, and developmental delay.

MR is superior to CT for demonstration of the abnormal convolutional pattern and thickened cortex seen in pachygyria, in addition to the associated anomalies. The aforementioned cell-sparse layer is best seen on T2-weighted images. Coronal images are useful in demonstrating the relative sparing of the temporal lobes.

Clinical References

1. Barkovich A, Chuang S, Norman D. MR of neuronal migration anomalies. AJR 1988;150:179–187.

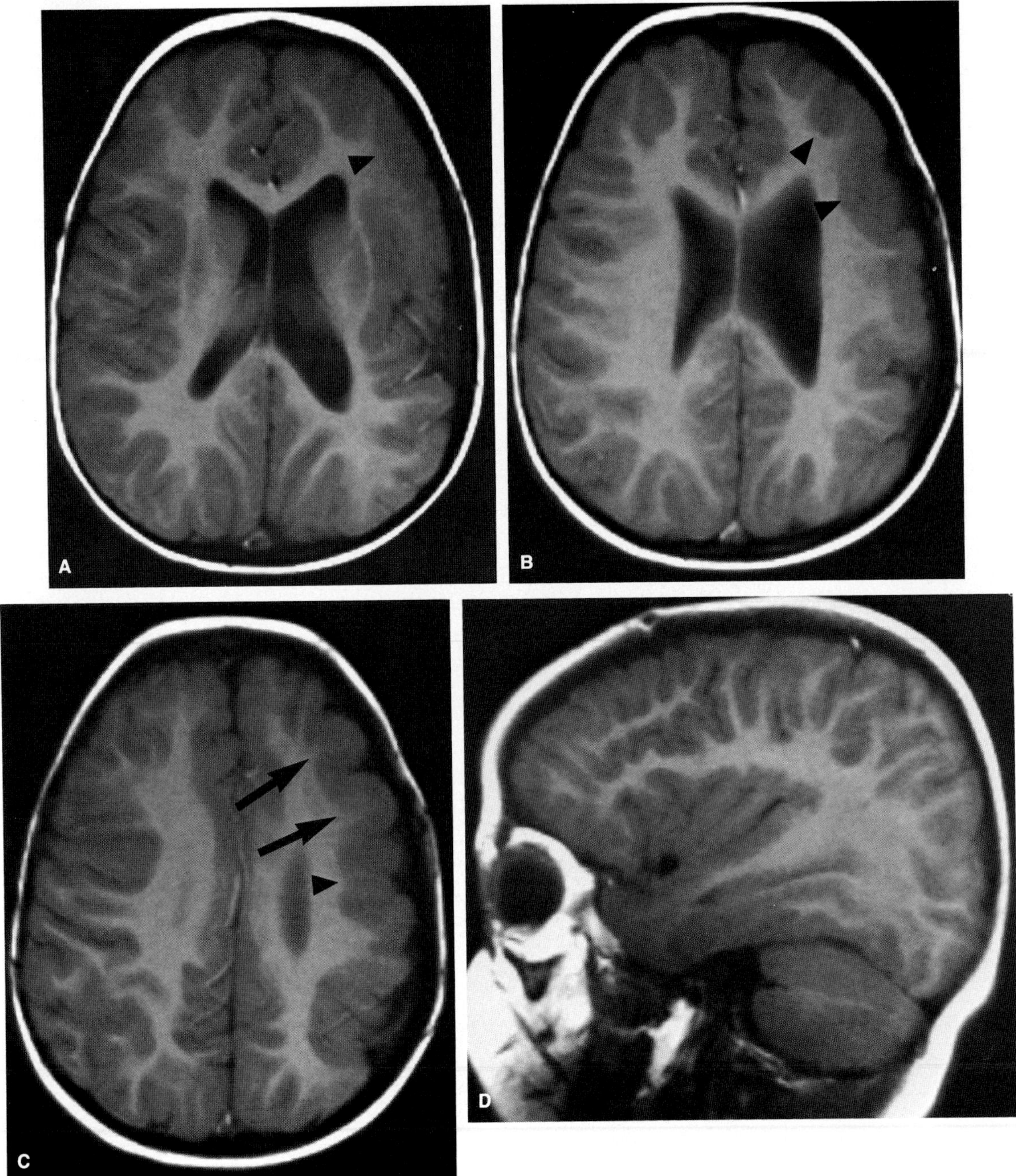

HISTORY

A 2-year-old with developmental delay, microcephaly, and right hemiparesis

FINDINGS

T1-weighted axial images at three different levels (*A to C*), T1-weighted sagittal images about 2.5 cm to the right (*D*) and left (*E*) of midline, demonstrate asymmetry of the cerebral hemispheres. The gyri (*arrows in C and E*) in the vascular territory of the left middle cerebral artery are broad and diminished in number. The cortical gray matter is abnormally thickened (*arrowheads in A to C and E*). The left lateral ventricle is mildly enlarged and the amount of white matter on the left is diminished. (*F and G*) Intermediate T2-weighted axial images at the same levels as *A* and *B* demonstrate multiple vessels draining into a large vein (*arrows in F and G*) that extends peripherally.

DIAGNOSIS

Polymicrogyria

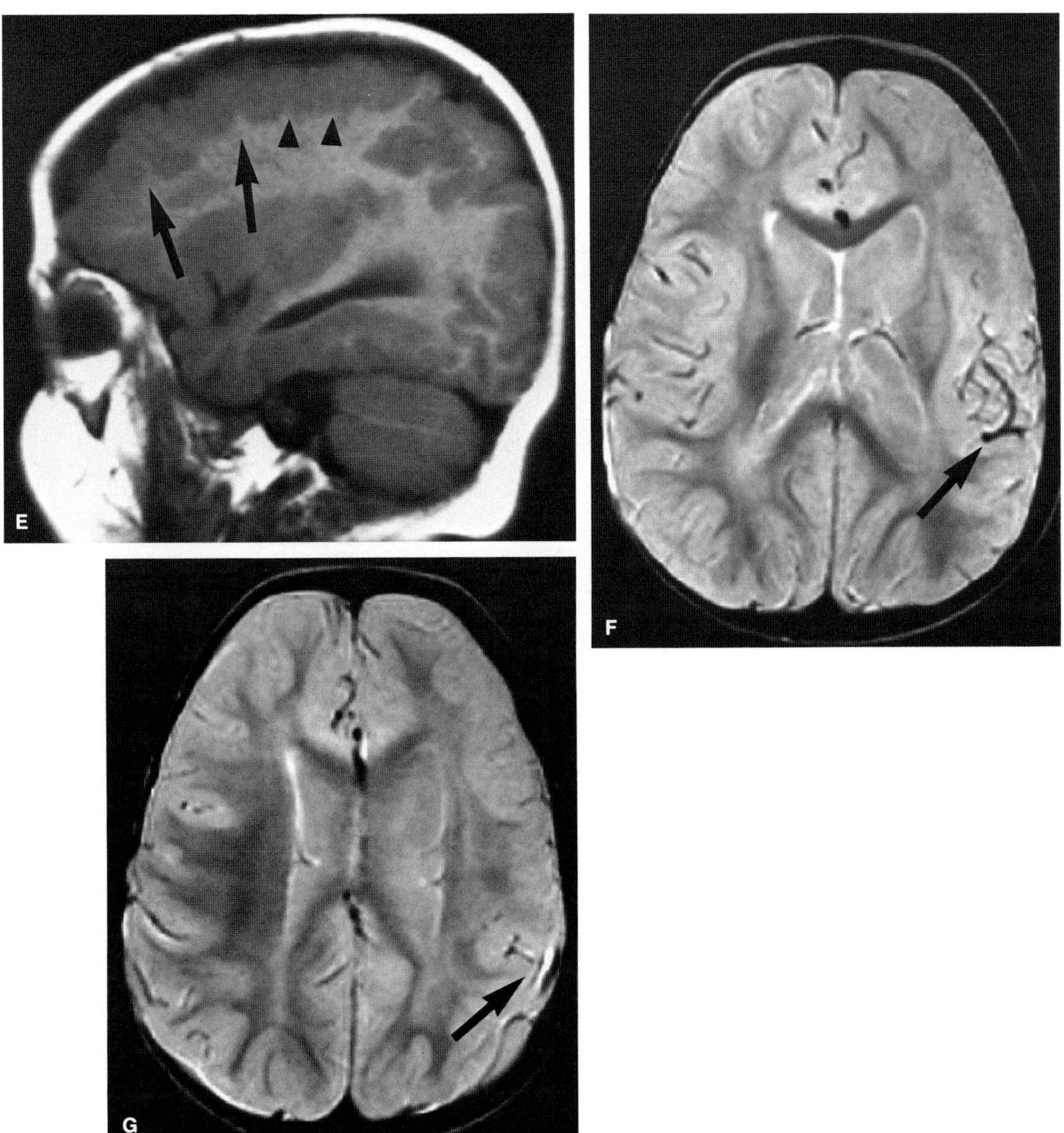

DISCUSSION

Neuronal migration abnormalities are congenital malformations of the brain characterized by ectopic location of neurons (gray matter).[1] These anomalies are separated into several discrete entities depending on the severity and timing of the arrest of neuronal migration and include lissencephaly, polymicrogyria, gray matter heterotopia, unilateral megalencephaly, and schizencephaly. Patients usually present with seizures, developmental delay, or mental retardation.

Cerebral cortex neurons are generated in the fetus in the germinal matrix of the subependyma along the lateral ventricles. The major neuronal migration from the germinal matrix to the final position in the peripheral cortex occurs from fetal weeks 8 through 16. Smaller waves of neuronal migration continue up to fetal week 25.[2] It is postulated that an ischemic, infectious, or metabolic insult during this period causes a neuronal migration abnormality, resulting in a cortex thickened by a large, disorganized layer of neurons.

Polymicrogyria is characterized by multiple abnormal, tiny indentations along the surface of the brain, thickened cortex, abnormal cortical histology (four layers instead of the normal six), and a decreased amount of white matter. On MR, polymicrogyria usually appears as a decreased number of broad, thick, smooth gyri because the abnormal convolutions on the surface of the brain are too small to be resolved. Polymicrogyria can be unilateral and is often seen in the middle cerebral artery distribution, supporting the theory of a vascular etiology. Anomalous venous drainage of the abnormal cortex is often seen as a network of vessels feeding a large vein in a deepened sulcus,[2] and should not be mistaken for a vascular malformation.

Pitfalls in Image Interpretation

Polymicrogyria and pachygyria can be difficult to differentiate on MR. Pachygyria is less common, usually bilateral, and within the cortex there is often a circumferential band of high signal intensity on T2-weighted images corresponding to a cell-sparse layer.[1]

Clinical References

1. Barkovich A, Chuang S, Norman D. MR of neuronal migration anomalies. AJR 1988;150:179–187.
2. Barkovich A. Abnormal vascular drainage in anomalies of neuronal migration. AJNR 1988;9:939–942.

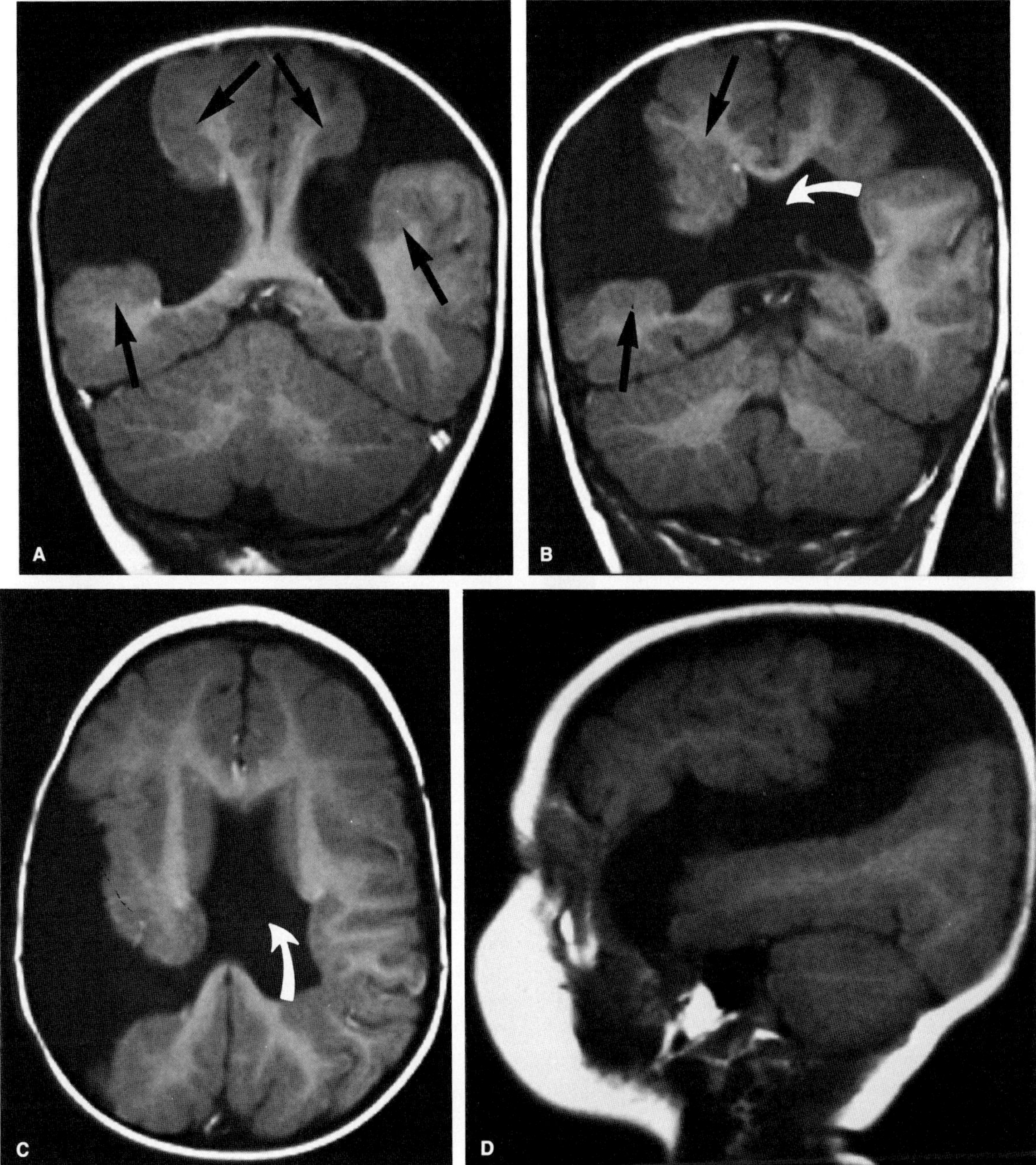

HISTORY

A 9-month-old infant with delay in motor development, decreased movement of the left arm and leg, and a generalized increase in limb tone—the last suggestive of bilateral brain involvement

FINDINGS

Bilateral CSF-filled clefts are noted on coronal (*A and B*) and axial (*C*) T1-weighted images. These spaces are lined by gray matter (*arrows in A and B*) and communicate with the ventricular system. The septum pellucidum is also absent (*curved white arrows* in *B and C*). (*D*) The large right-sided cleft, with its lining of gray matter, is also well depicted on a sagittal off-midline T1-weighted image. 3D TOF MRA, displayed in the craniocaudal (*E*) and AP (*F*) projections, reveals a loss of distal middle cerebral artery (MCA) branches on the right as well as bilateral displacement of MCA branches (*open arrows in F*).

DIAGNOSIS

Schizencephaly

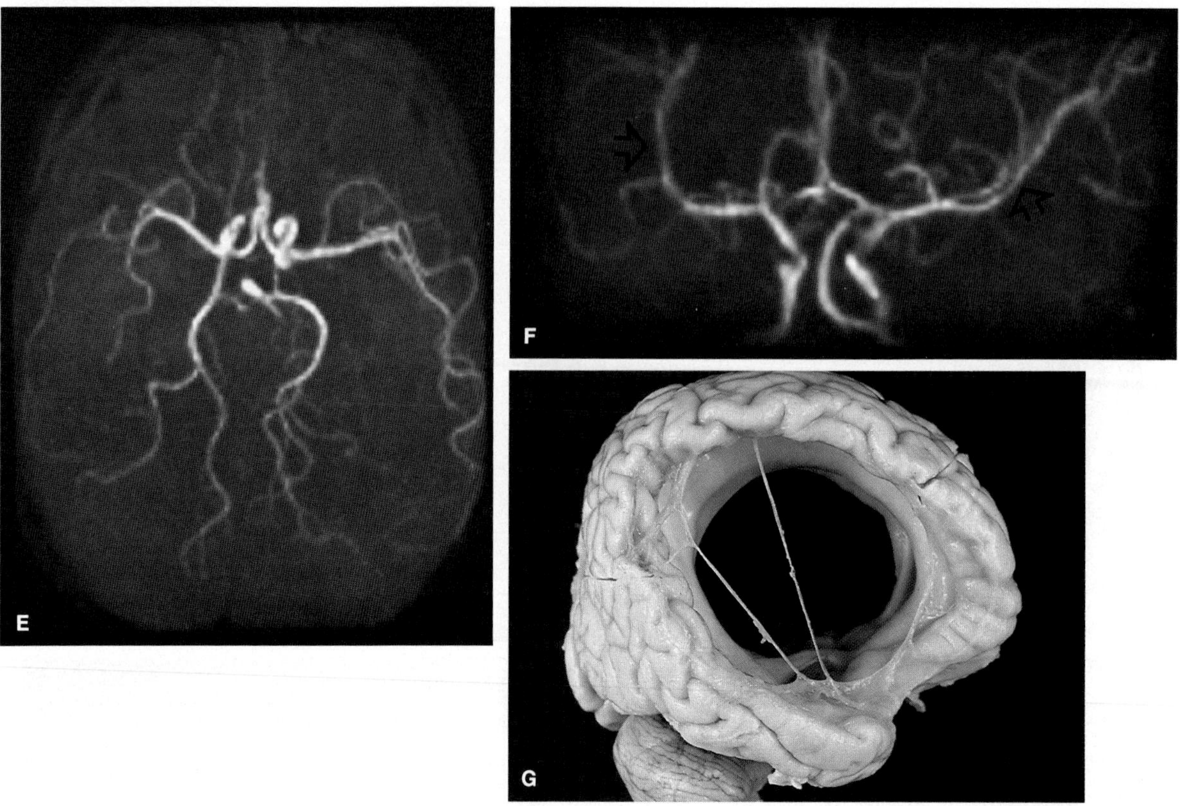

DISCUSSION

Schizencephaly is a disorder of cell migration, characterized by the presence of a gray matter–lined cleft. It has been hypothesized that the cleft develops as the result of an episode of hypotension in utero, causing infarction in a watershed area, specifically the germinal matrix along the wall of the lateral ventricle. Patients often present with intractable seizures. Motor dysfunction (ranging from weakness to spastic paralysis) and developmental delay are common. MR is more sensitive than CT in detection of both the primary lesion (the gray matter–lined cleft) and associated abnormalities, including pachygyria, polymicrogyria, and heterotopic gray matter.[1,2] The clefts, which extend from the cortex to the ventricles, can be unilateral or bilateral. The clefts vary widely with respect to separation of the two gray matter–lined walls, with a spectrum seen from actual fusion (fused lips or closed gap) to wide separation (wide gap). Neurologic disability can be mild (and intelligence normal) or severe with spastic diplegia, depending presumably on the amount of brain tissue involved. Septooptic dysplasia and schizencephaly frequently coexist. Both conditions are also associated with absence of the septum pellucidum. The pathogenesis of schizencephaly remains to be established, with evidence suggesting ischemia during the seventh week of gestation as the basis for this lesion.

In both the neurology and pathology literature, the term *schizencephaly* has fallen into disuse. This term originally referred to an entity believed to be developmental (in contradistinction to the result of a destructive event) in nature. It is now believed that virtually all clefts or cysts in the infant brain are caused by some type of destructive or vascular insult occurring in utero.

MR Technique

Under the age of 2, T1-weighted SE images provide sufficient tissue contrast to identify gray matter lining the cleft in schizencephaly. In older patients, T2-weighted SE images can be diagnostic. Irrespective of the specific technique chosen, thin-section imaging (less than 5 mm, to minimize partial volume effects) with good differentiation between gray and white matter (by choice of TE and TR) is required for the diagnosis of schizencephaly.

Pitfalls in Image Interpretation

Cerebral ischemia in a child or adult can produce, as an end result, porencephaly. In this condition, an abnormal

CSF space (due to destruction of brain tissue) exists, which communicates with the ventricular system but is not lined by gray matter.

Pathologic Correlate

(*G*) Gross pathologic specimen of schizencephaly is presented. In this case, which is severe in degree of involvement, there is a large defect in the cerebral hemispheres bilaterally, with absence also of midline structures.

Clinical References

1. Byrd SE, Osborn RE, Bohan TP, Naidich TP. The CT and MR evaluation of migrational disorders of the brain. II. Schizencephaly, heterotopia, and polymicrogyria. Pediatr Radiol 1989;19:219–222.
2. Barkovich AJ, Norman D. MR imaging of schizencephaly. AJR 1988;150:1391–1396.

(G from Okazaki H, Scheithauer B. Slide atlas of neuropathology. New York, Gower Medical Publishing, 1988. By permission of Mayo Foundation.)

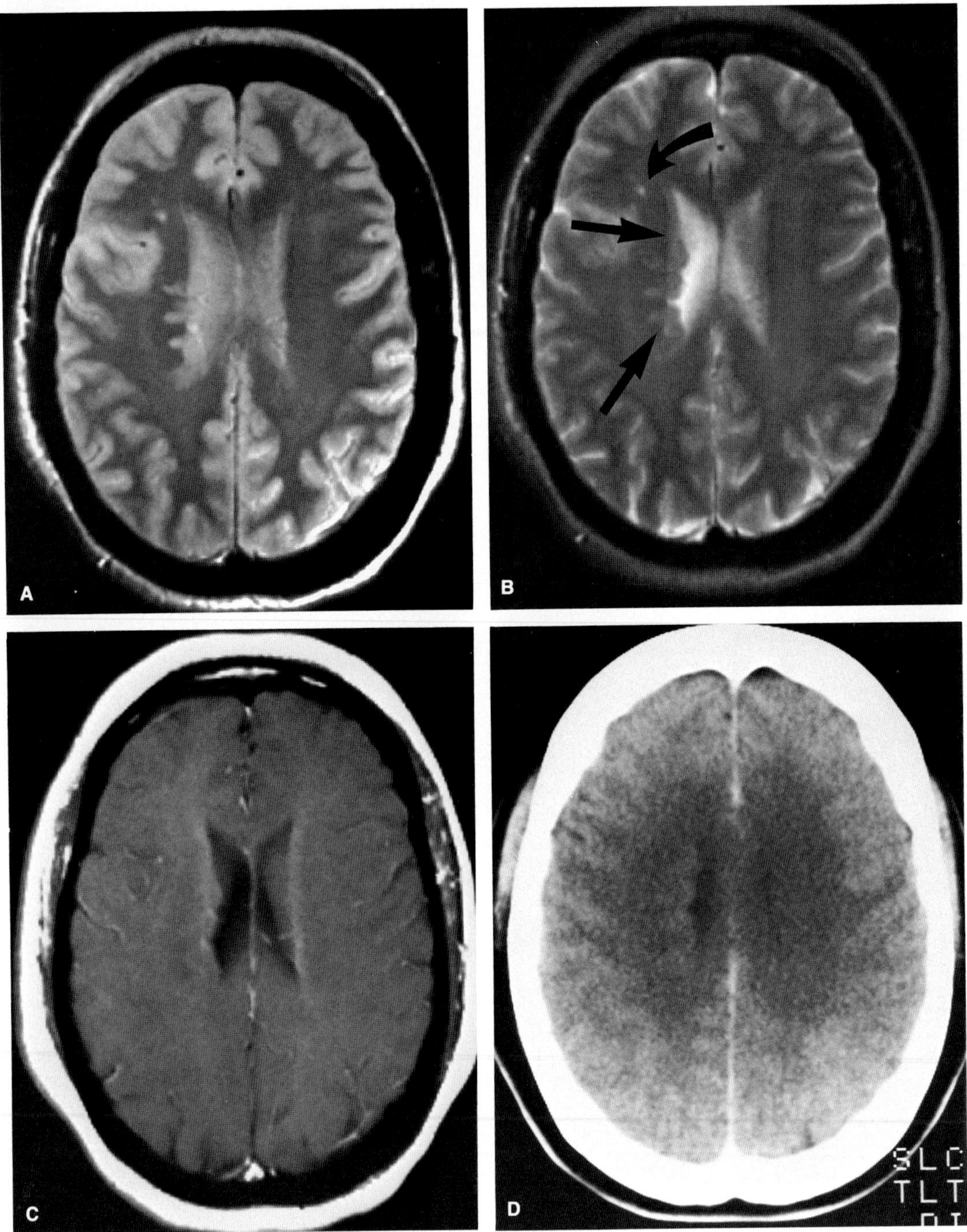

HISTORY

A 41-year-old patient with two seizures, separated by 1 year

FINDINGS

First (*A*) and second (*B*) echoes of the T2-weighted scan reveal abnormal soft tissue (*arrows in B*), isointense with gray matter (on all pulse sequences), seen adjacent to the posterior horn of the right lateral ventricle. These lesions project into the ventricle as small nodules. Incidental note is made of a small gliotic white matter focus (*curved arrow in B*), with signal intensity distinct from the periventricular mass, in the anterior forceps. (*C*) There is no abnormal enhancement on the postcontrast T1-weighted scan. (*D*) A hint of nodular densities is seen on the CT scan along the lateral wall of the right ventricle. No calcification is present.

DIAGNOSIS

Heterotopic gray matter

DISCUSSION

Displaced masses of nerve cells can be found in white matter anywhere from their embryologic site of development (periventricular) to their final destination after migration (cortex). In the most common form of heterotopia, these nests of ectopic neurons lie adjacent to the lateral ventricle. When involvement is focal, the location is often near the anterior and posterior horns, with projection of abnormal tissue as small nodules into the ventricular system. Pathologically, there is no associated calcification, permitting differentiation from subependymal nodules in tuberous sclerosis.

On MR, these lesions are isointense with gray matter on all pulse sequences.[1] Most cases are associated with seizures. Heterotopic gray matter may be nodular (periventricular) or laminar (white matter) in appearance. Late onset and mild symptoms are characteristic for isolated anomalies.[2]

MR Technique

MR is the preferred modality for diagnosis of heterotopic gray matter. Thin-section T1, mild T2, and heavily T2-weighted images should be acquired for complete evaluation. On all pulse sequences, the abnormal brain tissue (heterotopic gray matter) should be isointense with normal gray matter.

Pitfalls in Image Interpretation

Differentiation must be made from subependymal nodules in tuberous sclerosis, which are not characteristically isointense with gray matter on all pulse sequences. Cortical involvement and calcification are other differentiating features for the latter disease.

Clinical References

1. Smith AS, Weinstein MA, Quencer RM, et al. Association of heterotopic gray matter with seizures: MR imaging. Radiology 1988;168:195–198.
2. Canapicchi R, Padolecchia R, Puglioli M, et al. Heterotopic gray matter: neuroradiological aspects and clinical correlations. J Neuroradiol 1990;17:277–287.

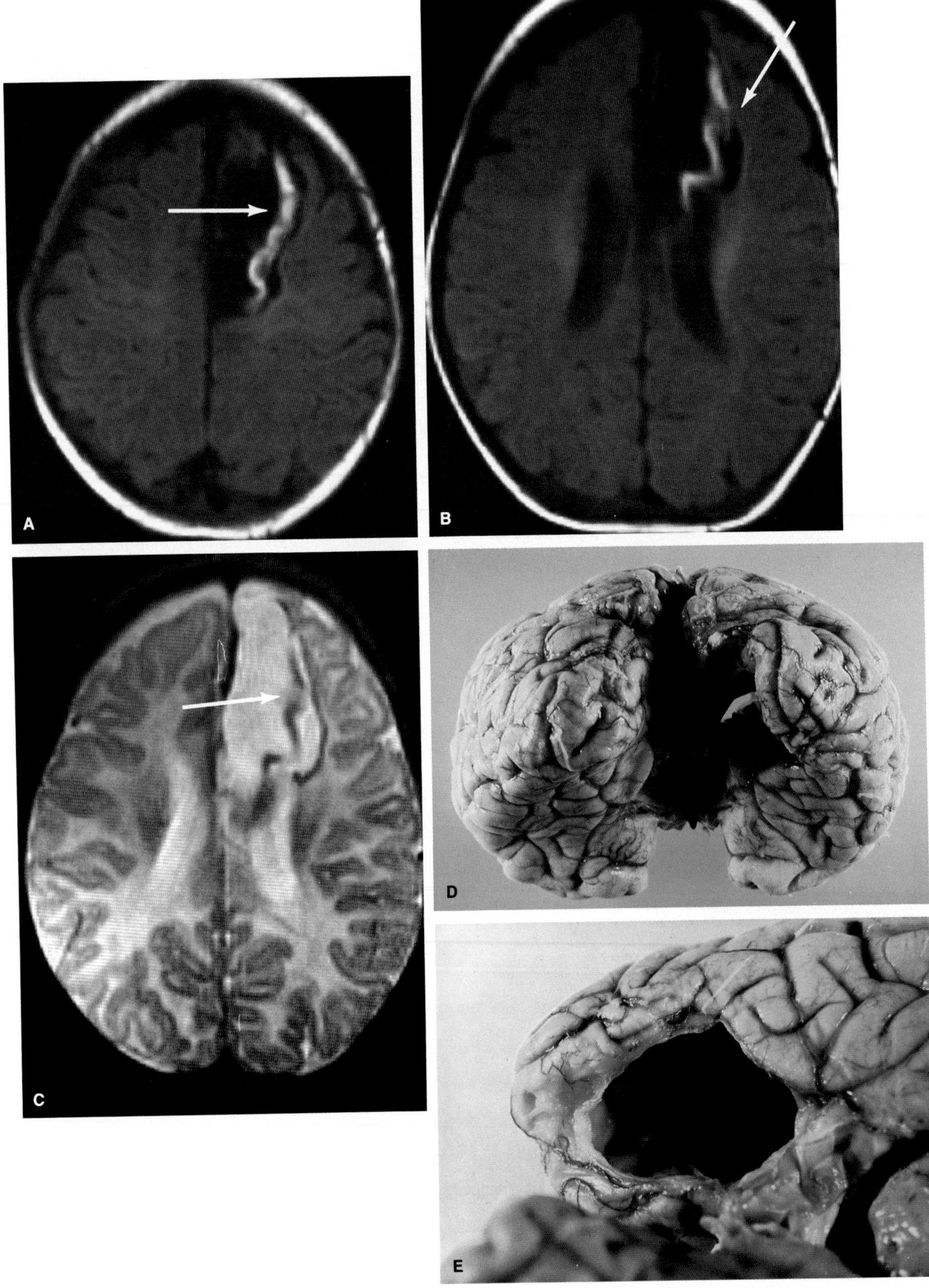
A
B
C
D
E

HISTORY

A 1-month-old with seizures

FINDINGS

(*A*) T1-weighted axial image through the level of the centrum semiovale demonstrates a low-signal-intensity, sharply marginated cavity in the medial left frontal lobe. The cavity communicates with the frontal subarachnoid space. On the adjacent cut (*B*), a T1-weighted axial image also, the lesion extends to, and communicates with, the left lateral ventricle. The lesion involves the vascular territory of the left anterior cerebral artery. The fluid within the cavity is isointense to CSF on both the T1-weighted images (*A and B*) and the T2-weighted axial image (*C*). Within the lateral aspect of the fluid-filled cavity there is a serpiginous structure (*thin white arrow*) that has high signal intensity on *A* and *B* and low signal intensity on *C*. This most likely represents a hemoglobin degradation product in this 1-month-old infant. A CT examination was not available to rule out the possibility that this represents calcification or, more specifically, the fatty matrix therein.

DIAGNOSIS

Porencephaly

DISCUSSION

The term *porencephaly* has been used and defined in many different ways. It has been used indiscriminately to describe any nonneoplastic cavity of the brain parenchyma, whatever the etiology, including vascular accidents, trauma, infection, and surgery.[1] However, the most widely accepted *strict* definition of porencephaly is a focal cavity resulting from brain destruction during the third trimester of fetal life.[2] The most common cause is an intrauterine vascular accident. Neuronal migration is already complete by the third trimester, and thus the insult does not cause histogenetic disorders such as agyria, pachygyria, and polymicrogyria. Because of the destruction of previously normal brain, this abnormality is also termed *encephaloclastic porencephaly.*"

Porencephaly may or may not communicate with the ventricular system or the subarachnoid space. A region of porencephaly often abuts the lateral ventricle, with the intact ependyma of the ventricular wall separating the two.

A unique feature of the reparative process after brain destruction during fetal life is the lack of gliosis due to an inability to mount a glial reaction in the immature brain. Therefore, necrotic tissue is completely reabsorbed, and the result is a well-demarcated cavity filled with CSF. On MR, porencephaly is isointense to CSF on all pulse sequences.

Pitfalls in Image Interpretation

Transcerebral porencephaly may mimic schizencephaly. However, the two can be differentiated with MR, as a schizencephalic cleft is lined by gray matter and porencephaly is lined by white matter.

Pathologic Correlate

(*D and E*) Gross specimens of a brain with porencephaly are shown. A large cavity extends from the surface of the brain down to, and communicating with, the lateral ventricle.

Clinical References

1. Ramsey R, Huckman M. Computed tomography of porencephaly and other cerebrospinal fluid-containing lesions. Radiology 1977;123:73–77.
2. Raybaud C. Destructive lesions of the brain. Neuroradiology 1983;25:265–291.

(D *and* E *courtesy of Daron G. Davis, MD.*)

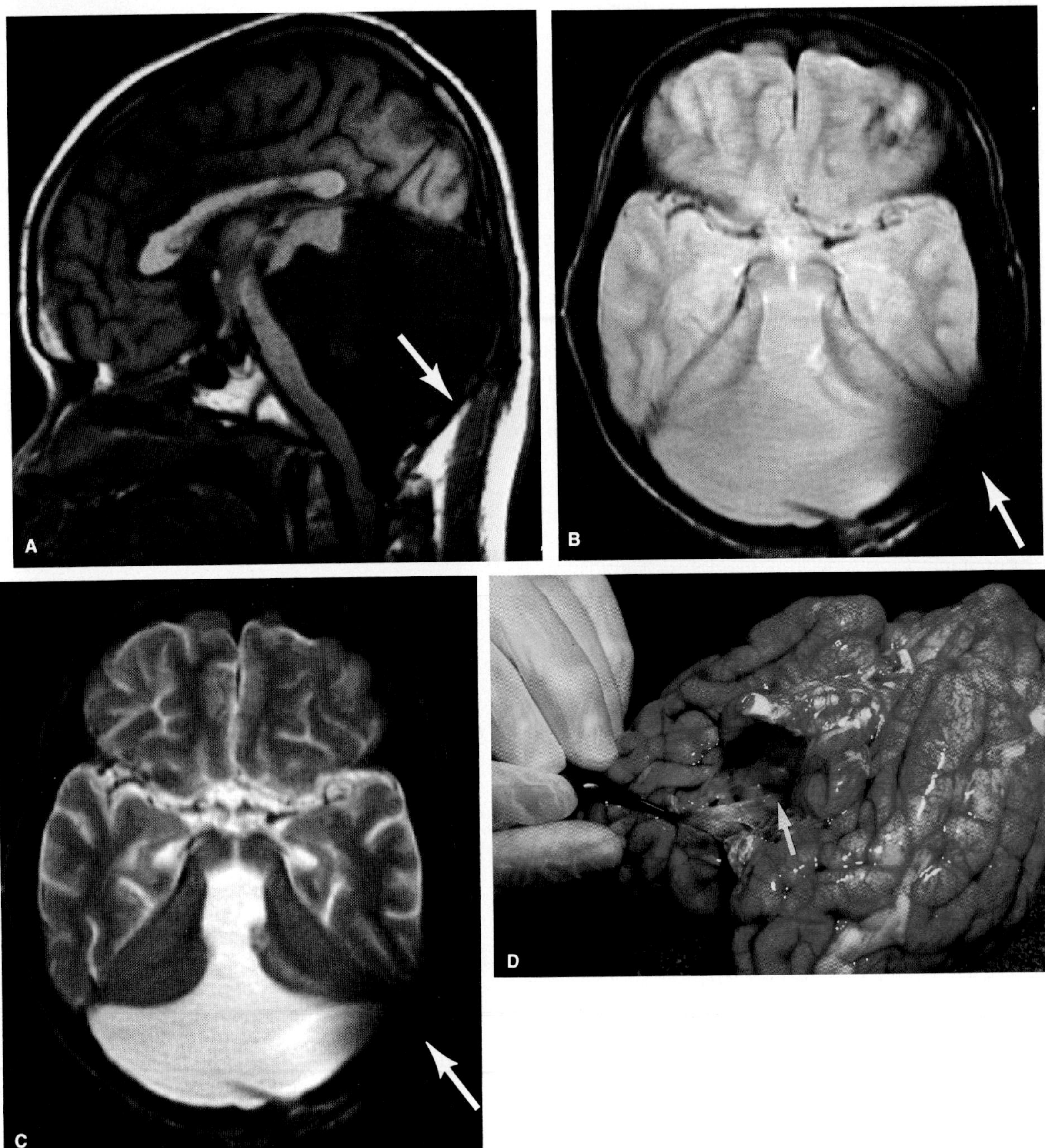

HISTORY

A 15-year-old mentally retarded boy with a history of hydrocephalus

FINDINGS

(*A*) An enlarged posterior fossa containing a large cyst with CSF signal intensity is identified on the sagittal T1-weighted image. Communication of this cyst with the fourth ventricle is seen on the first (*B*) and second (*C*) echoes of the axial T2-weighted sequence. The inferior cerebellar vermis is absent and the tentorium cerebelli is elevated. Scalloping of the inner table of the occipital bone is seen (*white arrow in A*). Metallic artifact (*white arrows in B and C*) arising from a piece of metal in the shunt tubing is seen on the left. No dilatation of the lateral or third ventricles was noted (*images not shown*).

DIAGNOSIS

Dandy-Walker malformation

DISCUSSION

The Dandy-Walker malformation is defined by the presence of three features: (1) high position of the tentorium, (2) dysgenesis or agenesis of the cerebellar vermis, and (3) cystic dilatation of the fourth ventricle that fills nearly the entire posterior fossa. An enlarged posterior fossa is a common finding. The cerebellar hemispheres are almost always hypoplastic. Scalloping of the inner table of the occipital bone is frequently seen.[1]

The classic Dandy-Walker malformation is associated with hydrocephalus in approximately 75% of patients. There is dysgenesis of the corpus callosum in about 25% of cases, with gray matter heterotopias identified in 10% of patients.

The fourth ventricular outlets (foramen of Magendie and Luschka) are inconsistently patent in these patients. It is theorized that the posterior fossa cyst is caused by delayed opening or obstruction of the median aperture (foramen of Magendie) with consequent enlargement of the fourth ventricle, which then bulges posteriorly to form the fourth ventricle–cisterna magna complex.[2]

MR Technique

Sagittal images are essential for definition of the structural abnormalities in the Dandy-Walker malformation.

Pathologic Correlate

(*D*) Gross appearance of the Dandy-Walker malformation is illustrated in this unfixed whole brain specimen from a different patient. Note the severe inferior vermian hypoplasia and large central cyst (*white arrow*), the latter occupying much of the posterior fossa.

Clinical References

1. Barkovich AJ, Kjos BO, Norman D, et al. Revised classification of posterior fossa cysts and cystlike malformations based on the results of multiplanar MR imaging. AJNR 1989;10:977–988.
2. Hirsch JF, Pierre-Kahn A, Tenier D, et al. The Dandy-Walker malformation: a review of 40 cases. J Neurosurg 1984; 61:515–522.

(D *courtesy of Daron G. Davis, MD.*)

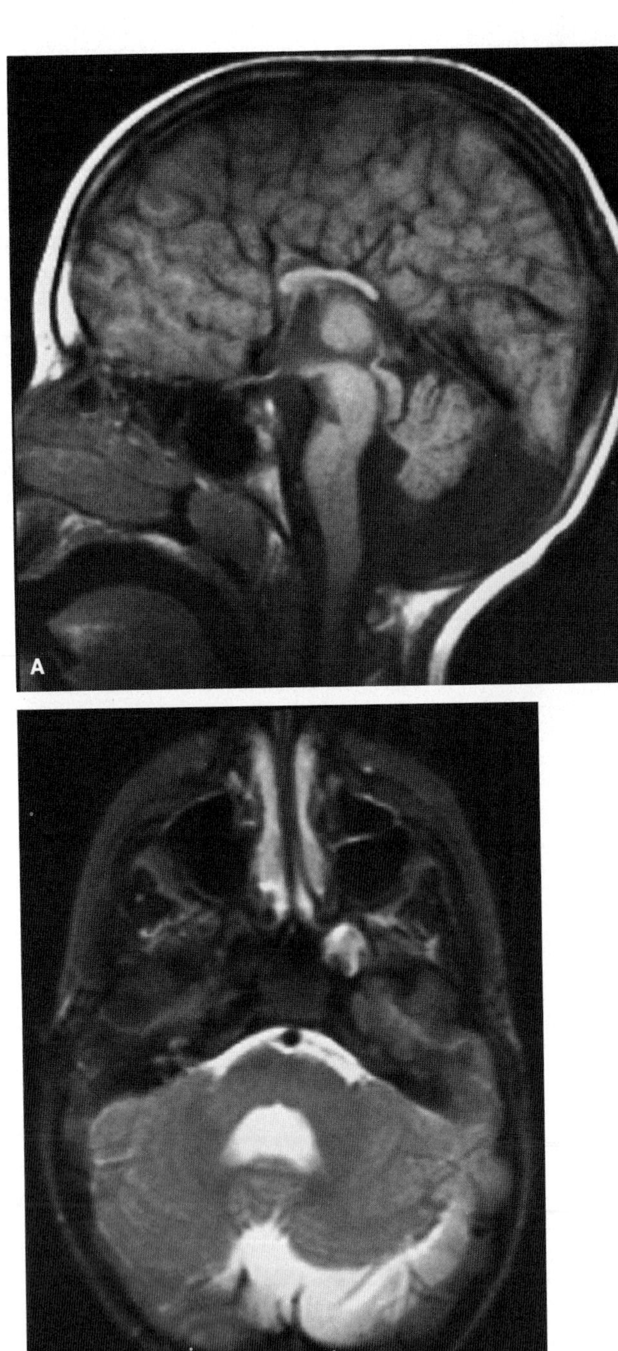
A
B
C

HISTORY

An 8-year-old child with a clinical diagnosis of cerebral palsy, delayed development, and difficulty walking

FINDINGS

(*A*) Midline sagittal T1-weighted image reveals partial agenesis of the corpus callosum, vermian hypoplasia, a large fourth ventricle, and a normal-size posterior fossa. The large fourth ventricle is confirmed on axial T1-weighted (*B*) and T2-weighted (*C*) images.

DIAGNOSIS

Dandy-Walker variant

DISCUSSION

Posterior fossa cystic malformations have been classically divided into three types: the Dandy-Walker malformation, the Dandy-Walker variant, and the mega cisterna magna. All present with developmental delay, the degree of which relates to the severity of supratentorial anomalies. In the Dandy-Walker variant, there is dysgenesis of the cerebellar vermis and cystic dilatation of the fourth ventricle, the latter without enlargement of the posterior fossa, in contradistinction to the Dandy-Walker malformation. In the mega cisterna magna, the posterior fossa is enlarged (because of the large cisterna magna), but the vermis and fourth ventricle are normal. Dysgenesis of the corpus callosum, with either partial or complete absence, is seen in about one fourth of all patients with posterior fossa cystic malformations. Recently, it has been postulated that these three disorders are not actually separate entities, but represent a continuum of developmental anomalies involving the posterior fossa. A new term, the *Dandy-Walker complex,* has been suggested to describe this continuum.[1]

MR Technique

In structural anomalies, imaging with T1-weighted sequences in all three planes (axial, sagittal, and coronal) is recommended. This can be accomplished by acquiring either three separate orthogonal image sets, or a single high-resolution 3D volume data set (using, for example, MP-RAGE). T2-weighted images are often of little benefit. MR is uniquely suited for study of congenital anomalies, unlike CT, because of its capability to acquire direct high-resolution images in any plane.[2]

Pitfalls in Image Interpretation

The differential diagnosis in patients with anomalies of the corpus callosum is large. Dysgenesis of the corpus callosum, with either complete or partial absence, can be seen in Chiari I and II malformations, migrational disorders (lissencephaly, gray matter heterotopias), encephaloceles, Dandy-Walker malformation, holoprosencephaly, Aicardi's syndrome, and lipoma.[3]

Clinical References

1. Barkovich AJ, Kjos BO, Norman D, Edwards MS. Revised classification of posterior fossa cysts and cystlike malformations based on the results of multiplanar MR imaging. AJR 1989;153:1289–1300.
2. Curnes JT, Laster DW, Koubek TD, et al. MRI of corpus callosal syndromes. AJNR 1986;7:617–622.
3. Barkovich AJ, Norman D. Anomalies of the corpus callosum: correlation with further anomalies of the brain. AJR 1988;151:171–179.

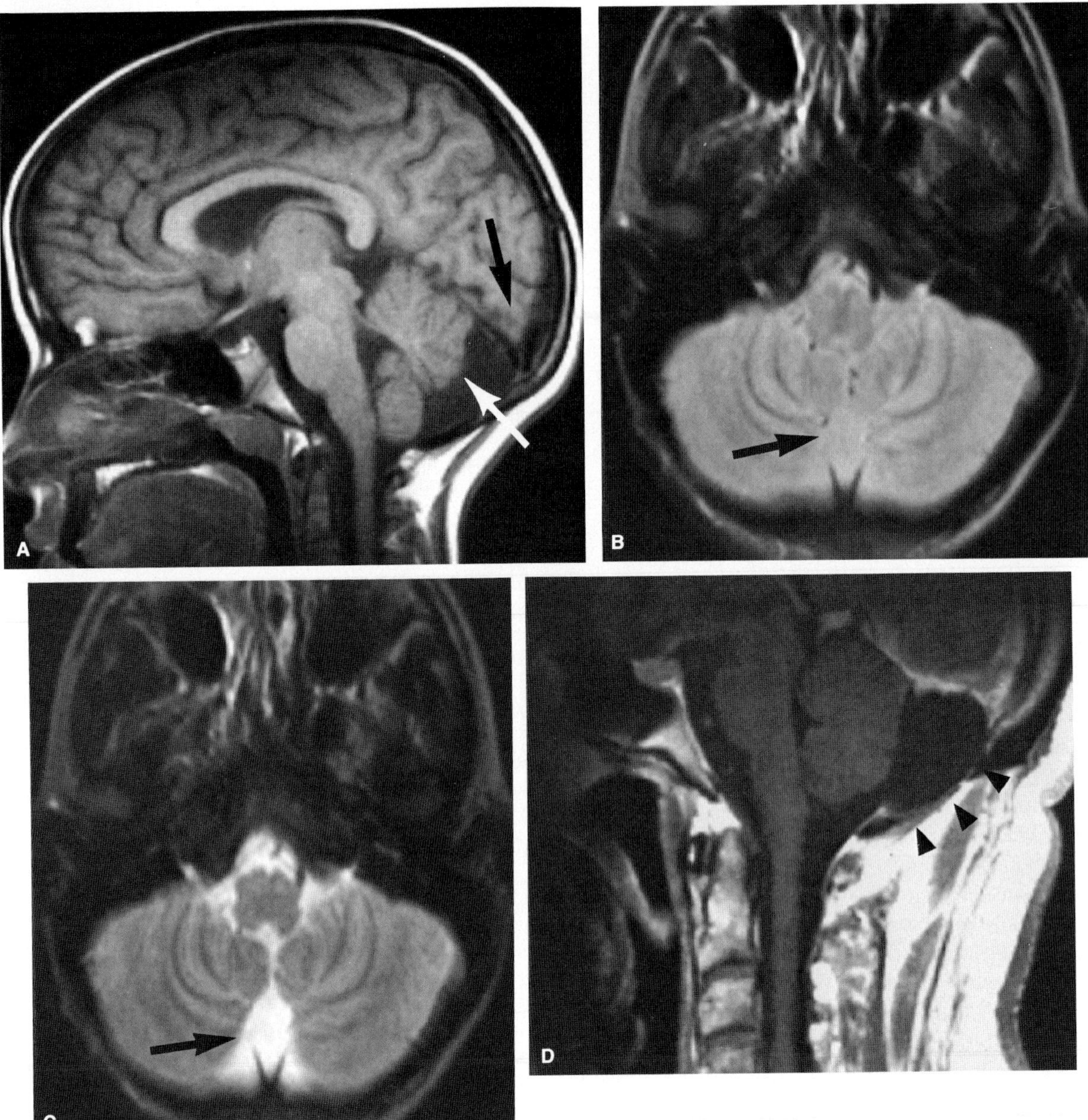

HISTORY

Noncontributory

FINDINGS

(*A*) T1-weighted sagittal image reveals a fluid collection in a retrocerebellar position. This collection has mass effect, with slight compression of the cerebellar vermis (*white arrow*). The vermis is normal in size, and there is no evidence for dysplasia. The posterior fossa is normal in size, and the angle between the straight sinus and the superior sagittal sinus is approximately 60° (*black arrow*), which is within the normal range of 50° to 75°. There are no supratentorial abnormalities. On the intermediate (*B*) and heavily (*C*) T2-weighted images, the fluid collection (*arrow*) is seen to lie in the midline and has the signal intensity of CSF. There is no direct communication between the fourth ventricle and the retrocerebellar fluid collection. (*D*) A similar retrocerebellar fluid collection is seen in an adult patient on a postcontrast T1-weighted sagittal image from a cervical spine examination. The inferior occipital bone is thin (*arrowheads*), indicative of scalloping caused by the retrocerebellar fluid collection.

DIAGNOSIS

Retrocerebellar arachnoid cyst

DISCUSSION

A posterior fossa arachnoid cyst is a collection of CSF located in a retrocerebellar location that does not communicate directly with the fourth ventricle.[1] Arachnoid cysts have a discrete cyst membrane, not always seen macroscopically, forming a separation from the vallecula. They most commonly occur in the midline in a retrovermian position. The size of the posterior fossa, and the position of the tentorium and straight sinus, remain normal with an arachnoid cyst.[1]

Posterior fossa arachnoid cysts are usually asymptomatic incidental findings on MR and are seen in patients of all ages. The fluid within an arachnoid cyst has the signal intensity of CSF on all pulse sequences. The vermis and cerebellar hemispheres are completely formed and of normal size. However, arachnoid cysts may have mass effect with compression of the cerebellar vermis or hemispheres. Rarely, ataxia may occur because of the compressive effect on the cerebellum. Scalloping of the inner table of the calvarium is a classic finding in an arachnoid cyst, but can also be seen with the Dandy-Walker malformation.

The cisterna magna is the normal CSF-containing space that lies posterior to the cerebellar hemispheres and vermis. An enlarged CSF space posterior to the cerebellum without mass effect or hypoplasia of the cerebellum has traditionally been referred to as a mega cisterna magna based on axial CT imaging. A mega cisterna magna cannot always be differentiated from an arachnoid cyst that is not producing mass effect. A revised classification of posterior fossa fluid collections based on MR findings[1] has suggested that mega cisterna magna is actually a mild form of a continuum of the Dandy-Walker malformations, and that the term *prominent cisterna magna* be reserved for those cases with a large retrocerebellar CSF space and cerebellar atrophy, rather than cerebellar hypoplasia.

Pitfalls in Image Interpretation

The differential diagnosis for a posterior fossa fluid collection includes the Dandy-Walker malformation complex. A retrocerebellar arachnoid cyst can be distinguished from the Dandy-Walker malformation with MR. The three hallmarks of the Dandy-Walker malformation are dysgenesis of the cerebellar vermis, high position of the tentorium due to enlargement of the posterior fossa, and cystic dilatation of the fourth ventricle.[1]

Clinical References

1. Barkovich A, Kjos, B, Norman D, et al. Revised classification of posterior fossa cysts and cystlike malformations based on the results of multiplanar MR imaging. AJR 1989; 153:1289–1300.

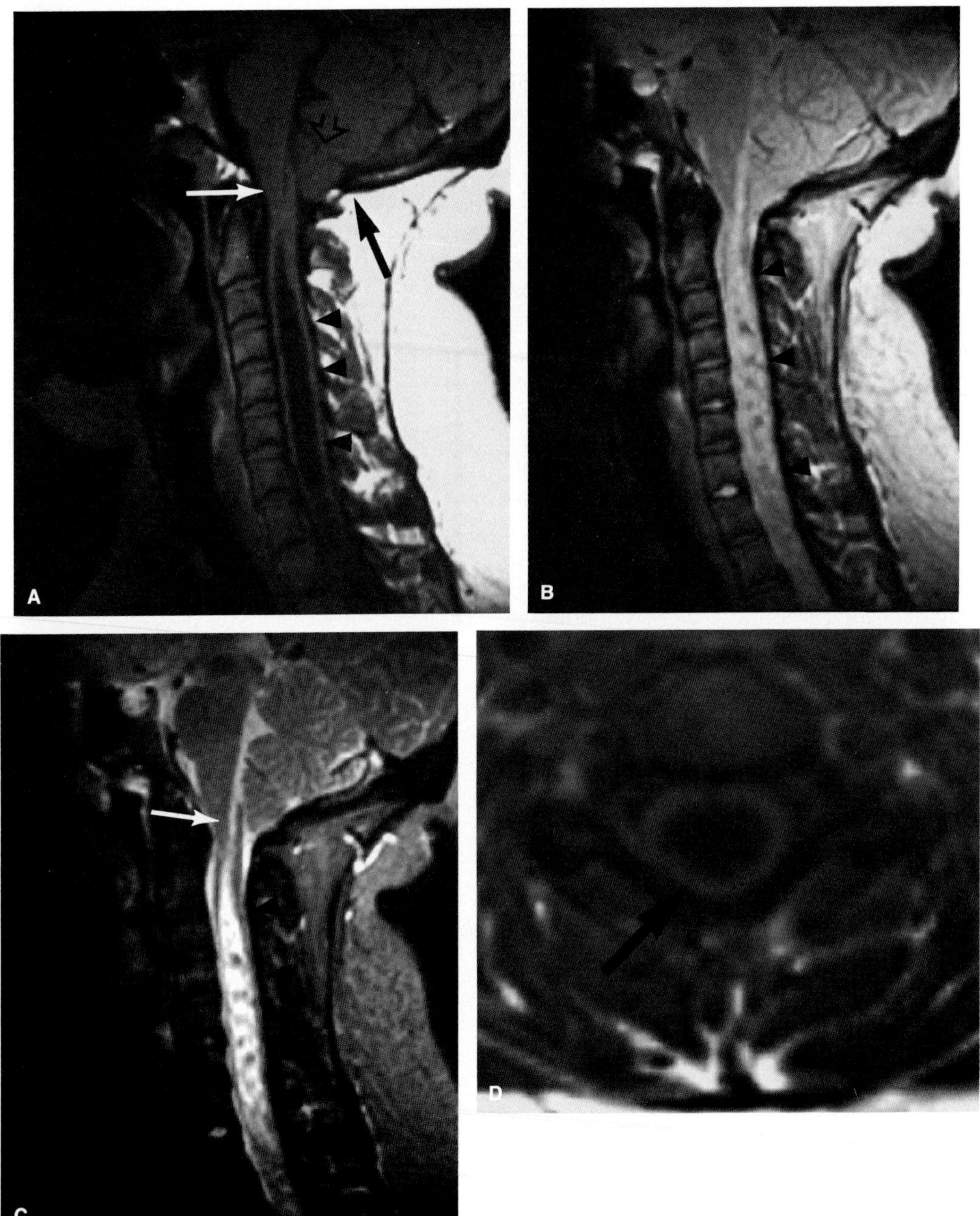

HISTORY

A 36-year-old with blurred vision

FINDINGS

(*A*) T1-weighted sagittal image demonstrates wedge-shaped cerebellar tonsils (*open arrow*), which are displaced 5 mm below the posterior lip of the foramen magnum (*black arrow*). On T1-weighted (*A*), intermediate T2-weighted (*B*), and heavily T2-weighted (*C*) sagittal images, within the spinal cord from the level of C2 extending inferiorly is a fluid collection (*arrowheads*) that has the signal intensity characteristics of CSF. (*D*) T1-weighted axial image at the level of C5 redemonstrates this abnormal fluid collection within the spinal cord (*arrow*). Communication (*white arrows in A and C*) between the spinal cord fluid collection and the fourth ventricle is demonstrated on the sagittal images. (*E*) Similar herniation of the cerebellar tonsils is noted on a T1-weighted coronal image from a different patient.

DIAGNOSIS

Chiari I malformation with associated syrinx

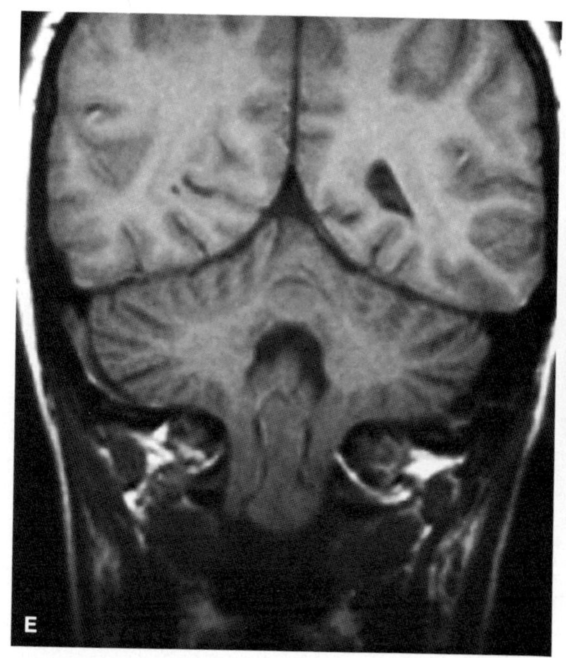

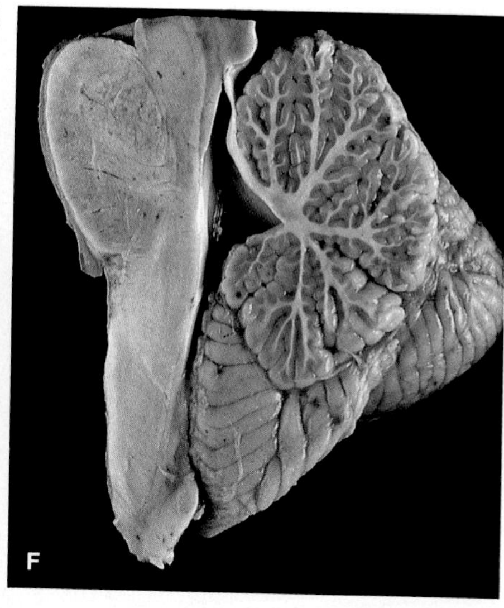

DISCUSSION

The Chiari I malformation is defined as congenital displacement of the cerebellar tonsils into the cervical spinal canal.[1] Studies using MR[1,2] have determined that downward herniation of the cerebellar tonsils more than 2 to 3 mm below the posterior lip of the foramen magnum is abnormal. Two thirds of cases have tonsillar herniation inferior to C1, but herniation beyond C3 is rare. In the Chiari I malformation, the cerebellar tonsils are usually pointed, or wedge-shaped. There may also be downward displacement of a portion of the cerebellar vermis, obliteration of the cisterna magna, and rarely cervicomedullary kinking.[1] The fourth ventricle retains its normal position, although it may be thinned.

Hydrocephalus is present in about one third of Chiari I malformation cases, and syringohydromyelia (syrinx) in about half. Bony craniocervical junction anomalies such as occipitalization of C1, basilar impression, and the Klippel-Feil deformity are also associated with the Chiari I malformation. The Chiari I malformation may be asymptomatic. When symptomatic, patients usually present in adulthood with cerebellar signs such as ataxia and nystagmus, or with signs of cranial nerve and brain stem compression such as vertigo, facial pain, sensorineural deafness, and bulbar palsy.[1]

MR Technique

Sagittal T1-weighted images well depict tonsillar herniation in the Chiari I malformation.

Pathologic Correlate

(*F*) Midsagittal gross specimen of the brain stem and cerebellum demonstrates downward herniation of the cerebellar tonsils, which are pointed. The fourth ventricle is normal in size and position. Symptoms associated with the Chiari I malformation may be due to direct compression of the tonsils and medulla or to an accompanying cervical syrinx.

Clinical References

1. Barkovich A, Wippold F, Sherman J, et al. Significance of cerebellar tonsillar position on MR. AJNR 1986;7:795–799.
2. Aboulezz A, Sartor K, Geyer C, et al. Position of cerebellar tonsils in the normal population and in patients with Chiari malformation: a quantitative approach with MR imaging. J Comput Assist Tomogr 1985;6:1033–1036.

(F *from Okazaki H, Scheithauer B. Slide atlas of neuropathology. New York, Gower Medical Publishing, 1988. By permission of Mayo Foundation.*)

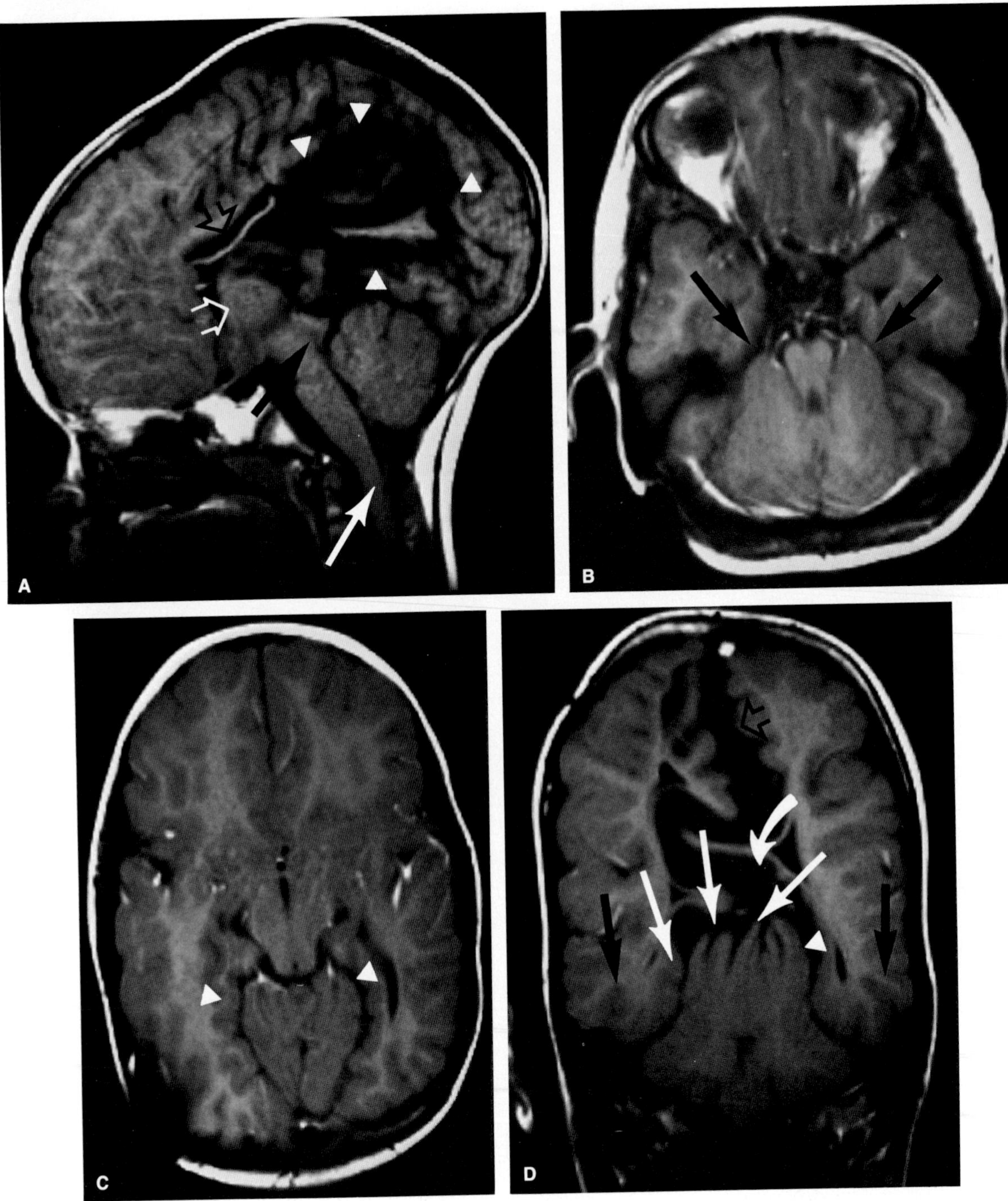

HISTORY

A 4-year-old with complex neurologic abnormalities, a ventriculoperitoneal shunt, and history of a myelomeningocele

FINDINGS

(*A*) T1-weighted sagittal image demonstrates elongation and inferior displacement of the fourth ventricle (*white arrow*), an abnormally shaped tectum (*black arrow*), a large massa intermedia (*open white arrow*), a small, thin anterior corpus callosum (*open black arrow*), absence of the posterior corpus callosum, and multiple widened CSF-containing spaces (*white arrowheads*). (*B*) T1-weighted axial image shows the inferior anterior cerebellum (*black arrows*) surrounding the brain stem.

T1-weighted axial image at a higher level (*C*) and T1-weighted coronal image (*D*) show abnormally wide margins of the tentorial incisura (*white arrowhead*), and an abnormally low position of the temporooccipital lobes (*black arrows in D*) in relation to the cerebellum.

In *D,* the interhemispheric fissure (*open black arrow*) is enlarged, and communicates with the supracerebellar cistern (*curved white arrow*) by way of an abnormal CSF-containing space. The falx cerebri is absent. The folia (*white arrows*) of the cerebellum are abnormally oriented in the sagittal plane.

DIAGNOSIS

Chiari II malformation

DISCUSSION

The Chiari II malformation is a complex congenital brain anomaly that is associated with myelomeningocele in nearly all cases. Its hallmark is dysgenesis of the hindbrain, with inferior displacement and elongation of the brain stem, cerebellar tonsils, vermis ("cerebellar peg"), and fourth ventricle. The inferior displacement of the medulla causes cervicomedullary kinking. The bony posterior fossa is small and the tentorial insertion is abnormally low, near the margin of the foramen magnum, which is widened. The tentorium is dysplastic, with a widened incisura, allowing cerebellar extension above the incisura ("cerebellar towering"). The cerebellum itself is often dysplastic, with abnormal orientation of the folia, and anterior migration around the brain stem. A cervical syrinx is present in 20% to 83% of cases.[1]

Multiple supratentorial abnormalities are also associated with the Chiari II malformation: obstructive hydrocephalus (98% of cases), anteroinferior pointing of the frontal horns of the lateral ventricles (50% to 90%),[2] dysgenesis of the corpus callosum (75%), absence of the septum pellucidum (40%), large massa intermedia (55% to 90%), fusion of the colliculi causing "tectal beaking" (60%),[1] interdigitation of cerebral gyri due to hypoplasia and fenestration of the falx, inferior displacement of the cerebral hemispheres in relation to the tentorium,[1] and stenogyria. (*Stenogyria* refers to multiple, small closely spaced gyri with histologically normal cortex, as opposed to *polymicrogyria,* in which there are multiple small gyri with abnormal cortical layers.) CSF-containing spaces are often present after ventriculoperitoneal shunting, sometimes communicating with widened cisterns or the interhemispheric fissure.[2] Infants with the Chiari II malformation and myelomeningocele also have craniolacunia (lacunar skull or *Lückenschädel*), which is no longer evident after 6 months of age.

The cause of Chiari II malformation is unclear but, because of the association with myelomeningocele, one theory speculates that the downward displacement of the intracranial contents is due to the fixation of the cord at the site of the spinal defect during fetal life.

Clinical References

1. El Gammel T, Mark E, Brooks B. MR imaging of Chiari II malformation. AJR 1988;150:163–170.
2. Wolpert S, Anderson M, Scott R, et al. Chiari II malformation: MR imaging evaluation. AJNR 1987;8:783–792.

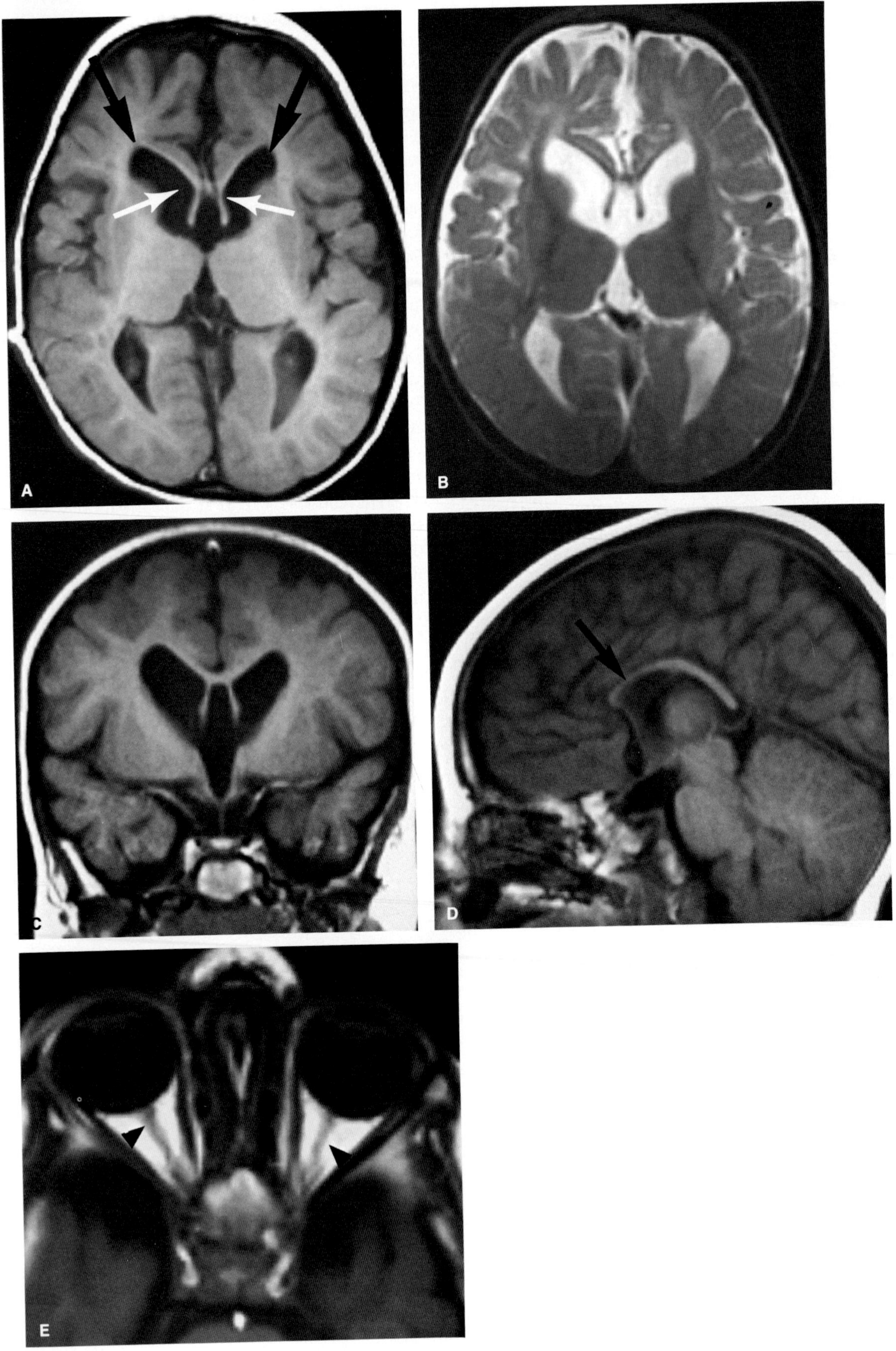
A
B
C
D
E

HISTORY

A 21-month-old infant with severe developmental delay

FINDINGS

The leaves of the septum pellucidum are incompletely formed and are widely separated on the T1-weighted (*A*) and T2-weighted (*B*) axial images, and the T1-weighted coronal image (*C*). Only the anterior portion of each leaf is present bilaterally (*white arrows in A*). The frontal horns of the lateral ventricles are large bilaterally (*arrows in A*). The bodies of the lateral ventricles, the ventricular atria, and the occipital horns are also enlarged on axial images (*not shown*) at higher levels. On the T1-weighted sagittal image (*D*), the anterior corpus callosum (*arrow*) is hypoplastic. There is little periventricular white matter, a finding best seen on the axial images. Myelination is delayed, with high signal intensity in the periventricular–subcortical white matter, especially anteriorly, noted in *B*. (*E*) T1-weighted axial image through the midorbits identifies the optic nerves (*arrowheads*), which are small bilaterally.

DIAGNOSIS

Septooptic dysplasia

DISCUSSION

Septooptic dysplasia is a congenital brain anomaly characterized by absence or hypoplasia of the septum pellucidum and hypoplasia of the optic nerves. However, this syndrome is not a single, homogeneous entity, and patients may present with a wide range of clinical symptoms including blindness (although vision may be normal), seizures, and hypothalamic-pituitary dysfunction.[1] The septum pellucidum may be only mildly dysplastic or entirely absent. About half the patients with septooptic dysplasia have associated schizencephaly.

Current theory suggests that there are two distinct subsets of septooptic dysplasia. Those patients with associated schizencephaly typically present with seizures, and usually have partial absence of the septum pellucidum. A vascular or infectious insult during fetal brain development could account for this subset of septooptic dysplasia.[1] Septooptic dysplasia without schizencephaly constitutes the second subset of patients, who commonly present with growth retardation and developmental delay. Anatomically, this second subset usually has complete absence of the septum pellucidum and diffuse white matter hypoplasia with accompanying ventriculomegaly.[1] This type of septooptic dysplasia probably represents a mild form of holoprosencephaly, a congenital midline defect caused by failure of the forebrain to divide into hemispheres.

MR Technique

The size of the intraorbital optic nerves is best evaluated using fat-suppression techniques. The suppression of signal from the abundant intraorbital fat minimizes chemical shift artifact, which can distort the apparent size of the optic nerves on conventional SE imaging.

Clinical References

1. Barkovich A, Fram E, Norman D. MR of septo-optic dysplasia. Radiology 1989;171:189–192.

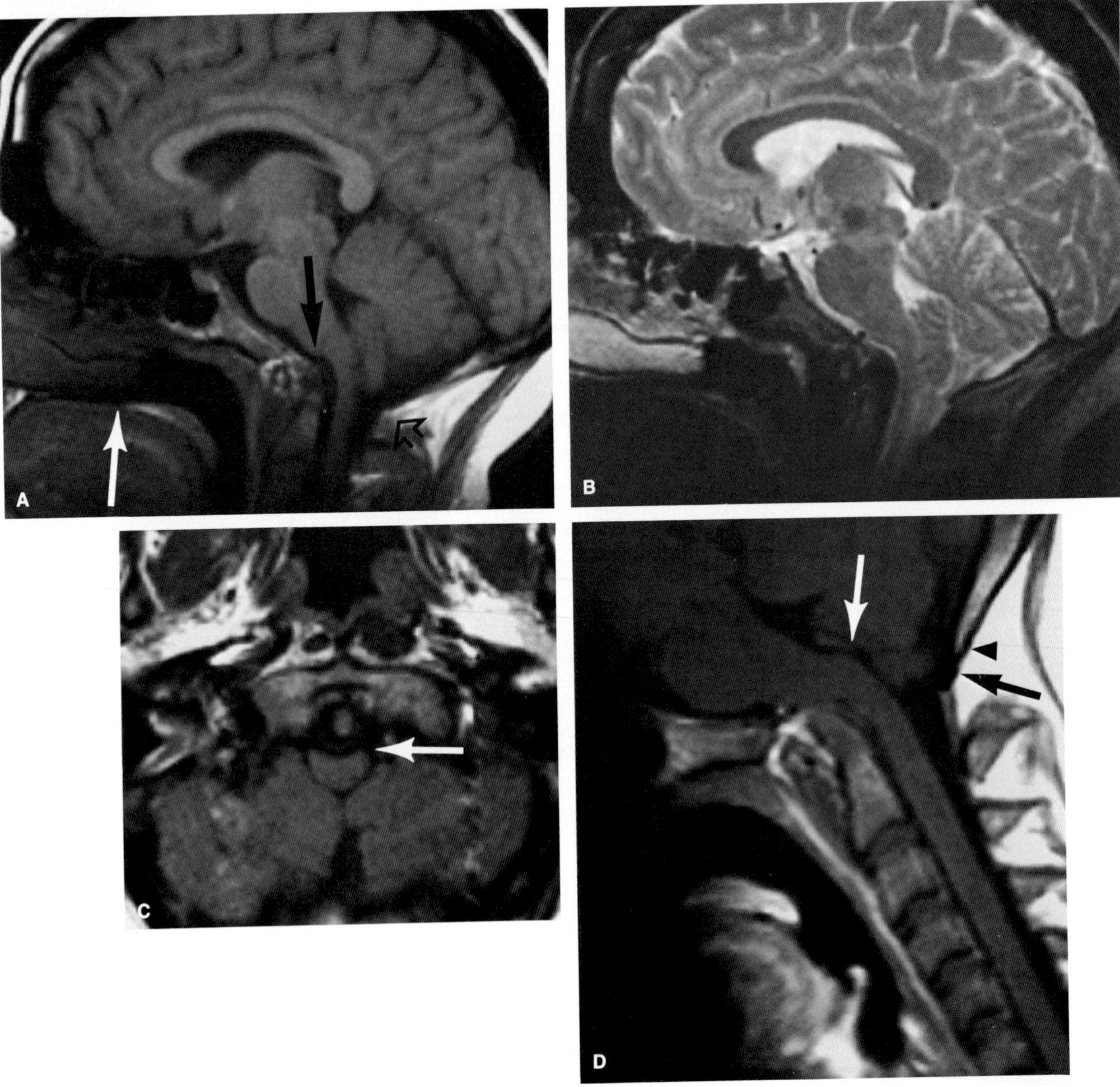

HISTORY

A 27-year-old with episodes of lightheadedness and headaches

FINDINGS

(*A*) The odontoid process (*arrow*) is abnormally positioned up within the foramen magnum, best seen on this T1-weighted sagittal image. The tip of the odontoid is located about 1 cm above an imaginary line drawn between the posterior edge of the hard palate (*white arrow*) and the posterior border of the foramen magnum (*open arrow*). (*B*) Similar findings are seen on the T2-weighted sagittal image. On the T1-weighted axial image (*C*) and T1-weighted sagittal image (*D*) obtained with the neck in flexion, the odontoid process (dens) is compressing and displacing the medulla (*white arrow*). In *D*, the posterior arch (*black arrow*) of the C1 vertebrae (atlas) lies directly adjacent to the occiput (*black arrowhead*), even with the neck in flexion.

DIAGNOSIS

Basilar invagination

DISCUSSION

Basilar invagination, or "basilar impression," is an osseous craniovertebral junction abnormality in which the odontoid process has an abnormal position relative to the foramen magnum. Basilar invagination is most commonly assessed radiographically by use of Chamberlain's line, which is drawn from the posterior edge of the hard palate to the posterior border of the foramen magnum. The normal odontoid should not extend more than 5 mm above Chamberlain's line.[1] The use of McGregor's line, which is drawn from the posterior edge of the hard palate to the undersurface of the occiput, is also common. The odontoid should not extend more than 7 mm above McGregor's line.[1]

Plain radiographs are adequate to evaluate the bony abnormalities of basilar invagination. The osseous abnormalities are also well seen with MR, where cortical bone has very low signal intensity and surrounds high-signal-intensity marrow on T1-weighted images. However, MR is also the modality of choice for evaluation of the resulting neuroanatomic distortion of the brain stem and spinal cord.[2]

Basilar invagination may be the result of primary bony anomalies of the craniovertebral junction and is often associated with assimilation (congenital fusion) of the posterior arch of C1 (atlas) to the occiput, as in this case. Basilar invagination also may be secondary to other diseases such as osteoporosis, osteomalacia, Paget's disease, fibrous dysplasia, achondroplasia, and osteogenesis imperfecta.[1] Platybasia may accompany basilar invagination and is defined as a flattened relationship between the anterior and middle cranial fossae, in which the basilar angle is greater than 140°.

Patients with primary basilar invagination may present with headaches, specific neurologic deficits, or symptoms related to vertebrobasilar artery compression.

Clinical References

1. Dolan K. Cervicobasilar relationships. Radiol Clin North Am 1977;15:155–166.
2. Smoker W, Deyes W, Dunn V, et al. MRI versus conventional radiologic examinations in the evaluation of the craniovertebral and cervicomedullary junction. Radiographics 1986; 6:953–94.

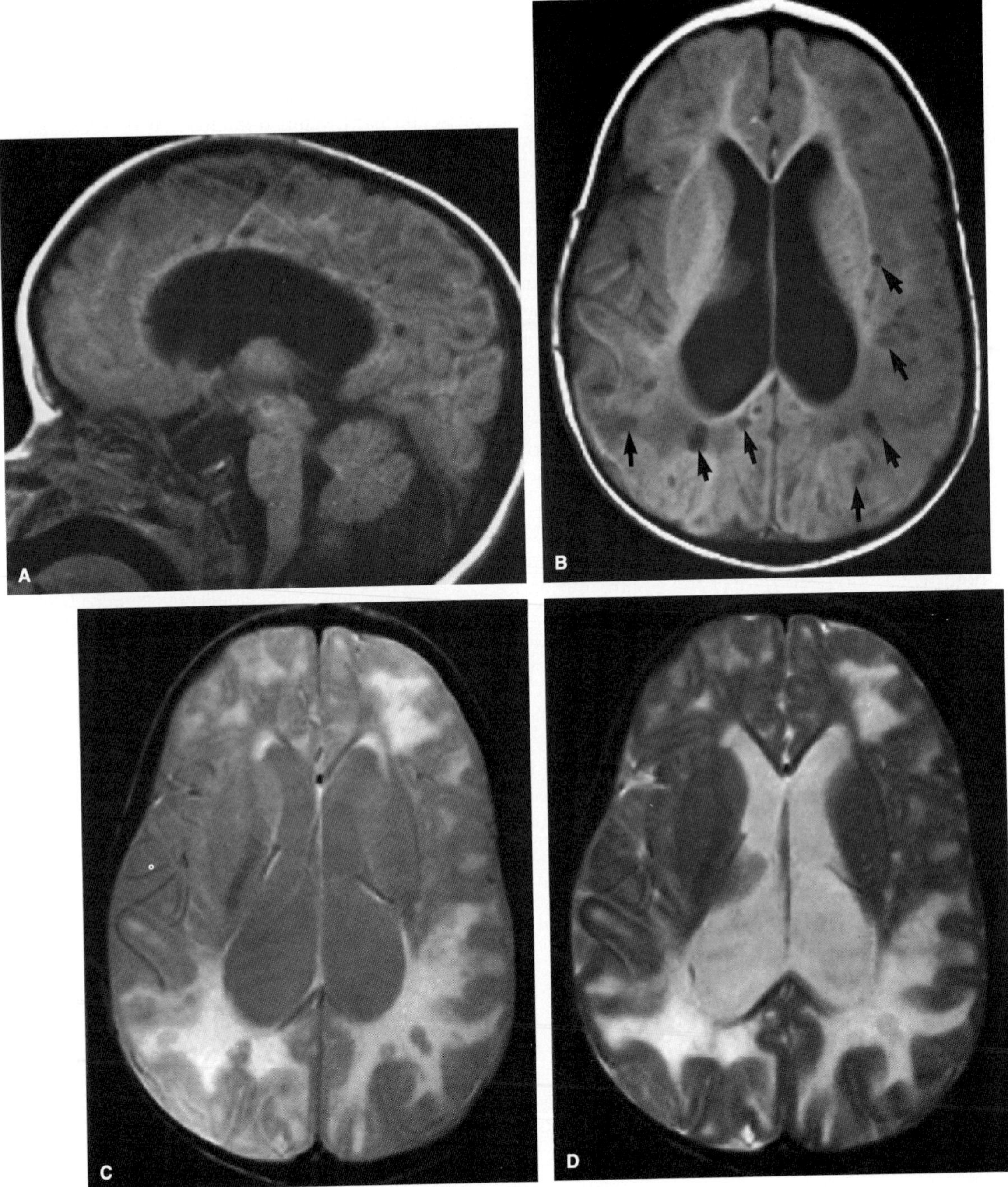

HISTORY

A 2-year-old with increasing head circumference

FINDINGS

Sagittal (*A*) and axial (*B*) T1-weighted images demonstrate numerous small round and oval lesions (*arrows in B*) of decreased signal intensity predominantly in the white matter. Moderate ventriculomegaly is noted. No abnormal contrast enhancement was seen (*images not shown*). First (*C*) and second (*D*) echoes of the axial T2-weighted sequence show diffuse abnormal hyperintensity throughout the white matter.

DIAGNOSIS

Hurler's syndrome

DISCUSSION

The mucopolysaccharidoses are inborn errors of metabolism and are divided into six subtypes.[1] The most common form, Hurler's disease, is caused by a defect in the enzyme, α-L-iduronidase. Clinical features include mental retardation, deafness, short stature, corneal clouding, coarse facial features, and death by the teen years.[2]

MR features of Hurler's disease include ventriculomegaly, J-shaped sella, cavitated lesions within the white matter, and diffuse cerebral white matter disease (as reflected by hyperintensity on T2-weighted images). This abnormal hyperintensity is thought to represent gliosis and demyelination. The pathologic literature refers to small perivascular lacunes or pits visible on the cut surface of the white matter in patients with mucopolysaccharidoses. These cysts contain mononuclear cells and a viscous fluid. The mononuclear cells have been termed *gargoyle* cells because they contain vacuoles filled with mucopolysaccharide.

Clinical References

1. Kulkarni MV, Williams JC, Yeakley JW, et al. Magnetic resonance imaging in the diagnosis of the cranio-cervical manifestations of the mucopolysaccharidoses. Magn Reson Imaging 1987;5:317–323.
2. Rauch RA, Friloux LA, Lott IT. MR imaging of cavitary lesions in the brain with Hurler/Scheie. AJNR 1989;10:S1–S3.

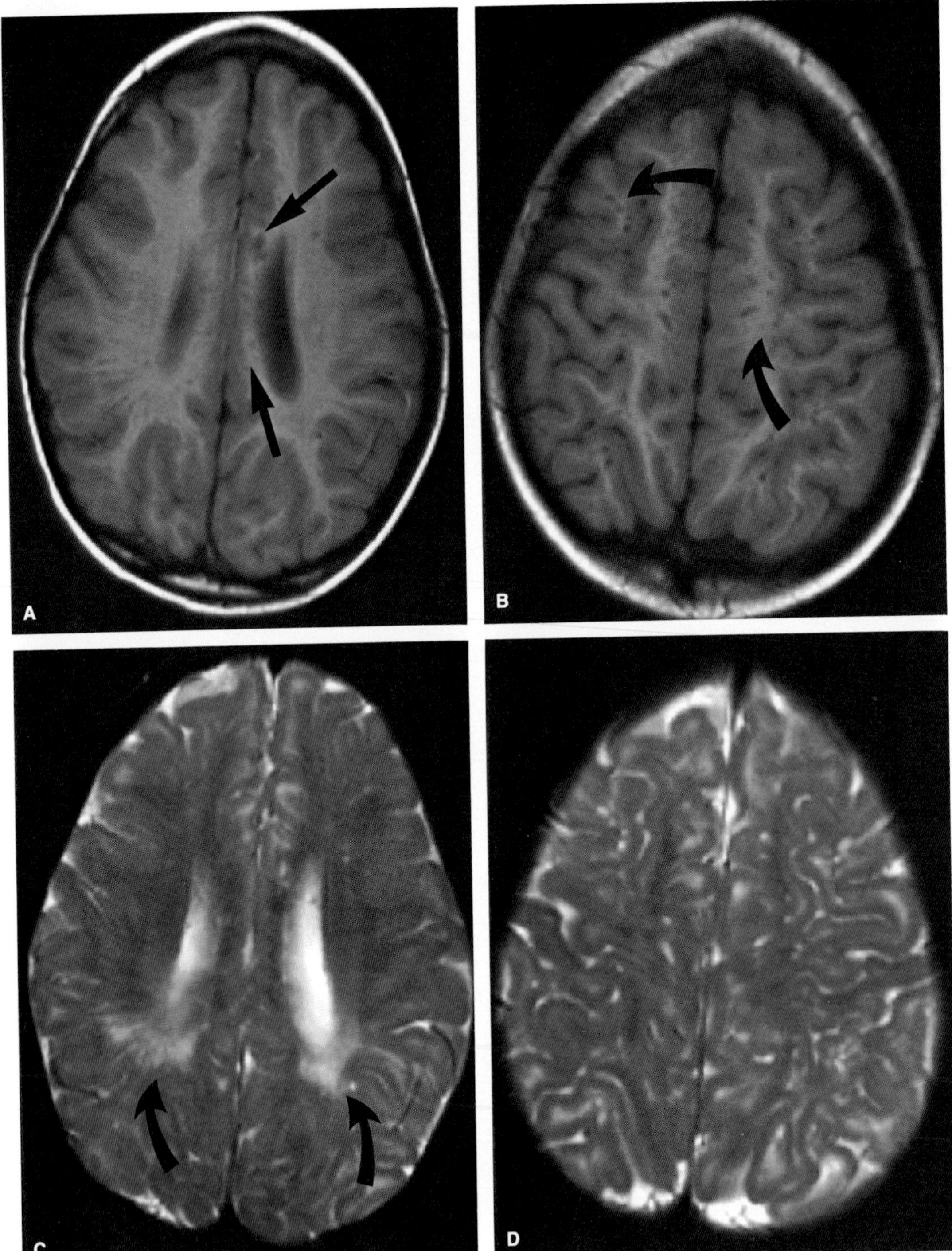
A
B
C
D

HISTORY

A 4-year-old boy with developmental delay and decreased audition

FINDINGS

T1-weighted (*A and B*) and T2-weighted (TE = 90 msec) (*C and D*) images reveal multiple punctate abnormalities within both the corpus callosum (*arrows in A*) and peripheral white matter (*curved arrows in B*). The signal intensity of these lesions is compatible with CSF. The white matter is diffusely abnormal (it should be darker or of lower signal intensity) except in the immediate periventricular region anteriorly on the T2-weighted scan, suggesting delayed myelination or damage to myelin. There is prominent abnormal hyperintensity in the periatrial white matter (*curved arrows in C*) on the T2-weighted scan. Mild cerebral atrophy is also present.

DIAGNOSIS

Hunter's syndrome (mucopolysaccharidosis type II)

DISCUSSION

In each of the mucopolysaccharidoses, there is a genetic deficiency of a specific enzyme involved in the catabolism of mucopolysaccharides.[1] These disorders are included within the larger group of lysosomal storage diseases. The enzyme deficiencies lead to abnormal accumulation of mucopolysaccharides in tissue, producing both neurologic and skeletal abnormalities.[2] All patients have coarse facial features (gargoylism), with both skeletal and multiple organ involvement.

The lysosomal storage diseases consist of the sphingolipidoses (which include the gangliosidoses [Tay-Sachs disease], Krabbe's disease, Fabry's disease, Gaucher's disease, Niemann-Pick disease, and Farber's disease), mucopolysaccharidoses, mucolipidoses, oligosaccharidoses, and glycogenoses. At least seven subtypes of mucopolysaccharidoses are recognized: Hurler's, Hunter's, Sanfilippo's, Morquio's, Scheie's, Maroteaux-Lamy, and Sly's diseases.

Hunter's syndrome resembles Hurler's, but is X-linked, with slower progression and longer survival, and lacks corneal clouding. Gross pathologic features of the mucopolysaccharidoses include cerebral atrophy and prominent perivascular spaces, which are reflected by this patient's MR.

Pitfalls in Image Interpretation

In every head MR examination, the relative signal intensity of gray and white matter should be compared. By this process, a diffuse abnormality of the brain can be recognized, as in the current case on T2-weighted images. Inherited metabolic diseases (which include both the storage diseases and the leukodystrophies) characteristically cause such global changes. The cystic CSF spaces and mild cerebral atrophy support the diagnosis of chronic disease.

Clinical References

1. Becker LE, Yates AJ. Inherited metabolic disease. In: Davis RL, Robertson DM, eds. Textbook of neuropathology, 2nd ed. Baltimore, Williams & Wilkins, 1991.
2. Adams RD, Victor M. The inherited metabolic diseases of the nervous system. In: Adams RD, Victor M, eds. Principles of neurology, 4th ed. New York, McGraw-Hill, 1989.

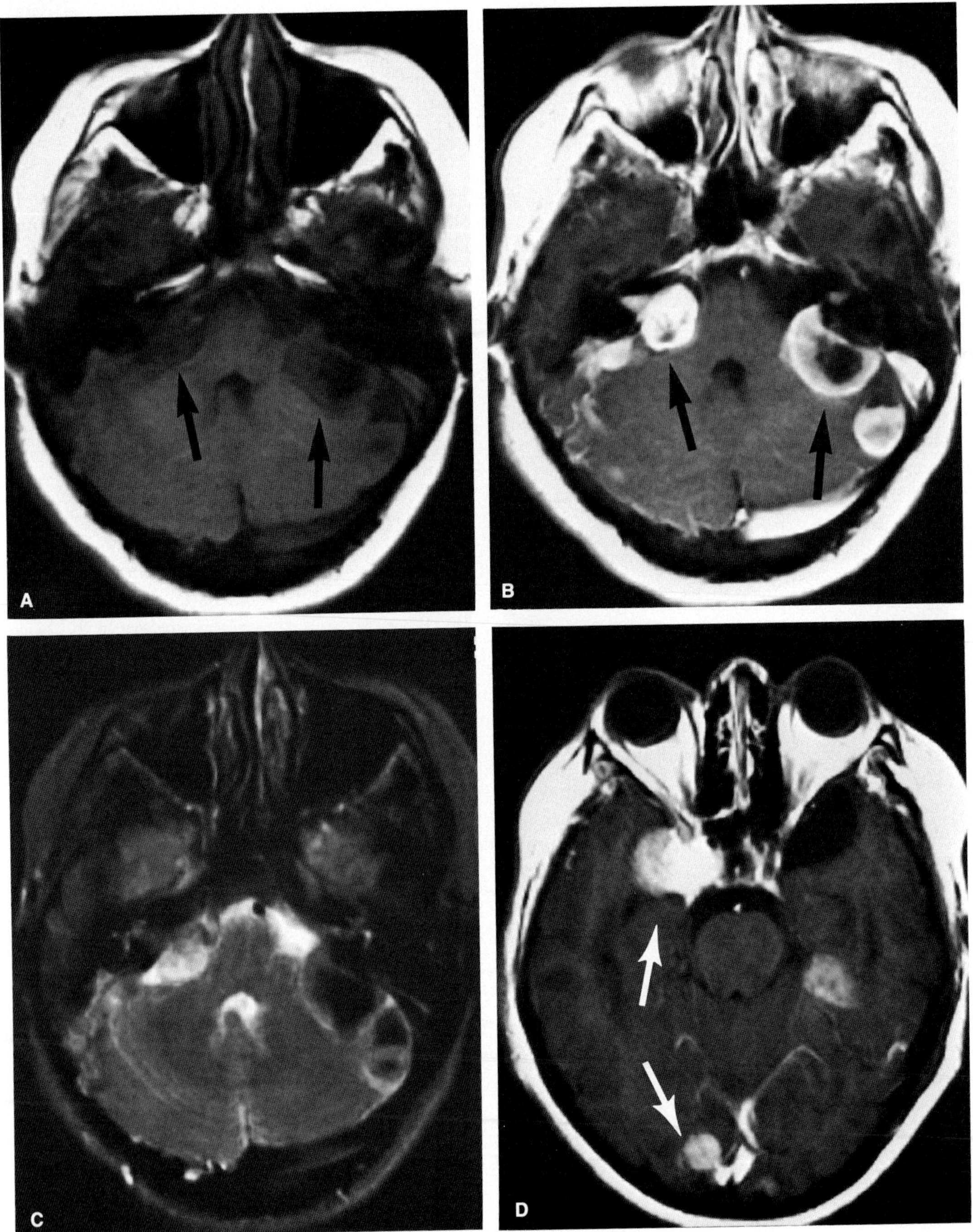

HISTORY

A 48-year-old woman with deteriorating neurologic function and a known congenital syndrome

FINDINGS

Precontrast (*A*) and postcontrast (*B*) axial T1-weighted images show bilateral enhancing extraaxial cerebellopontine angle masses (*black arrows*). (*C*) These masses are of varying signal intensity on the axial T2-weighted study. (*D*) Two other enhancing extraaxial masses (*white arrows*) are seen on a postcontrast axial T1-weighted image at a different anatomic level.

DIAGNOSIS

Neurofibromatosis type 2

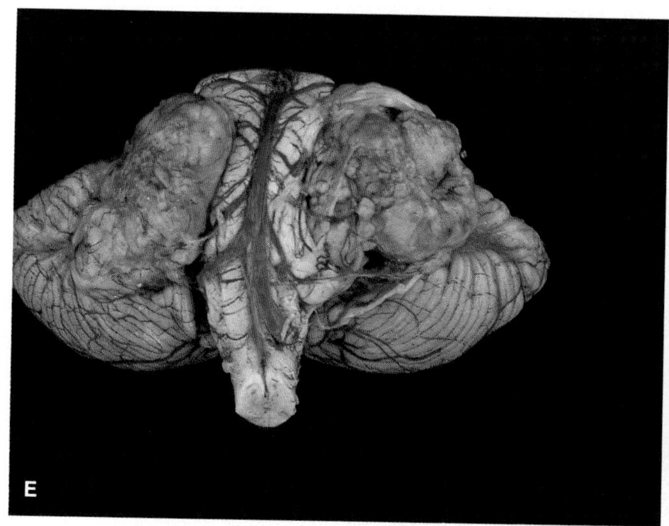

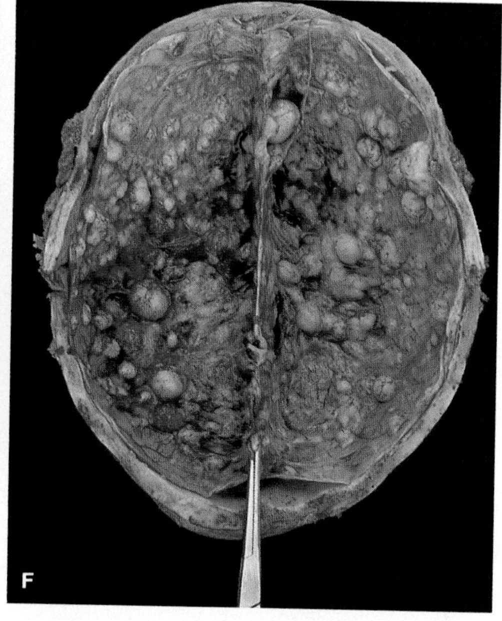

DISCUSSION

Neurofibromatosis is an autosomal dominant syndrome, with a prevalence of 1 per 2000 to 3000 population. Two distinct syndromes are described.[1]

Neurofibromatosis type 1 (von Recklinghausen's disease) is characterized by cutaneous café au lait spots, axillary freckles, hamartomas of the iris, and multiple subcutaneous nodules. The subcutaneous nodules represent peripheral nerve tumors of Schwann cell and fibroblast origin. Tumors also arise in the spinal canal. The gene responsible for neurofibromatosis type 1 is located on the long arm of chromosome 17. This is the more common form of the disease (12 to 20 times more frequent than type 2). Optic nerve gliomas are bilateral in 10% to 20% of cases and are the most frequent intracranial tumor associated with neurofibromatosis type 1, with an incidence of 10% to 70%.[2] A primary glioma occurs in 10% to 15% of patients with neurofibromatosis type 1.

Neurofibromatosis type 2 (bilateral acoustic neurofibromatosis) is characterized by the presence of bilateral acoustic neuromas which usually develop between 10 and 30 years of age. Cranial nerve tumors, cranial and spinal meningiomas, paraspinal neurofibromas, and spinal cord ependymomas are commonly found. Café au lait spots and subcutaneous nodules may also be found. This syndrome is believed to result from the deletion of genetic material from chromosome 22 and has an incidence of 1 in 50,000.

MR Technique

IV contrast is necessary to demonstrate small intracanalicular tumors of the seventh and eighth cranial nerves.

Pathologic Correlate

(*E*) A case of neurofibromatosis type 2, with bilateral acoustic neuromas, is illustrated by a gross brain stem specimen. Note the compression of the pons by the masses bilaterally. (*F*) In another specimen, innumerable small, partially confluent, meningiomas are seen, viewed from above with the skull removed.

Clinical References

1. Bognanno JR, Edwards MK, Lee TA, et al. Cranial MR imaging in neurofibromatosis. AJR 1988;151:381–388.
2. Aoki S, Barkovich AJ, Nishimura K, et al. Neurofibromatosis types 1 and 2: cranial MR findings. Radiology 1989;172:527–534.

(E *and* F *from Okazaki H, Scheithauer B. Slide atlas of neuropathology. New York, Gower Medical Publishing, 1988. By permission of Mayo Foundation.)*

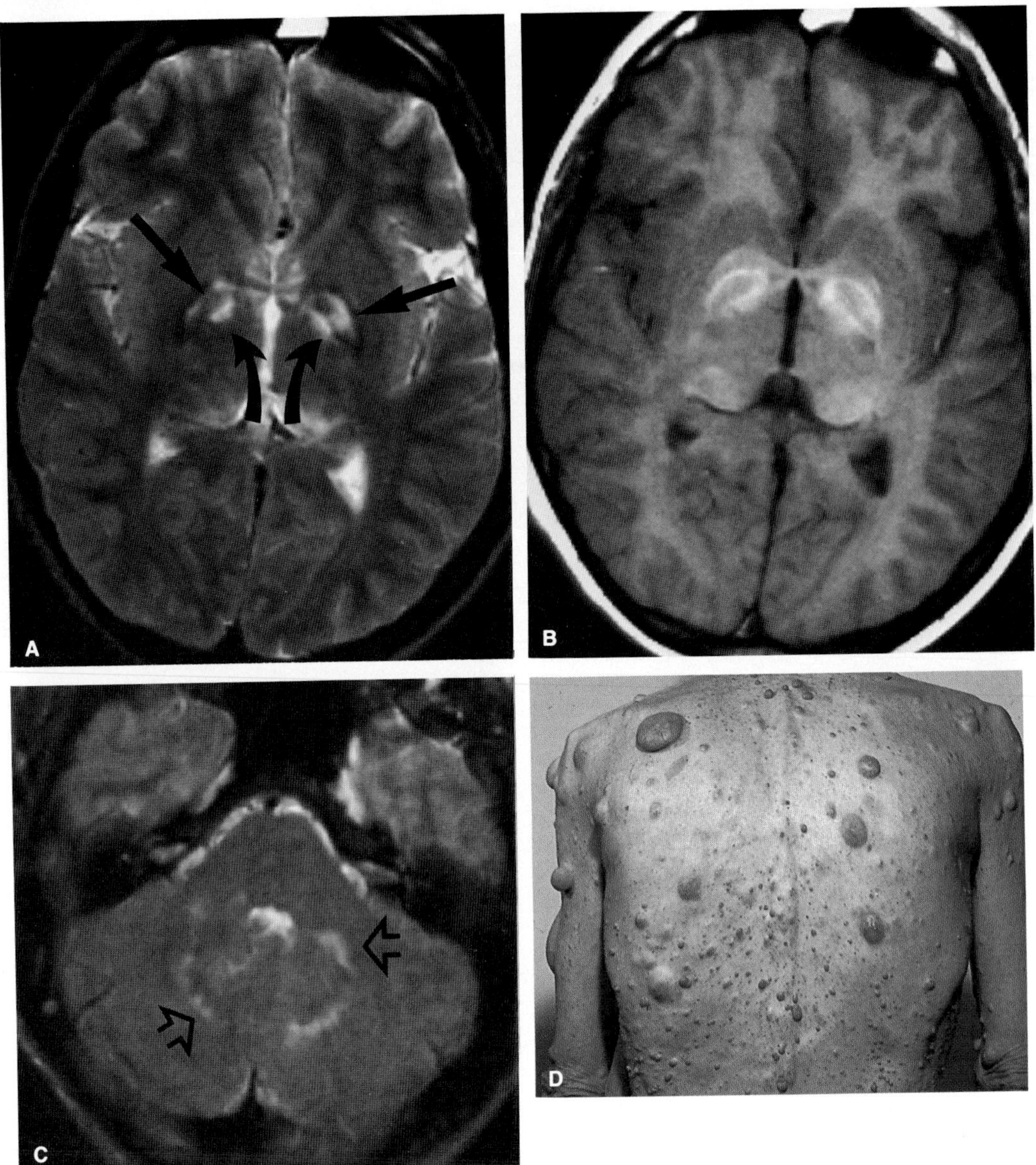

HISTORY

A 12-year-old patient with an inherited neurocutaneous disorder

FINDINGS

(*A*) Axial T2-weighted image (TE = 90 msec) at the level of the basal ganglia reveals symmetric abnormal hyperintensity in the globus pallidus (*arrows*) and posterior limb of the internal capsule (*curved arrows*). (*B*) The axial T1-weighted image at the same level demonstrates abnormal high signal intensity in a slightly more extensive area. There is no apparent mass effect. Also present, but less prominent, is abnormal high signal intensity in the thalami on the T2-weighted image. (*C*) A T2-weighted image at the level of the pons reveals abnormal hyperintensity (*open arrows*) bilaterally in the cerebellar white matter.

DIAGNOSIS

Neurofibromatosis type 1

DISCUSSION

Most patients with neurofibromatosis type 1 demonstrate lesions of increased signal intensity in the brain on T2-weighted images.[1] These abnormalities are seen most commonly in the basal ganglia (specifically globus pallidus), brain stem, and cerebellar white matter. The pathologic basis and clinical consequence of such abnormalities are unknown, although these lesions most likely represent hamartomas or heterotopias.

Abnormal hyperintense foci on T1-weighted scans, involving the globus pallidus and internal capsule bilaterally (usually symmetrically) with extension across the anterior commissure, have also been described.[2] The same lesions on T2-weighted scans appear smaller and less prominent. There is typically no associated mass effect or abnormal contrast enhancement.

Pitfalls in Image Interpretation

In the presence of bilateral basal ganglia abnormalities, as described above with abnormal hyperintensity on both T1- and T2-weighted examinations, the diagnosis of neurofibromatosis should be considered. The pathologic basis for these lesions is unclear, with caution indicated in the use of this sign. Clearly, this signal intensity pattern is not unique, with extracellular methemoglobin also resulting in such an appearance. Abnormal high-intensity foci in the basal ganglia on T2-weighted scans, without accompanying high intensity on T1-weighted scans, may be a more common finding in neurofibromatosis, although this appearance is even less specific.

Pathologic Correlate

(*D*) Typical clinical appearance of an adult with fully developed type I (peripheral or cutaneous) neurofibromatosis is illustrated. Innumerable nodular neurofibromas are noted. Early manifestations of von Recklinghausen's disease, not illustrated, include multiple café au lait spots of varying size.

Clinical References

1. Goldstein SM, Curless RG, Donovan Post MJ, Quencer RM. A new sign of neurofibromatosis on magnetic resonance imaging of children. Arch Neurol 1989;46:1222–1224.
2. Mirowitz SA, Sartor K, Gado M. High intensity basal ganglia lesions on T1 weighted MR images in neurofibromatosis. AJR 1990;154:369–373.

(D *from Okazaki H, Scheithauer B. Slide atlas of neuropathology. New York, Gower Medical Publishing, 1988. By permission of Mayo Foundation.)*

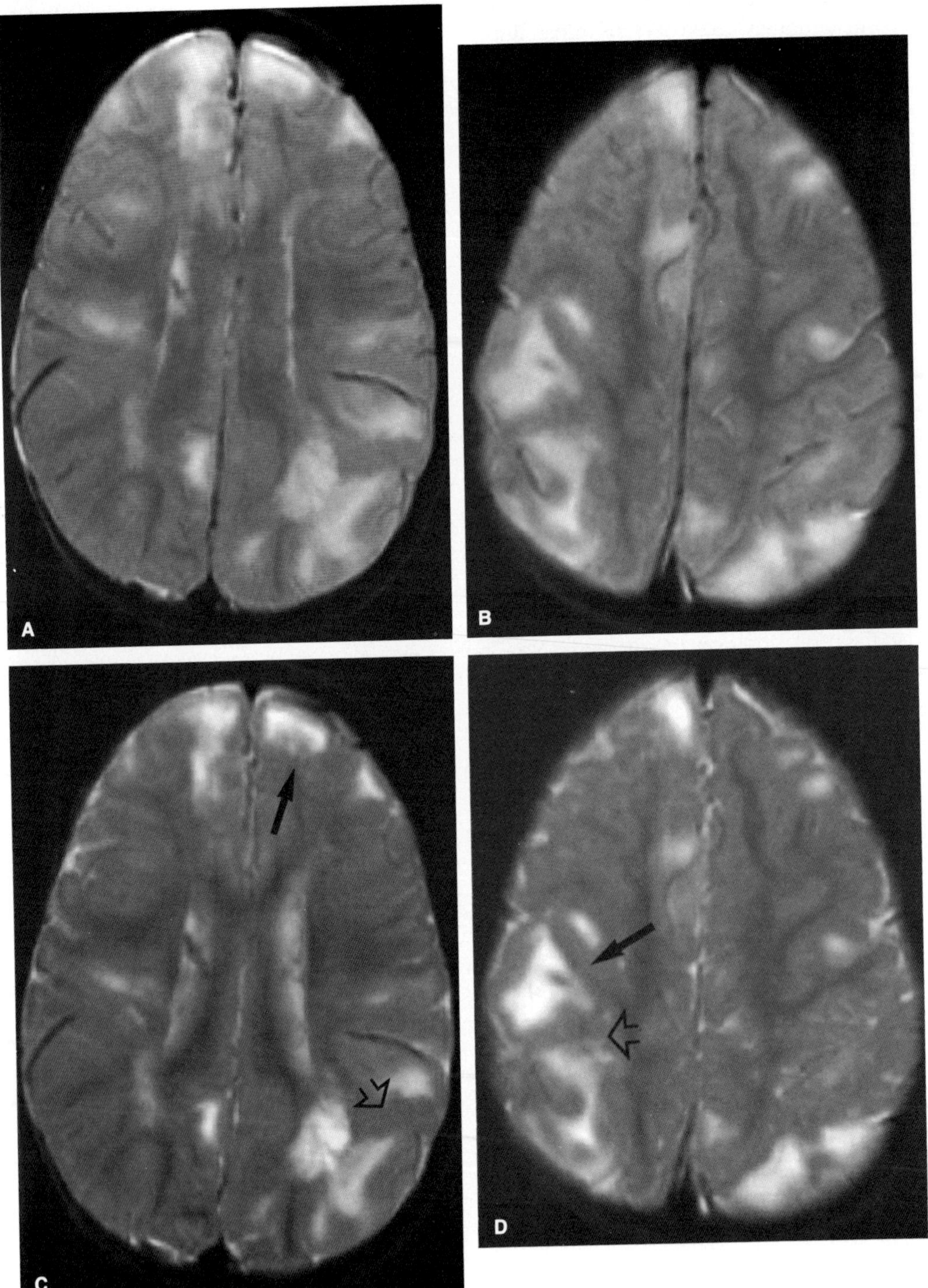

HISTORY

A 19-month-old infant with seizures and mental retardation

FINDINGS

Multiple high-signal-intensity parenchymal lesions are seen on intermediate (*A and B*) and heavily (*C and D*) T2-weighted images, involving both cortical and subcortical regions. In most, there is involvement of both gray and white matter. In several instances, the abnormality (*arrows in C and D*) appears confined to the subcortical white matter core of an expanded gyrus (a "gyral core" lesion). In *C* and *D,* involvement of two adjacent gyri in this fashion, with sparing of normal intervening cortex lining a sulcus (a "sulcal island") can also be seen (*arrow*). Some lesions are noted involving the deep white matter and periventricular region, although these are

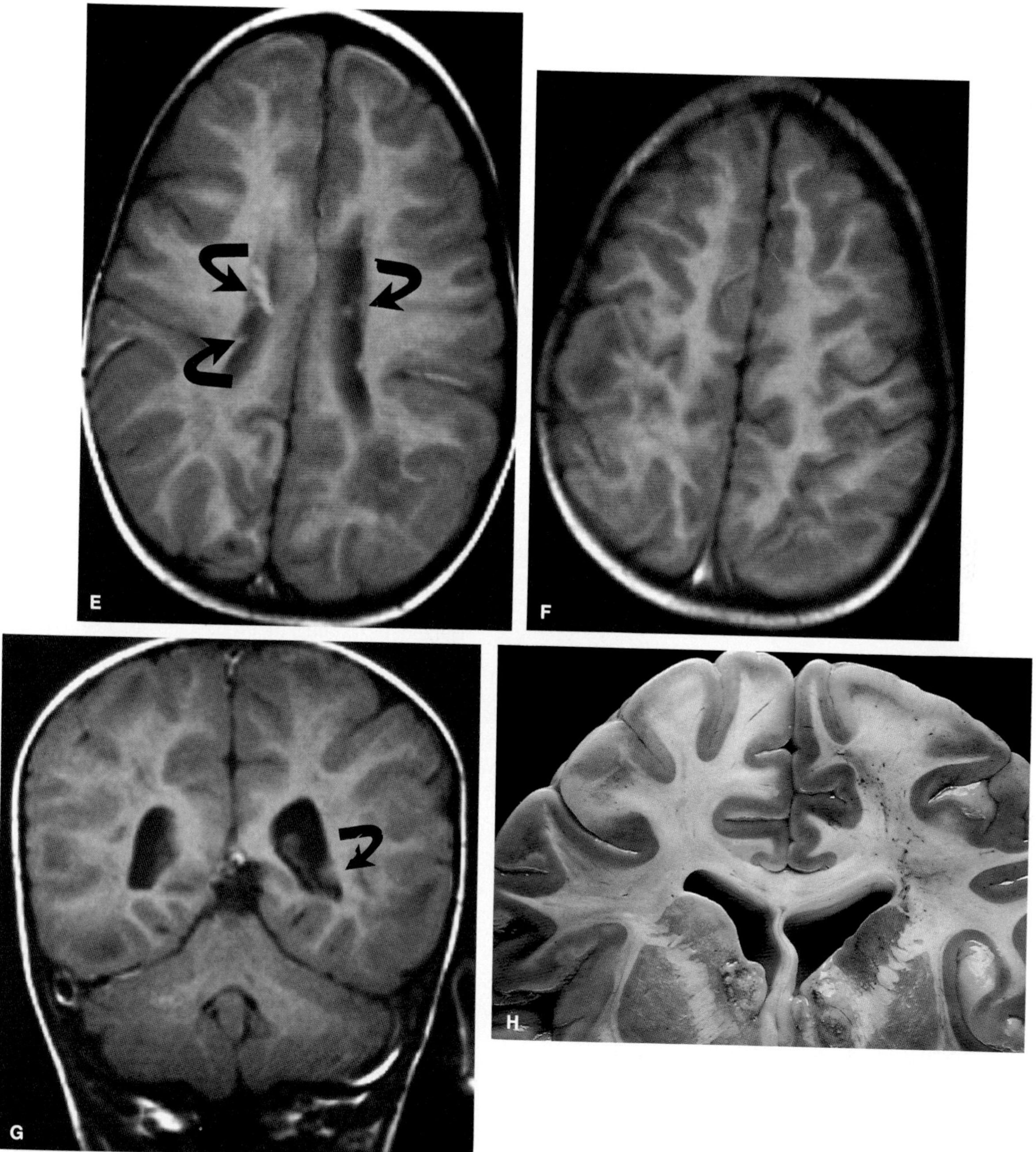

smaller and less numerous than peripheral abnormalities. (*E to G*) The parenchymal lesions are low signal intensity, but in general less well visualized on T1-weighted images. Multiple subependymal nodules (*curved arrows in E and G*) are best identified on T1-weighted images.

DIAGNOSIS

Tuberous sclerosis

DISCUSSION

CT findings in tuberous sclerosis include calcified subependymal nodules, parenchymal hypointensity, peripheral calcifications, ventricular dilatation (due to atrophy), and (less commonly) giant cell astrocytoma. MR has replaced CT as the diagnostic modality of choice, with the combination of parenchymal lesions and subependymal nodules being pathognomonic.[1,2] The parenchymal lesions represent tubers (pathologically these are hamartomas) that contain more unbound water than normal brain.

Tuberous sclerosis is one of the neurocutaneous syndromes, with autosomal dominant inheritance (dominant mutation of chromosome 9). Cutaneous lesions include leaf-shaped hypopigmented spots (trunk and limbs) and adenoma sebaceum, the latter distributed over the cheeks, chin, and forehead in a butterfly pattern. Individual adenomas are pinkish and vary from 1 to 10 mm. There may also be a patch of rough, thickened, yellow skin over the lumbosacral region (shagreen patch). Mental retardation and infantile epilepsy are common. Brain tumors occur in 2% to 5% of cases, the most common being a subependymal giant-cell astrocytoma. The classic location of such a tumor is within the wall of the lateral ventricle. When large, these may cause blockage of the foramen of Monro and resultant hydrocephalus.

MR Technique

Parenchymal lesions in tuberous sclerosis are best identified on T2-weighted images, whereas subependymal nodules are well depicted on T1-weighted images. Enhancement of a large lesion raises the question of neoplasia, specifically a giant cell astrocytoma.

Pitfalls in Image Interpretation

Cortical tubers can be differentiated, on the basis of subcortical involvement, from ischemic lesions such as those encountered in lupus erythematosus and cerebral infarction. Calcified subependymal nodules should not be confused with normal subependymal veins.

Pathologic Correlate

(*H*) Coronal gross section through the frontal horns in a case of tuberous sclerosis is presented for correlation. Subependymal nodules are seen buried at the inferior angle of each frontal horn, a characteristic location. Another common appearance of subependymal hamartomatous lesions is that of melted candle wax drippings ("candle guttering") along the walls of the lateral ventricles.

Clinical References

1. Nixon JR, Houser OW, Gomez MR, Okazaki H. Cerebral tuberous sclerosis: MR imaging. Radiology 1989;170:869–873.
2. McMurdo SK, Moore SG, Brant-Zawadzki M, et al. MR imaging of intracranial tuberous sclerosis. AJNR 1987;8:77–82.

(H from Okazaki H, Scheithauer B. Slide atlas of neuropathology. New York, Gower Medical Publishing, 1988. By permission of Mayo Foundation.)

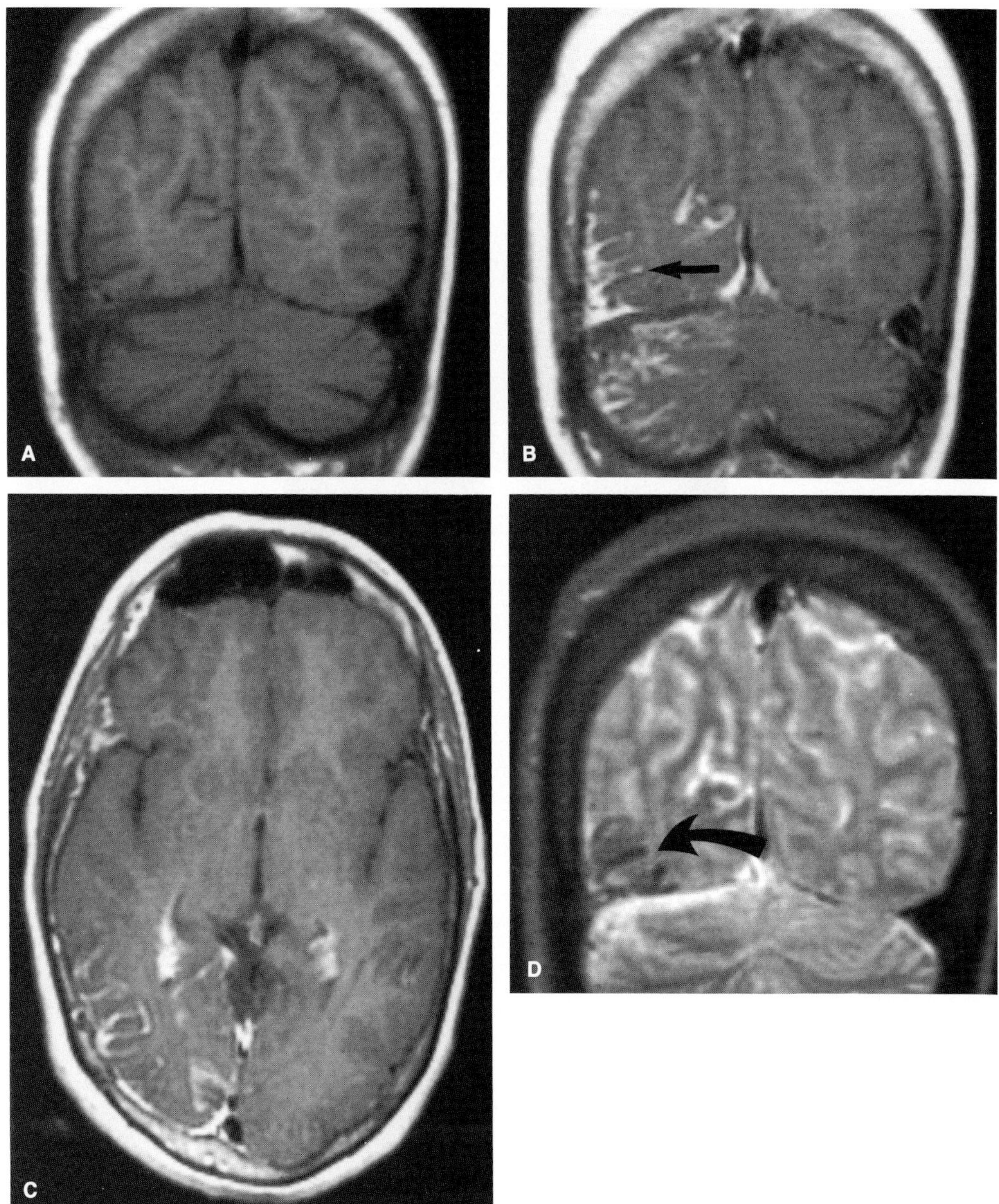

HISTORY

A 28-year-old patient with a facial nevus

FINDINGS

Precontrast (*A*) and postcontrast (*B*) coronal T1-weighted images demonstrate leptomeningeal enhancement (*arrow in B*) in the right posterior parietal lobe and the right cerebellar hemisphere. (*C*) Axial T1-weighted postcontrast image shows leptomeningeal enhancement along with atrophic changes in the right parietal and occipital lobes. (*D*) Coronal T2-weighted image demonstrates very low signal intensity (*curved arrow*) in a gyriform pattern in the posterior parietal lobe. This is in a slightly different location than the leptomeningeal enhancement seen in *B* and *C*.

DIAGNOSIS

Sturge-Weber syndrome

DISCUSSION

Encephalotrigeminal angiomatosis (Sturge-Weber syndrome) is a rare, nonfamilial neurocutaneous syndrome characterized by the following features: port-wine stain,

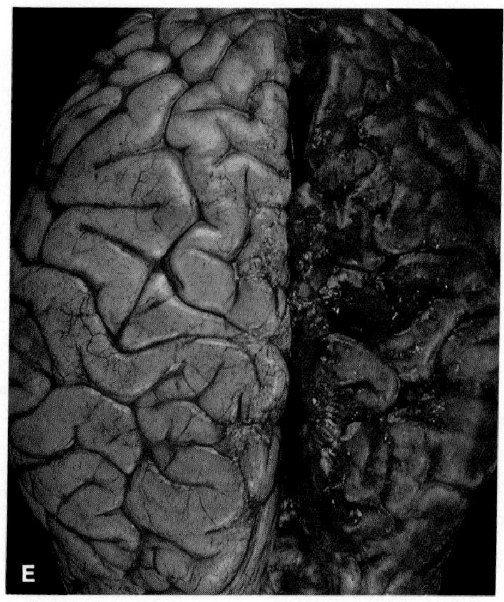

leptomeningeal angiomatosis, cerebral atrophy, choroidal angioma, buphthalmos (congenital enlarged globe and glaucoma), seizures, mental retardation, hemiparesis, and hemiatrophy. The intracranial lesion is usually ipsilateral to the facial nevus. Calcifications are frequently noted in the brain parenchyma adjacent to the leptomeningeal abnormality. CT is more sensitive for the detection of calcification than MR. The gyriform pattern of low signal intensity seen in *D* is presumably secondary to the magnetic susceptibility of calcium, although this finding can also be seen with hemosiderin deposition. Pathologically, calcification occurs in a pericapillary distribution, typically in the fourth layer of the atrophied cerebral cortex, and is thought to be related to chronic tissue hypoxia.

The basic venous abnormality in this syndrome is a lack of superficial cortical veins overlying the area of cerebral atrophy. Enlarged internal cerebral veins, basal vein of Rosenthal, deep medullary veins, and subependymal veins may be seen. These patients have venous angiomatosis of the leptomeninges, and enhancement of these abnormal vessels (*A and C*) is seen after administration of a gadolinium chelate.

An overlap with the Klippel-Trenaunay syndrome has been reported. This is a disease characterized by the triad of port-wine nevus, varicose veins, and limb overgrowth.

MR Technique

Contrast enhancement is necessary to demonstrate the full extent of leptomeningeal abnormality.

Pitfalls in Image Interpretation

The enhancement of the leptomeninges should not be confused with the gyriform enhancement secondary to blood–brain barrier breakdown seen in subacute stroke.

Pathologic Correlate

(*E*) Gross appearance of the superior surface of this unfixed brain specimen shows unilateral diffuse leptomeningeal angiomatosis. The neurologic deficits in the Sturge-Weber syndrome are thought to be secondary to the presence of this capillary-venous malformation (angioma) within the leptomeninges.

Clinical References

1. Elster AD, Chen MYM. MR Imaging of Sturge-Weber syndrome: role of gadopentetate dimeglumine and gradient-echo techniques. AJNR 1990;11:685–689.
2. Sperner J, Schmauser, Bittner R, et al. MR-imaging findings in children with Sturge-Weber syndrome. Neuropediatrics 1990;21:146–152.
3. Wasendo JJ, Rosenbloom SA, Duchesneau PM, et al. The Sturge-Weber syndrome: comparison of MR and CT characteristics. AJNR 1990;11:131–134.

(E *from Okazaki H, Scheithauer B. Slide atlas of neuropathology. New York, Gower Medical Publishing, 1988. By permission of Mayo Foundation.)*

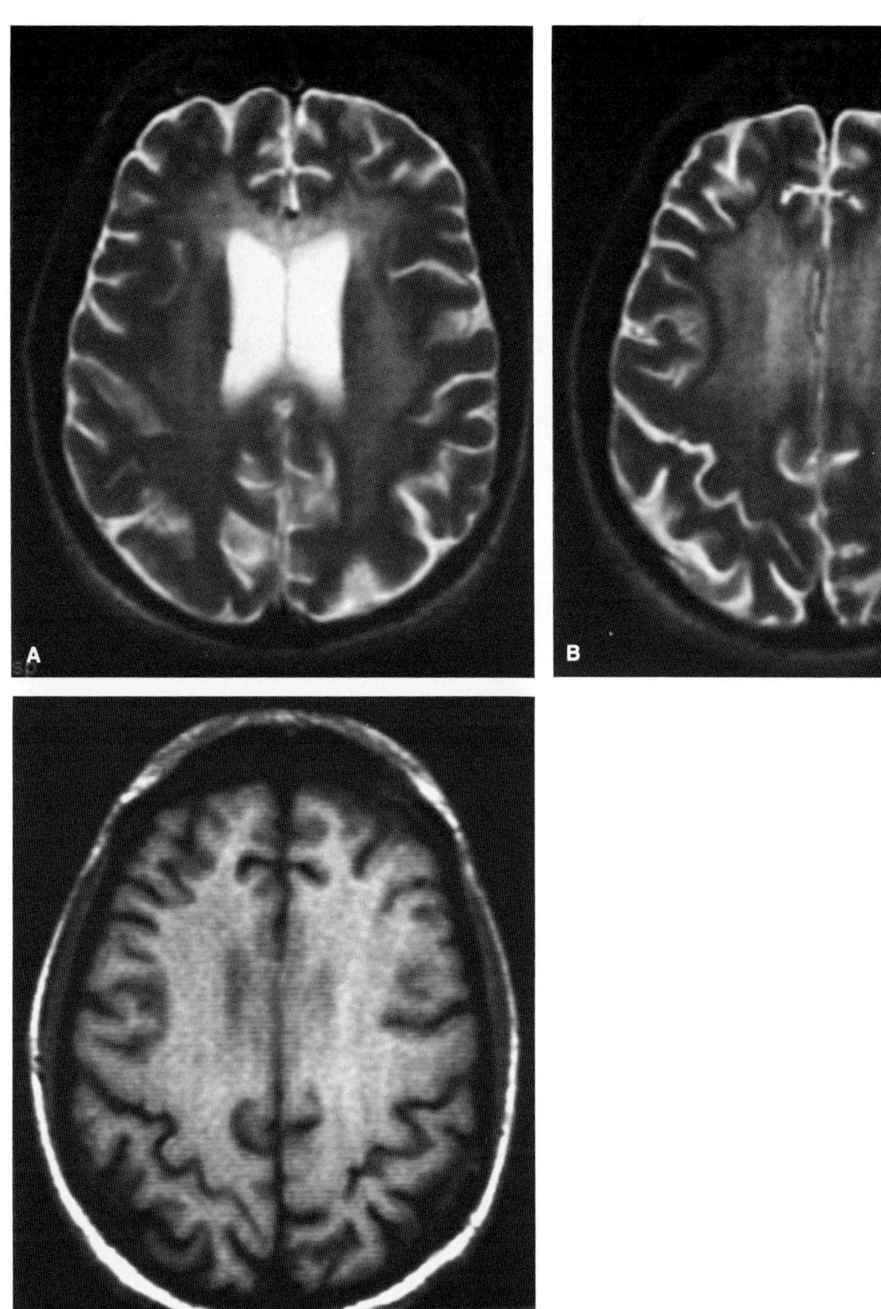

HISTORY

A 29-year-old HIV-positive man

FINDINGS

(*A and B*) Axial T2-weighted images identify abnormal diffuse high signal intensity in a symmetric pattern in the white matter of the centrum semiovale. (*C*) The axial T1-weighted image reveals only mild cortical atrophy. No abnormal contrast enhancement was noted (*images not shown*).

DIAGNOSIS

HIV encephalitis

DISCUSSION

About 30% of patients with acquired immunodeficiency syndrome (AIDS) have evidence of white matter disease on MR. This is usually secondary to direct involvement of the brain by human immunodeficiency virus (HIV). Pathologically, the hallmark of HIV encephalitis is the presence of multinucleate giant cells located primarily in the white matter and less commonly in the gray matter. Diffuse, abnormal high signal intensity is seen primarily in the periventricular white matter on T2-weighted images secondary to a direct neurotropic effect of the HIV.[1]

Progressive multifocal leukoencephalopathy (PML) is a viral demyelinating disease of the CNS seen in AIDS and other immunocompromised patients. It is a result of infection with a papovavirus (subtype JC virus), which attacks oligodendrocytes. PML is seen in 2% to 4% of all patients with AIDS. On MR imaging, PML is manifested as focal areas of demyelination predominantly in the white matter, which are typically asymmetric. This disease progresses relentlessly, usually leading to the patient's death within 6 months.[2]

Clinical References

1. Olsen WL, Longo FM, Mills CM, et al. White matter disease in AIDS: findings at MR imaging. Radiology 1998;169:445–448.
2. Mark AS, Atlas SW. Progressive multifocal leukoencephalopathy in patients with AIDS: appearance on MR images. Radiology 1989;173:517–520.

(A to C courtesy of William Yuh, MD.)

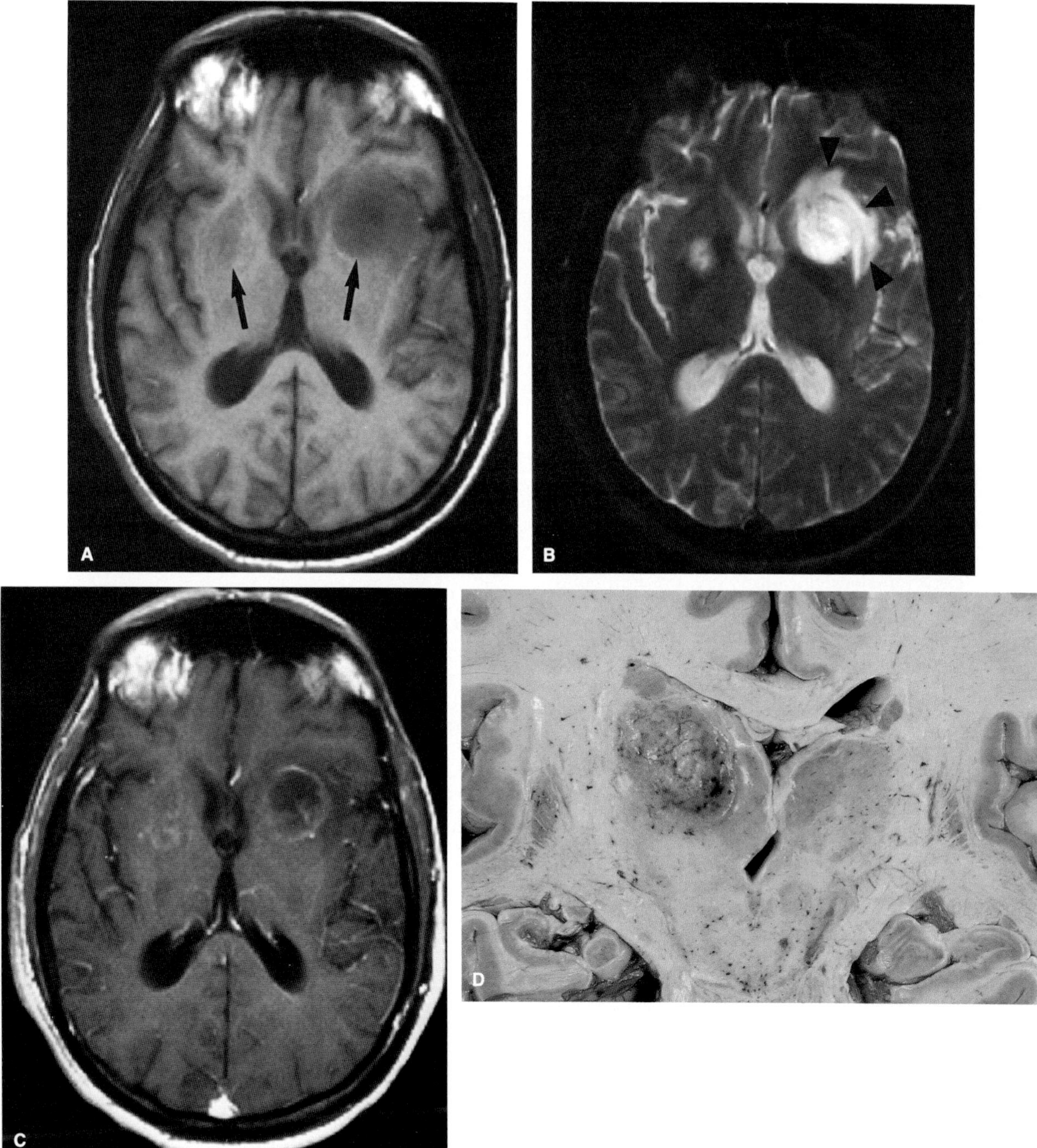

HISTORY

A 35-year-old HIV-positive man with headaches

FINDINGS

(*A*) T1-weighted axial image demonstrates low-signal-intensity lesions (*arrows*) in the basal ganglia bilaterally. On the T2-weighted axial image (*B*), the lesions have high signal intensity with a round mass–like appearance. The irregular high signal intensity (*arrowheads*) surrounding the mass in the left basal ganglia, particularly laterally, represents edema. (*C*) Postcontrast T1-weighted axial image reveals ring enhancement of the lesions. The edema surrounding the mass in the left basal ganglia has low signal intensity on T1-weighted images and is more easily separated from the mass itself after contrast infusion.

DIAGNOSIS

Toxoplasmosis

DISCUSSION

Toxoplasma gondii is a ubiquitous obligate intracellular protozoan that causes a mild self-limited infection consisting of mild lymphadenopathy and fever in the immunologically intact adult. A large number of normal adults, between 25% and 70% of the US population, have been exposed to toxoplasmosis and have chronic seropositive titers for antibodies to the organism. The most common modes of transmission are thought to be through insufficiently cooked meat or from cat feces.[1]

Toxoplasmosis is an important pathogen in the fetus and in people with compromised immune systems. Toxoplasmosis can be transmitted transplacentally (congenital toxoplasmosis) to the fetus during an acute infection in a pregnant woman. Congenital toxoplasmosis causes either diffuse or focal encephalitis resulting in brain destruction. The infection results in intracranial calcifications scattered throughout the brain that can be detected most easily with CT. This is in contradistinction to congenital infection with cytomegalovirus (CMV), in which the intracranial calcifications are predominantly periventricular.

Toxoplasmosis is the most common intracranial opportunistic infection in patients with AIDS. In AIDS, there is compromise of cell-mediated immunity that allows for reactivation of latent infection or for a more fulminant, acquired toxoplasmosis infection. Lesions are usually located in the basal ganglia and in the cerebral hemispheres at the gray-white matter junction. On MR, toxoplasmosis usually appears as nodular or ring-enhancing lesions on postcontrast T1-weighted images. The lesions have variable signal intensity on T2-weighted images, and are usually surrounded by high-signal-intensity edema.

Pitfalls in Image Interpretation

The differential diagnosis for multiple ring-enhancing lesions in an immune-compromised patient includes lymphoma, which may look identical to toxoplasmosis.[2] AIDS patients with brain lesions are usually treated empirically with antitoxoplasma medication (pyrimethamine and sulfadiazine) and are monitored with serial MR. Decrease in the size or number of lesions should be detected in 2 to 4 weeks if the lesions are due to toxoplasmosis. The differential diagnosis for ring-enhancing lesions in an adult should also always include metastatic disease.

Pathologic Correlate

(*D*) Fresh-cut coronal pathologic specimen shows a toxoplasmosis lesion in the thalamus causing mass effect on the lateral ventricle. Toxoplasmosis lesions have a necrotic center and may have a hemorrhagic border, as in this specimen.

Clinical References

1. Ramsey R, Geremia G. CNS complications of AIDS: CT and MR findings. AJR 1988;151:449–454.
2. Balakrishnan J, Becker P, Kumar A, et al. Acquired immunodeficiency syndrome: correlation of radiologic and pathologic findings in the brain. Radiographics 1990; 10:201–215.

(D from Okazaki H, Scheithauer B. Slide atlas of neuropathology. New York, Gower Medical Publishing, 1988. By permission of Mayo Foundation.)

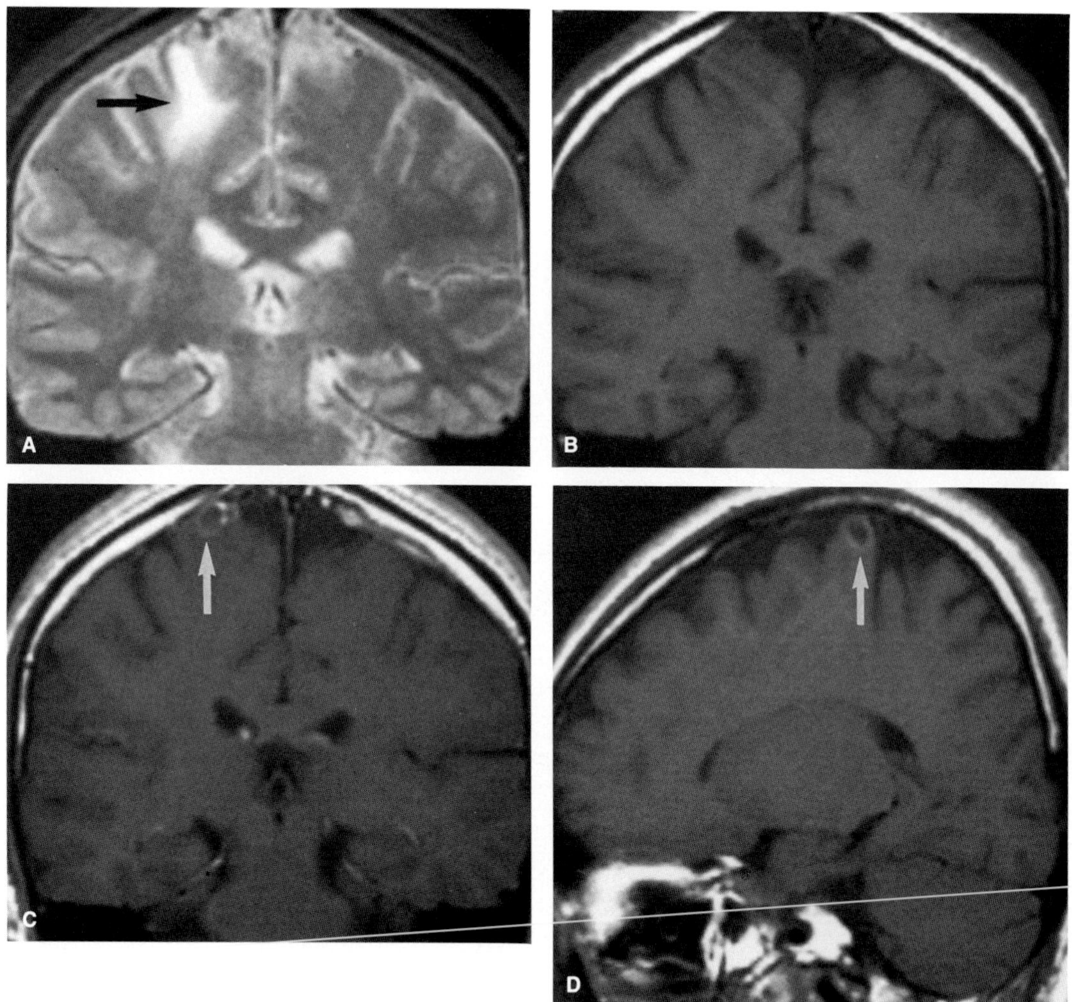

HISTORY

A 27-year-old man with new-onset seizures

FINDINGS

(*A*) T2-weighted coronal image reveals increased signal intensity (*arrow*) consistent with edema high along the convexity in the posterior right frontal lobe. (*B*) Coronal precontrast T1-weighted image reveals only subtle abnormal low signal intensity in this region. On coronal (*C*) and sagittal (*D*) postcontrast T1-weighted images a small ring enhancing lesion (*white arrow*) is demonstrated in the right frontal lobe.

DIAGNOSIS

Neurocysticercosis

DISCUSSION

Neurocysticercosis is an infection of the CNS caused by the larval stage of the pork tapeworm, *Taenia solium*. It is an endemic disease in underdeveloped countries and is seen in immigrants to the United States. This bloodborne organism has a predilection for localizing in muscle and skin, where it is typically asymptomatic, and in the CNS. Viable parenchymal larvae survive for about 5 years. With the death of the parasite, there is resultant cyst degeneration and a pronounced host inflammatory reaction with larvae in the CNS.

CT is useful in identifying parenchymal calcifications associated with neurocysticercosis, but intraventricular cysts are often difficult to identify by CT. Parenchymal cysts most commonly involve the gray–white matter junction. Typically, the cysts are isointense to CSF on T1- and T2-weighted sequences.[1,2] High signal intensity on T2-weighted scans, representing brain edema, is frequently observed surrounding the parenchymal cysts. Contrast-enhanced studies commonly show small ring-enhancing masses (*curved arrows in C and D*).

Patients with parenchymal cysts may present with seizures, while those with intraventricular cysts generally have symptoms related to obstructive hydrocephalus. The interval between infection and clinical manifestation is usually 4 to 5 years. The treatment is the drug praziquantel, which is a heterocyclic pyrazinoisoquinoline oral anthelmintic agent. Steroids are often given to decrease the inflammatory reaction.

MR Technique

IV contrast is necessary to demonstrate the small ring-enhancing cyst wall and permits a more specific diagnosis.

Pitfalls in Image Interpretation

A solitary metastasis or small brain abscess can mimic the appearance of neurocysticercosis.

Clinical References

1. Teitelbaum GP, Otto RJ, Lin M, et al. MR imaging of neurocysticercosis. AJR 1989;153:857–866.
2. Martinez HR, Rangel-Guerra R, Elizondo G, et al. MR imaging in neurocysticercosis: a study of 56 cases. AJNR 1989;10:1011–1019.

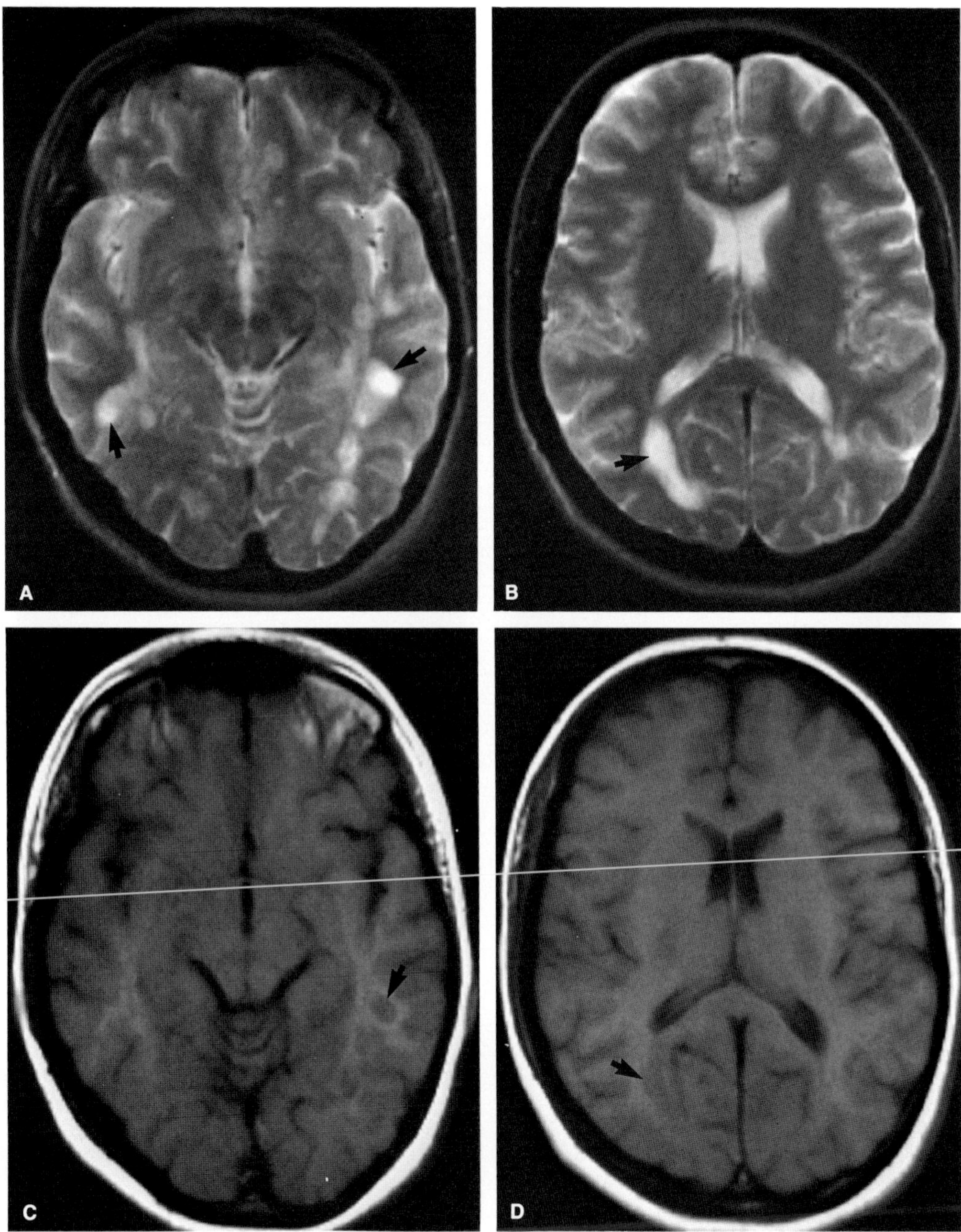

HISTORY

A 40-year-old patient with seizures

FINDINGS

(*A and B*) T2-weighted (TR/TE = 3000/90) images at two levels reveal hyperintense parenchymal abnormalities (*arrows*) in the deep white matter, primarily posteriorly, some of which are periventricular in location, specifically adjacent to the occipital horn. (*C and D*) Precontrast T1-weighted images, at the same anatomic levels, reveal corresponding areas (*arrows*) of subtle abnormal low signal intensity. (*E and F*) These postcontrast images demonstrate abnormal enhancement (*curved arrows*) within at least two of these regions. The enhancement seen in *F* is linear and appears to follow either Virchow-Robin spaces

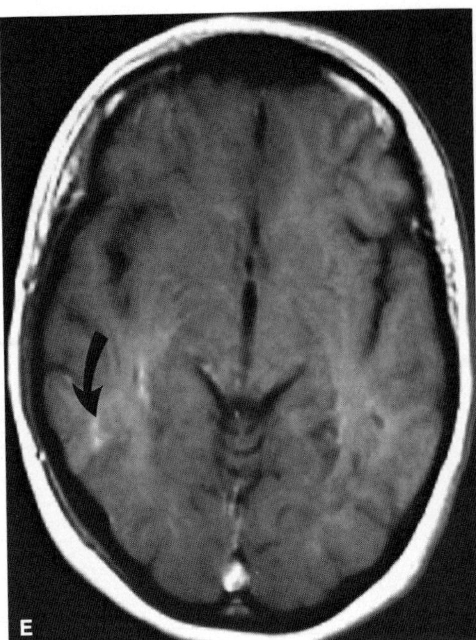

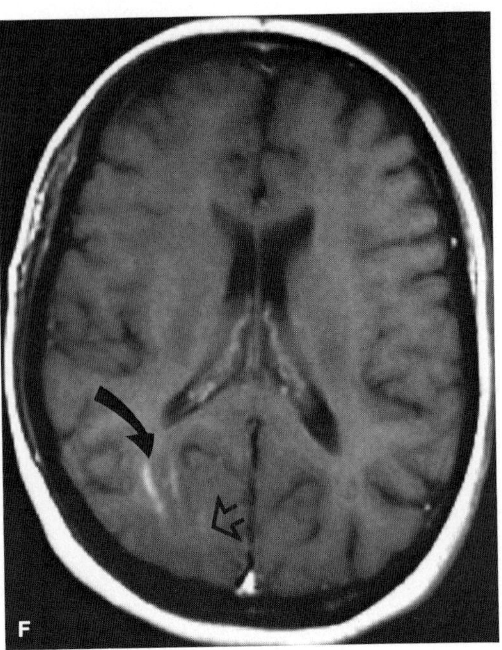

or white matter tracts to an area of parenchymal involvement (*open arrow*).

DIAGNOSIS

Neurosarcoidosis

DISCUSSION

Two main patterns of brain involvement with sarcoidosis have been classically described. The most common is a granulomatous leptomeningitis involving either the meninges diffusely or focally at the skull base. Clinical symptoms include cranial nerve palsies, meningeal signs, and hypothalamic syndromes. The second pattern is that of parenchymal involvement by granulomatous lesions, typically accompanied by leptomeningeal disease. Symptoms in this form of disease are that of an intracranial mass lesion. Parenchymal lesions most likely result from spread of leptomeningeal disease along Virchow-Robin spaces.

Imaging studies confirm the predilection for meningeal disease (diffuse or focal) in neurosarcoidosis, although involvement of the brain parenchyma has been noted in up to half of cases.[1] Disease involvement (listed from most common to least) of the hypothalamus/pituitary, periventricular white matter, optic chiasm, and ependyma has been described. In the only large study of its type,[1] periventricular lesions were noted to enhance following gadolinium chelate administration in six of eight patients. Hydrocephalus is not uncommon. Vasogenic edema is elicited by some parenchymal lesions, but need not be present. Spread along Virchow-Robin spaces, demonstrated by contrast enhancement of adjacent parenchyma, has been observed.[2] Enhanced MR is the preferred technique for detection and evaluation of CNS sarcoidosis, with CT less sensitive for both parenchymal and meningeal involvement.

MR Technique

Intravenous contrast enhancement markedly improves the sensitivity of MR for detection of meningeal disease in neurosarcoidosis.

Pitfalls in Image Interpretation

Although most patients under the age of 50 with periventricular white matter disease on MR have multiple sclerosis, neurosarcoidosis should be considered in the differential diagnosis.[3] In patients with diffuse leptomeningitis on MR, the differential diagnosis is broad. In addition to sarcoidosis, this appearance can be produced by trauma (with subarachnoid and subdural blood), tuberculosis, fungal diseases, bacterial meningitis, and tumor (meningeal carcinomatosis, leukemia, and lymphoma).

Clinical References

1. Sherman JL, Stern BJ. Sarcoidosis of the CNS: comparison of unenhanced and enhanced MR images. AJR 1990; 155;1293–1301.
2. Williams DW, Elster AD, Kramer SI. Neurosarcoidosis: gadolinium enhanced MR imaging. J Comput Assist Tomogr 1990;14:704–707.
3. Smith AS, Meisler DM, Weinstein MA, et al. High signal periventricular lesions in patients with sarcoidosis: neurosarcoidosis or multiple sclerosis? AJR 1989;153:147–152.

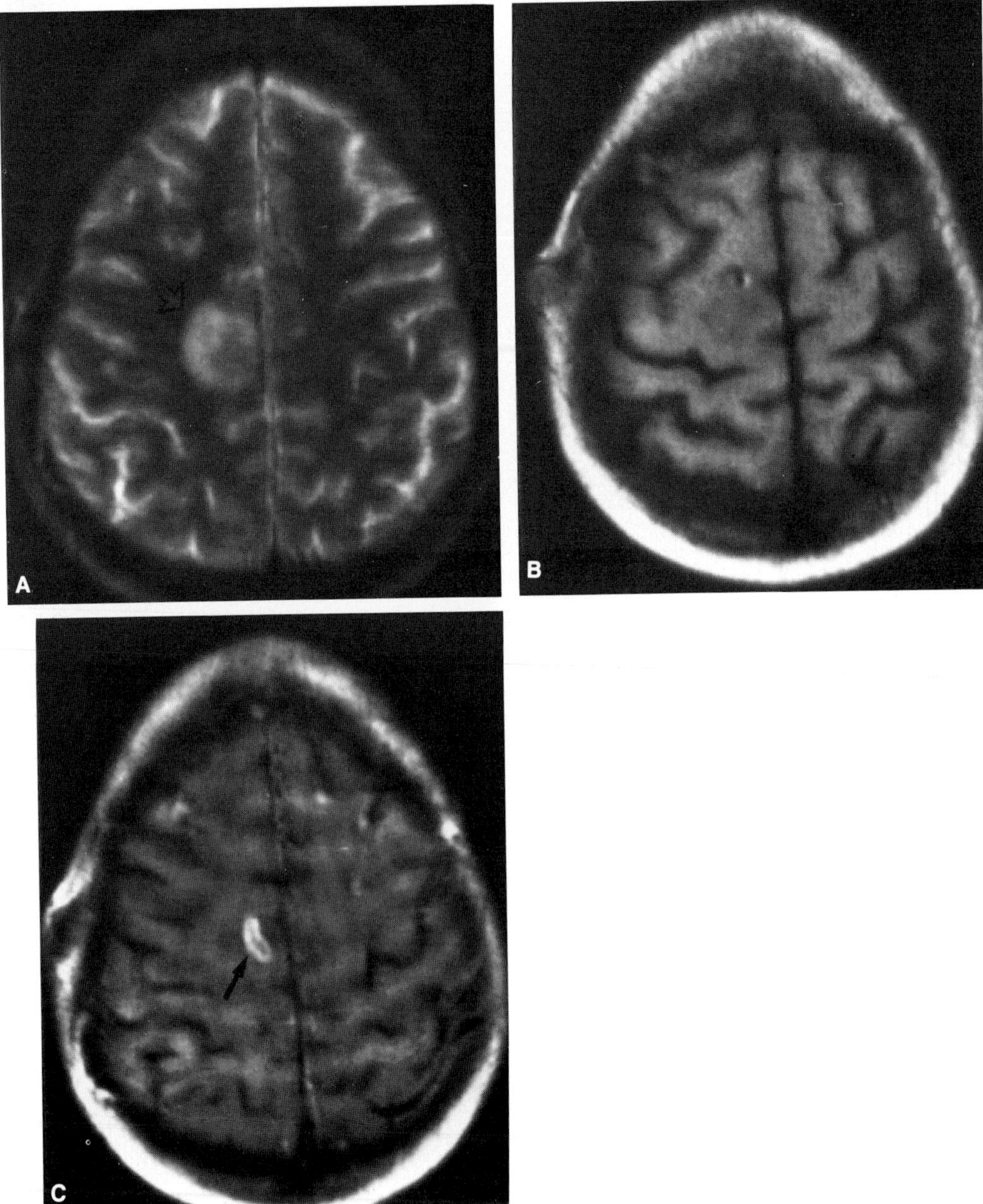

HISTORY

A 27-year-old patient with known tuberculous meningitis

FINDINGS

(*A*) T2-weighted image delineates a lesion at the corticomedullary junction with high signal intensity peripherally (*open arrow*) and relative isointensity centrally. (*B*) Corresponding T1-weighted image reveals only subtle low signal intensity. (*C*) Postcontrast T1-weighted image shows the central portion of the lesion to enhance (*arrow*).

DIAGNOSIS

Intracranial tuberculoma

DISCUSSION

In developing countries, tuberculomas constitute up to 40% of space occupying brain lesions. Most are solitary, although multiple lesions are not uncommon. Serial imaging permits objective assessment of treatment (antituberculous drugs) efficacy.[1] Complete lesion resolution, as assessed by MR, can occur after prolonged therapy (over months to a year or more). Granulomas are seen as ring-enhancing nodules on postcontrast MR.[2] On T2-weighted MR, the center of the lesion can have a variable appearance, from hypointense to hyperintense, the latter presumed to represent liquefaction necrosis. The "capsule," as visualized by contrast enhancement, is often thicker for a tuberculoma than a pyogenic abscess. MR is superior to CT for detection of tuberculomas, in particular those located within the brain stem.

Granulomas may be the result of direct extension of infection from CSF or hematogenous spread. As might be expected from the latter route of dissemination, lesions are most common in a periventricular location and at the corticomedullary junction. By CT, tuberculomas are seen in the minority of patients with tuberculous meningitis. Parenchymal infection may also occur without meningitis.

MR Technique

Contrast enhancement with a gadolinium chelate is advised. Only in this instance is MR superior to CT in the evaluation of active intracranial tuberculosis.

Pitfalls in Image Interpretation

The differential diagnosis in this case is that of a solitary enhancing intraparenchymal lesion, and must include metastatic disease, primary neoplasm, and infection. A history of travel or residence in Third World countries would make a tuberculoma more likely, although even then other entities including cysticercosis should be considered. In the case of a solitary pontine lesion,[3] a tuberculoma must also be considered, in addition to more common abnormalities, including astrocytoma, infarction, and demyelinating disease.

Clinical References

1. Gupta RK, Jena A, Singh AK, et al. Role of magnetic resonance (MR) in the diagnosis and management of intracranial tuberculomas. Clin Radiol 1990;41:120–127.
2. Chang KH, Han MH, Roh JK, et al. Gd-DTPA-enhanced MR imaging in intracranial tuberculosis. Neuroradiology 1990; 32:19–25.
3. Talamas O, Del Brutto OH, Garcia-Ramos G. Brainstem tuberculoma. Arch Neurol 1989;46:529–135.

(A to C from Runge VM. Clinical magnetic resonance imaging. Philadelphia, JB Lippincott, 1990.)

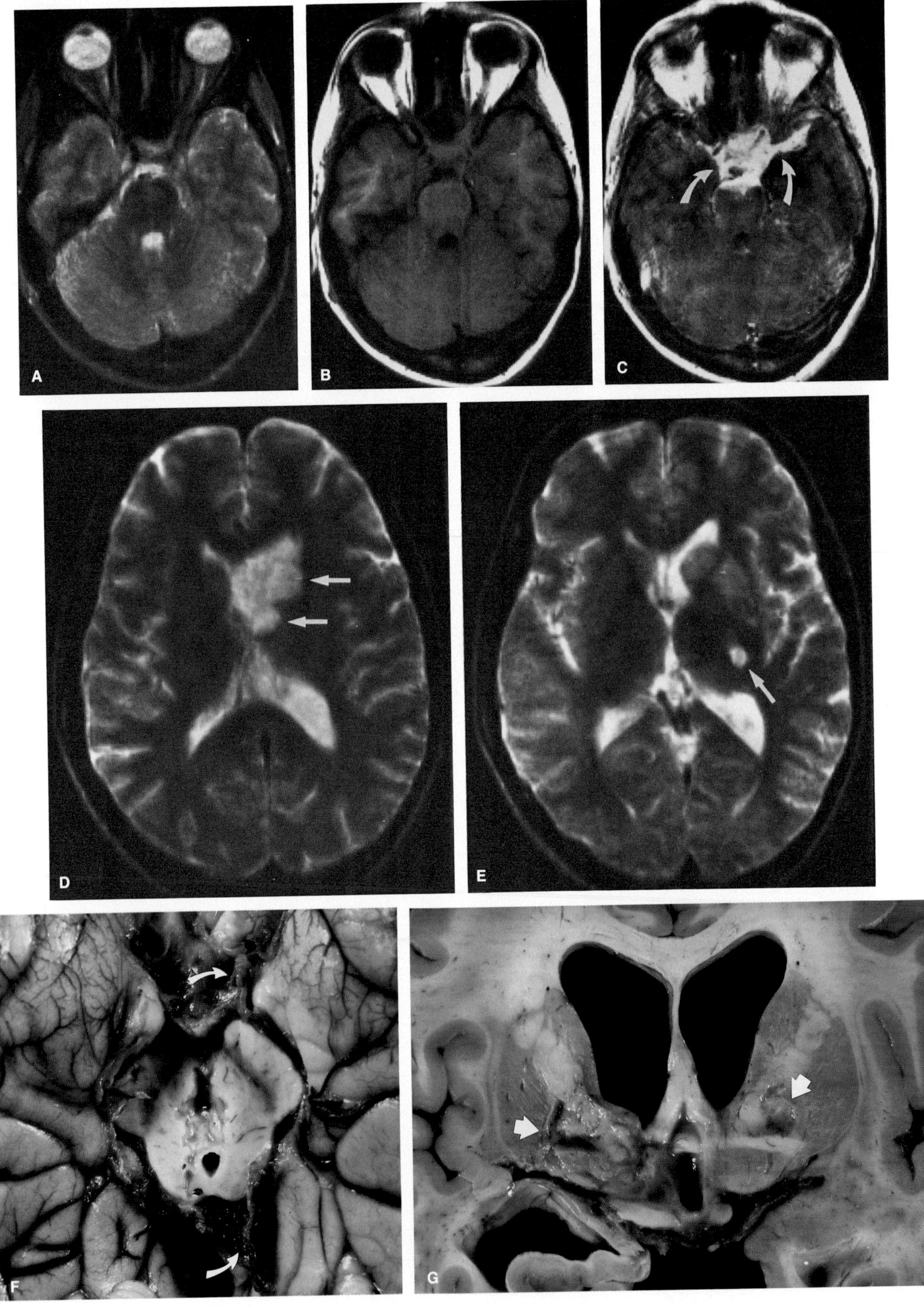
A
B
C
D
E
F
G

HISTORY

A 27-year-old with right hemiparesis

FINDINGS

(*A*) The T2-weighted image at the level of the pons is unremarkable. (*B*) The precontrast T1-weighted image raises the question of abnormal thickening of the basal meninges, particularly surrounding the optic chiasm. (*C*) The postcontrast T1-weighted image demonstrates thick confluent prominent enhancement (*curved arrows*) of the meninges in the prepontine space and supracellular cistern. (*D and E*) Precontrast T2-weighted images demonstrate infarction involving the caudate and thalamus (*arrows in D*), as well as the posterior limb of the left internal capsule (*arrow in E*).

DIAGNOSIS

Tuberculous meningitis

DISCUSSION

CNS involvement with tuberculosis occurs in less than 0.5% of cases in the United States. Tuberculous meningitis is the most common presentation, and traditionally has had the highest incidence in infants and children. As a result of basal meningitis, arteries that course through the basal cisterns can become involved either directly or indirectly, resulting in thrombosis and infarction. The small perforating branches which supply the basal ganglia are most often affected. Communicating hydrocephalus can result due to blockage of the basal cisterns by inflammatory exudate.

Contrast-enhanced T1-weighted MR reveals the characteristic basal meningeal inflammation seen with tuberculous meningitis.[1] Before the clinical introduction of gadolinium chelates, MR was unable to visualize the basal exudate in many cases. After hydrocephalus and basal meningeal disease, infarction is the third most common finding on imaging in tuberculous meningitis. T2-weighted pulse sequences are used to delineate ischemic changes, although these can be difficult to differentiate with certainty from parenchymal inflammatory foci. Ischemia and inflammatory changes are, however, sometimes both present in the same lesion histologically. MR is superior to CT for definition of parenchymal signal abnormalities, particularly those in the brain stem and temporal lobes. MR may also more clearly define ischemic involvement in the basal ganglia and diencephalon.[2]

MR Technique

Precontrast T1- and T2-weighted images are needed in patients with meningitis to delineate ischemia, edema, and subacute hemorrhage.[3] Contrast-enhanced T1-weighted images are required to define active inflammation of the meninges, and also more precisely identify focal lesions. With contrast enhancement, MR is superior to CT in patients with suspected meningitis.

Pathologic Correlate

Whole (base view) (*F*) and cut (coronal) (*G*) specimens from a different patient demonstrate the basal meningitis and secondary infarction of the basal ganglia that can occur in CNS tuberculosis. There is thickening of the meninges (*curved arrows in F*) both anterior and posterior to the cerebral peduncles and lacunar infarction (*arrows in G*) involving the globus pallidus bilaterally.

Clinical References

1. Offenbacher H, Fazekas F, Schmidt R, et al. MRI in tuberculous meningoencephalitis: report of four cases and review of the neuroimaging literature. J Neurol 1991; 238:340–344.
2. Schoeman J, Hewlett R, Donald P. MR of childhood tuberculous meningitis. Radiology 1988;30:473–477.
3. Chang KH, Han MH, Roh JK, et al. Gd-DTPA-enhanced MR imaging of the brain in patients with meningitis: comparison with CT. AJR 1990;154:809–816.

(A *to* E *from Runge VM. Clinical magnetic resonance imaging. Philadelphia, JB Lippincott, 1990;* F *and* G *courtesy of Daron G. Davis, MD.*)

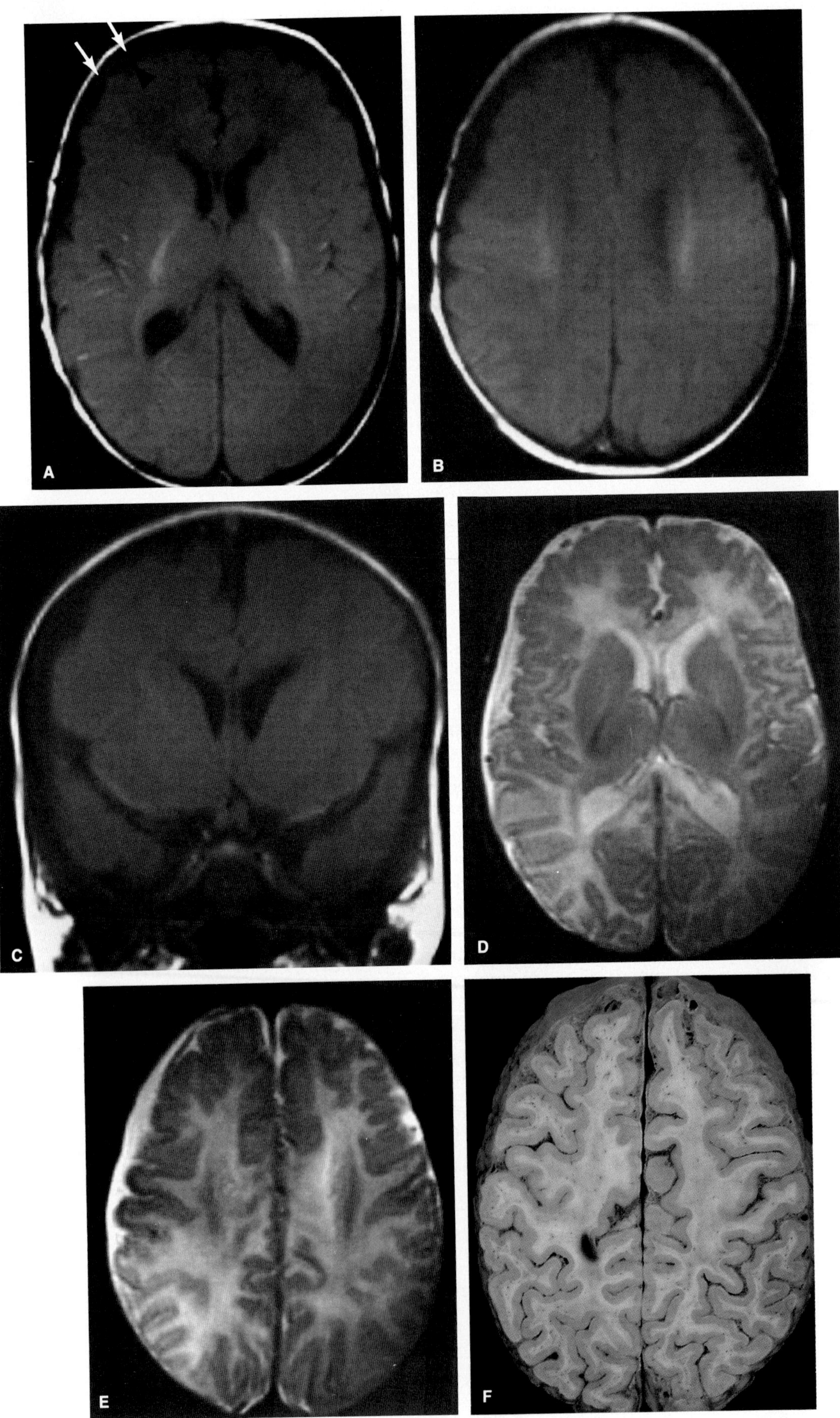
A
B
C
D
E
F

HISTORY

A 1-month-old infant with seizures

FINDINGS

(*A and B*) T1-weighted axial images at two different levels demonstrate extraaxial fluid collections adjacent to the frontal lobes bilaterally, the right larger than the left. The fluid collections are located between the brain and the dura (*white arrows in A*), and thus lie in the subdural space. The signal intensity of the subdural fluid is slightly higher than CSF on T1-weighted images. Within the subdural fluid on the right, there are linear foci of intermediate signal intensity (*arrowhead in A*) bridging the space between the brain and dura, probably due to purulent material or thickened membranes. (*C*) The subdural fluid extends over the high convexity of the cerebral hemispheres, best seen on this T1-weighted coronal image. (*D and E*) T2-weighted axial images show that the subdural fluid is isointense to slightly hyperintense compared with CSF. The brain appears normal.

DIAGNOSIS

Bacterial meningitis

DISCUSSION

Meningitis is defined as inflammation of the meninges of the brain or spinal cord. Bacterial meningitis is usually caused by hematogenous spread of pyogenic organisms, most commonly *Streptococcus pneumoniae, Neisseria meningitidis,* and *Haemophilus influenzae* in the general population. *Escherichia coli,* other gram-negative rods, and group B streptococci are common in neonates. This patient had *S. pneumoniae* in the CSF obtained by lumbar puncture.

Acute bacterial meningitis is rapidly lethal without treatment. Despite the use of antibiotics, acute bacterial meningitis is often accompanied by short- and long-term complications including cerebral infarction, brain edema, deafness, intellectual impairment, ventriculomegaly, and the development of subdural effusions.[1] Subdural effusions are most common in children with meningitis due to *H. influenzae,* although they can be seen with any organism, including viruses.[2] Subdural collections are more easily seen by MR than CT because of the lack of artifact from the adjacent skull. On MR, subdural effusions associated with meningitis are usually bilateral and are located in the frontoparietal extraaxial space. They are usually slightly hyperintense compared with CSF on all pulse sequences.

Uncomplicated meningitis may produce no detectable abnormalities on MR. Severe cases cause abnormal enhancement of the leptomeninges after contrast infusion, which is better detected by MR than CT.

Pitfalls in Image Interpretation

A simple subdural effusion must be differentiated from a subdural empyema. Subdural empyemas are uncommon extracerebral pyogenic infections that are usually secondary to previous trauma or otorhinologic infection. They are rarely associated with meningitis. Empyemas are more proteinaceous than a simple effusion and thus will have a higher signal intensity on T1-weighted images.

Pathologic Correlate

(*F*) An axial cross section of a gross specimen from a patient with pneumococcal meningitis. Thick, neutrophilic exudate fills the subdural and subarachnoid space, including the sulci, particularly in the frontal lobes.

Clinical References

1. Cockrill H, Dreisbach J, Lowe B, et al. Computed tomography in leptomeningeal infections. AJR 1978;130:511–515.
2. Sze G, Zimmerman R. The magnetic resonance imaging of infections and inflammatory diseases. Radiol Clin North Am 1988;26:839–859.

(F from Okazaki H, Scheithauer B. Slide atlas of neuropathology. New York, Gower Medical Publishing, 1988. By permission of Mayo Foundation.)

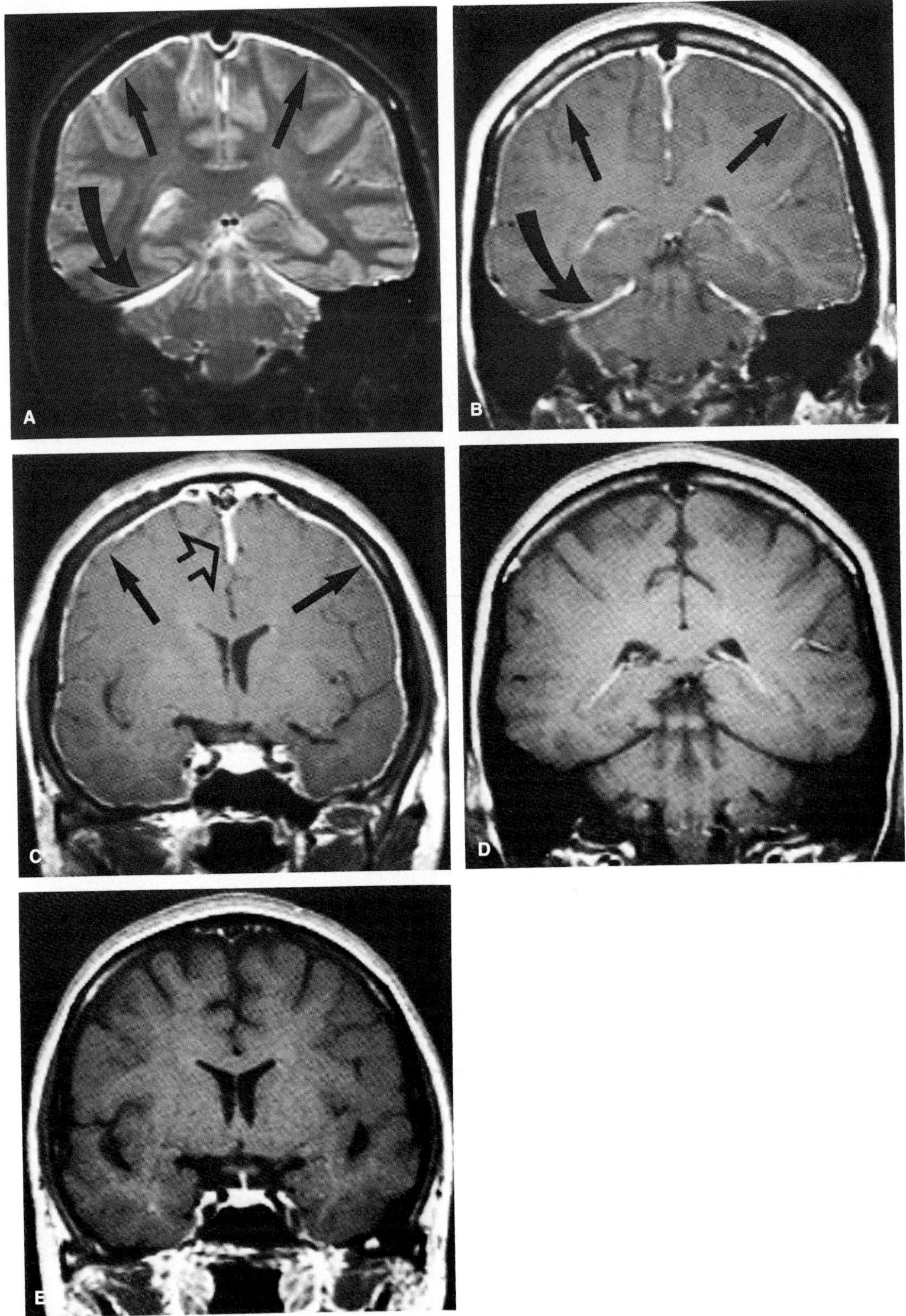
A
B
C
D
E

HISTORY

A 30-year-old patient presenting to the emergency department with severe headache, vomiting, and photophobia

FINDINGS

(*A*) Coronal T2-weighted (TE = 70 msec) scan reveals abnormal fluid along both the tentorium (*curved arrow*) and convexity (*arrows*). (*B and C*) Coronal postcontrast T1-weighted scans at two levels demonstrate abnormal enhancement of the tentorium (*curved arrow in B*), falx (*open arrow in C*), and dura (*circumferential arrows in B and C*). Four months later, following treatment, the MR examination is within normal limits. (*D and E*) Coronal postcontrast T1-weighted scans reveal no abnormal enhancement. The cortical sulci are now well seen as a result of resolution of generalized pressure effects.

DIAGNOSIS

Viral meningitis

DISCUSSION

Contrast-enhanced MR has been shown to be far more sensitive than enhanced CT for identification of meningeal disease due to infection.[1] Abnormal leptomeningeal enhancement correlates with inflammatory cell infiltration. Additional possible complications, such as ventriculitis and cerebritis, are also more effectively identified. Mild leptomeningitis, ependymitis, and cerebritis may not, however, demonstrate abnormal enhancement.

Associated changes, including infarction, edema, subacute hemorrhage, and subdural fluid collections are well depicted by precontrast T2-weighted images, with greater sensitivity than CT.[2]

MR Technique

IV gadolinium chelate administration is necessary to identify meningeal inflammation on MR. Unenhanced MR is insensitive and may reveal only abnormal extraaxial fluid.

Pitfalls in Image Interpretation

Generalized meningeal enhancement can also be due to a diffuse chemical arachnoiditis that may follow surgery (with bleeding into the subarachnoid space).

Clinical References

1. Mathews VP, Kuharik MA, Edwards MK, et al. Gd-DTPA-enhanced MR imaging of experimental bacterial meningitis: evaluation and comparison with CT. AJNR 1988;9:1045–1050.
2. Chang KH, Han MH, Roh JK, et al. Gd-DTPA-enhanced MR imaging of the brain in patients with meningitis: comparison with CT. AJR 1990;154:809–816.

(A *to* E *courtesy of Clifford Wolf, MD.*)

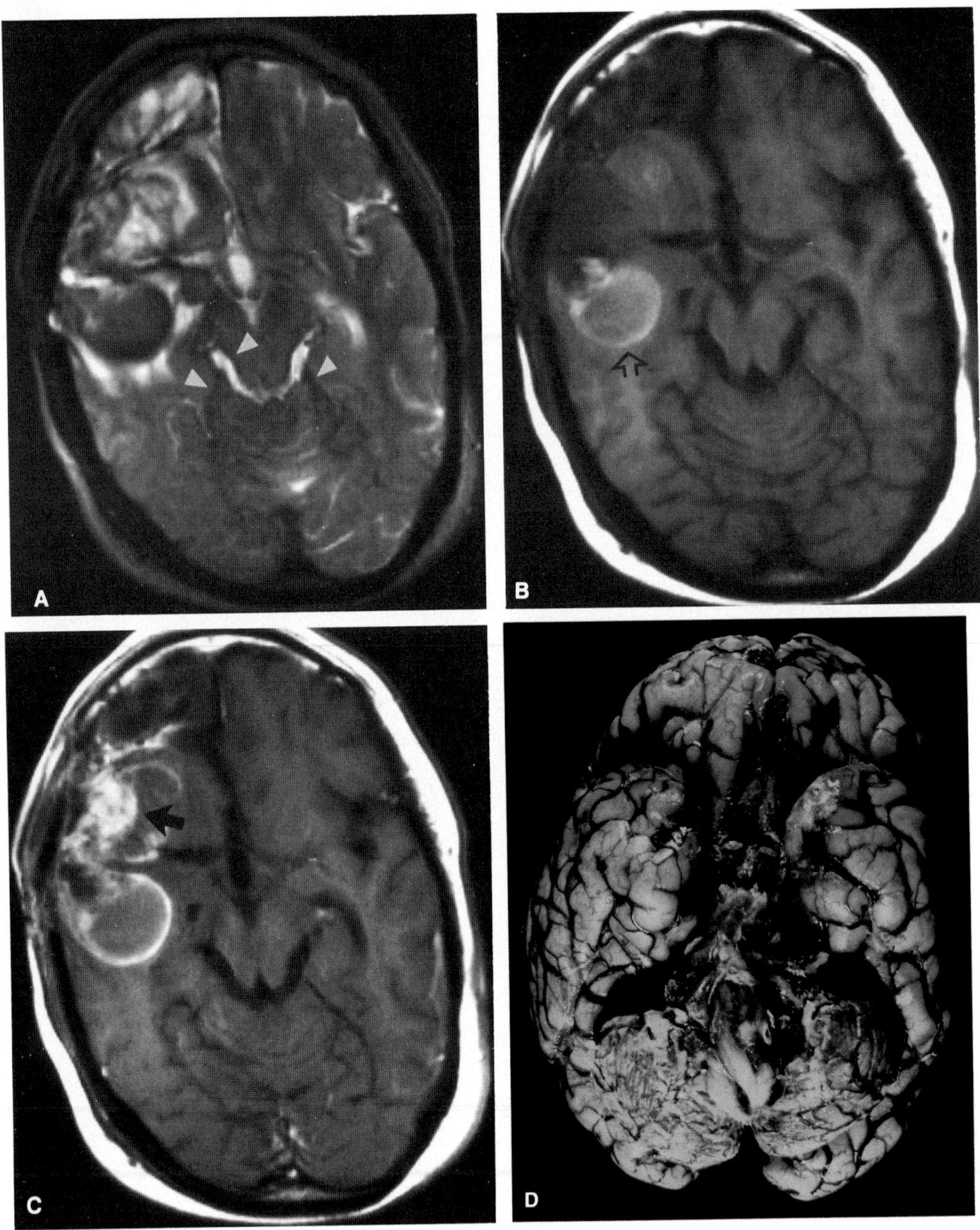

HISTORY

A 36-year-old patient with three previous surgeries for resection of an oligodendroglioma

FINDINGS

(*A*) This T2-weighted image (TR/TE = 3000/90) is presented primarily for discussion of the origin of the hypointensity (*arrowheads*) noted lining the brain stem and cerebellar folia. There has been a previous right frontal and temporal craniotomy, with underlying brain changes. (*B*) On the precontrast T1-weighted image, a collection of abnormal hyperintensity (*open arrow*) indicating the presence of hemorrhage is noted. (*C*) The postcontrast T1-weighted image shows multiple areas of abnormal contrast enhancement, with the central mass of enhancing tissue (*arrow*) representing recurrent tumor.

DIAGNOSIS

Superficial siderosis

DISCUSSION

Superficial siderosis is caused by hemosiderin deposition in the leptomeninges from chronic subarachnoid hemorrhage.[1] Sources of recurrent bleeding include neoplasm (ependymoma, oligodendroglioma) and neonatal intraventricular hemorrhage.[2] Microscopically, most of the hemosiderin is contained within macrophages.

In superficial siderosis, there are characteristic findings on high field (1.5 T) MR scans. T1-weighted images are typically normal. T2-weighted images, however, reveal hypointensity of the pial and arachnoid membranes. The cerebellum is a common site for hemosiderin deposition, with more prominent hypointensity typically observed. Hemosiderin deposits can also be well demonstrated on GRE scans. Intraventricular siderosis is seen most commonly secondary to neonatal hemorrhage but can also be observed as a result of hemorrhage from aneurysms and vascular malformations. Images in the current case were acquired at 1 T, with this and lower field strengths less sensitive in detection of abnormal hemosiderin deposition, particularly on SE images.

The clinical syndrome of superficial siderosis becomes manifest only with heavy hemosiderin deposition. Such patients can have sensorineural hearing loss, pyramidal tract signs, cerebellar dysfunction, and progressive mental deterioration. Cranial nerves II, V, VII, and VIII (with the latter particularly sensitive to injury) can be affected, with the severity of nerve injury proportional to the proximal (glial) length of the nerve. Although the clinical syndrome of superficial siderosis is rare, lesser degrees of abnormal hemosiderin deposition with little or no clinical symptoms are frequent.

MR Technique

At high field (1.5 T), T2-weighted SE images can be used for detection of superficial siderosis. GRE imaging is more sensitive, however, and can provide delineation of this disease at lower field strengths. Hypointensity is observed as the result of an increase in magnetic susceptibility caused by heterogeneous distribution of hemosiderin.

Pathologic Correlate

(*D*) Gross pathologic specimen from a different patient, also with recurrent subarachnoid hemorrhage due to an oligodendroglioma, is presented for comparison. Note the yellow–rusty brown staining on the surface of the brain caused by hemosiderin deposition.

Clinical References

1. Kwartler JA, De La Cruz A, Lo WW. Superficial siderosis of the central nervous system. Ann Otol Rhinol Laryngol 1991;100:249–250.
2. Gomori JM, Grossman RI, Goldberg HI, et al. High-field spin-echo MR imaging of superficial and subependymal siderosis secondary to neonatal intraventricular hemorrhage. Neuroradiology 1987;29:339–342.

*(*A *to* C *from Runge VM. Clinical magnetic resonance imaging. Philadelphia, JP Lippincott, 1990;* D *courtesy of Daron G. Davis, MD.)*

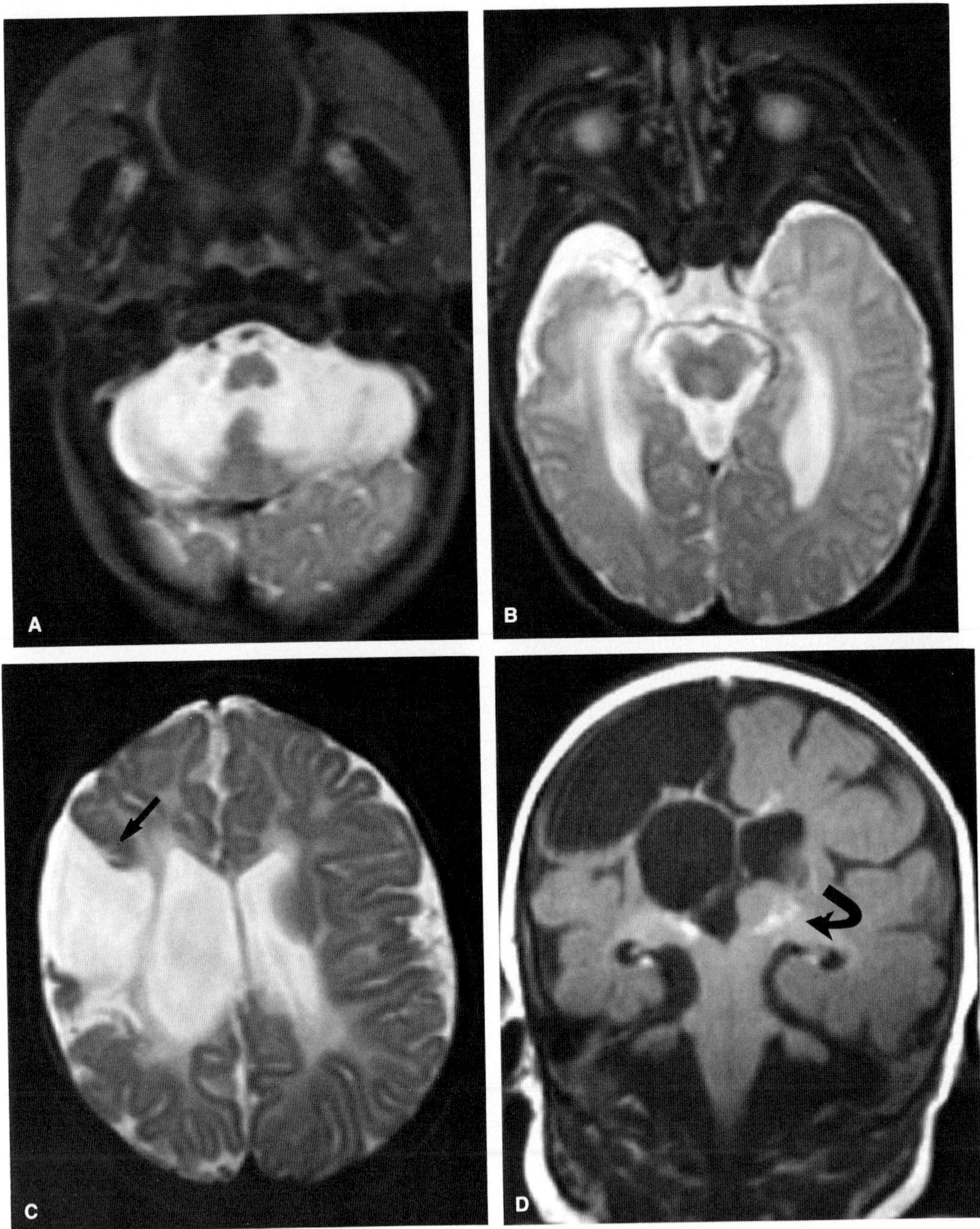

HISTORY

A 6-month-old infant who was noted at birth to have microcephaly and a vesiculopustular rash

FINDINGS

(*A to C*) T2-weighted SE images (TR/TE = 3500/90) at three anatomic levels are presented. (*A*) At the level of the medulla, loss of brain tissue is noted in the cerebellar hemispheres bilaterally. (*B*) The cerebral peduncles are small, and there is generalized brain underdevelopment. (*C*) At the level of the lateral ventricles, a large area of cystic encephalomalacia is noted on the right (*arrow*), with compensatory dilatation of the right lateral ventricle. The white matter demonstrates abnormal increased signal intensity, consistent with delayed myelinization. (*D*) The coronal T1-weighted image, which is slightly degraded by motion artifact, once again depicts brain underdevelopment (specifically the brain does not completely fill the bony calvarium). The ventricles are large bilaterally. Again seen is loss of cerebellar hemispheric brain tissue. The markedly increased signal intensity in the basal ganglia region (*curved arrow*) could be explained by dystrophic calcification.

DIAGNOSIS

Herpes encephalitis (type 2)

DISCUSSION

The imaging findings of neonatal herpes simplex encephalitis have been well described on CT.[1] Early in the disease course, there may be patchy or widespread low attenuation (edema) primarily confined to white matter. These areas increase rapidly in size and prominence, and are accompanied by a transient increase in attenuation of cortical gray matter (the latter possibly due to marked vasodilatation and resultant increased cerebral blood volume). Atrophic changes appear rapidly in neonatal herpes simplex encephalitis. Late findings on CT include extensive, diffuse white matter low attenuation (multicystic encephalomalacia) with cortical atrophy. Calcification can assume a variety of patterns from punctate to gyral. In one CT study, the cerebellum was involved in more than half of the patients.[1]

The findings on MR in neonatal herpes simplex encephalitis are not well described, although they can be predicted from the known evolution of the disease, with early localized or generalized edematous changes evolving to multicystic encephalomalacia.[2] Imaging findings and final outcome are consistent with a severe widespread necrotizing meningoencephalitis.

MR Technique

In the neonate, the T2 of normal brain tissue is prolonged owing to increased water content and the lack of myelinization. The use of a long TR (3500 to 4000 msec) is important to provide sufficient contrast for visualization of gray and white matter parenchymal abnormalities. In this context, FSE techniques (which allow the use of a long TR and yet can be obtained in a substantially shorter scan time than conventional techniques) are advantageous.

Pitfalls in Image Interpretation

Early findings on MR in neonatal herpes simplex encephalitis can be subtle. Normal cerebral white matter on T1-weighted images in neonates is of low signal intensity, with the abnormality in herpes encephalitis seen as simply one of degree (greater hypointensity). T2-weighted scans are similarly limited, since neonatal white matter normally exhibits very high signal intensity because of the absence of myelination and high water content. The findings on CT early in the disease course are similarly subtle. For this reason, it is important to check neonatal MR scans closely with regard to gray and white matter signal intensity. Gray matter involvement, seen early in disease evolution, can lead to loss of gray–white matter contrast on MR. This finding can be bilateral and somewhat symmetric, thus also being difficult to detect.[3]

Clinical References

1. Noorbehesht B, Enzmann DR, Sullender W, et al. Neonatal herpes simplex encephalitis: correlation of clinical and CT findings. Radiology 1987;162:813–819.
2. Taccone A, Gambaro G, Ghiorzi M, et al. Computed tomography (CT) in children with herpes simplex encephalitis. Pediatr Radiol 1988;19:9–12.
3. Enzmann D, Chang Y, Augustyn G. MR findings in neonatal herpes simplex encephalitis type II. J Comput Assist Tomogr 1990;14:453–457.

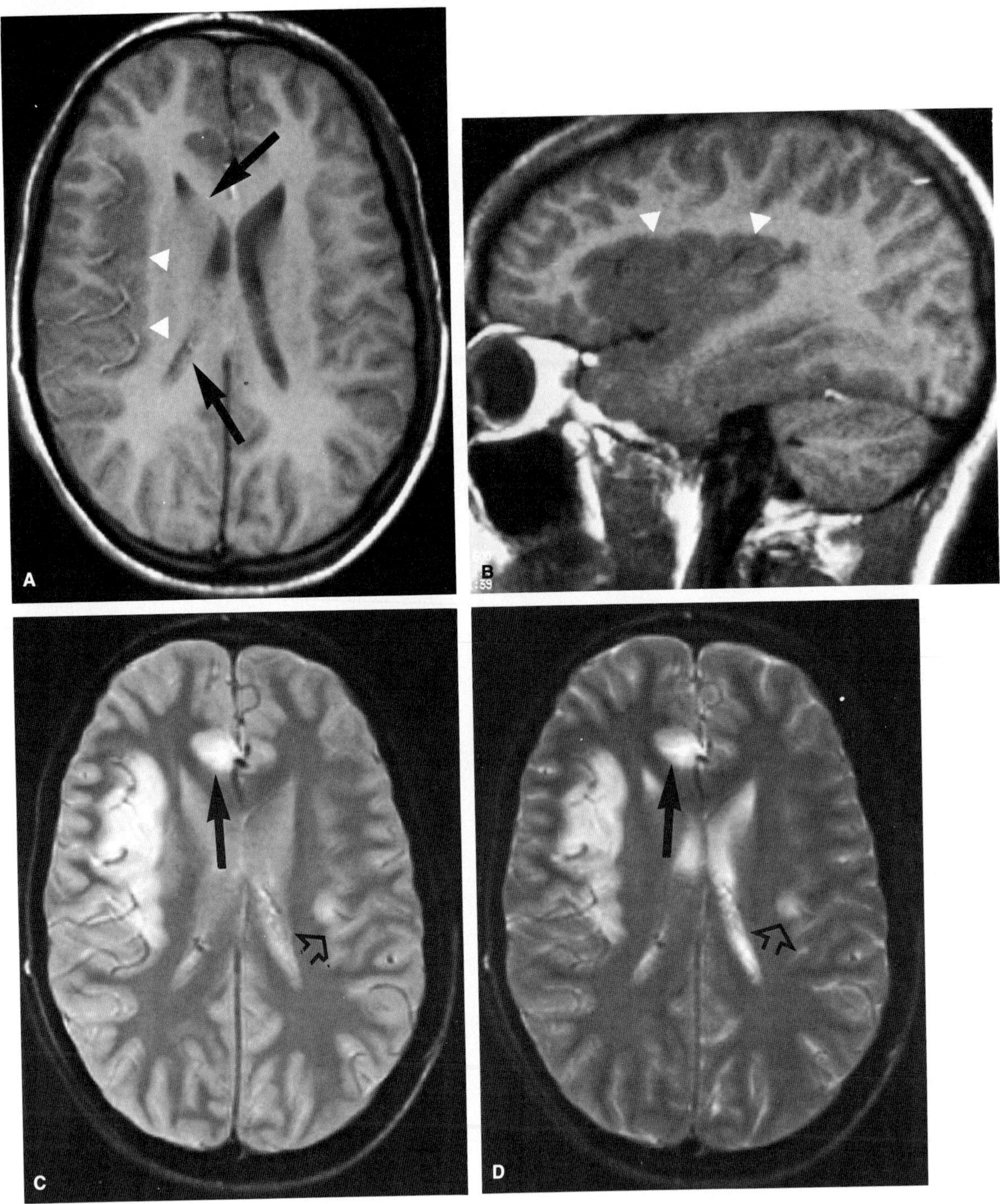

HISTORY

A 16-year-old patient with lethargy and new onset of seizures

FINDINGS

T2-weighted axial (*A*) and sagittal (*B*) images demonstrate low signal intensity and swelling of the insular cortex (*white arrowheads*), and the directly adjacent subcortical white matter. The corresponding region has high signal intensity on the intermediate (*C*) and heavily (*D*) T2-weighted axial images. In addition, there is abnormal high signal intensity in the medial right frontal cortex (*arrow*) and the left insular cortex (*open arrow*). Mass effect is identified, with partial obliteration of the right lateral ventricle (*black arrows in A*). (*E*) On the postcontrast T1-weighted axial image there is abnormal meningeal enhancement adjacent to the right insular cortex

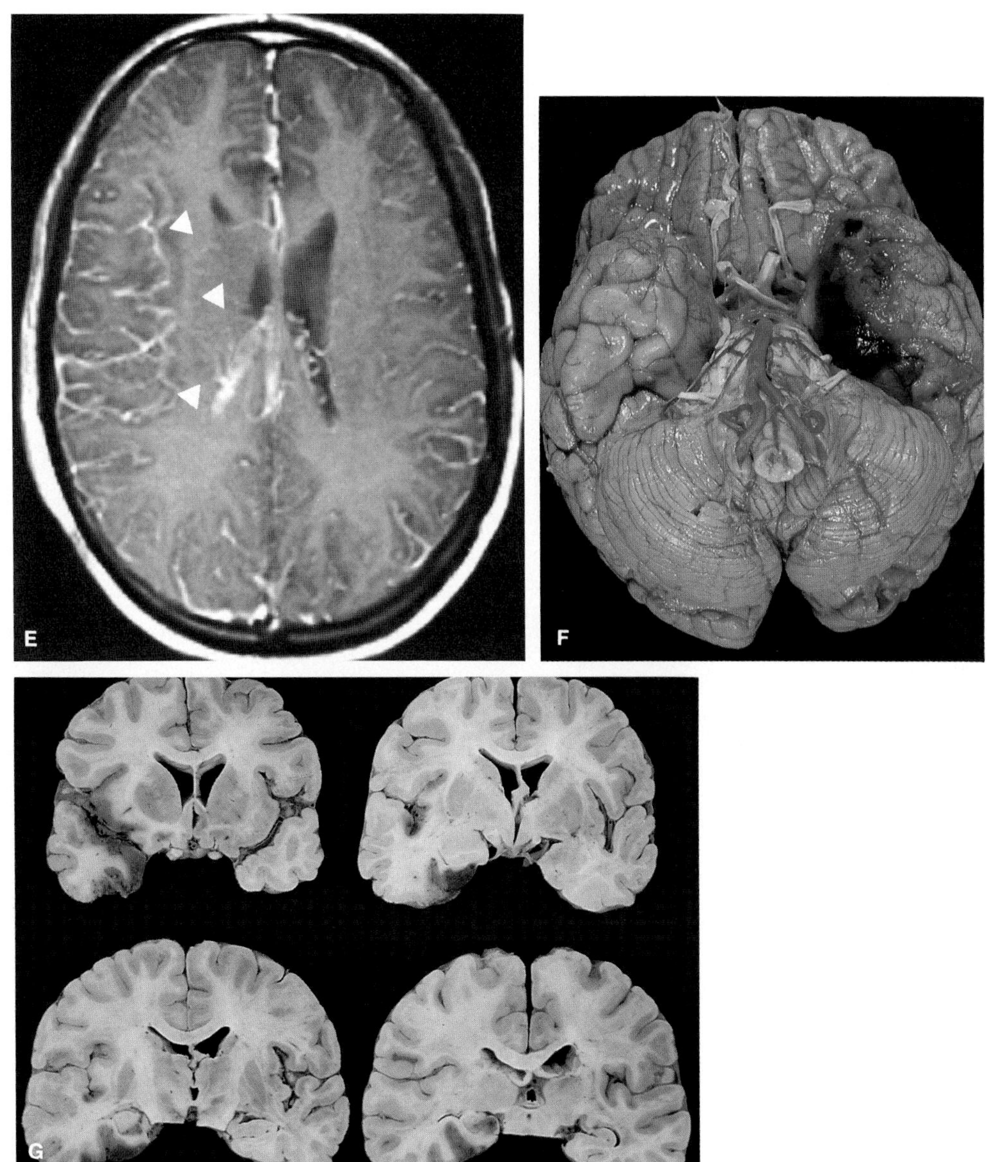

(*white arrowheads*). Abnormal low signal intensity is also seen in the cortex of the right temporal lobe (*black arrows in B*).

DIAGNOSIS

Herpes encephalitis (type 1)

DISCUSSION

Herpes encephalitis may result from CNS infection with either herpes simplex virus type 1 (HSV-1) or type 2 (HSV-2). In the neonate, encephalitis is a primary infection usually due to HSV-2 acquired during vaginal delivery. In older children and adults, HSV-1 is the most common cause of sporadic viral encephalitis in the United States.[1] Nearly every adult has had exposure to HSV-1, which causes cold sores. Encephalitis results from reactivation of latent infection in the trigeminal ganglion, with spread along the branches of the trigeminal nerve (cranial nerve V) that innervate the meninges of the middle and anterior cranial fossa. As a result, herpes encephalitis most commonly affects the temporal and inferior frontal lobes.

The clinical symptoms of herpes encephalitis typically evolve over several days. Patients may present with headache, fever, seizures, expressive or receptive aphasia, behavioral changes, and confusion. Early diagnosis of herpes encephalitis is critical to prevent the hemorrhage and necrosis seen in advanced disease.[2] Mortality is as high as 70% in cases not treated with the antiviral drug acyclovir.[1]

MR is much more sensitive than CT for detection of the early inflammatory changes in herpes encephalitis. Abnormal high signal intensity on T2-weighted images in both the cortex and white matter of the involved areas of the brain can be seen as early as the second day after the onset of illness.[2] Herpes encephalitis is commonly unilateral initially, but subsequent bilateral involvement is not unusual.

Pitfalls in Image Interpretation

The differential diagnosis for unilateral abnormal high signal intensity on T2-weighted images localized to the temporal and inferior frontal lobes, with mass effect, includes low-grade glioma and infarction. Follow-up examinations to detect contralateral disease or improvement after acyclovir therapy are often useful in confirming the diagnosis of herpes encephalitis. In addition, herpes encephalitis usually spares the putamen.

Pathologic Correlate

Unfixed brain (*F*) and multiple fixed coronal (*G*) sections from a different subject demonstrate the typical gross appearance of herpes encephalitis. There is hemorrhagic necrosis of the cortex of the right inferior frontal lobe, insula, and temporal lobe. The petechial hemorrhagic component of the necrosis in herpes encephalitis is not usually seen with MR.

Clinical References

1. Lester J, Carter M, Reynolds T. Herpes encephalitis: MR monitoring of response to acyclovir therapy. J Comput Assist Tomogr 1988;12:941–943.
2. Schroth G, Kretzschmar K, Gawehn J, et al. Advantage of magnetic resonance imaging in the diagnosis of cerebral infections. Neuroradiology 1987;29:120–126.

(F and G from Okazaki H, Scheithauer B. Slide atlas of neuropathology. New York, Gower Medical Publishing, 1988. By permission of Mayo Foundation.)

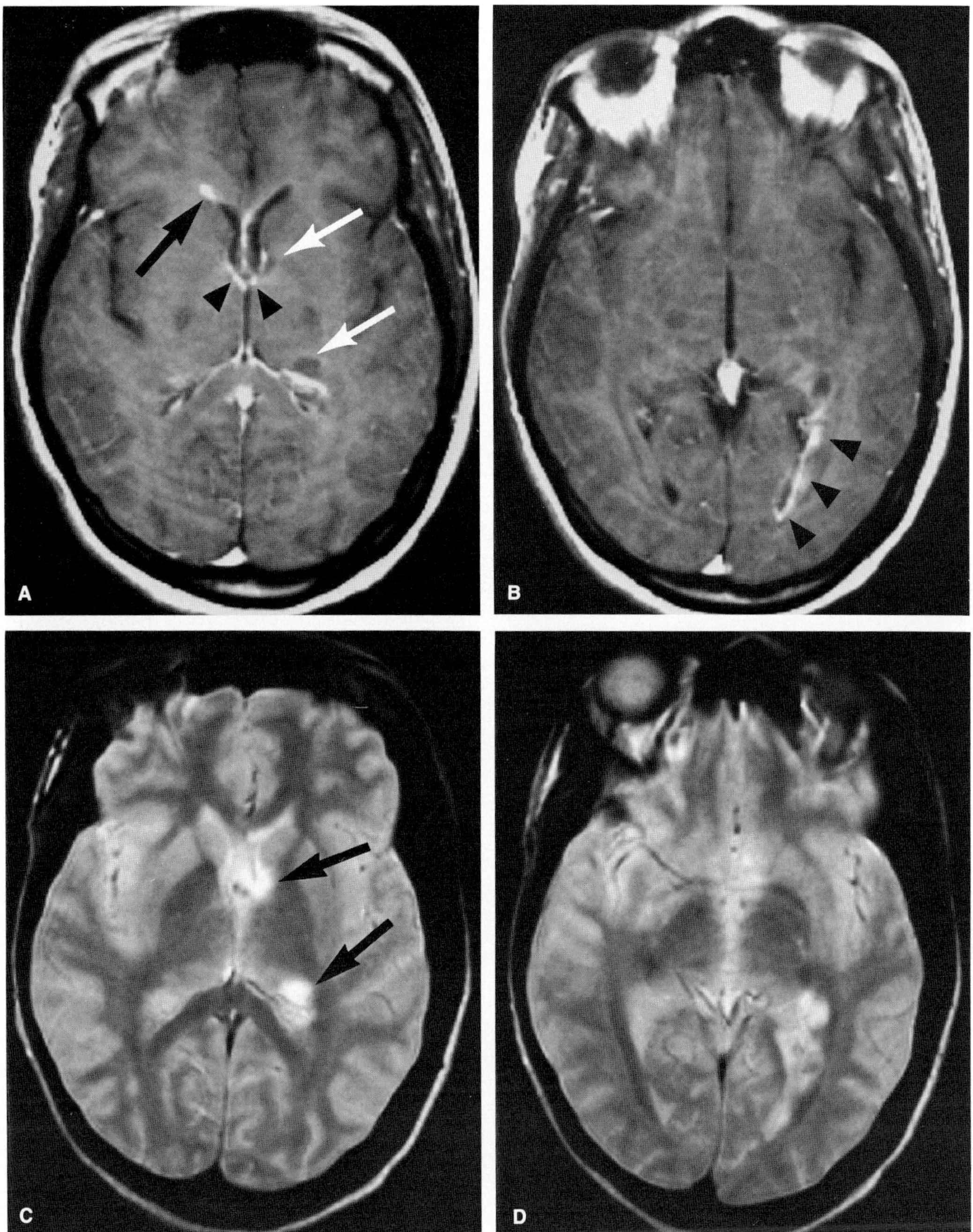

HISTORY

A 25-year-old with 1 week of nausea, vomiting, fever, and a rash

FINDINGS

(*A and B*) Postcontrast T1-weighted axial images demonstrate abnormal enhancement of the ventricular lining of the right frontal horn (*arrow in A*), near the foramen of Monro bilaterally (*arrowheads in A*), and of the ependyma of the left ventricular atrium and occipital horn (*arrowheads in B*). In addition, there are subtle low-signal-intensity lesions with peripheral enhancement in the brain parenchyma directly adjacent to the abnormal ventricles (*white arrows in A*). (*C*) Intermediate T2-weighted axial image at the same level as *A* shows these lesions (*arrows*) to have increased signal intensity. (*D*) Intermediate T2-weighted image at the same level as *B* shows irregular contour of the left ventricular atrium and occipital horn, with abnormal high signal intensity in the periventricular white matter.

DIAGNOSIS

Ependymitis (ventriculitis), secondary to measles

DISCUSSION

Ependymitis is inflammation of the ependymal lining of the cerebral ventricles, and is also referred to as ventriculitis. Ependymitis is an uncommon complication of meningitis or encephalitis, and is usually bacterial in origin.[1] Ependymitis can also occur following intraventricular shunt placement, surgery, intrathecal chemotherapy, bacteremia, and contiguous extension of otitis media or paranasal sinusitis.[1]

On MR, ependymitis is manifested by abnormally increased signal intensity of the ventricular lining and CSF on T2-weighted images. The CSF also has an abnormally high signal intensity on T1-weighted images and there often is enhancement of the affected ventricular walls after contrast infusion.[1] Abnormalities in periventricular white matter are common.

Measles may be complicated by the direct effects of the virus on the brain and meninges or by postinfectious encephalomyelitis. Postinfectious encephalomyelitis occurs in approximately 1 in 1000 cases of measles and is thought to be an autoimmune demyelinating disease.[2] Neurologic signs and symptoms usually appear 3 to 21 days after the measles rash and include headache, vomiting, fever, and stupor. Involvement of the spinal cord may cause flaccid paraplegia and absence of deep tendon reflexes.

Pitfalls in Image Interpretation

The differential diagnosis for enhancement of the ependymal lining of the ventricles includes intraventricular metastatic disease. Ependymal tumor deposits usually have a nodular pattern.

Clinical References

1. Barloon T, Yuh W, Knepper L, et al. Cerebral ventriculitis: MR findings. J Comput Assist Tomogr 1990;14:272–275.
2. Johnson R. The pathogenesis of acute viral encephalitis and postinfectious encephalomyelitis. J Infect Dis 1987;155: 359–364.

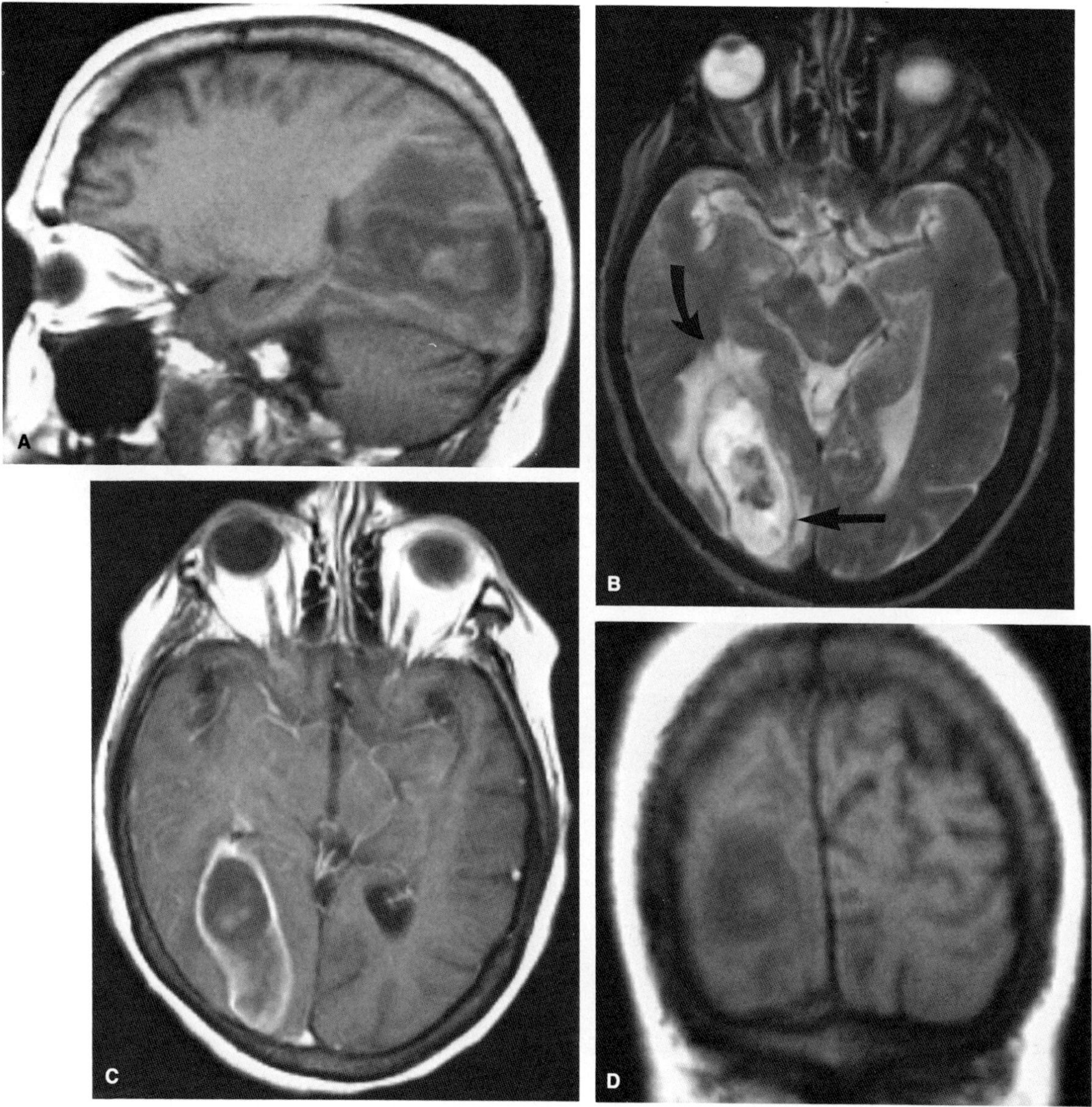

HISTORY

A 65-year-old woman with a visual field cut and altered mental status

FINDINGS

Precontrast sagittal T1-weighted (*A*) and axial T2-weighted (*B*) images identify a right occipital mass with surrounding edema (*curved arrow in B*). There is a distinct circumferential low-signal-intensity rim (*arrow in B*) on the T2-weighted image. (*C*) Ring enhancement is noted on the contrast-enhanced axial T1-weighted scan. Comparison of precontrast (*D*) and postcontrast (*E*) coronal T1-weighted images demonstrates a thick uniform enhancing rim. (*F*) The enhanced CT image is comparable to *C,* with relatively poor demonstration of cerebral edema compared with the T2-weighted image (*B*).

DIAGNOSIS

Brain abscess

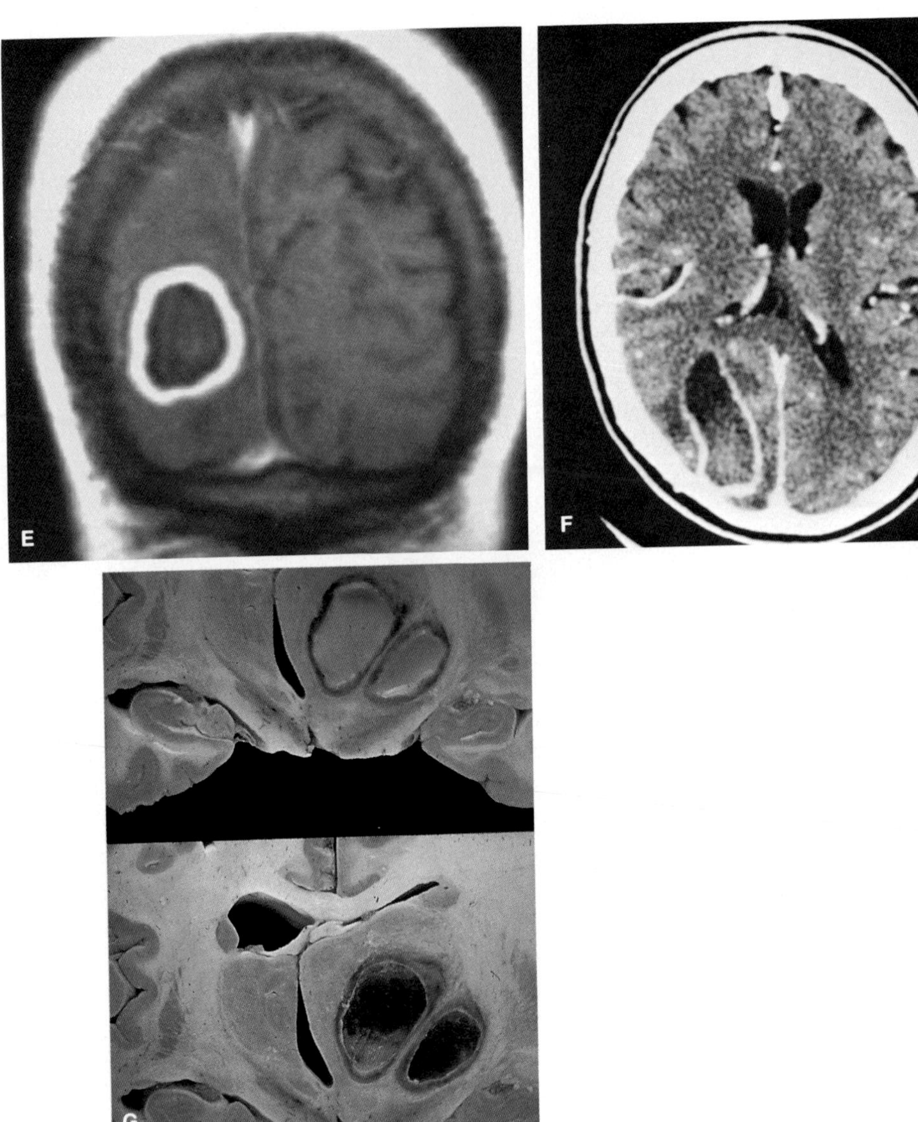

DISCUSSION

Features characteristic of a pyogenic cerebral abscess on MR include (1) central necrosis; (2) visualization of the abscess capsule (hypointense on T2-weighted scans); (3) surrounding vasogenic edema; and (4) extraparenchymal spread, to the CSF in the ventricular system or the subarachnoid space. Only the first three features are illustrated here.[1] The necrotic contents may be heterogeneous in signal characteristics. Lesions are classically located at the corticomedullary junction and demonstrate a smooth, well-defined, enhancing rim. The medial edge of this rim may be thinner than that demonstrated laterally, presumably on the basis of greater vascularity for gray matter as compared with white matter. Experimentally, untreated cerebral infection progresses from cerebritis to capsule stages, with contrast enhancement present even in early cerebritis, as a result of blood–brain barrier disruption. In the early stages of evolution, a brain abscess may be missed on MR unless IV contrast is administered.[2] Cultures for the lesion illustrated were positive for gram-positive cocci.

Because of early diagnosis and rapid detection of treatment failures or complications, the era of CT brought a marked improvement in survival of patients with brain abscess.

MR Technique

IV contrast administration is recommended for assessment of lesion activity and for identification of early brain infection.

Pitfalls in Image Interpretation

A high-grade astrocytoma, large solitary necrotic metastasis, or granuloma can mimic the appearance of a brain abscess.

Pathologic Correlate

(*G*) Two well-encapsulated abscesses on coronal gross section. The upper view was photographed with pus still within the cavities and the lower view with the pus drained, more clearly depicting the cavities and their walls. In a mature brain abscess, the layer of granulation tissue at the periphery evolves into a thick collagenous wall, containing the infection and preventing further spread.

Clinical References

1. Haimes AB, Zimmerman RD, Morgello S, et al. MR imaging of brain abscesses. AJNR 1989;10:279–291.
2. Runge VM, Clanton JA, Price AC, et al. Evaluation of contrast-enhanced MR imaging in a brain abscess model. AJNR 1985;6:139–147.

(G from Okazaki H, Scheithauer B. Slide atlas of neuropathology. New York, Gower Medical Publishing, 1988. By permission of Mayo Foundation.)

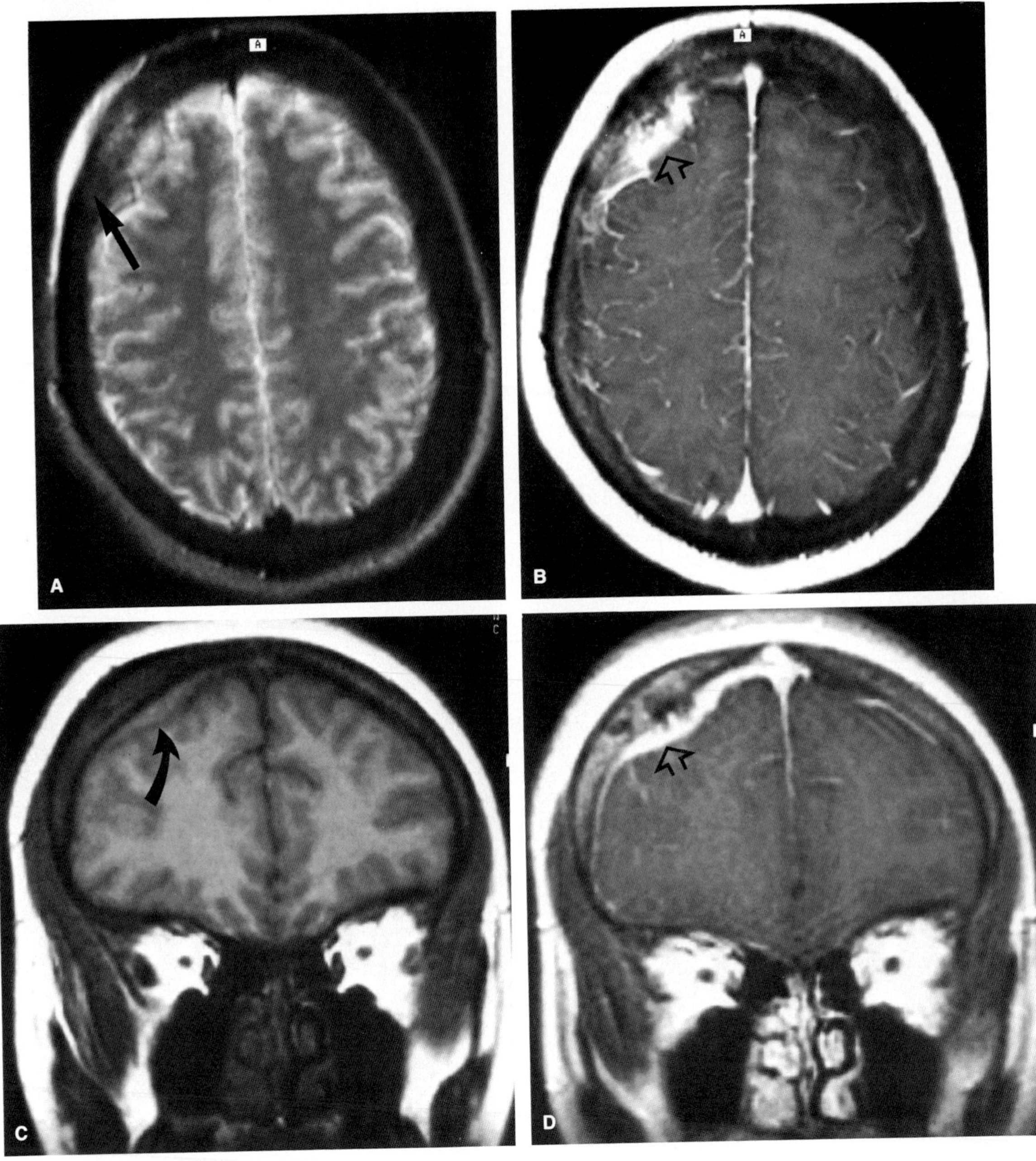

HISTORY

A 24-year-old inmate with progressive right-sided headache, fever, and vomiting for 3 weeks. Blood cultures were positive for *Salmonella* organisms.

FINDINGS

(*A*) T2-weighted axial section demonstrates abnormal high signal intensity (*arrow*), corresponding to subcutaneous soft tissue edema in the right frontal region. There is also a subtle abnormal increase in signal intensity of the adjacent diploic space (between the inner and outer tables of the skull). (*B*) Postcontrast axial T1-weighted scan confirms involvement of the marrow. An enhancing extraaxial mass (*open arrow*) is also identified. Comparison of precontrast (*C*) and postcontrast (*D*) coronal scans better demonstrates this mass (*open arrow in D*). Note the hypointense rim, corresponding to the dura (*curved arrow in C*), separating the lesion from normal brain. (*E*) Enhanced CT reveals only a small extraaxial enhancing abnormality (*open arrow*). (*F*) Bone windows reveal adjacent permeative destruction of bone (*arrowheads*).

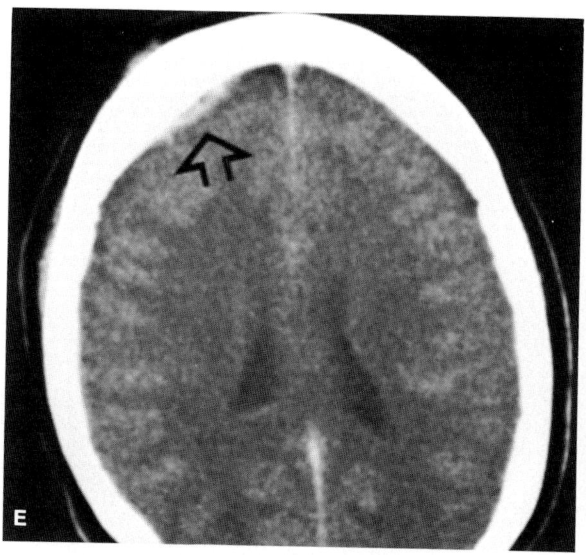

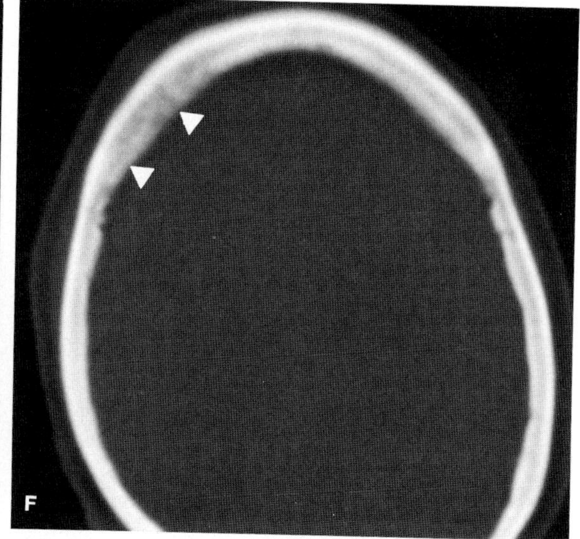

DIAGNOSIS

Epidural abscess (empyema), with accompanying osteomyelitis

DISCUSSION

MR depicts extraaxial empyemas as "mildly hyperintense relative to CSF and hypointense relative to white matter on short TR pulse sequences and hyperintense relative to CSF and white matter on long TR pulse sequences."[1] This appearance, as well as the presence of contrast enhancement, permits differentiation from sterile effusions. In an epidural empyema, the displaced dura can be identified on both T1- and T2-weighted images as a hypointense interface between the lesion and brain. This feature is absent in subdural empyemas. Contrast-enhanced MR is superior to CT for identification, definition of extent, and characterization of extraaxial empyemas.[1] Early diagnosis significantly improves prognosis, with MR strongly recommended when intracranial infection is clinically suspected. IV contrast enhancement is required for specific definition of active inflammation involving the meninges.[2]

MR Technique

IV contrast administration substantially improves detection of epidural and subdural inflammation on MR. Coronal scans in many instances improve the detection of dural disease when compared with axial scans because of reduced partial volume effects.

Pitfalls in Image Interpretation

The size of lesions adjacent to the skull is underestimated by CT as compared with MR. Caution is indicated with respect to assessment of temporal changes in lesion size, when comparing two images (one MR, one CT) of different dates.

Clinical References

1. Weingarten K, Zimmerman RD, Becker RD, et al. Subdural and epidural empyemas: MR imaging. AJNR 1989;10:81–87.
2. Chang KH, Han MH, Roh JK, et al. Gd-DTPA-enhanced MR imaging of the brain in patients with meningitis: comparison with CT. AJR 1990;154:809–816.

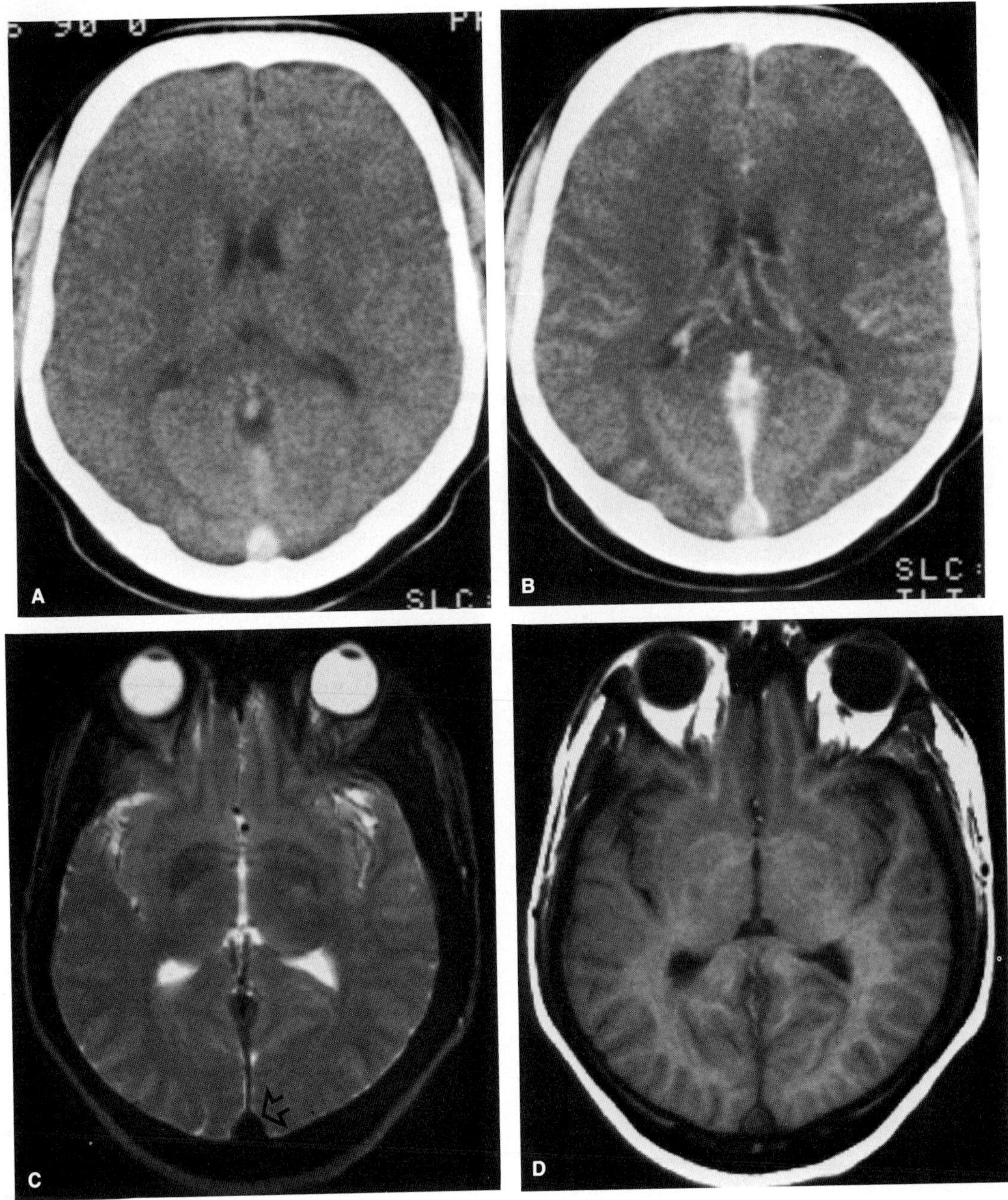

HISTORY

A 19-year-old man with Ewing's sarcoma, now on chemotherapy following tumor excision and presenting with signs of infection of his Hickman catheter

FINDINGS

The superior sagittal sinus is hyperdense on precontrast CT (*A*), with a suggestion of peripheral enhancement on postcontrast CT (*B*). On the T2-weighted image (*C*), low signal intensity (*open arrow*) is noted within the superior sagittal sinus, with intermediate signal intensity on the T1-weighted scan (*D*). On the basis of these findings alone, the venous system could be patent. However, the postcontrast T1-weighted scan (*E*) reveals a lack of enhancement centrally (*short arrow*) due to thrombus, with peripheral venous congestion (*curved arrow*). (*F*) On a slightly lower section, thrombosis of the straight sinus can also be noted (*long arrow*). (*G*) An MR venogram in the craniocaudal projection, performed using 2D TOF technique, confirms lack of flow in the straight and superior sagittal sinuses.

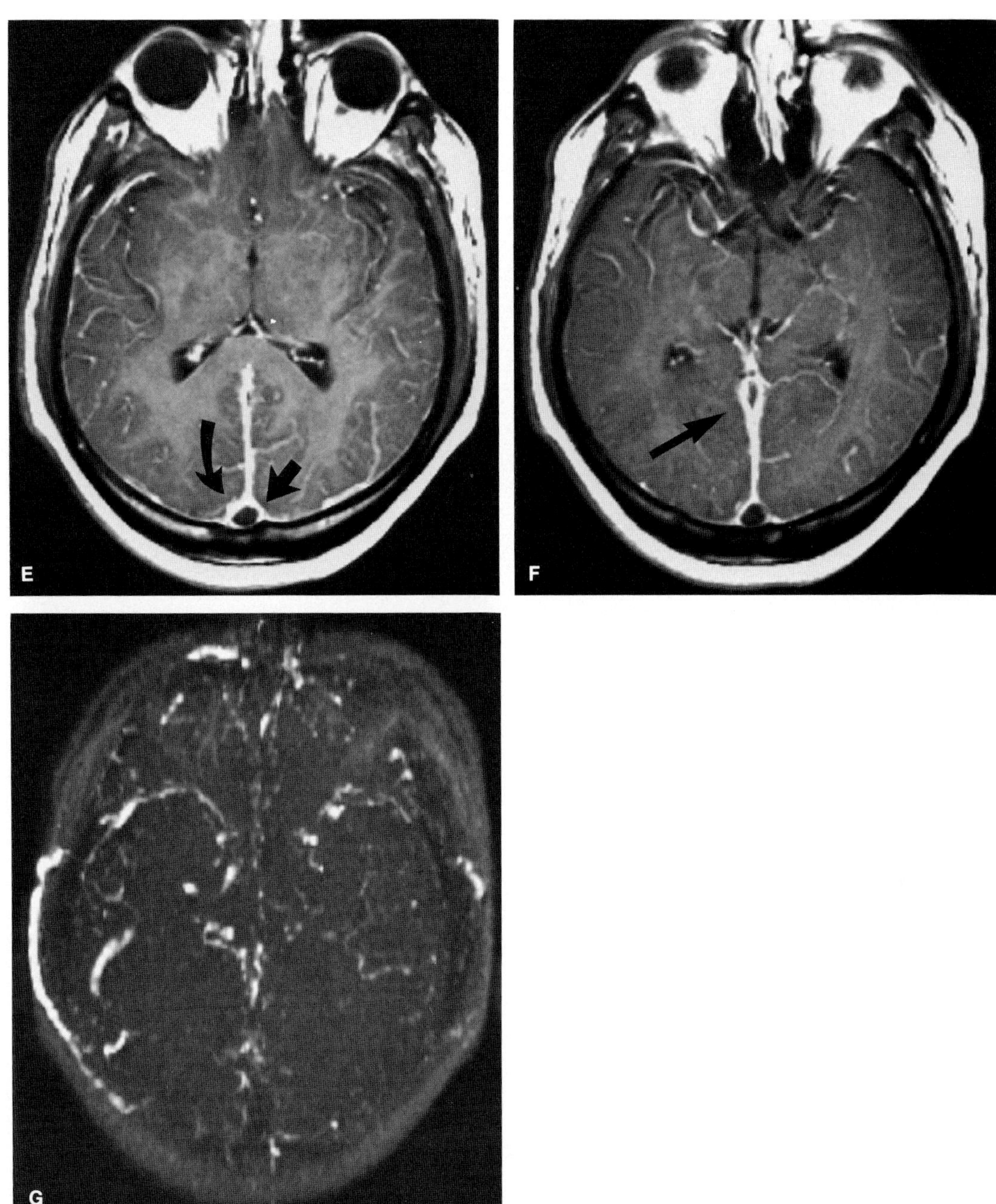

DIAGNOSIS

Superior sagittal sinus thrombosis

DISCUSSION

Dural sinus thrombosis may present without obvious cause or may be precipitated by certain disease states including infection, dehydration, trauma, hematologic abnormalities, and neoplasm. Symptoms due to increased intracranial pressure may be noted, such as headache and lethargy. Treatment is with anticoagulants. Morbidity and mortality are high, particularly with associated cerebral infarction.

Abnormalities identified on CT include the "empty" delta sign following contrast administration (due to enhancement of collateral channels surrounding the thrombosed sinus) and hemorrhagic infarction.

MR has been advocated as the modality of choice for definitive diagnosis of sinus thrombosis. Flow-related effects allow diagnosis on conventional MR, with MRA providing a direct assessment of flow.[1]

MR Technique

Phase imaging, flow-sensitive 2D GRE imaging (as used in the present case), and PC^2 imaging all represent MR techniques sensitive to slow flow and thus suitable for use in confirmation of dural sinus thrombosis.

Pitfalls in Image Interpretation

Acute thrombosis (as illustrated in this case) at high field strength (1.5 T) can lead to decreased intravascular signal intensity, which should not be mistaken to represent vessel patency.

Clinical References

1. Padayachee TS, Bingham JB, Graves MJ, et al. Dural sinus thrombosis: diagnosis by magnetic resonance angiography and imaging. Neuroradiology 1991;33:165–167.
2. Tsuruda JS, Shimakawa A, Pelc NJ, Saloner D. Dural sinus occlusion: evaluation with phase-sensitive gradient-echo MR imaging. AJNR 1991;12:481–488.

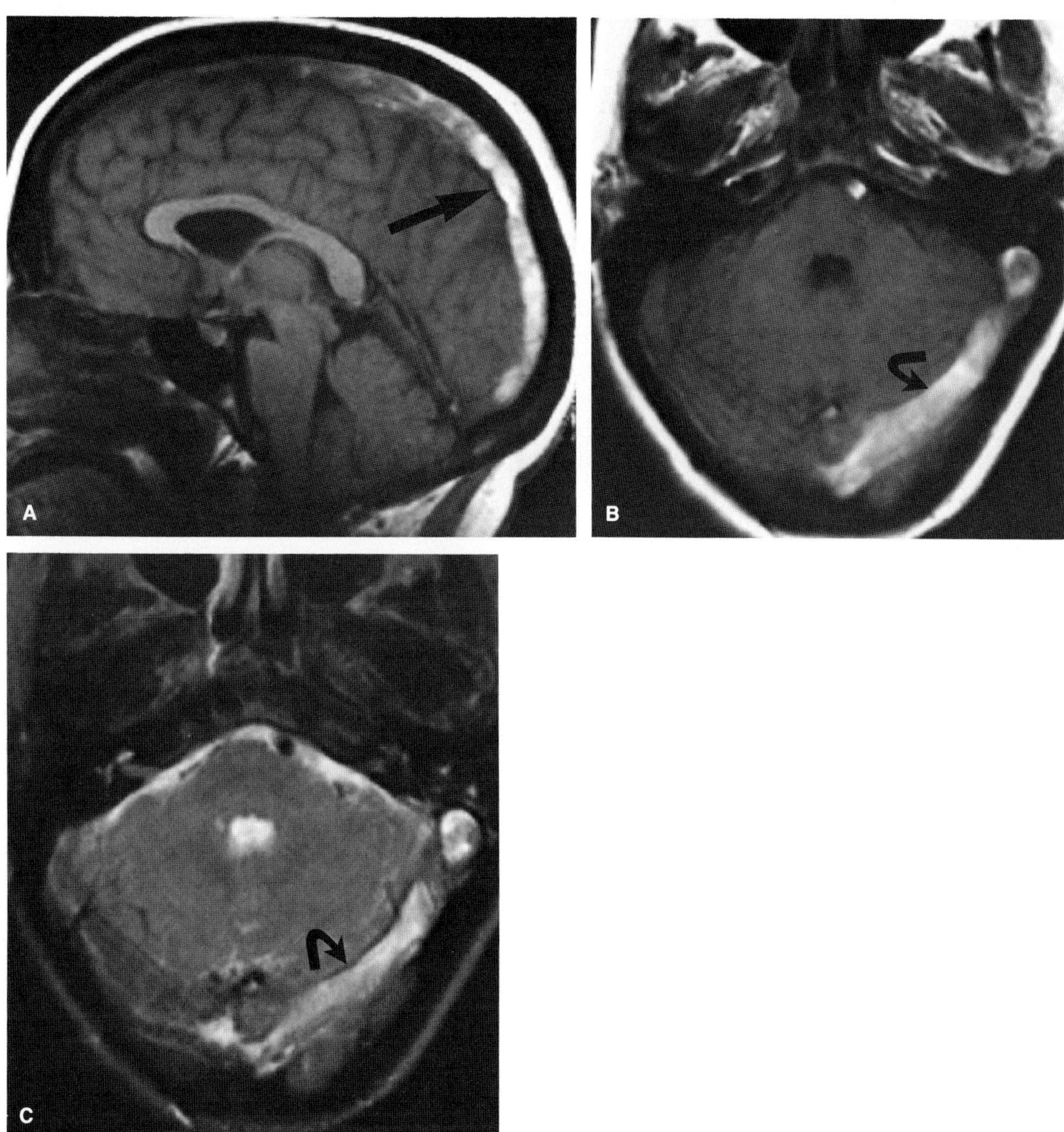

HISTORY

A 42-year-old woman with systemic lupus erythematosus, papilledema, and a 3-week history of nonremitting, bilateral temporal headaches

FINDINGS

Abnormal hyperintensity is noted on sagittal (*A*) and axial (*B*) T1-weighted images in both the superior sagittal sinus (*arrow in A*) and the left transverse sinus (*curved arrow in B*). Both venous sinuses were of uniform hyperintensity on images (*not shown*) obtained in two perpendicular planes (sagittal and axial). The left transverse sinus is dominant in this patient, with no right transverse sinus identified. (*C*) The axial T2-weighted image (TE = 90 msec) also demonstrates that the left transverse sinus is of uniform hyperintensity (*curved arrow*). No pulsation artifacts (which would indicate patency) attributable to the transverse sinus can be identified. Higher axial T2-weighted scans (*not shown*) revealed the superior sagittal sinus to be consistently hyperintense. Unenhanced CT (*not shown*) was interpreted as within normal limits. In retrospect, the attenuation of the superior sagittal sinus was slightly high and thus questionably abnormal.

DIAGNOSIS

Superior sagittal and transverse sinus thrombosis

DISCUSSION

Second MR 3 months later (*not shown*) in this patient revealed recanalization, with patency of both the superior sagittal and transverse sinuses. Observation of such recanalization by MR has been previously documented.[1] Before the advent of antibiotics, the most frequent cause of cerebral venous thrombosis was systemic or localized infection, in particular chronic otitis media. Today, most such occlusions are nonseptic, occurring in patients with a primary disease (such as systemic lupus erythematosus) that alters clotting factors or blood constituents. Leading high-risk states include postpartum and malignancy. Symptoms depend on the specific vessels involved, rapidity of thrombosis, and collateralization of flow. Headache, nausea and vomiting, papilledema, and meningeal signs are common.

Flowing blood can appear hyperintense on both SE and GRE imaging as a result of wash-in of unsaturated spins between RF excitations. This TOF effect, also known as flow-related enhancement, can be employed to verify vessel patency.[2] Sequential acquisition GRE imaging in particular has been used to diagnose superior sagittal sinus occlusion.[3] One pitfall, illustrated by this case, is high signal intensity within a clot due to methemoglobin.

A more definitive technique of differentiating between flow and thrombus is the use of phase images, which can be acquired simultaneously with conventional magnitude images and require no additional scan time.[4] Moving blood demonstrates a phase shift relative to static tissue. However, very slow flow velocities (below 2.5 cm/s) may go undetected by phase imaging. Interpretation of phase images in addition to standard-magnitude SE images substantially improves diagnostic confidence with respect to detection of intravascular thrombosis.

Pitfalls in Image Interpretation

Extracellular methemoglobin, a principal component in this subacute clot, is presumed to be responsible for the high signal intensity observed on all pulse sequences. To exclude the possibility of flow-related phenomena, imaging in two planes must document the same abnormal signal intensity. On a single image, intravascular signal from flowing blood may be indistinguishable from vascular occlusion caused by tumor or thrombus.

Clinical References

1. Morikawa E, Yoshida S, Basugi N, et al. Sequential magnetic resonance images of a case of cerebral sinus thrombosis: imaging of the thrombosed sinus and its recanalization. No To Shinkei 1988;40:357–363.
2. Kucharczyk W, Kelly WM, Davis DO, et al. Intracranial lesions: flow-related enhancement on MR images using time-of-flight effects. Radiology 1986;161:767–772.
3. Daniels DL, Czervionke LF, Hendrix LE, et al. Gradient recalled echo MR imaging of superior sagittal sinus occlusion. Neuroradiology 1989;31:134–136.
4. Nadel L, Braun IF, Kraft KA, et al. Intracranial vascular abnormalities: value of MR phase imaging to distinguish thrombus from flowing blood. AJR 1991;156:373–380.

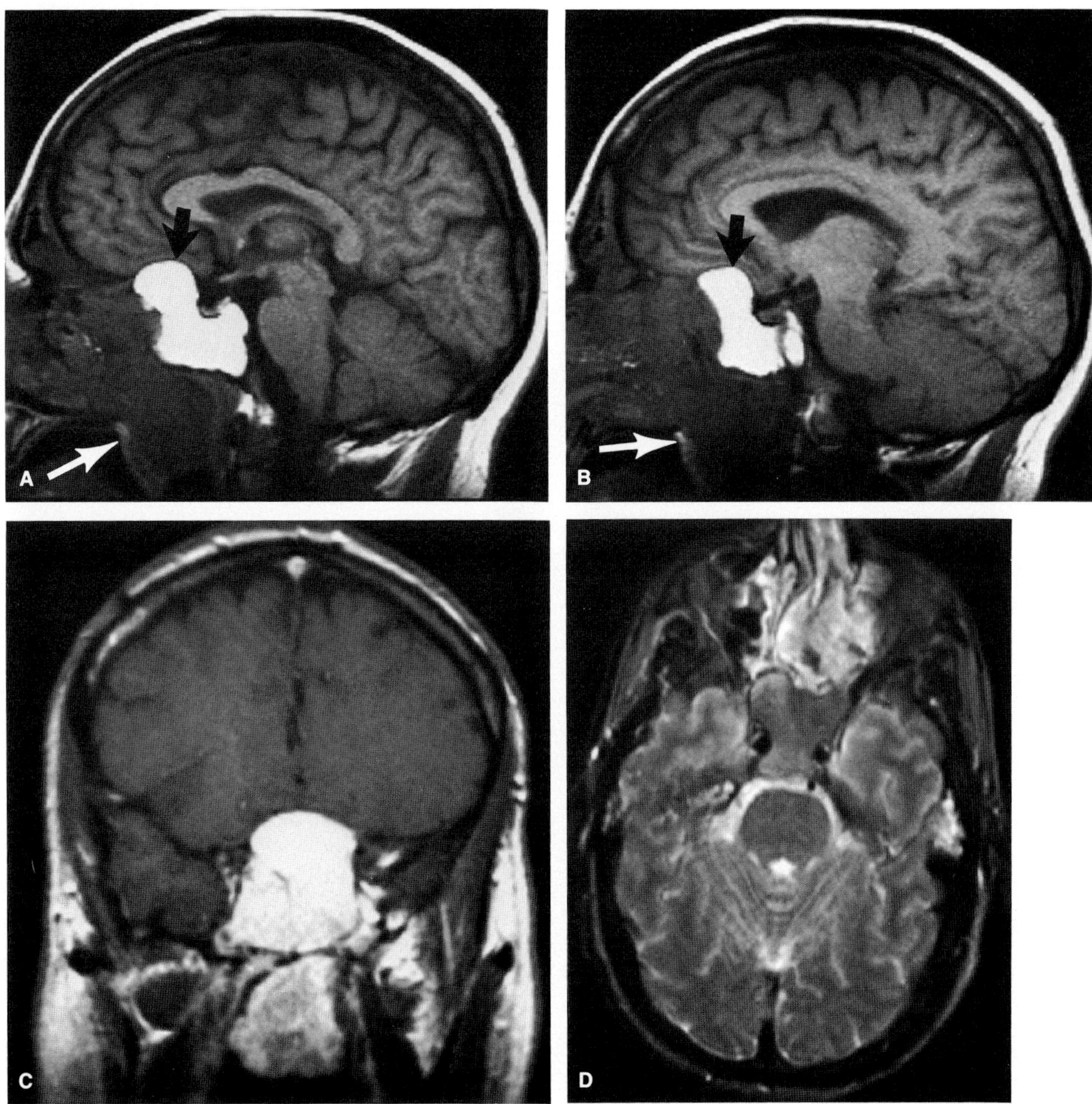

HISTORY

A 38-year-old man with a 20-year history of chronic sinus complaints who noted an increase in nasal congestion

FINDINGS

(*A and B*) Sagittal T1-weighted images demonstrate a large soft-tissue-intensity mass (*white arrows*) in the ethmoid air cells and nasopharynx. This mass extends posteriorly to the anterior wall of the sphenoid sinus and superiorly into the frontal sinus. (*C*) On the coronal T1-weighted postcontrast image the mass demonstrates homogeneous enhancement. (*D*) Axial precontrast T2-weighted image shows that the mass is of increased signal intensity. A high-signal-intensity (precontrast on T1-weighted images) expansile lesion (*black arrows in A and B*) is present in the sphenoid sinus, consistent with a mucocele.

DIAGNOSIS

Esthesioneuroblastoma

DISCUSSION

Olfactory neuroblastoma (esthesioneuroblastoma) is a malignant neoplasm that arises from the olfactory neuroepithelium lining the roof of the nasal vault. They constitute 3% of all nasal neoplasms. Two thirds of patients are between 10 and 39 years, although the reported age range is 3 to 88 years. It is a highly malignant tumor and hematogenous metastases are seen in 10% to 18% of cases.[1]

Findings on MR are nonspecific as with most nasal cavity masses. The typical appearance is that of a large destructive nasoethmoid soft tissue mass, with or without extension into the cranial vault, orbits, or paranasal sinuses. These tumors arise either just above or below the cribriform plate.[2] Frontal lobe abscess can result secondary to free communication between the ethmoid air cells and the intracranial compartment.

Current treatment consists of surgical excision and radiation therapy. Five-year survival rates have been reported as high as 50%.

Pitfalls in Image Interpretation

The differential diagnosis for nasoethmoid masses is broad and includes primary squamous cell carcinoma, metastasis, adenoid cystic carcinoma, osteogenic sarcoma, fibrous dysplasia, and chronic infection.

Clinical References

1. Regenbogen VS, Zinreich SJ, Kim KS, et al. Hyperostotic esthesioneuroblastoma: CT and MR findings. J Comput Assist Tomogr 1988;12:52–56.
2. Schroth D, Gawehn J, Marquardt B, et al. MR imaging of esthesioneuroblastoma. J Comput Assist Tomogr 1986;10: 316–319.

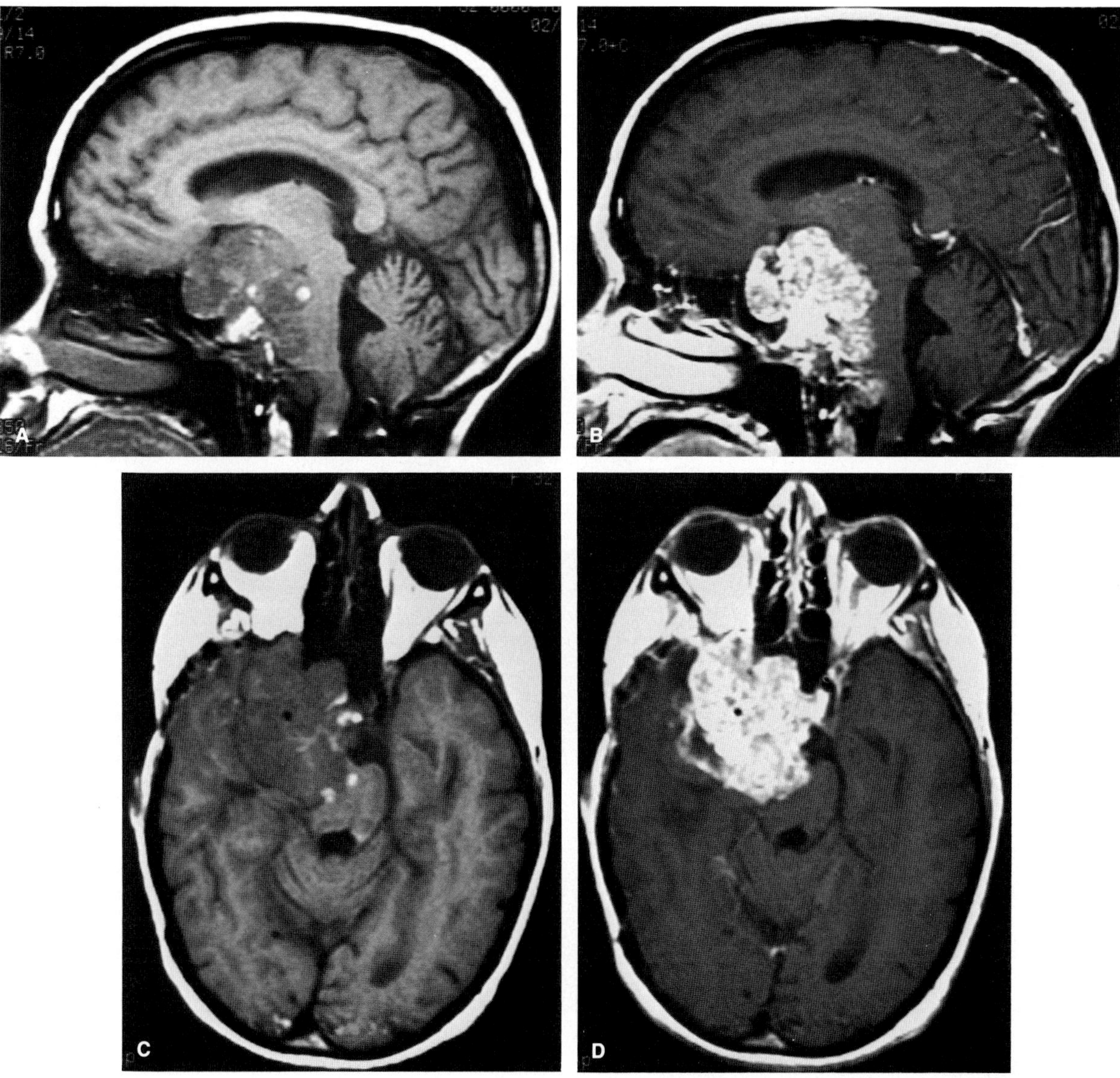

HISTORY

A 42-year-old woman with multiple cranial nerve palsies

FINDINGS

(*A*) On the sagittal T1-weighted image, a large extraaxial mass of predominantly decreased signal intensity is identified anterior to the brain stem and extending into the suprasellar cistern. The normal high signal intensity of the clivus (which occurs due to the presence of marrow fat) is absent. Several punctate foci of increased signal intensity are seen within the mass on this T1-weighted image (*A*). (*B*) On the sagittal T1-weighted postcontrast image the mass demonstrates heterogeneous enhancement. Abnormal soft tissue is seen extending to the right orbital apex on the precontrast (*C*) and postcontrast (*D*) axial T1-weighted images. A significant amount of mass effect is present on the right pons. The temporal horn of the right lateral ventricle is displaced by the mass on precontrast (*E*) and postcontrast (*F*) coronal T1-weighted images. (*G*) The mass is of moderately increased signal intensity on the axial T2-weighted image.

DIAGNOSIS

Clivus chordoma

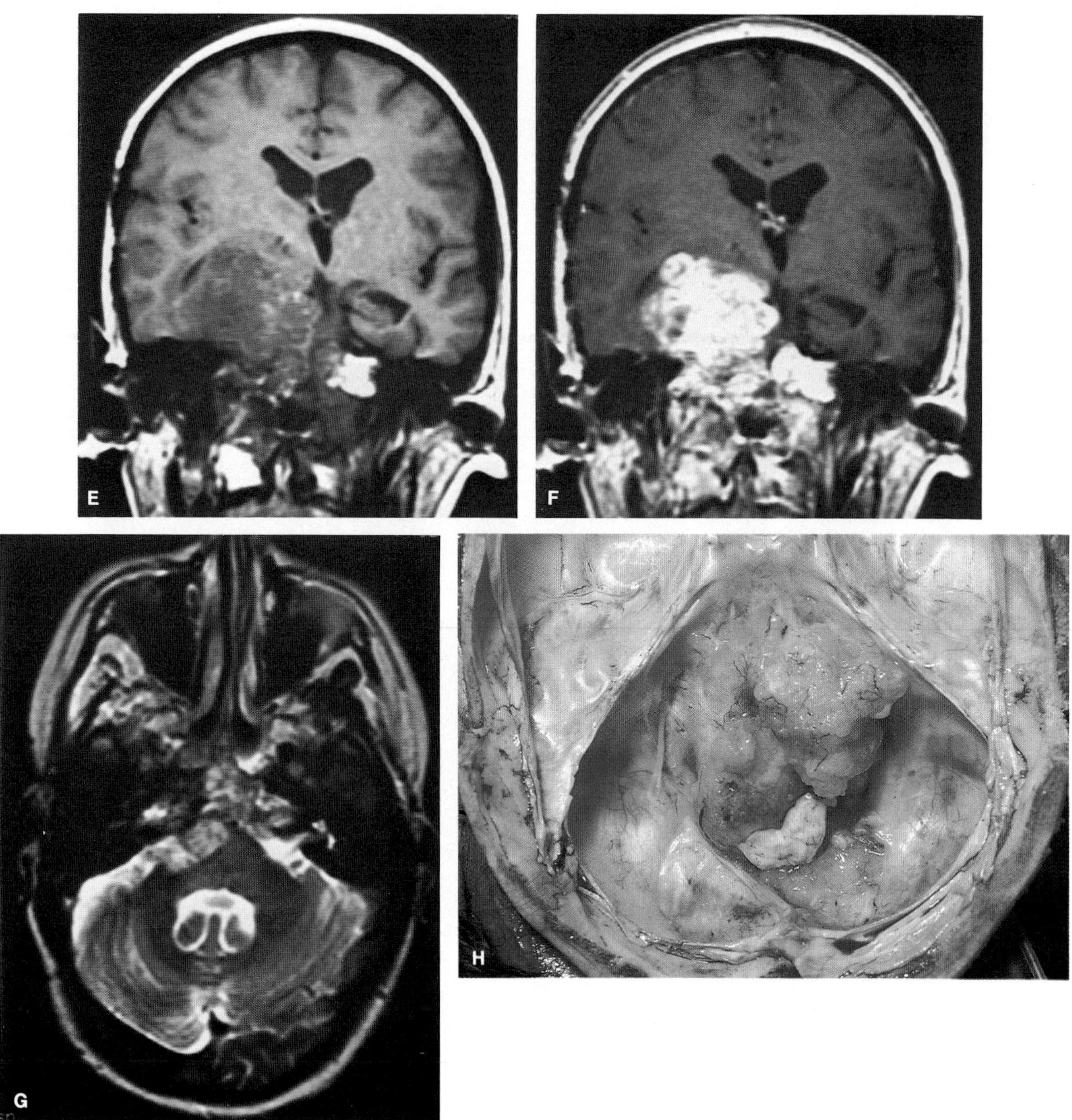

DISCUSSION

Chordomas are rare, slow-growing primary bone tumors that originate from remnants of the primitive notochord. The primitive notochord extends from Rathke's pouch to the clivus, continuing caudally to the vertebral bodies. Remnants of the notochord can occur at any location along this tract.[1]

Approximately 35% of chordomas are intracranial, and most of these arise from the clivus; 50% are sacrococcygeal and 15% arise from within a vertebral body. Within the calvarium they may involve the posterior or middle fossa by extension through the dura. Most of these tumors cause extensive destruction of bony structures. These tumors rarely metastasize to distant sites, but they are locally aggressive, and total surgical resection is rarely possible. Although locally invasive, they are histologically benign. Macroscopically, chordomas are soft gelatinous tumors that frequently result in destruction of the clivus and skull base. They occur most commonly in men in the third and fourth decades. Patients present with headaches, facial pain, progressive cranial nerve palsies, and nasal stuffiness.[2]

Calcification is identified in 50% to 60% of cases on CT. On MR imaging, chordomas are usually well-defined, extraaxial tumors that show isointensity or mild hypointensity on T1-weighted images and moderate to extremely high intensity on T2-weighted images. About

70% of chordomas have septations of low signal intensity separating lobulated areas of higher signal intensity on T2-weighted images. Chordomas typically enhance after the administration of a gadolinium chelate.

Pitfalls in Image Interpretation

These tumors can occasionally be located predominantly suprasellar, and chordoma should be in the differential diagnosis of suprasellar masses.

Pathologic Correlate

(*H*) Gross image of a clivus chordoma in situ shows a glassy mucoid tumor with gross permeation and destruction of bone. The lesion has expanded into both the nasopharynx and foramen magnum.

Clinical References

1. Sze G, Uichanco LS, Brant-Zawadzki MN, et al. Chordomas: MR imaging. Radiology 1988;166:187–191.
2. Oot RF, Melville GE, New PF, et al. The role of MR and CT in evaluating clival chordomas and chondrosarcomas. AJR 1989;151:567–575.

*(*A *to* G *courtesy of William Yuh, MD;* H *from Okazaki H, Scheithauer B. Slide atlas of neuropathology. New York, Gower Medical Publishing, 1988. By permission of Mayo Foundation.)*

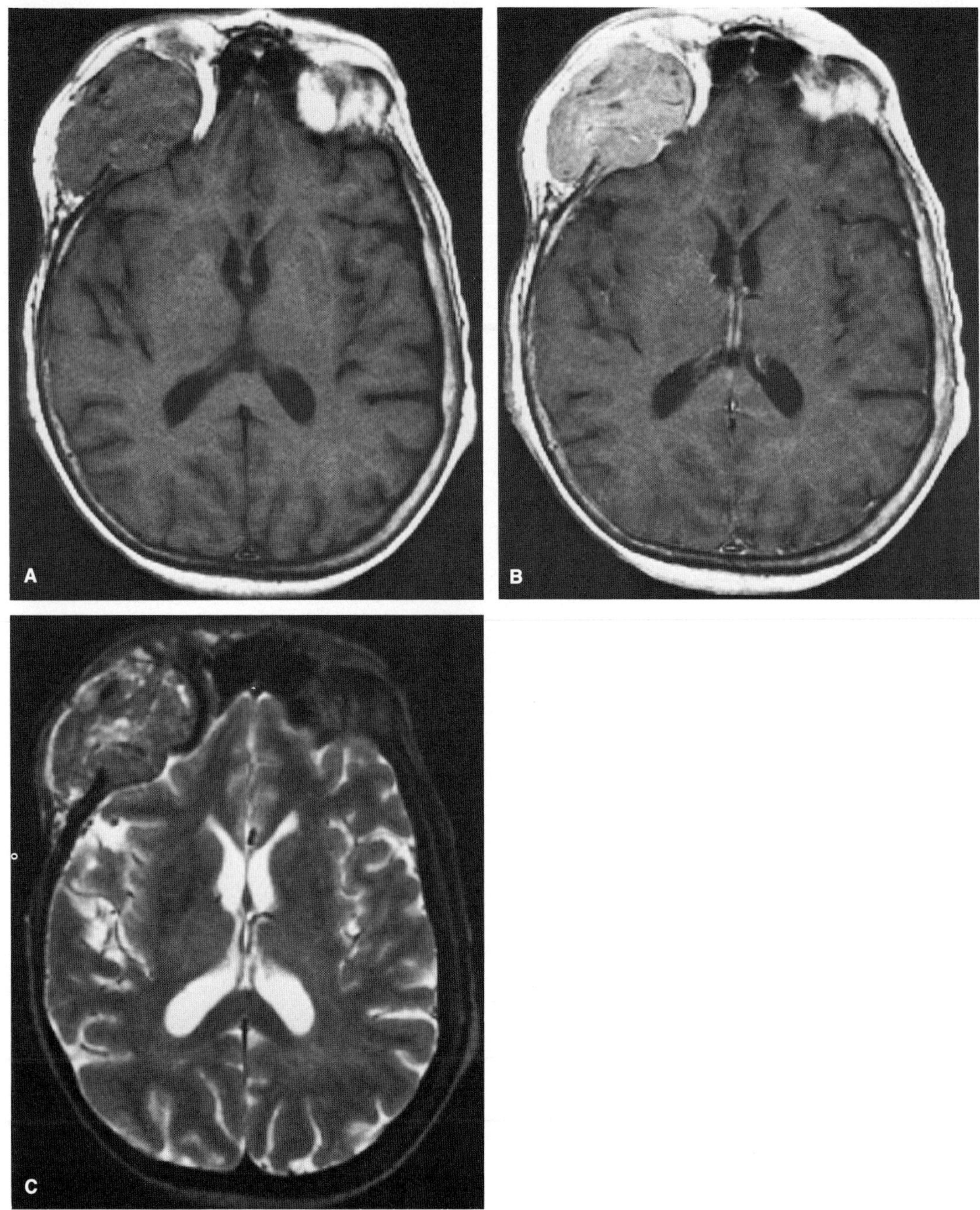
A
B
C

HISTORY

Elderly man with a history of renal cell carcinoma

FINDINGS

A large oval enhancing calvarial mass is identified on axial precontrast (*A*) and postcontrast (*B*) T1-weighted images. (*C*) This lesion is of intermediate signal intensity on the axial T2-weighted image. Although the mass produces some compression of the right frontal lobe, no definite invasion is appreciated.

DIAGNOSIS

Calvarial metastasis

DISCUSSION

The normal diploic space does not enhance, except for the diploic veins and the meninges near pacchionian granulations. The intradiploic space sometimes appears inhomogeneous with areas of increased and decreased signal intensity on nonenhanced studies; however, it should appear symmetric from side to side. Gross asymmetry is highly suggestive of calvarial disease, even in the absence of appreciable destruction of the outer or inner table. Calvarial metastases typically enhance with IV gadolinium chelate administration.[1]

Diploic veins appear as linear foci of low to moderate signal intensity on nonenhanced MR images. These foci normally demonstrate postcontrast enhancement.

Intracranial structures that normally enhance include the pituitary gland, infundibulum, cavernous sinus, choroid plexus, and nasal mucosa.

MR Technique

IV contrast enhancement can improve the detection of calvarial metastases, but close comparison of precontrast and postcontrast images is often required.

Pitfalls in Image Interpretation

Recognition of hyperintense foci (representing normal fat) on nonenhanced T1-weighted images is required to prevent mistaking calvarial fatty marrow for pathologic enhancement.

Clinical References

1. West MS, Russell EJ, Breit R, et al. Calvarial and skull base metastases: comparison of nonenhanced and Gd-DTPA-enhanced MR images. Radiology 1990;174:85–91.

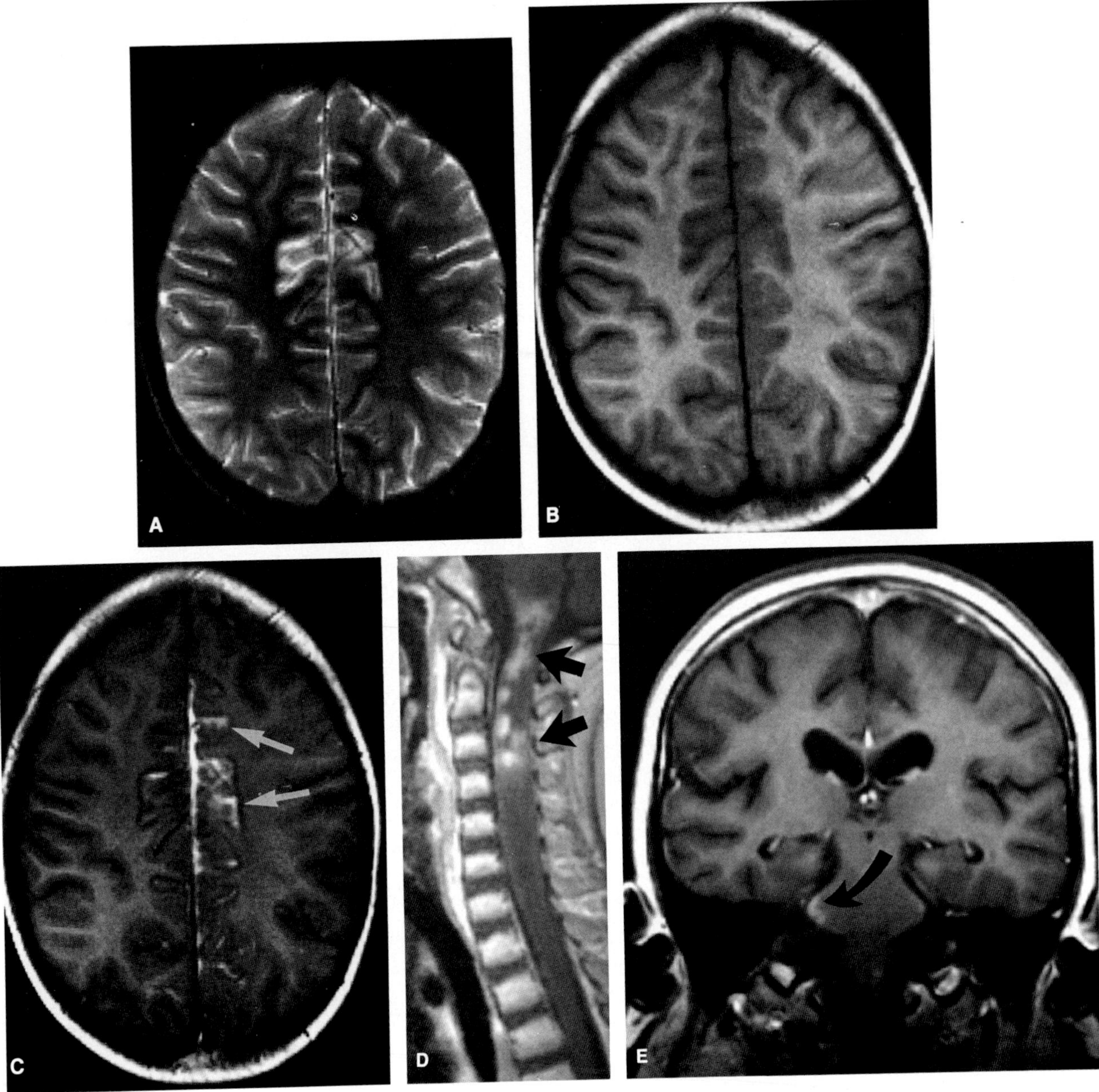

HISTORY

Two pediatric patients, previously in remission, but now with recurrence of leukemia

FINDINGS

PATIENT 1: On the T2-weighted scan (*A*), there is mild abnormal hyperintensity along several sulci in the midline. (*B*) The precontrast T1-weighted image is unremarkable. (*C*) The T1-weighted postcontrast image reveals abnormal enhancement along both the falx and meninges, the latter within several sulci (*white arrows*) both to the right and left of midline.

PATIENT 2: (*D*) The postcontrast T1-weighted sagittal midline image of the cervical spine reveals abnormal soft tissue enhancement (*arrows*) within an expanded upper cervical cord. Also noted is abnormal uniform hyperintensity of bone marrow within the cervical and thoracic spine due to previous radiation therapy. (*E*) A coronal postcontrast T1-weighted image, from MR of the head, demonstrates abnormal enhancement at the origin of the right fifth cranial nerve (*curved arrow*).

DIAGNOSIS

Leptomeningeal (patients 1 and 2) and parenchymal (patient 2) metastases in leukemia

DISCUSSION

Detection of neoplastic involvement of the leptomeninges relies principally on the evaluation of CSF cytology. However, large CSF volumes and multiple samples may be required for diagnosis. Subarachnoid tumor seeding carries a poor prognosis.

Primary brain tumors with a propensity for leptomeningeal metastases include medulloblastoma, ependymoma, germinoma, pineoblastoma, glioblastoma multiforme, oligodendroglioma, and retinoblastoma. Subarachnoid seeding is also common with certain visceral neoplasms (eg, carcinoma of the breast and lung) and nonvisceral neoplasms (eg, melanoma, lymphoma, and leukemia).

CT in patients with leptomeningeal metastases may reveal indirect signs of tumor spread, including hydrocephalus and obliteration of the sylvian fissures or basal cisterns. Contrast administration can demonstrate direct tumor involvement, with abnormal smooth or nodular enhancement.[1] The most common sites of involvement include the quadrigeminal plate, perimesencephalic, and superior cerebellar cisterns, as well as the ventricular ependyma and high parietal subarachnoid space. Intramedullary tumor recurrence, as seen in patient 2, has also been previously described.[2] Neither enhanced CT nor enhanced MR is as sensitive as cytopathology, with the inaccuracy of these modalities perhaps due to the lack of macroscopic invasion of the meninges in some patients.[1]

Pitfalls in Image Interpretation

Abnormal enhancement of the leptomeninges is not specific for tumor involvement in immunosuppressed patients. Other entities that must be considered include infection and inflammation, with the latter seen both postoperatively and following trauma.

Clinical References

1. Yousem DM, Patrone PM, Grossman RI. Leptomeningeal metastases: MR evaluation. J Comput Assist Tomogr 1990; 14:255–261.
2. Nielsen H. Fatal intramedullary tumor of the cervical spinal cord during remission of acute lymphoblastic leukemia. J Neurooncol 1989;7:315–317.

(A to C from Runge VM. Clinical magnetic resonance imaging. Philadelphia, JB Lippincott, 1990.)

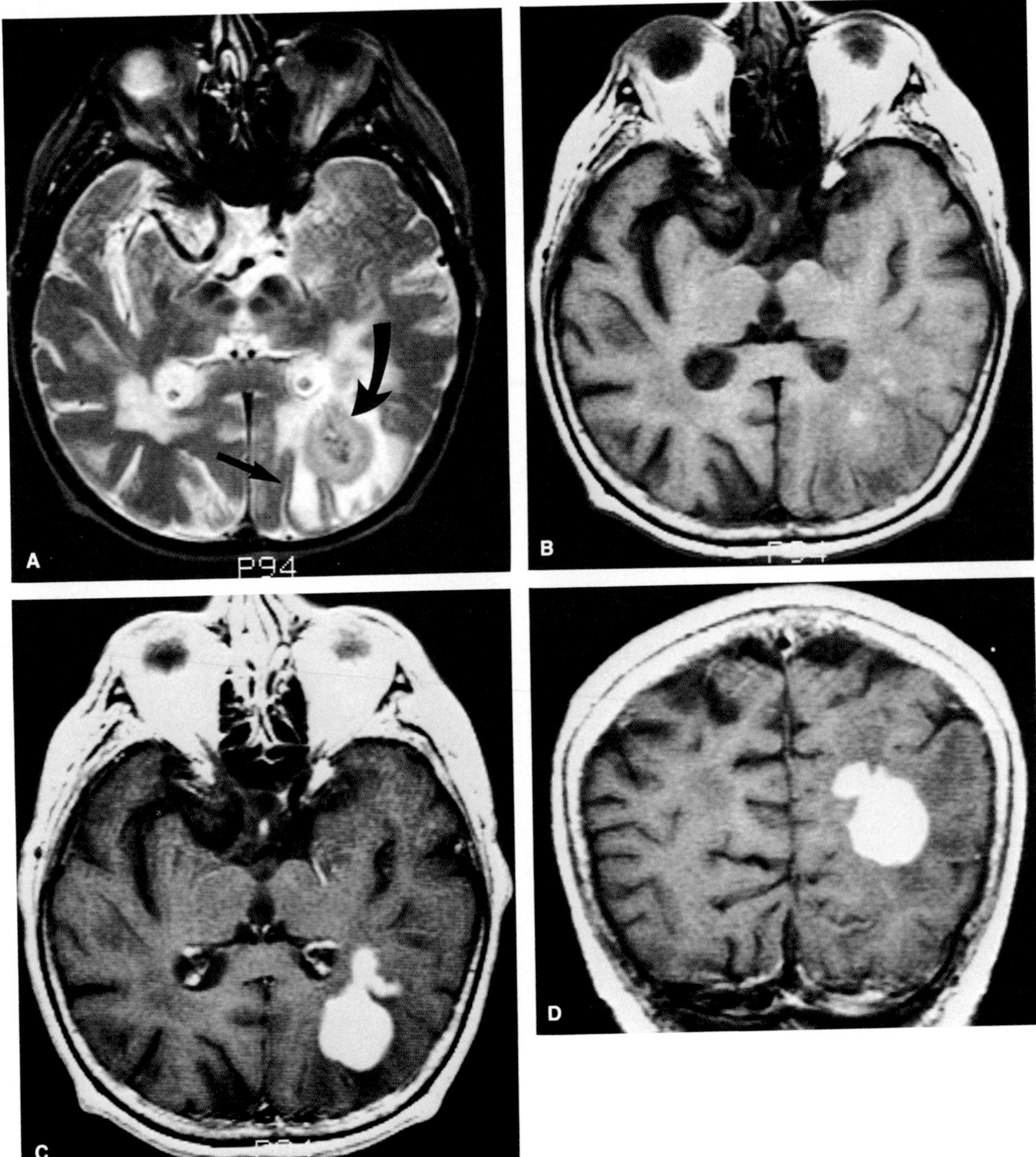

HISTORY

A 76-year-old patient with dementia

FINDINGS

(*A*) The T2-weighted axial scan (TE = 90) reveals a left parietal mass (*curved arrow*), which is predominantly isointense with gray matter. There is extensive surrounding abnormal hyperintensity due to edema (*arrow*). (*B*) Slight mass effect on the left atrium of the lateral ventricle is best appreciated on the precontrast T1-weighted axial scan. Intense homogeneous enhancement of the lesion is noted on postcontrast axial (*C*) and coronal (*D*) T1-weighted images.

DIAGNOSIS

Primary cerebral lymphoma

DISCUSSION

Primary CNS lymphoma is a rare tumor, representing less than 2% of all primary CNS malignancies.[1] Most CNS lymphomas are primary in origin. Development of these tumors in immunodeficiency disorders, whether congenital or acquired, is well recognized. In particular, organ transplantation with intensive immunosuppressive therapy is associated with the occurrence of cerebral lymphomas. Immunosuppression is also thought to be responsible for the well-documented occurrence of CNS lymphomas with HIV infection. In patients with AIDS, however, secondary CNS involvement by lymphoma is almost as frequent as primary lymphoma. Most tumors are of B-cell origin, in common with most nodal and visceral non-Hodgkin's lymphomas.

Most cases of lymphoma are seen in adult life. Stereotactic needle biopsy is preferred for diagnosis. Radiation, combined with steroid therapy, is effective short term. Despite the typical marked initial response to treatment, most patients experience relapse, with median survival less than 24 months. Clinical symptoms in this patient are not inconsistent with a brain tumor. In approximately 5% of patients, dementia proves to be secondary to an intracranial tumor and thus is potentially reversible.

On CT, primary CNS lymphoma is typically of increased density, with homogeneous contrast enhancement.[1] Ringlike enhancement has been described, with a thick enhancing wall being a possible differential point from an abscess (in immunosuppressed patients). Prominent peritumoral edema is common. Tumor nodules are generally large (average diameter of 4 cm in one series). Location in the central white matter is not a hallmark of primary CNS lymphoma (this is a common misconception), with only 30% of lesions in one study located in deep central structures. Multiple lesions and subependymal spread are seen in a minority of cases. Most lesions display mass effect on angiographic study.

In a large study of AIDS patients with suspected toxoplasmosis, primary CNS lymphoma, or progressive multifocal leukoencephalopathy (the three most common focal CNS lesions) by MR, 71% of solitary lesions were lymphomas. Thus, empiric treatment for toxoplasmosis is unlikely to be successful in AIDS patients with a solitary lesion on MR.[2] A focal enhancing mass with subependymal spread (as assessed by either MR or CT) and high attenuation on unenhanced CT are the most reliable features for identification of primary CNS lymphoma and thus differentiation from toxoplasmosis in AIDS patients.[3] In AIDS, lesions are commonly smaller than 2 cm in size, frequently multiple, and often located in the temporal lobes or basal ganglia.[4] In non-AIDS patients, the lesions are typically larger (greater than 2 cm) and solitary, with preferential location in the deep parietal lobe.

Pitfalls in Image Interpretation

Misdiagnosis in primary lymphoma is common, with only 11% of patients in one CT series correctly diagnosed prospectively. If there are multiple lesions, the scan is often misinterpreted to represent metastatic disease. With solitary lesions, the most common misdiagnosis is meningioma. With ring-enhancing lesions in immunosuppressed patients, misdiagnosis as an abscess or glioma is possible.

Clinical References

1. Jack CR Jr, Reese DF, Scheithauer BW. Radiographic findings in 32 cases of primary CNS lymphoma. AJR 1986;146:271–276.
2. Ciricillo SF, Rosenblum ML. Use of CT and MR imaging to distinguish intracranial lesions and to define the need for biopsy in AIDS patients. J Neurosurg 1990;73:720–724.
3. Dina TS. Primary central nervous system lymphoma versus toxoplasmosis in AIDS. Radiology 1991;179:823–828.
4. Schwaighofer BW, Hesselink JR, Press GA, et al. Primary intracranial CNS lymphoma: MR manifestations. AJNR 1989;10:725–729.

(A to D *courtesy of Mark Osborne, MD.*)

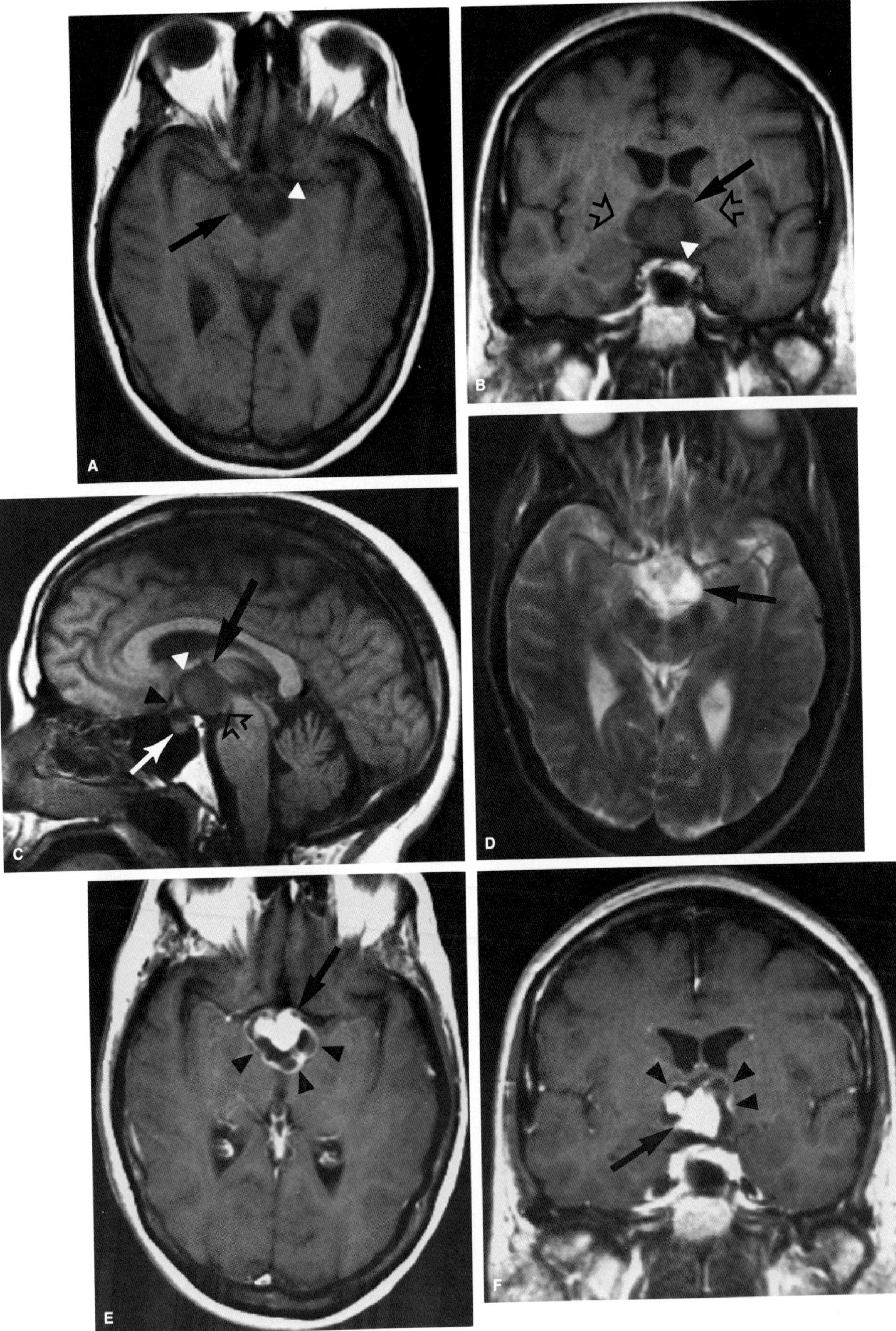
A
B
C
D
E
F

HISTORY

A 52-year-old woman with fatigue and blurred vision

FINDINGS

T1-weighted axial (*A*), coronal (*B*), and sagittal (*C*) images demonstrate an irregular, multilobulated mass (*black arrow*) about 2.5 cm in diameter in the suprasellar region. The mass has both cystic and soft tissue components, with the signal intensity of the cystic fluid being only slightly greater than that of CSF. A soft tissue component (*white arrowhead*) is isointense to gray matter. On the T2-weighted axial image (*D*), the cystic fluid (*black arrow*) has very high signal intensity. Postcontrast T1-weighted axial (*E*) and coronal (*F*) images show intense enhancement of the margins (*black arrowheads*) of the mass, and its soft tissue component (*black arrow*).

The mass compresses the optic chiasm (*black arrowhead in C*) anteriorly and the mamillary body (*open arrow in C*) posteriorly. The thalami (*open arrows in B*) and hypothalami are displaced laterally. The pituitary gland (*white arrow in C*) is normal.

DIAGNOSIS

Craniopharyngioma

DISCUSSION

Craniopharyngiomas are usually complex, heterogeneous masses with both a cystic and solid component. In most cases, the signal intensity of the cystic fluid is lower than brain and higher than CSF on T1-weighted images, reflecting a low cholesterol and protein content.[1] On T2-weighted images the signal intensity of the cystic fluid is almost always very high, greater than CSF, no matter what its protein and cholesterol composition. The borders of a craniopharyngioma, particularly the low-signal-intensity cystic component, may be indistinct on noninfused images, often as a result of volume averaging of adjacent structures. The use of IV gadolinium chelate infusion is helpful in delineating the exact borders of these tumors, and for identifying solid components.[1]

Adults with craniopharyngioma commonly complain of visual disturbances or have symptoms of hypopituitarism due to compression of the optic apparatus, hypothalamus, or pituitary by the suprasellar mass.[2] The anterior pituitary is a very vascular gland which receives its blood supply through the hypothalamic-hypophyseal portal vessels, which travel in the pituitary stalk. The hypothalamus secretes several hormones, including thyroid-stimulating hormone (TSH)–releasing hormone (TRH), which pass to the anterior pituitary by means of this portal system. TRH causes the release of TSH from the pituitary, which stimulates the secretion of thyroid hormones by the thyroid gland. Compression of the hypothalamus or pituitary may disrupt this pathway and cause hypothyroidism, commonly manifested as sluggishness (fatigue) and obesity.

Pitfalls in Image Interpretation

Craniopharyngioma is the most common suprasellar mass presenting in an adult but the differential diagnosis includes hypothalamic glioma, meningioma, metastatic disease, aneurysm, chordoma, and sarcoidosis, in addition to teratoma, Rathke's pouch cyst, epidermoid, and pituitary macroadenoma.

Clinical References

1. Pigeau I, Sigal R, Halimi P, et al. MRI features of craniopharyngiomas at 1.5 Tesla. J Neuroradiol 1988;15:276–287.
2. Pusey E, Kortman K, Flannigan B, et al. MR of craniopharyngiomas: tumor delineation and characterization. AJNR 1987;8:439–444.

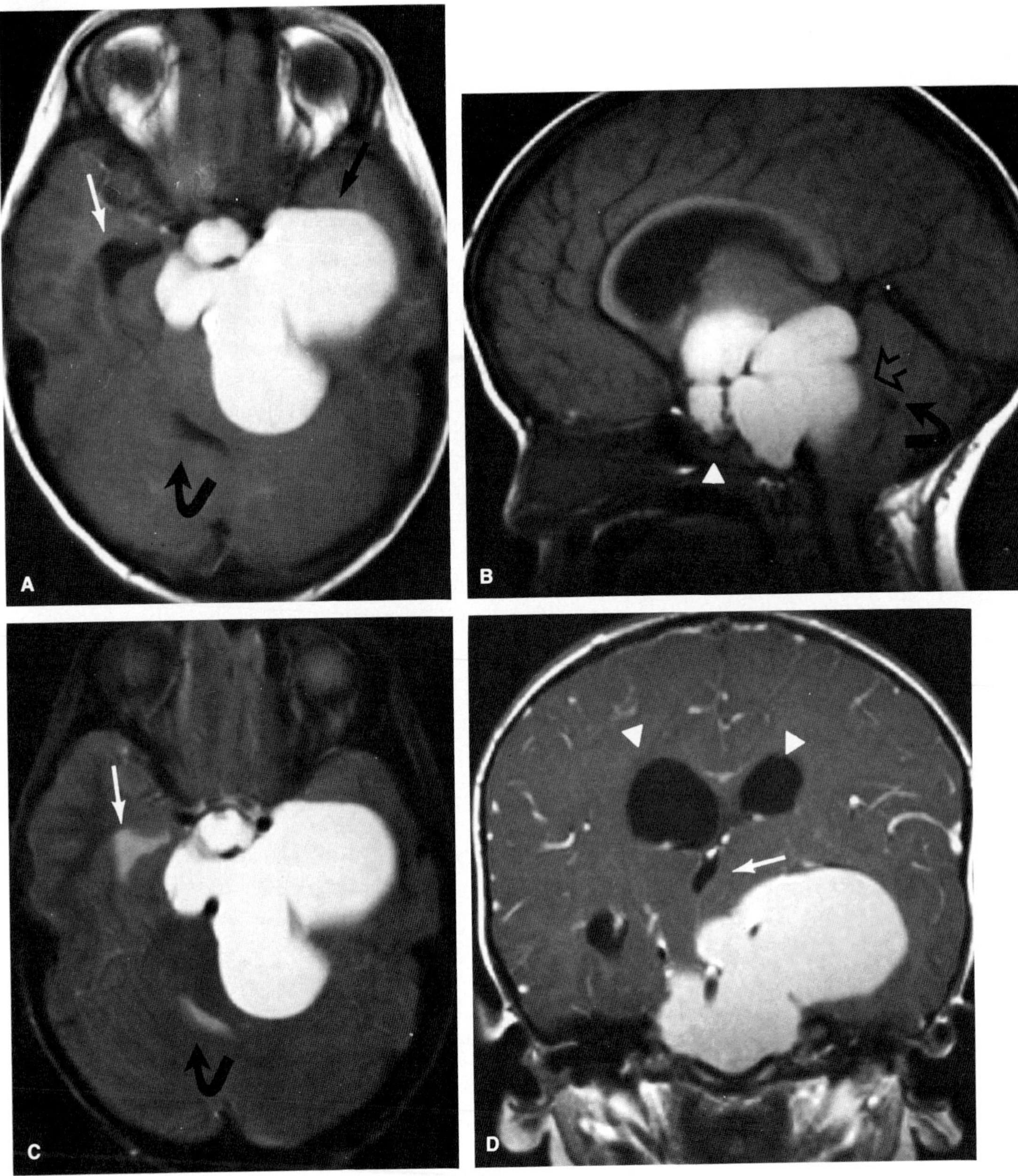

HISTORY

A 7-year-old with short stature, recent lethargy, and headache

FINDINGS

T1-weighted (*A and B*) and heavily T2-weighted (*C*) images identify a large lobulated mass that occupies the sella (*white arrowhead in B*) and suprasellar cistern, with extension into the left temporal fossa (*straight black arrow in A*), and the posterior fossa, where there is mass effect with displacement of the brain stem posteriorly (*open arrow in B*) and compression of the fourth ventricle (*curved arrows in A to C*). (*D*) The postinfusion T1-weighted image demonstrates no apparent enhancement. The third ventricle (*white arrow in D*), right temporal horn (*white arrows in A and C*), and the lateral ventricles (*white arrowheads in D*) are dilated. The mass has homogeneous high signal intensity, seen on *A* to *C*.

DIAGNOSIS

Craniopharyngioma

DISCUSSION

Craniopharyngiomas are slow-growing benign tumors arising from remnants of Rathke's pouch. Seventy percent are both intrasellar and suprasellar in location, with an additional 20% located solely in the suprasellar region. Craniopharyngioma is the most common suprasellar tumor in any age group and may occur from birth to the seventh decade. Two peaks in incidence are present, one in childhood and one in young adults (about 10 and 35 years of age). Presenting symptoms include headache, visual disturbances, and dysfunction of the pituitary or hypothalamus. Children often present with growth failure.

Craniopharyngiomas may have soft tissue and fluid components, both of which have various appearances on T1- and T2-weighted images. The soft tissue component usually is heterogeneous on T1-weighted images, and demonstrates high signal intensity on T1-weighted images with enhancement after IV gadolinium chelate infusion. The fluid component, in most cases, has very high signal intensity, greater than CSF, on T2-weighted images. Signal intensity on T1-weighted images of the fluid component varies from low to high, reflecting biochemical composition. High signal intensity on T1-weighted images is associated with a high protein, cholesterol, or methemoglobin content. Signal intensity on T1-weighted images is believed to correlate most closely with protein content.[1]

The presence and extent of tumor is best defined by MR.[2] CT is superior to MR for detecting calcifications, however, and thus is more specific for diagnosis.[2] Calcification is seen by CT in 80% of pediatric cases and 40% of adult cases.

Pitfalls in Image Interpretation

Differential diagnosis includes teratoma, Rathke's pouch cyst, epidermoid, and hemorrhagic pituitary macroadenoma. MR underestimates calcification, which is most common in craniopharyngiomas.

Clinical References

1. Pigeau I, Sigal R, Halimi P, et al. MRI features of craniopharyngiomas at 1.5 Tesla. J Neuroradiol 1988;15:276–287.
2. Pusey E, Kortman K, Flannigan B, et al. MR of craniopharyngiomas: tumor delineation and characterization. AJNR 1987;8:439–444.

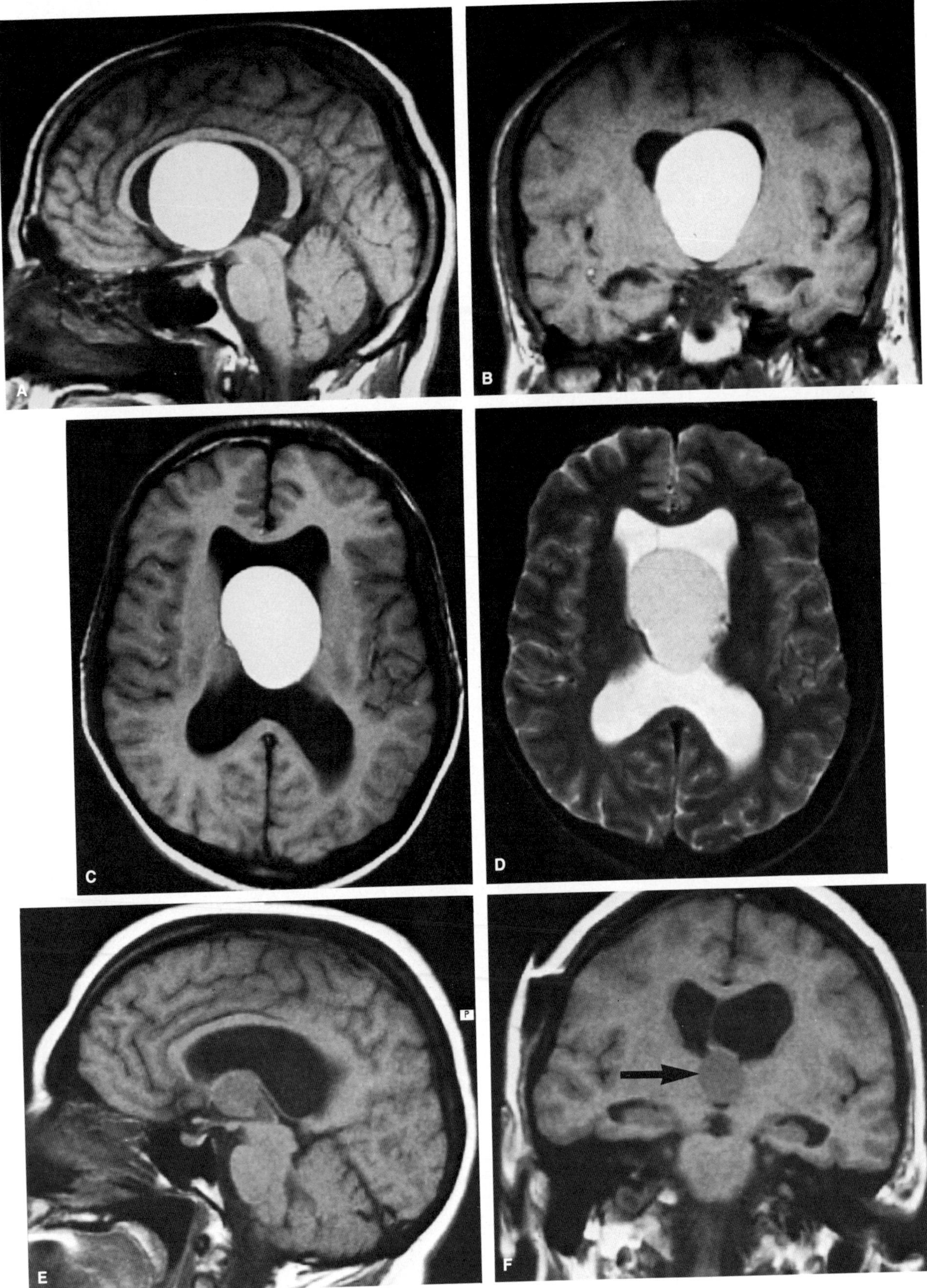
A
B
C
D
P
E
F

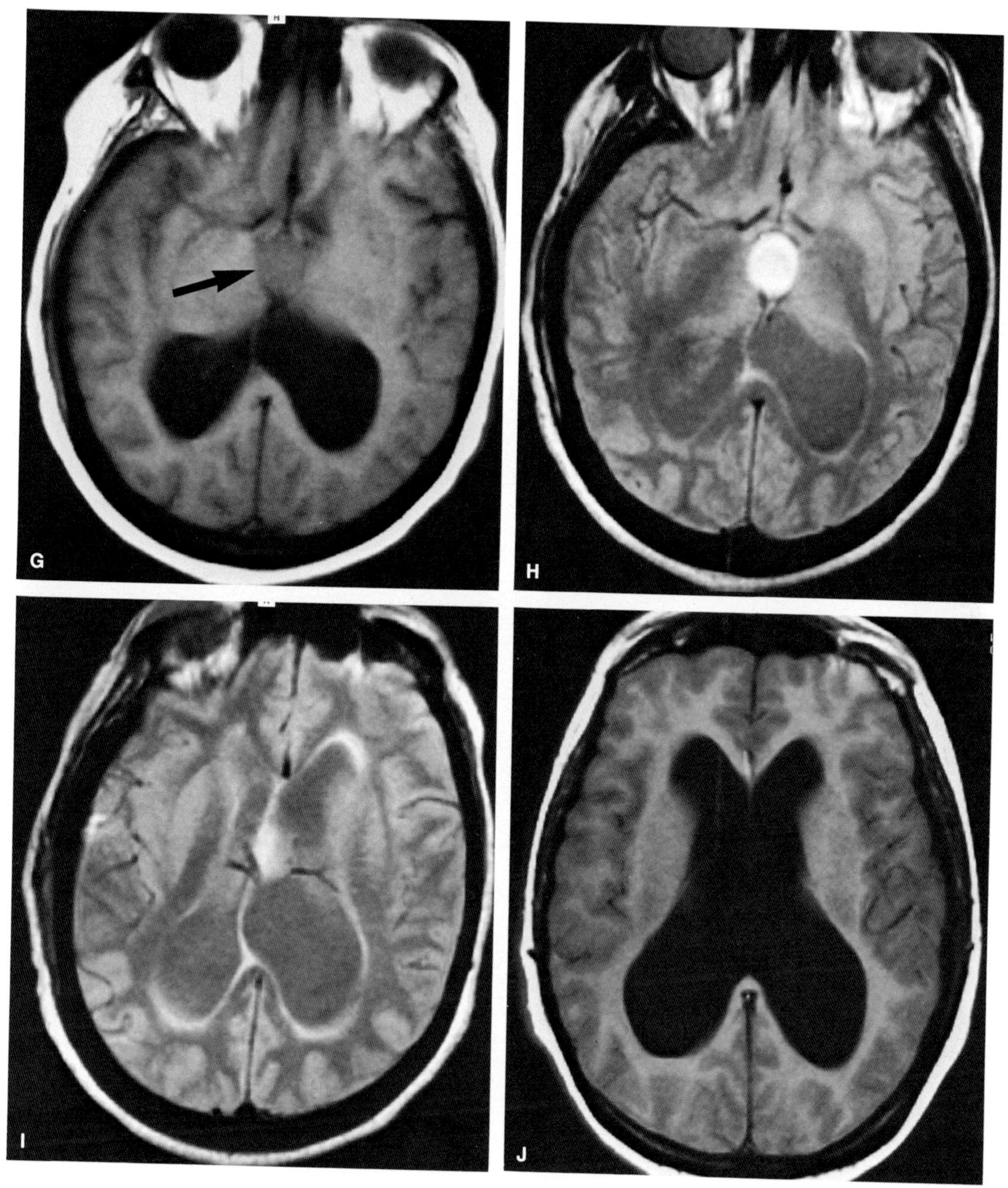

HISTORY

Three different patients with the same intracranial pathology

FINDINGS

PATIENT 1: A large round mass of increased signal intensity is identified in the anterior third ventricle on sagittal (*A*), coronal (*B*), and axial (*C*) T1-weighted images. No abnormal contrast enhancement was noted (*images not shown*). This mass is of slightly lower signal intensity than CSF on the axial T2-weighted image (*D*). The lateral ventricles are enlarged.

PATIENT 2: Sagittal (*E*), coronal (*F*), and axial (*G*) T1-weighted images reveal a 1.5-cm isointense mass (*arrows in F and G*) in the inferior third ventricle. No contrast enhancement was noted (*images not shown*). (*H*) This mass is of increased signal intensity on the first echo of the axial T2-weighted sequence. (*I*) Transependymal flow is identified surrounding the lateral ventricles on the first echo of the axial T2-weighted sequence.

PATIENT 3: Marked dilatation of the lateral ventricles is seen on the axial T1-weighted image (*J*). A 1-cm isointense mass (*arrow*) is identified in the anterior third ventricle

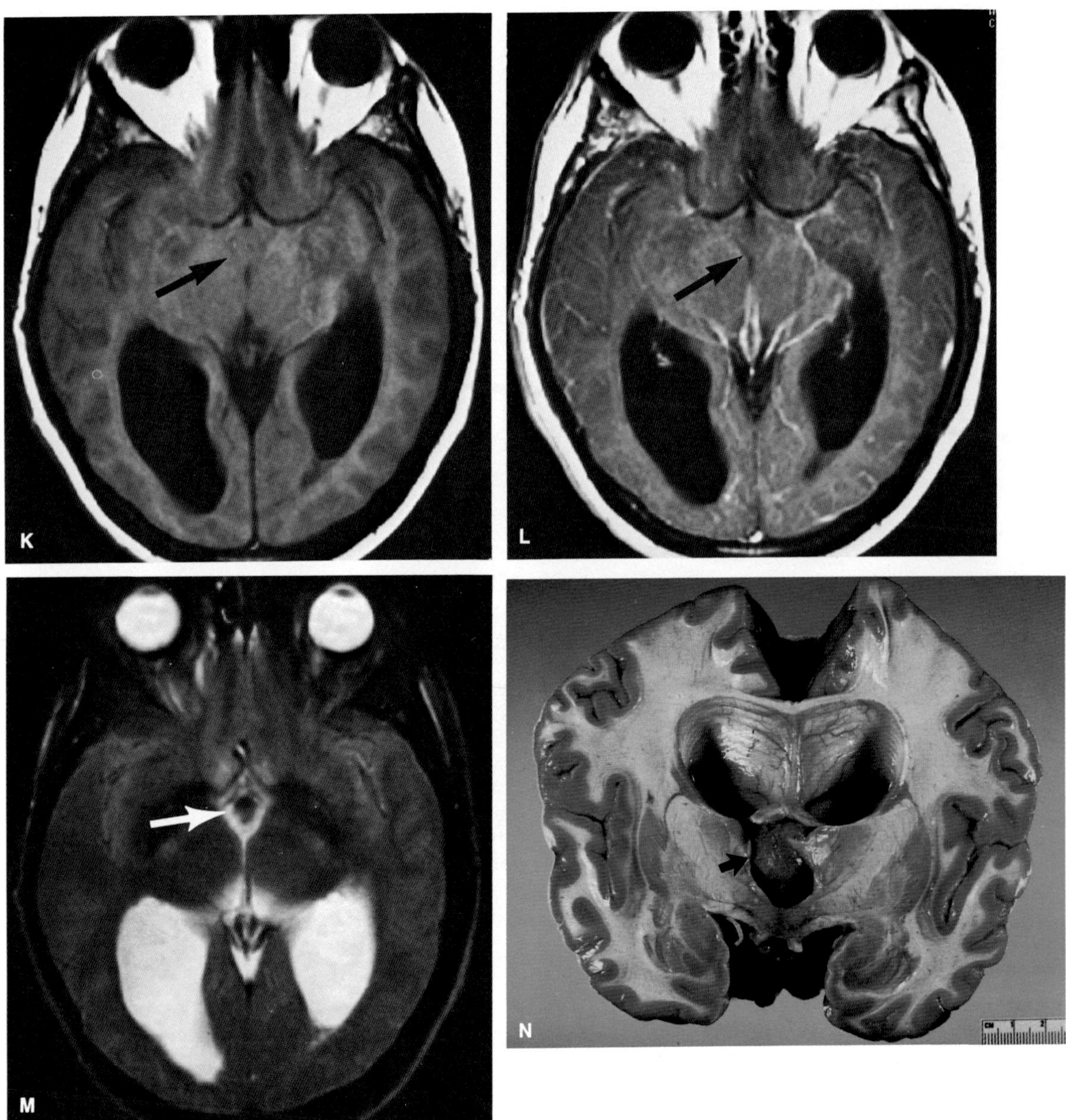

on the axial T1-weighted image (*K*). No contrast enhancement is identified on the postcontrast axial T1-weighted image (*L*). This mass is more clearly demonstrated as a relatively low-signal-intensity lesion within the anterior third ventricle on the axial T2-weighted image (*M*).

DIAGNOSIS

Colloid cyst

DISCUSSION

Colloid cysts are rare tumors of the third ventricle. They are congenital lesions and enlarge slowly, and usually do not become symptomatic until adulthood when they result in hydrocephalus. Size of these lesions varies from a few millimeters to several centimeters. The location of the colloid cyst in the anterior third ventricle allows it to obstruct one or both foramina of Monro. Patients usually present with headaches, which occasionally are intermittent and positional. Colloid cysts originate from the primitive neuroepithelium of the tela choroidea.[1] Histologically, these cysts have a thin, fibrous capsule with an epithelial lining. Colloid cysts contain principally secretory and breakdown products from the epithelial lining of the cyst, including fat, old blood, foamy cells, cholesterol crystals, hemosiderin-laden macrophages, and CSF.[2]

Colloid cysts are usually of increased signal intensity on T1-weighted images, but they can be isointense

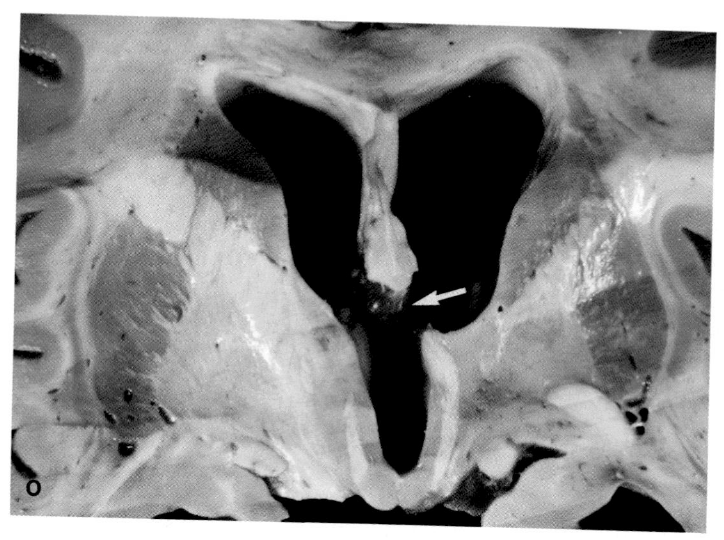

or even hypointense on T1-weighted images. On T2-weighted images these cysts are usually of increased signal intensity. On CT, a colloid cyst appears as a round lesion of decreased to increased attenuation in the anterosuperior third ventricle. Surrounding brain edema is rare.

Pathologic Correlate

Two cases are presented. (*N*) A smoothly marginated, spherical, 2-cm tumor is identified in the anterior third ventricle (*arrow*). There is dilatation of the lateral and third ventricles. (*O*) The lesion is smaller (*arrow*), without gross ventricular enlargement, and located as anticipated in the anterosuperior aspect of the third ventricle.

Clinical References

1. Maeder PP, Holtas SL, Basibuyuk LN, et al. Colloid cysts of the third ventricle: correlation of MR and CT findings with histology and chemical analysis. AJNR 1990;11:575–581.
2. Waggenspack GA, Guinto FC. MR and CT of masses of the anterosuperior third ventricle. AJR 1989;152:609–614.

(N *and* O *courtesy of Daron G. Davis, MD.)*

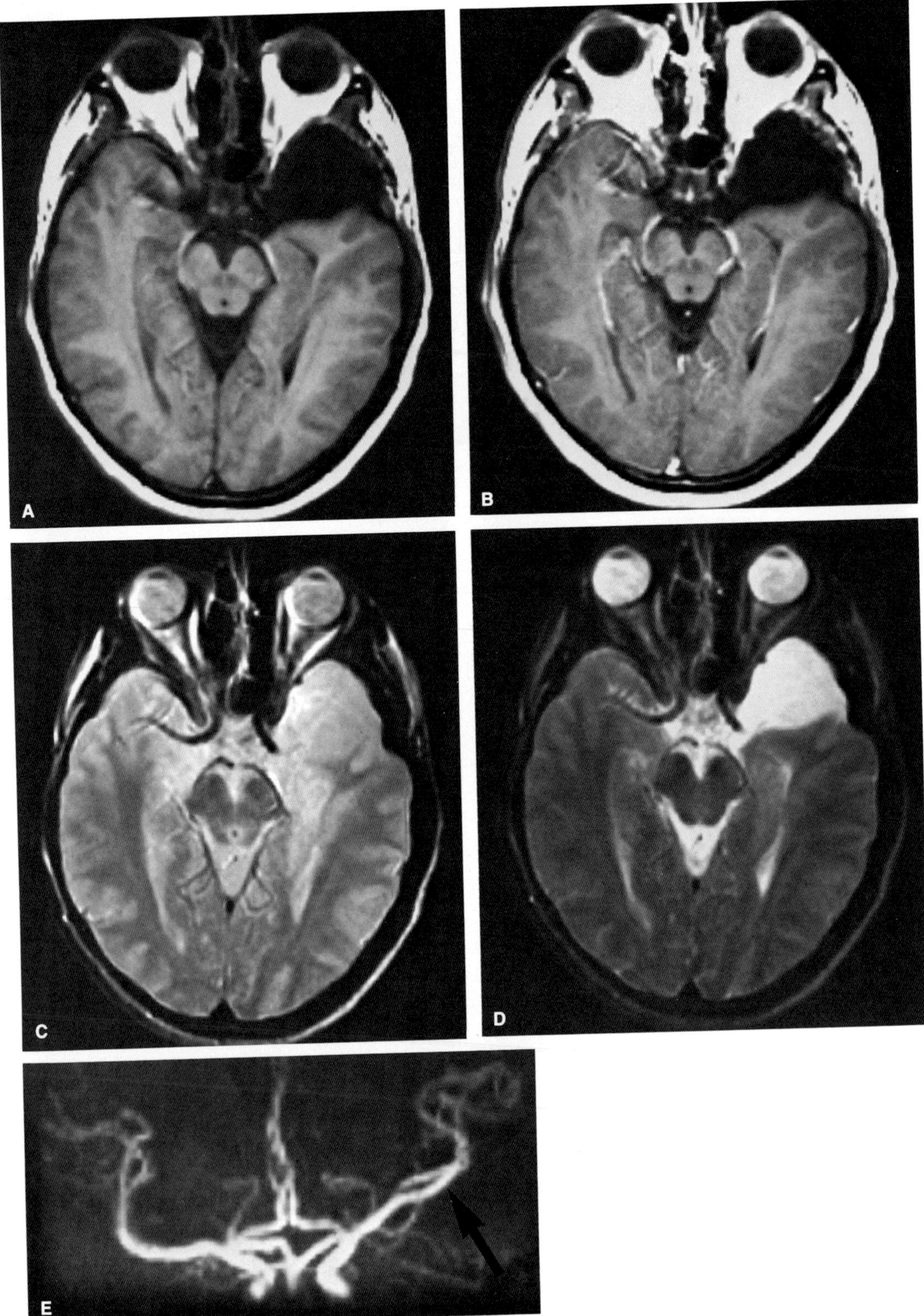
A
B
C
D
E

HISTORY

A 42-year-old man with a 29-year history of migraine headaches

FINDINGS

A large nonenhancing lesion of low signal intensity is identified in the left temporal fossa on precontrast (*A*) and postcontrast (*B*) axial T1-weighted images. The left temporal lobe is displaced, but not invaded by this mass. This lesion is of CSF signal intensity on the first (*C*) and second (*D*) echoes of the T2-weighted sequence. (*E*) MRA (AP projection) reveals displacement (elevation) of the left middle cerebral artery (*arrow*) by the mass.

DIAGNOSIS

Temporal fossa arachnoid cyst

DISCUSSION

Arachnoid cysts are common benign CSF-filled lesions, representing approximately 1% of intracranial masses. There are multiple causes for the development of arachnoid cysts including an inflammatory process in the subarachnoid space secondary to head trauma, leptomeningitis, and primary subarachnoid hemorrhage. Most of these lesions are thought to be congenital, originating secondary to malformation of the meninges.[1] They occur in specific locations, including the middle cranial fossa (the most common location), over the convexity of the brain, retrocerebellar, and in the perimesencephalic cisterns. Hypogenesis of the temporal lobe is a common finding in middle cranial fossa arachnoid cysts. They present at any age, are frequently asymptomatic, but can become symptomatic as a result of mass effect. Patients present with seizures, headaches, or focal neurologic signs.[2]

Arachnoid cysts are of CSF signal intensity on all pulse sequences, and do not demonstrate enhancement with a gadolinium chelate. Intrathecal contrast penetrates into these cysts on delayed scans.

Epidermoid tumors typically have signal characteristics only slightly different from CSF on SE MR images, pointing out the need for close image inspection. Diffusion-weighted images have proved useful in differentiation between epidermoid tumors and arachnoid cysts.[3]

Clinical References

1. Atlas SW. MRI of brain and spine. New York, Raven Press, 1991:364.
2. Robertson SJ, Wolpert SM, Runge VM. MR imaging of middle cranial fossa arachnoid cysts: temporal lobe agenesis syndrome revisited. AJNR 1989;10:1007–1010.
3. Tsuruda JS, Chew WM, Moseley ME, et al. Diffusion-weighted MR imaging of the brain: value of differentiating between extraaxial cysts and epidermoid tumors. AJNR 1990;11:925–931.

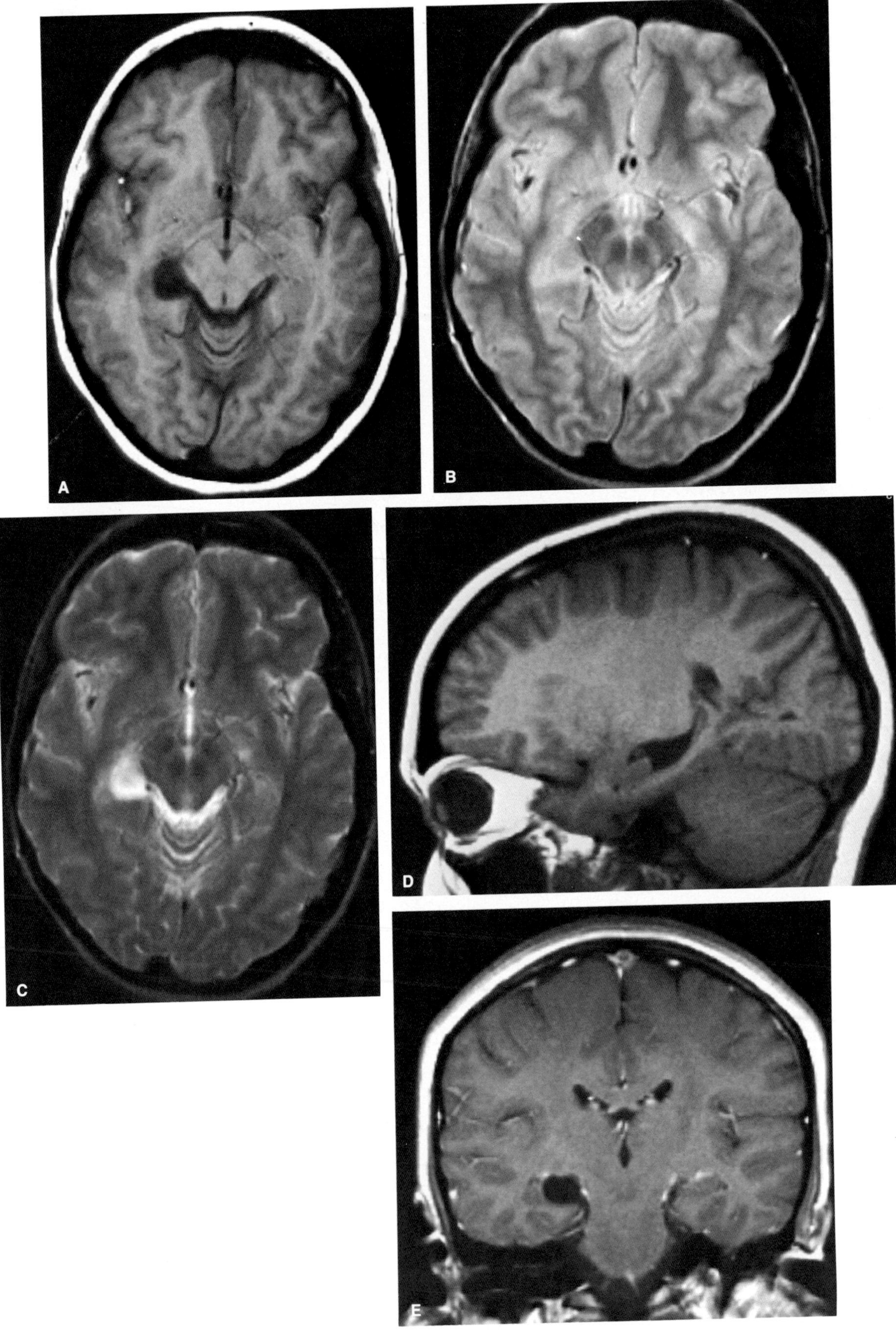
A
B
C
D
E

HISTORY

A 20-year-old woman in whom a questionable tumor was seen on CT

FINDINGS

A 2-cm lesion of CSF signal intensity on all pulse sequences is present in the right choroidal fissure on axial T1-weighted (*A*), intermediate T2-weighted (*B*), and heavily T2-weighted (*C*) images. The cystic mass is clearly delineated on sagittal precontrast (*D*) and coronal postcontrast (*E*) T1-weighted images. No surrounding gliosis is seen. No abnormal contrast enhancement was noted.

DIAGNOSIS

Choroidal fissure arachnoid cyst

DISCUSSION

Cystic masses of the CNS are categorized in several ways. The most important is whether the lesion is neoplastic. Contrast enhancement, a detectable cyst wall, associated soft tissue mass, heterogeneous appearance, and surrounding gliosis or edema are all findings inconsistent with a simple benign cystic mass and raise the possibility of neoplasm. Nonneoplastic cystic lesions expanding the choroidal fissure have a characteristic appearance. These cysts are sharply demarcated from adjacent brain tissue with no visible wall, or surrounding gliosis or edema. The signal intensity of these cysts is identical to CSF on all pulse sequences, and no contrast enhancement is present.[1]

The choroidal fissure is the CSF space between the fimbria of the hippocampus and diencephalon. It is a narrow fissure that curves posterosuperiorly from the anterior temporal lobe to the atrium of the lateral ventricle. Developmental errors can occur at the time of formation of the primitive choroid plexus anywhere along the choroid fissure, thus forming a cyst. These cysts may be either neuroepithelial or arachnoid in origin. Neuroepithelial cysts are lined by epithelium; arachnoid cysts are usually not lined by epithelium and form between layers of arachnoid or between the dura and the arachnoid.

MR Technique

Coronal images often more clearly reveal the location of a choroidal fissure arachnoid cyst, depicting expansion of the fissure as it courses through the temporal lobe.

Pitfalls in Image Interpretation

The characteristic MR appearance of cerebrospinal cysts is important to recognize, so that these lesions are not confused with a neoplastic process, such as an intraaxial cystic tumor.

Clinical References

1. Sherman JL, Camponovo E, and Citrin CM. MR imaging of CSF-like choroidal fissure and parenchymal cysts of the brain. AJR 1990;155:1069–1075.

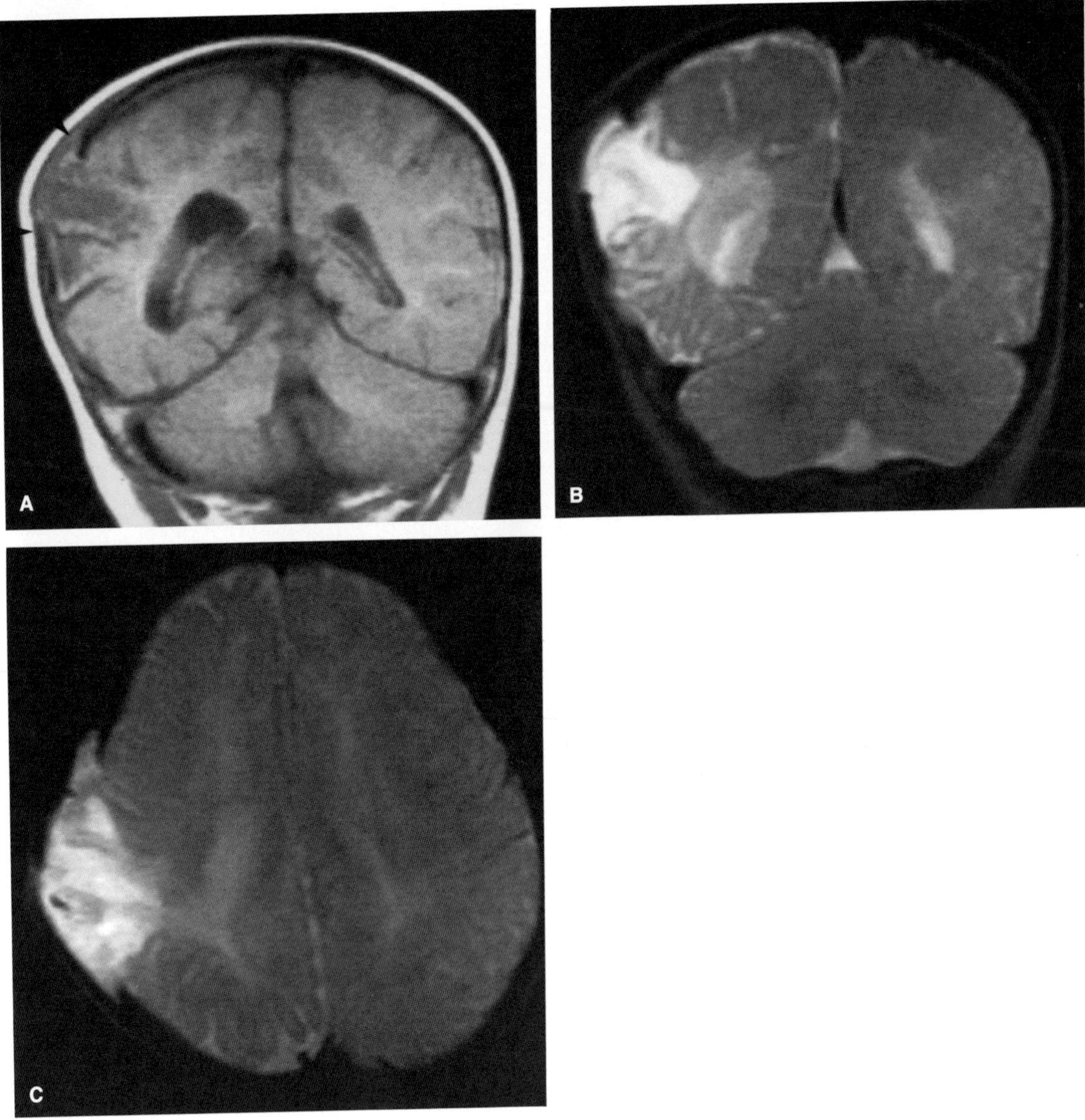

HISTORY

A 7-month-old infant with a history of a skull fracture

FINDINGS

(*A*) Coronal T1-weighted image demonstrates a soft tissue mass representing herniated brain extending through the right parietal bone (*arrows*). The normal low signal intensity associated with cortical bone is lost at the point of brain herniation. The mass is of predominantly increased signal intensity on coronal (*B*) and axial (*C*) T2-weighted images, representing a combination of CSF and brain tissue.

DIAGNOSIS

Posttraumatic leptomeningeal cyst

DISCUSSION

Leptomeningeal cysts are rare complications of skull fractures in infancy and early childhood, usually involving the parietal bone.[1–3] The trauma produces a tear in the dura in addition to the skull fracture, allowing the leptomeninges to herniate through the dural defect preventing normal bony apposition and healing. The essential feature is the dural tear. Pulsation of the brain gradually pushes more leptomeninges through the dural tear. Subarachnoid fluid becomes trapped along with herniated brain, forming a cyst. The growing cyst gradually erodes the edges of the bone and compresses the underlying cortex, leading to atrophy. Diagnosis is made in some cases years after the initial injury. A leptomeningeal cyst can also occur following craniotomy.

MR Technique

The dural defect may be difficult to visualize in a single plane, with imaging in both the axial and coronal planes recommended.

Clinical References

1. Cook PG, Norman PF. Case report: intradiploic leptomeningeal cyst of the frontal bone occurring as a complication of head injury in an adult. Clin Radiol 1988;39:214–215.
2. Halliday AL, Chapman PH, Heros RC. Leptomeningeal cyst resulting from adulthood trauma: case report. Neurosurgery 1990;26:150–153.
3. Palaoglu S, Beskonakli E, Senel K, et al. Intraosseous location of posterior fossa post-traumatic leptomeningeal cyst. Neuroradiology 1990;32:78.

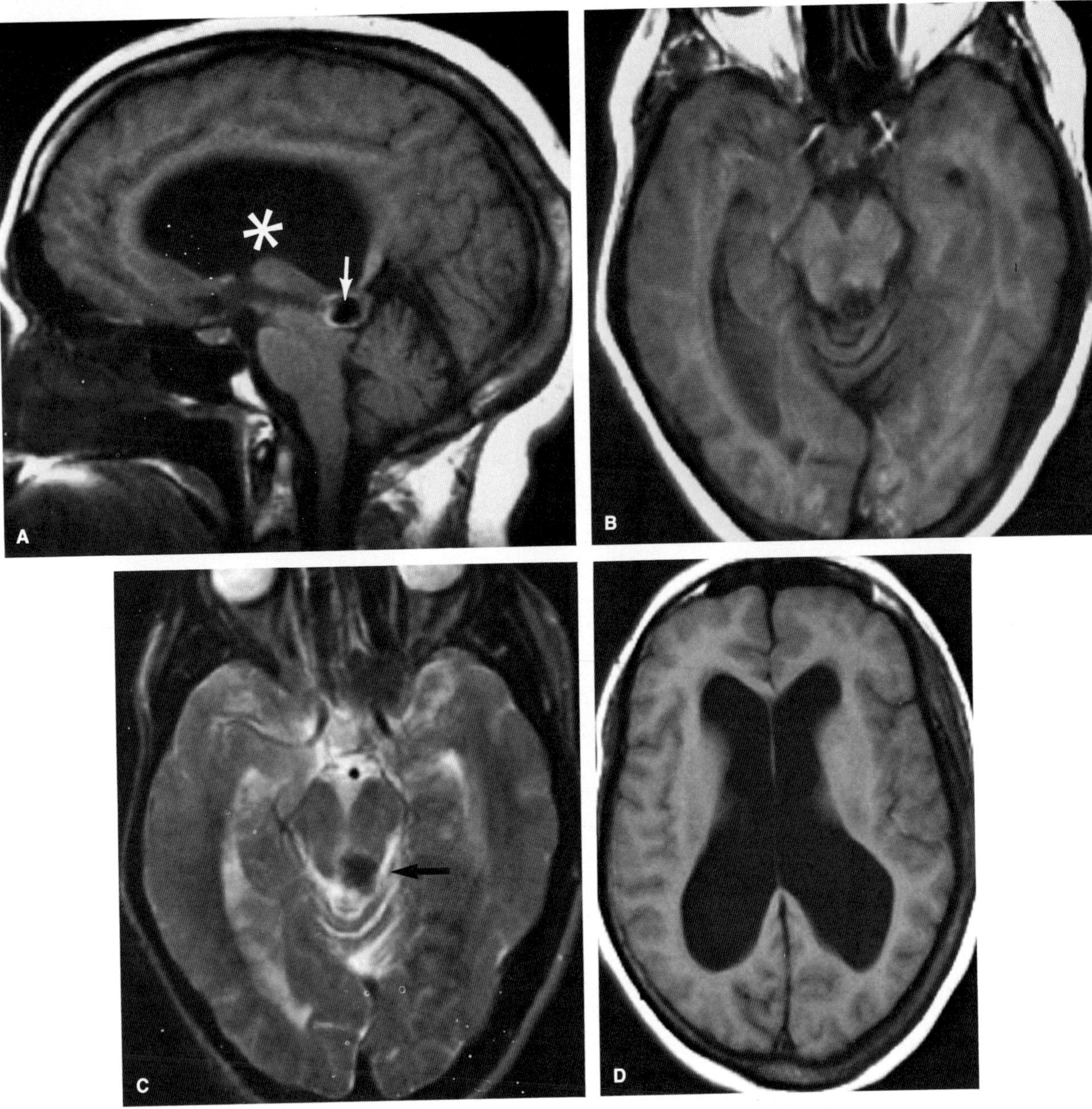

HISTORY

A 62-year-old woman with ataxia

FINDINGS

(*A*) On the T1-weighted sagittal image there is a well-demarcated, very low signal intensity mass (*white arrow*) in the expected region of the pineal gland. There is high signal intensity surrounding the mass on this noninfused image. The third ventricle (*asterisk*) is abnormally large. (*B*) The T1-weighted axial image demonstrates compression of the left side of the tectum by the low-signal-intensity mass. (*C*) The T2-weighted axial image (*arrow*) also shows the mass to be low signal intensity. There is no edema in the midbrain. The lateral ventricles are abnormally dilated on the T1-weighted axial image (*D*) at a more cephalad level. A noninfused CT (*not shown*) of the brain demonstrated a 1-cm dense calcification in the region of the pineal gland.

DIAGNOSIS

Pineocytoma

DISCUSSION

Pineal region neoplasms are uncommon tumors, accounting for approximately 3% to 8% of intracranial tumors in children, and 0.4% to 1% in adults.[1] These tumors can be divided into four major groups: (1) germ cell tumors, (2) pineal parenchymal tumors, (3) gliomas, and (4) meningiomas. Most masses arising from the stroma of the pineal gland itself are germ cell tumors, especially in children. Gliomas and meningiomas are usually large masses that arise from contiguous structures and secondarily invade the pineal gland.

Pineal parenchymal tumors include pineoblastomas and pineocytomas, and constitute only 5% of all tumors of the pineal region.[2] They arise from the neuroepithelial cells of the pineal gland. Pineoblastomas are highly malignant neoplasms and, like germ cell tumors of the pineal gland, usually occur in the first two decades of life. Pineocytomas are benign, well-demarcated, noninvasive, slow-growing tumors that commonly present in adulthood and have no sex predilection.[3] Pineocytomas are usually heterogeneous on MR, enhance after contrast infusion and contain calcification, sometimes with chunky pieces of calcium.[3] Patients with pineal tumors may present with symptoms due to obstructive hydrocephalus (eg, ataxia), Parinaud's syndrome (paralysis of upward gaze) due to compression of the tectum, or endocrinologic abnormalities, seen most commonly with germ cell tumors.[1]

Pitfalls in Image Interpretation

MR is often nonspecific in determining the tissue type of pineal region tumors. Differentiation is usually made according to the patient's age and sex, and the involvement of adjacent structures. The most common calcified neoplasm arising from, and confined to, the pineal gland parenchyma in an elderly female is a pineocytoma. Germ cell tumors have a decidedly male predominance and usually occur in the first two decades of life.

Clinical References

1. Tein R, Barkovich A, Edwards M. MR imaging of pineal tumors. AJR 1990;155:143–151.
2. Muller-Forell W, Schroth G, Egan P. MR imaging in tumors of the pineal region. Neuroradiology 1988;30:224–231.
3. Ganti S, Hilal S, Stein B, et al. CT of pineal region tumors. AJR 1986;146:451–458.

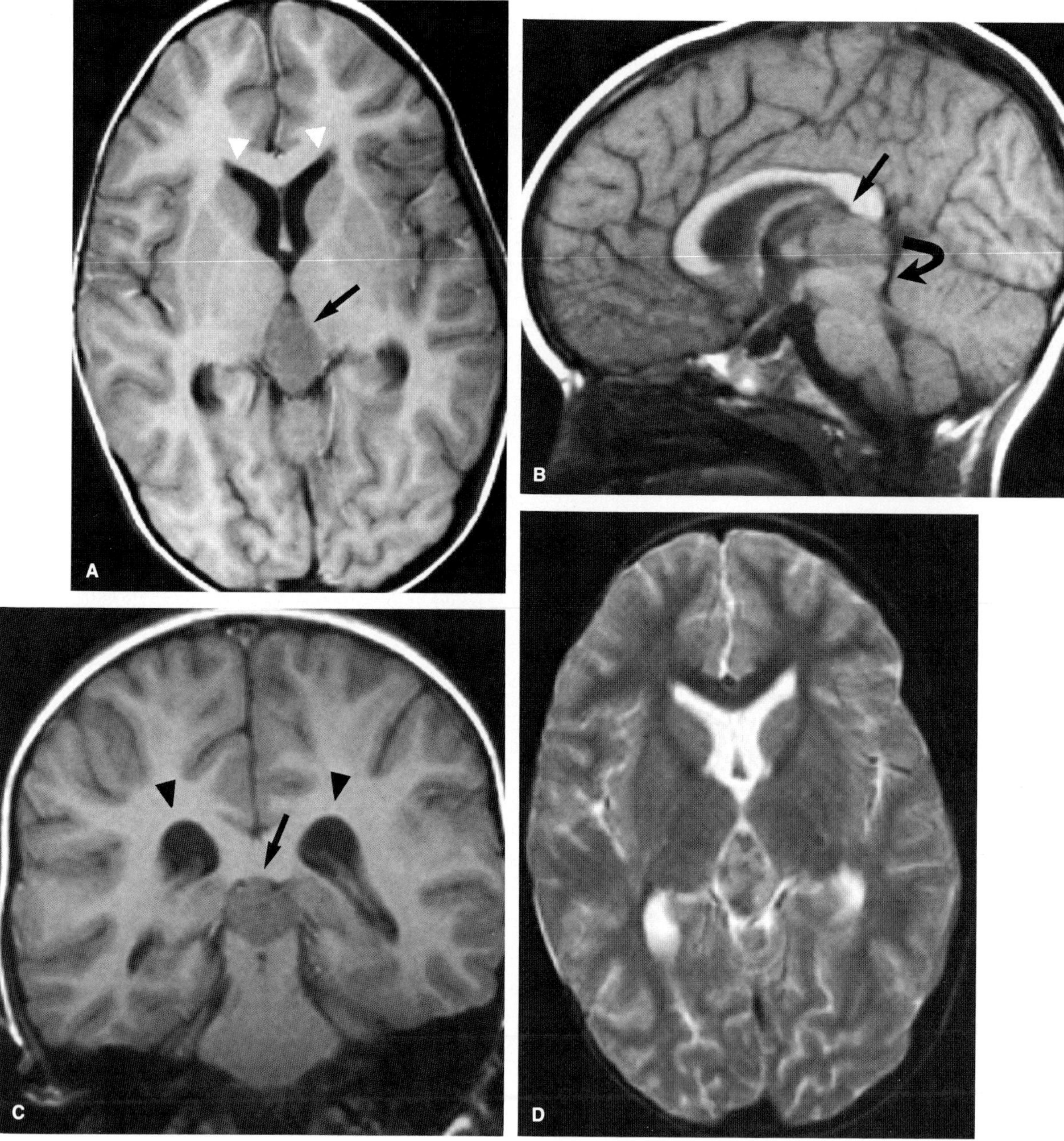

HISTORY

A 5-year-old with headaches, nausea, and vomiting for 2 weeks. Physical examination revealed papilledema. The medical history is pertinent in regard to a left enucleation and radiation to the right globe for bilateral retinoblastomas.

FINDINGS

T1-weighted axial (*A*), sagittal (*B*), and coronal (*C*) images demonstrate a soft tissue mass (*black arrow*) with homogeneous signal intensity, equal to that of gray matter, in the expected location of the pineal gland. The tectum (*curved black arrow in B*) is compressed and deformed by the mass. (*D*) Signal intensity of the mass on the T2-weighted axial image is heterogeneous, but predominantly equal to that of gray matter. The frontal horns (*white arrowheads in A*) and the atria (*arrowheads in C*) of the lateral ventricles are mildly enlarged. The lesion demonstrated marked homogeneous postcontrast enhancement (*images not shown*).

DIAGNOSIS

Pineal retinoblastoma

DISCUSSION

Ectopic retinoblastoma in the region of the pineal gland associated with bilateral ocular retinoblastomas is referred to as "trilateral retinoblastoma." This rare syndrome is genetically transferred, and approximately 66% of patients have family histories of retinoblastoma.[1] Ocular tumors in patients with trilateral retinoblastoma usually occur around the age of 6 months. The pineal retinoblastoma subsequently occurs several years later, after successful treatment of the retinal tumors by enucleation or radiation. The pineal tumor causes headache, hydrocephalus, vomiting, papilledema, and ataxia. Parinaud's syndrome, or paralysis of conjugate upward gaze caused by compression of the superior colliculi, may be present. Leptomeningeal spread from pineal retinoblastomas is common and is a poor prognostic factor.

There is phylogenic evidence of vestigial photoreceptor tissue in the pineal gland.[1] It is well known that in lower vertebrates the pineal gland is a photoreceptor organ with functions similar to those of the retina in humans.[2] Thus, the pineal gland is sometimes referred to as the "third eye." A pineal retinoblastoma is histologically identical to an ocular retinoblastoma. It is theorized that trilateral retinoblastoma is due to the combination of a genetic mutation that targets all photoreceptor tissue and inherited impaired host resistance to the carcinogenic effects of these genes.[1]

On MR, a pineal retinoblastoma is usually isointense or hypointense on T1-weighted images, and isointense to hyperintense on T2-weighted images compared with gray matter. The tumor enhances homogeneously after contrast infusion.

Pitfalls in Image Interpretation

The differential diagnosis for a pineal tumor includes pineoblastoma, pineocytoma, metastases, and germ cell tumors. However, a pineal mass in a patient with a history of bilateral ocular retinoblastomas is pathognomonic for a trilateral retinoblastoma. Pineal retinoblastoma is considered a rare variant of pineoblastoma by some investigators.

Clinical References

1. Johnson D, Chandra R, Fisher W, et al. Trilateral retinoblastoma: ocular and pineal retinoblastomas. J Neurosurg 1985;63:367–370.
2. Mafee M, Goldberg M, Greenwald M, et al. Retinoblastoma and simulating lesions: role of CT and MR imaging. Radiol Clin North Am 1987;25:667–682.

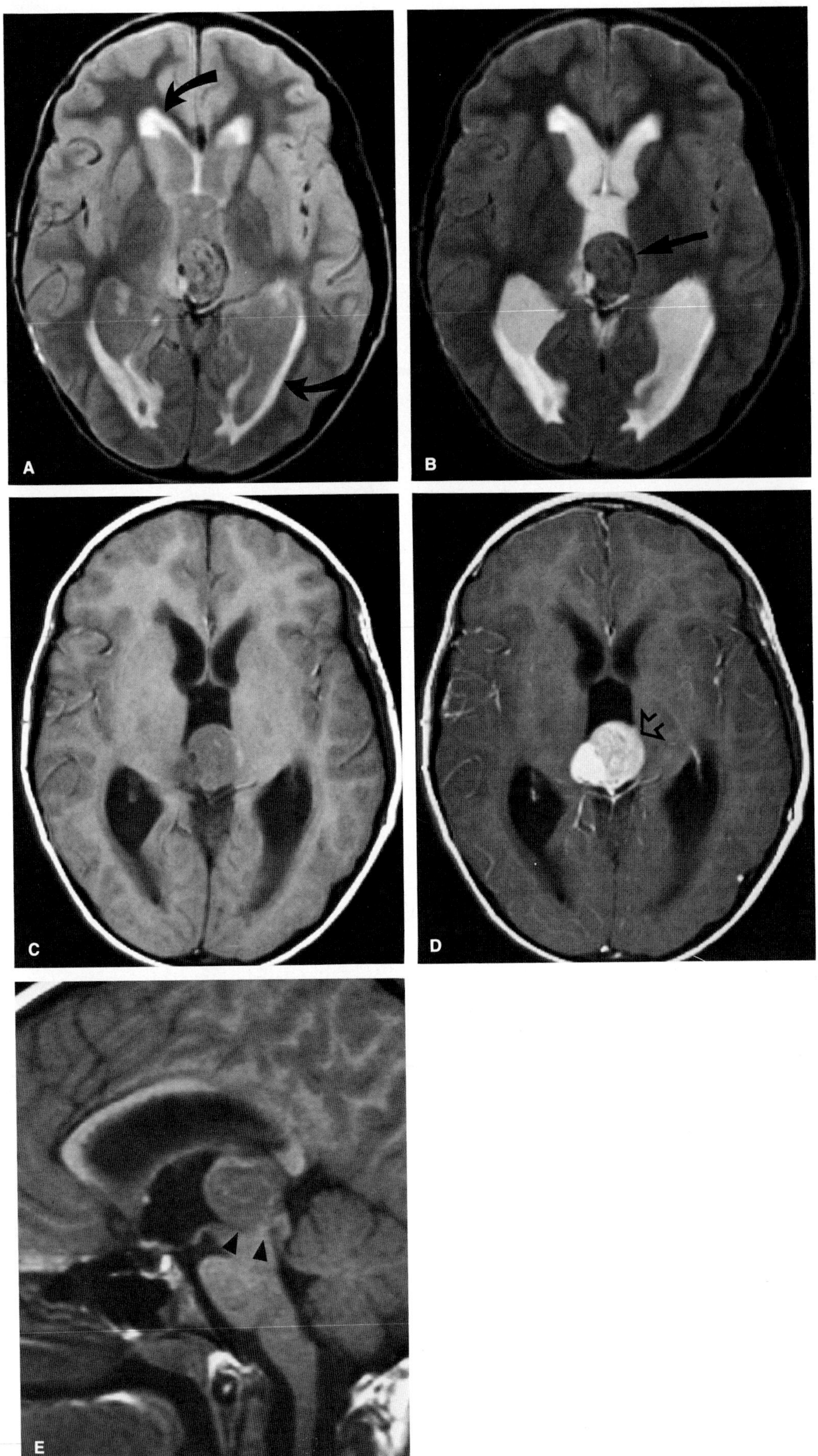
A
B
C
D
E

HISTORY

A 9-year-old boy with increasing headache, nausea, and vomiting for several weeks. There was papilledema on ophthalmologic examination.

FINDINGS

(*A and B*) Axial T2-weighted (TE = 45 and 90 msec) images reveal a 2 × 2 cm mass (*arrow in B*), which is predominantly isointense with white matter (a small portion of the tumor on the right side exhibits hyperintense characteristics), bordering the posterior portion of the third ventricle. The third and lateral ventricles are dilated, with a smooth cap of periventricular high signal intensity, best seen on the intermediate echo, corresponding to transependymal flow (*curved arrows in A*). Comparison of precontrast (*C*) and postcontrast (*D*) T1-weighted images reveals intense lesion enhancement (*open arrow in D*). (*E*) The sagittal unenhanced T1-weighted "scout" image localizes the lesion to the pineal region, and demonstrates aqueductal compression (*arrowheads*) with obstruction of the third and lateral ventricles. The fourth ventricle is normal in size.

DIAGNOSIS

Mixed germ cell tumor, with both germinoma and embryonal carcinoma elements, causing obstructive hydrocephalus

DISCUSSION

MR is sensitive for detection of pineal region tumors and provides accurate lesion localization. However, signal intensity characteristics are nonspecific with respect to tumor type.[1] IV contrast enhancement is important in particular for detection of tumor seeding by way of CSF fluid pathways.

Germ cell tumors of the brain develop most commonly in central neuraxis sites, in particular the pineal and hypothalamic (suprasellar) regions. Both germinomas and tumors of totipotential cells (endodermal sinus tumor and embryonal carcinoma, teratoma, and choriocarcinoma) are thought to arise from germ cell precursors. These lesions occur principally in the first three decades of life, with a preponderance in males. All are prone to seeding by way of the CSF. Germinomas are the most common type of germ cell tumor, being also the most frequent tumor encountered at the site of the pineal gland. Germinomas are markedly radiosensitive with survival extending to one or two decades with responsive lesions. Embryonal carcinomas and endodermal sinus tumors are highly malignant. Mature teratomas, if completely excised, carry a good prognosis. The occurrence of mixed germ cell tumors, with various cellular elements, is common.

MR Technique

Intermediate T2 weighting (TR≈2500/TE≈45) assists in identification of soft tissue abnormalities immediately adjacent to CSF in either the ventricular system or subarachnoid space.

Pitfalls in Image Interpretation

Two perpendicular planes are often needed for precise anatomic localization of intracranial masses. A protocol that begins with a multislice sagittal "scout" scan (used in patient positioning and later for clinical interpretation), followed by axial imaging, suffices in many instances.

Clinical References

1. Tien RD, Barkovich AJ, Edwards MSB. MR imaging of pineal tumors. AJR 1990;155:143–151.

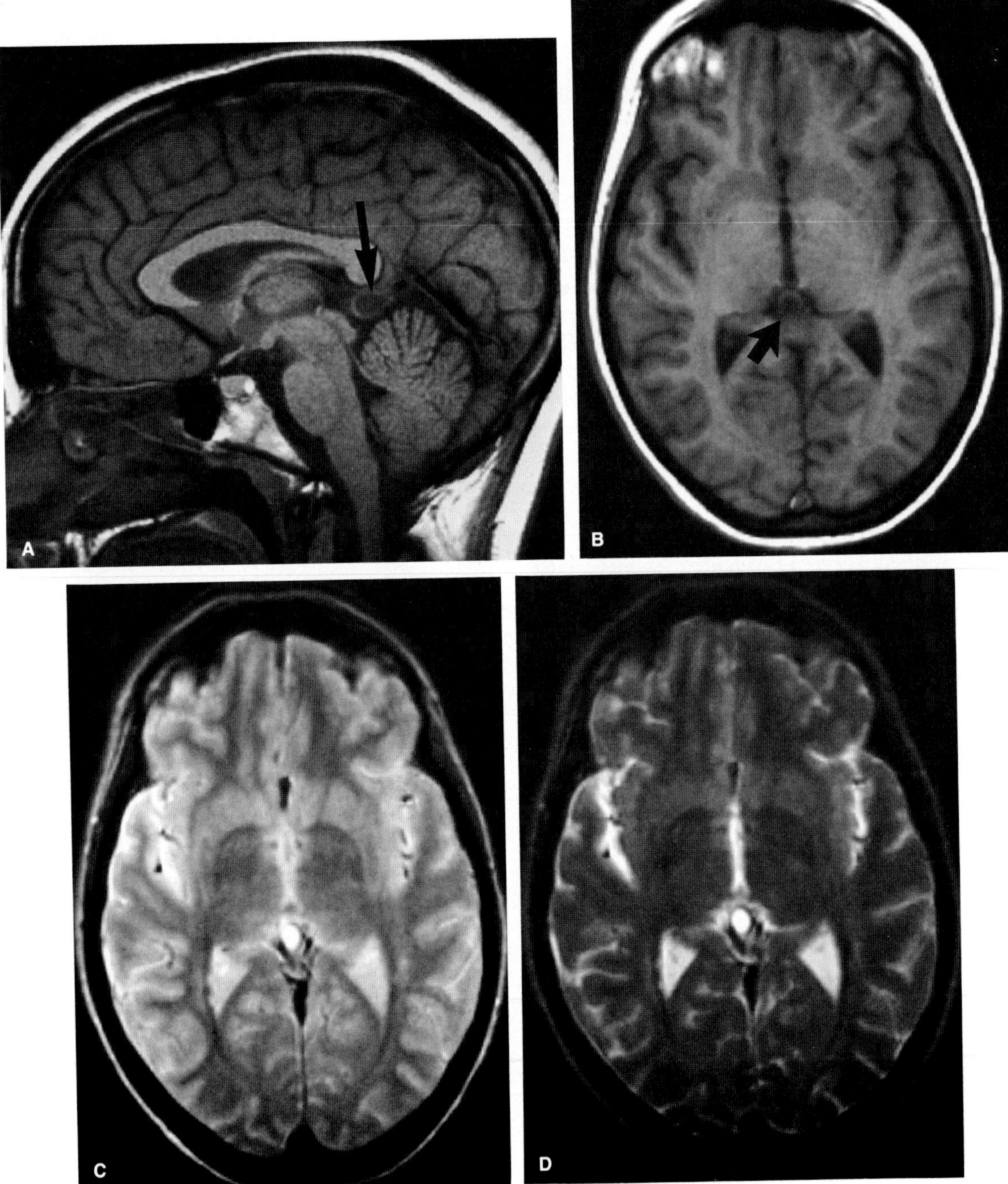

HISTORY

Noncontributory

FINDINGS

T1-weighted sagittal (*A*) and axial (*B*) images identify a small round cystic lesion (*arrows*) of decreased signal intensity in the expected location of the pineal gland. The wall of this cyst is thin and smooth. The fluid within the lesion is hyperintense to CSF on the first (*C*) and second (*D*) echoes of the axial T2-weighted sequence. There is no mass effect.

DIAGNOSIS

Pineal cyst

DISCUSSION

Pineal cysts are benign lesions that are almost always asymptomatic. Rarely, they can bleed internally or cause aqueductal compression and result in hydrocephalus. These cysts are a common finding at autopsy with an incidence reported as high as 40%. On MR imaging, pineal cysts are round and smoothly marginated. They rarely measure more than 15 mm in diameter. The cyst walls are thin and usually measure less than 2 mm in thickness. A cyst can occupy a portion of the pineal gland or replace the entire structure.

The contents of a pineal cyst are homogeneous, and are usually isointense to CSF on all pulse sequences. Occasionally, pineal cysts can be hyperintense to CSF on T2-weighted images, as illustrated in this case. This divergence from CSF signal intensity is best delineated on intermediate T2-weighted sequences. Increased signal intensity on T2-weighted images may be secondary to lack of fluid motion within the cyst, high protein content, or old hemorrhage; it does not indicate neoplastic involvement.[1]

The contents of a pineal cyst do not enhance, but the margins of the cyst, which represent the residual normal pineal gland, do enhance. The pineal gland enhances because of the absence of the blood–brain barrier.

MR Technique

Pineal cysts are best visualized on sagittal images.

Pitfalls in Image Interpretation

A pineal cyst must be differentiated from a cystic neoplasm. Size, enhancing characteristics, and the presence or absence of mass effect are important differentiating features.

Clinical References

1. Lee DH, Norman D, Newton TH. MR imaging of pineal cysts. J Comput Assist Tomogr 1987;11:586–590.

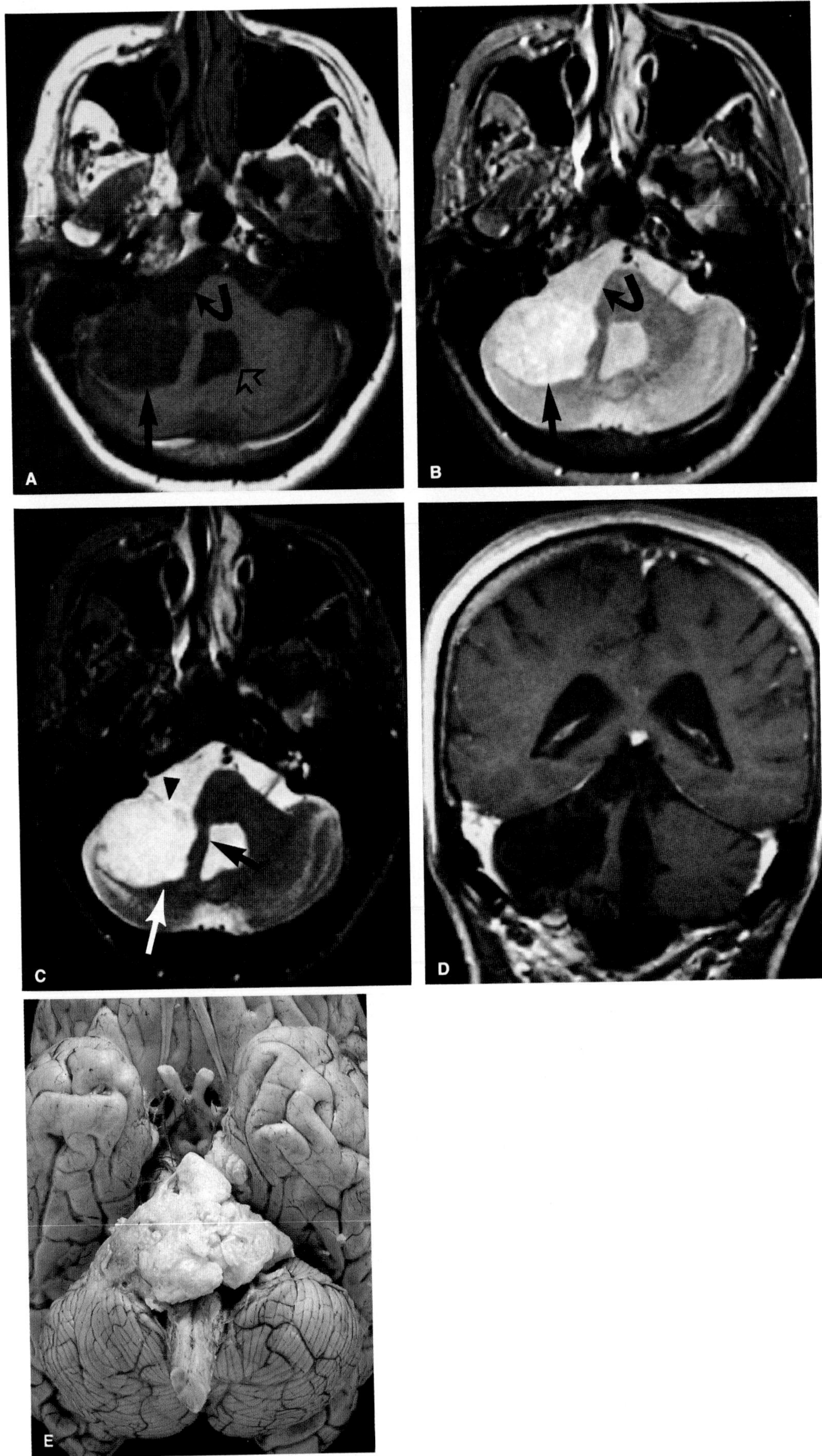
A
B
C
D
E

HISTORY

A 51-year-old patient with new onset of ataxia, spasticity of the right leg, numbness of the right side of the face, diminished hearing on the right, and remote history of posterior fossa surgery

FINDINGS

(*A*) T1-weighted axial image demonstrates an irregular, well-demarcated extraaxial mass (*arrow*) in the right cerebellopontine angle (CPA) cistern. The mass has slightly higher signal intensity than CSF in the CPA cistern (*curved arrow*), and the fourth ventricle (*open arrow*). (*B*) On the intermediate T2-weighted image the signal intensity of the mass (*arrow*) is heterogeneous, but definitely higher than CSF (*curved arrow*). (*C*) The difference in signal intensity between the lesion and CSF is not apparent on the heavily T2-weighted image. The lesion is severely compressing the right middle cerebellar peduncle (*arrow*) and right cerebellar hemisphere (*white arrow*), and is causing the right seventh and eighth nerve complex (*arrowhead*) to be stretched. The distortion of these structures is best appreciated by comparing them to the corresponding normal structures on the left side. (*D*) Postcontrast T1-weighted coronal image shows no enhancement of the mass.

DIAGNOSIS

Epidermoid

DISCUSSION

Intracranial epidermoids, or epidermoid cysts, are benign congenital lesions that form from incomplete cleavage of neural ectoderm from cutaneous ectoderm at the time of closure of the neural tube. This results in retention of ectopic ectodermal cells in the neural groove.[1] Epidermoids slowly increase in size by progressive desquamation of epithelial cells from the tumor lining. These tumors are pliable, allowing them to extend into and conform to subarachnoid spaces in which they are located. As a result, epidermoids usually are not large enough to cause symptoms until adulthood, at which time patients present with neurologic signs caused by local compression. Eighty percent of epidermoids are intradural, and the CPA cistern and the middle cranial fossa are the most common locations.[2] Epidermoid is the third most common CPA tumor, following acoustic neuroma and meningioma.

The interior of an epidermoid contains keratin and solid cholesterol crystals, which are epithelial breakdown products.[3] These components cause the signal intensity of an epidermoid to be slightly greater than CSF on both T1- and T2-weighted images. This is opposed to an arachnoid cyst, the main consideration in the differential diagnosis, which has signal intensity identical to CSF on all pulse sequences. Because both an arachnoid cyst and an epidermoid may have identical low density on CT, MR is the procedure of choice for differentiating between the two.

Complete surgical resection of an epidermoid is frequently not possible because of its tendency to insinuate within and around adjacent structures. Thus, residual or "recurrent" tumor is not unusual.

MR Technique

Intermediate T2-weighted images are the most useful for determining the hyperintensity of an epidermoid in comparison with CSF.

Pathologic Correlate

(*E*) Basal view of a gross brain specimen demonstrates a large prepontine epidermoid that originates from the right CPA cistern. Epidermoids have an irregular shape and contour, unlike arachnoid cysts, which usually are smooth.

Clinical References

1. Yuh W, Barloon T, Jacoby C, et al. MR of fourth-ventricular epidermoid tumors. AJNR 1988;9:794–796.
2. Tampieri D, Melanson D, Ethier R. MR imaging of epidermoid cysts. AJNR 1989;10:351–356.
3. Steffey D, DeFilipp G, Spera T, et al. MR imaging of primary epidermoid tumors. J Comput Assist Tomogr 1988;12:438–440.

(E *from Okazaki H, Scheithauer B. Slide atlas of neuropathology. New York, Gower Medical Publishing, 1988. By permission of Mayo Foundation.*)

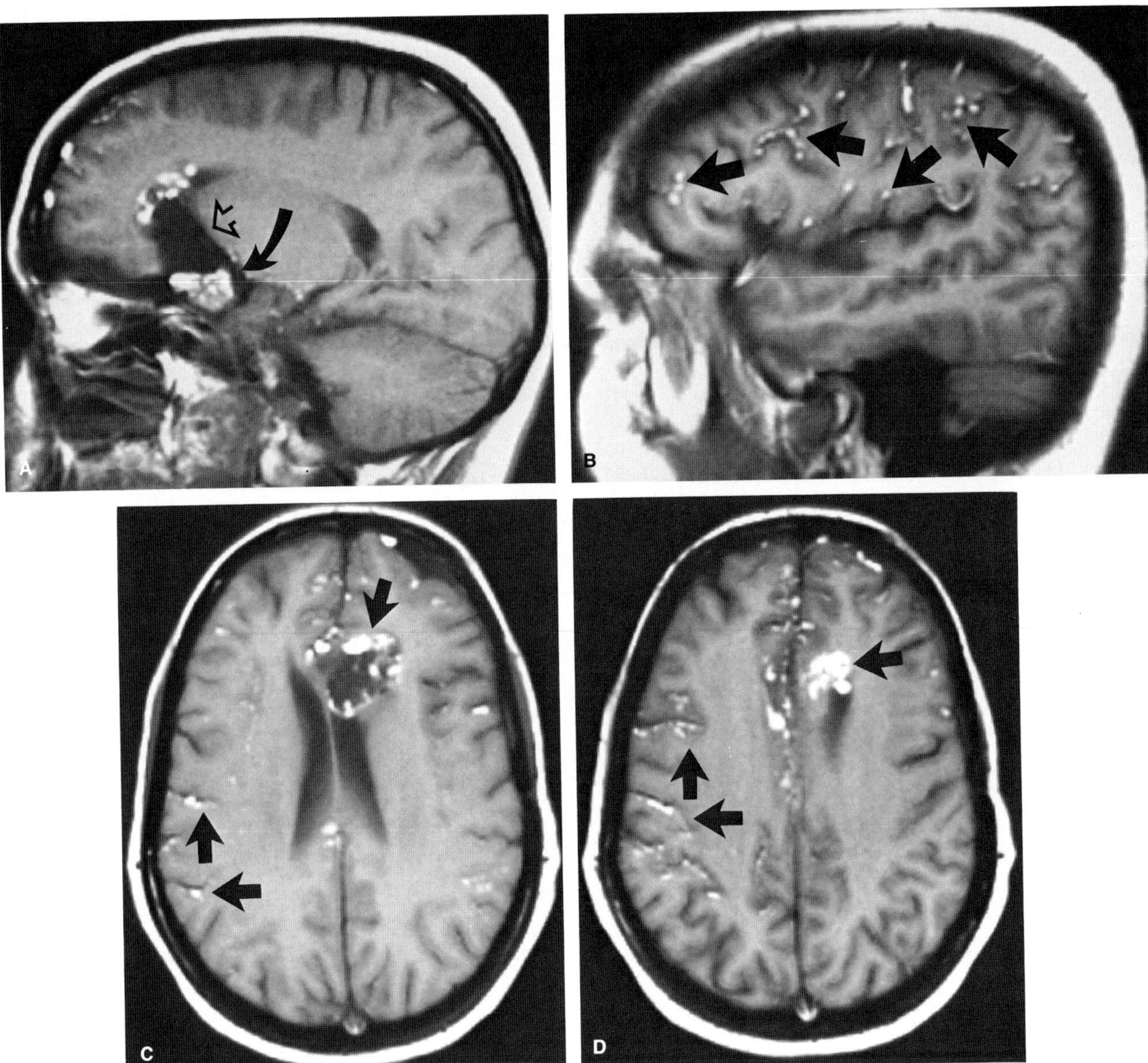

HISTORY

A 33-year-old patient, 6 months after intracranial surgery, who presented for routine follow-up without symptoms

FINDINGS

(*A and B*) Precontrast T1-weighted sagittal images demonstrate a postsurgical defect in the left parasellar and suprasellar region (*open arrow in A*), with a 2-cm residual hyperintense mass (*curved arrow in A*) and multiple hyperintense globules (*arrows in B*) that appear to lie in the subarachnoid space. Again noted on precontrast T1-weighted axial images (*C and D*) are scattered small foci of high signal intensity (*arrows*) lying principally in the operative defect and within the brain sulci. The signal intensity of these lesions paralleled that of fat on heavily T2-weighted images (*not shown*). (*E and F*) Intermediate T2-weighted images (TE = 45 msec) from a low-bandwidth pulse sequence demonstrate most of the foci with hypointense superior margins (*small black arrows*) and hyperintense inferior margins (*small white arrows*), in the direction of the readout gradient, as a result of chemical shift artifact. On CT (*not shown*), these abnormalities were of low attenuation.

DIAGNOSIS

Ruptured intracranial dermoid

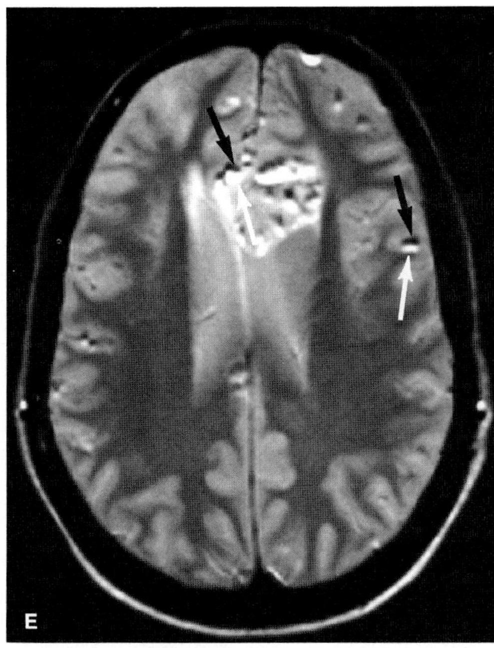

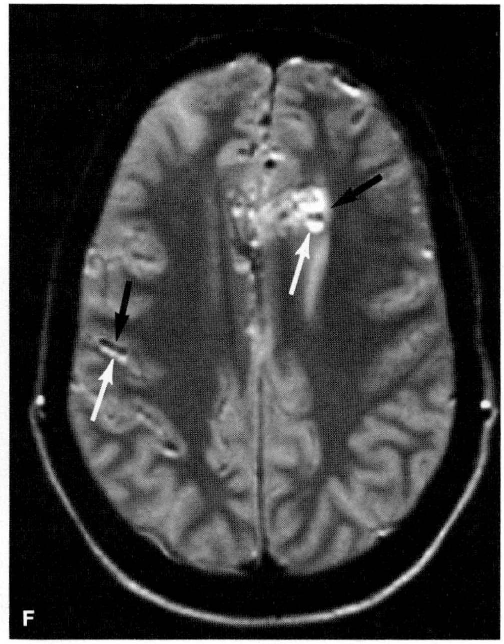

DISCUSSION

Intracranial dermoids are rare congenital tumors, which present in the first two to three decades of life and occur in the midline near the cerebellar vermis, pons, or sella turcica. These lesions, like epidermoids, are thought to arise as a result of the inadvertent inclusion of ectodermal tissue during neural tube closure. In common with epidermoids, the dermoid cyst has a lining of squamous epithelial cells. However, dermoids are distinguished by the presence of skin appendages and hair follicles. The term *pearly tumor* arises from the glistening white appearance of the fibrous capsule in intact lesions. Clinical presentation is variable. On rupture, patients can present with meningeal signs, seizures, transient ischemic attacks (due to vasospasm), or (rarely) hydrocephalus.[1] In contradistinction to early reports that suggested that rupture was uniformly fatal, many cases are now reported with survival. After rupture, spread of fatty material can be observed in both the subarachnoid space and the ventricular system. On CT, the fat content gives rise to hypodensity with negative attenuation values. Frequently, the fat is mobile, which can be demonstrated by changing the position of the patient's head and rescanning. This also accounts for the redistribution of fatty material that can be observed on follow-up scans. On MR, the signal intensity of the fatty material within a dermoid can be observed to parallel that of subcutaneous fat. Lesions are typically strongly hyperintense on T1-weighted scans, but this appearance varies, depending on the fat content. Other compartments such as hair may predominate, or fat can even be absent. Sulcal widening by fat, although rare, has been described as a pathognomonic sign for a ruptured dermoid.

Diagnostically, MR is superior to CT in patients with a ruptured dermoid because it provides improved identification of (1) fat within the subarachnoid space, (2) involvement of extraaxial structures, and (3) vascular compromise.[2]

In the clinical case presented, the primary dermoid cyst lay (preoperatively) in the left parasellar region, with rupture leading to spread into the subarachnoid space.

Pitfalls in Image Interpretation

The high signal intensity of fat on T1-weighted images in a lesion such as a dermoid must be differentiated from the appearance of methemoglobin. Although the use of fat suppression techniques permits definitive differentiation, sufficient clues may at times be derived from comparison with T2-weighted images or close inspection for chemical shift effects. The high signal intensity of a lesion on T1-weighted images is also not a reliable criterion for differentiation of a dermoid from an epidermoid tumor, with the latter reported rarely to demonstrate such signal intensity change.[2]

Clinical References

1. Wilms G, Casselman J, Demaerel PH, et al. CT and MRI of ruptured intracranial dermoids. Neuroradiology 1991;33: 149–151.
2. Smith AS, Benson JE, Blaser SI, et al. Diagnosis of ruptured intracranial dermoid cyst: value of MR over CT. AJNR 1991;12:175–180.

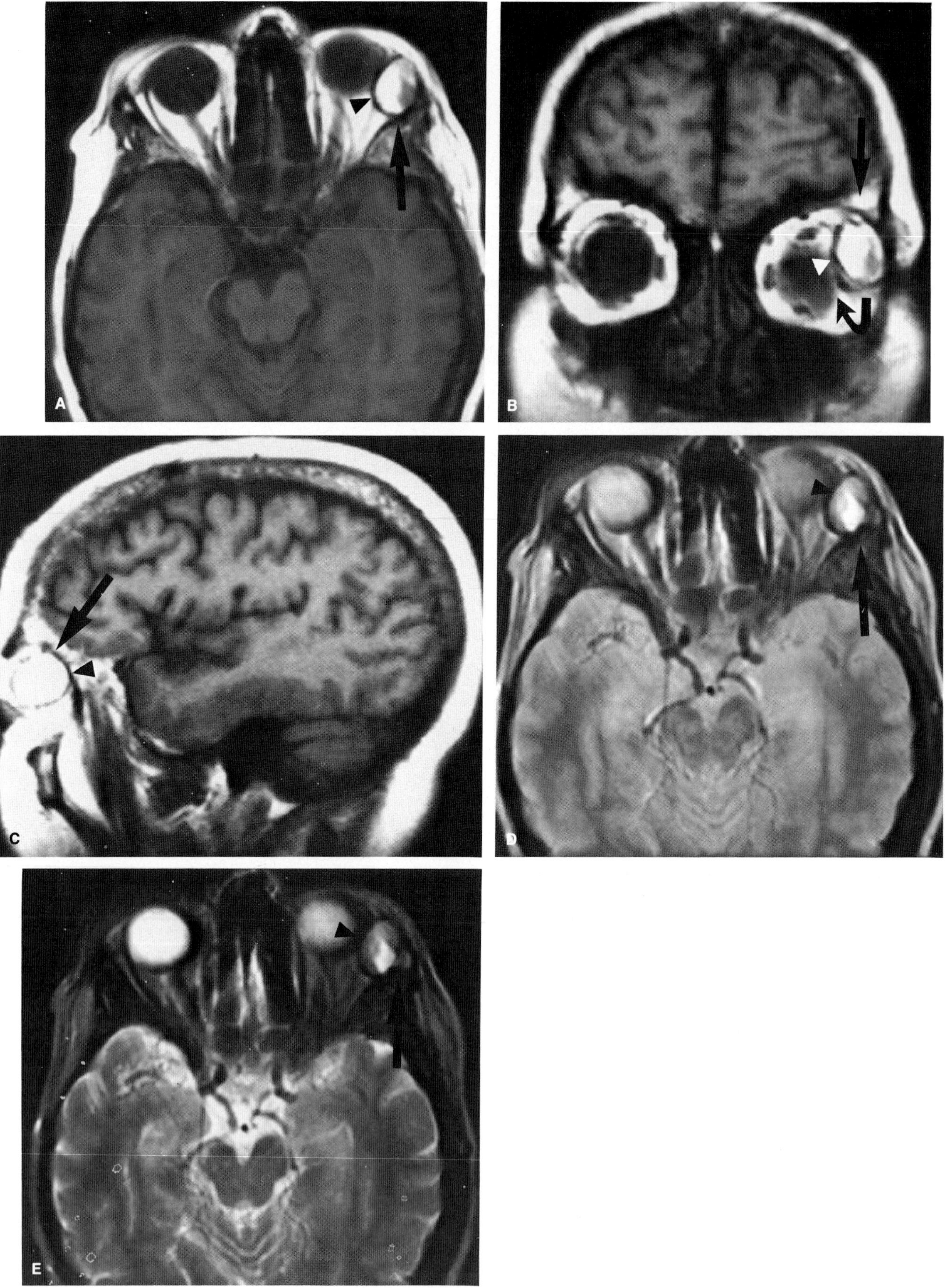
A
B
C
D
E

HISTORY

A 61-year-old with a firm, nontender palpable mass just superior and lateral to the left globe

FINDINGS

T1-weighted axial (*A*), coronal (*B*), and sagittal (*C*) images, and intermediate (*D*) and heavily (*E*) T2-weighted axial images demonstrate a 1.5-cm, well-circumscribed ovoid mass (*black arrows in A through E*) located anterolaterally in the left orbit. The mass is heterogeneous, although the signal intensity of the predominant component (*black arrowheads in A and C to E; white arrowhead in B*) is equal to fat on all images. The lesion did not enhance after IV contrast infusion (*images not shown*). The left globe and lateral rectus muscle (*curved black arrow in B*) are displaced medially, reflecting the extraconal location of the mass. The left globe is mildly proptotic.

DIAGNOSIS

Intraorbital dermoid

DISCUSSION

Dermoids are the most common orbital tumor in childhood, and are the most common congenital orbital lesion regardless of age. These tumors are usually discovered in the first year of life as a palpable, superficial, nontender nodule in the region of the lacrimal gland. Dermoids in older children and adults tend to be deeper within the orbit, and cause proptosis or displacement of the globe.[1] Rupture of a dermoid is not uncommon, and may cause granulomatous inflammation with calcification and scar development, although the lesion is often asymptomatic.[1]

Orbital dermoids result from sequestration of ectodermal elements along the suture lines of the orbital bones during embryonic development.[2] They most commonly occur at the frontozygomatic suture, in the superior temporal quadrant of the orbit. Dermoids contain fat and one or more dermal appendages such as sebaceous glands, hair follicles, and sweat glands, which accounts for their heterogeneous radiologic appearance. Epidermoids are similar in origin and location but are homogeneous masses that do not contain these dermal elements.

On MR, orbital dermoids are well-circumscribed spheric lesions with heterogeneous signal intensity, often with layering.[3] However, the lipid component dominates the MR appearance with high signal intensity on T1-weighted images and following the signal intensity of fat on all pulse sequences. The presence of fat in an orbital mass is virtually pathognomonic for a dermoid, since orbital lipomas, liposarcomas, and hemorrhagic soft tissue masses are rare.[1]

Pitfalls in Image Interpretation

The differential diagnosis for an orbital mass not involving the globe includes hemangioma, lymphangioma, lymphoma/leukemia, metastases, abscess, pseudotumor, rhabdomyosarcoma, optic nerve glioma, optic sheath meningioma, and neurofibroma.

Clinical References

1. Nugent R, Lapointe J, Rootman J, et al. Orbital dermoids: features on CT. Radiology 1987;165:475–478.
2. Mafee M, Putterman A, Valvassori G, et al. Orbital space-occupying lesions: role of computed tomography and magnetic resonance imaging. Radiol Clin North Am 1987; 25:529–559.
3. Sullivan J, Harms S. Surface-coil MR imaging of orbital neoplasms. AJNR 1985;7:29–34.

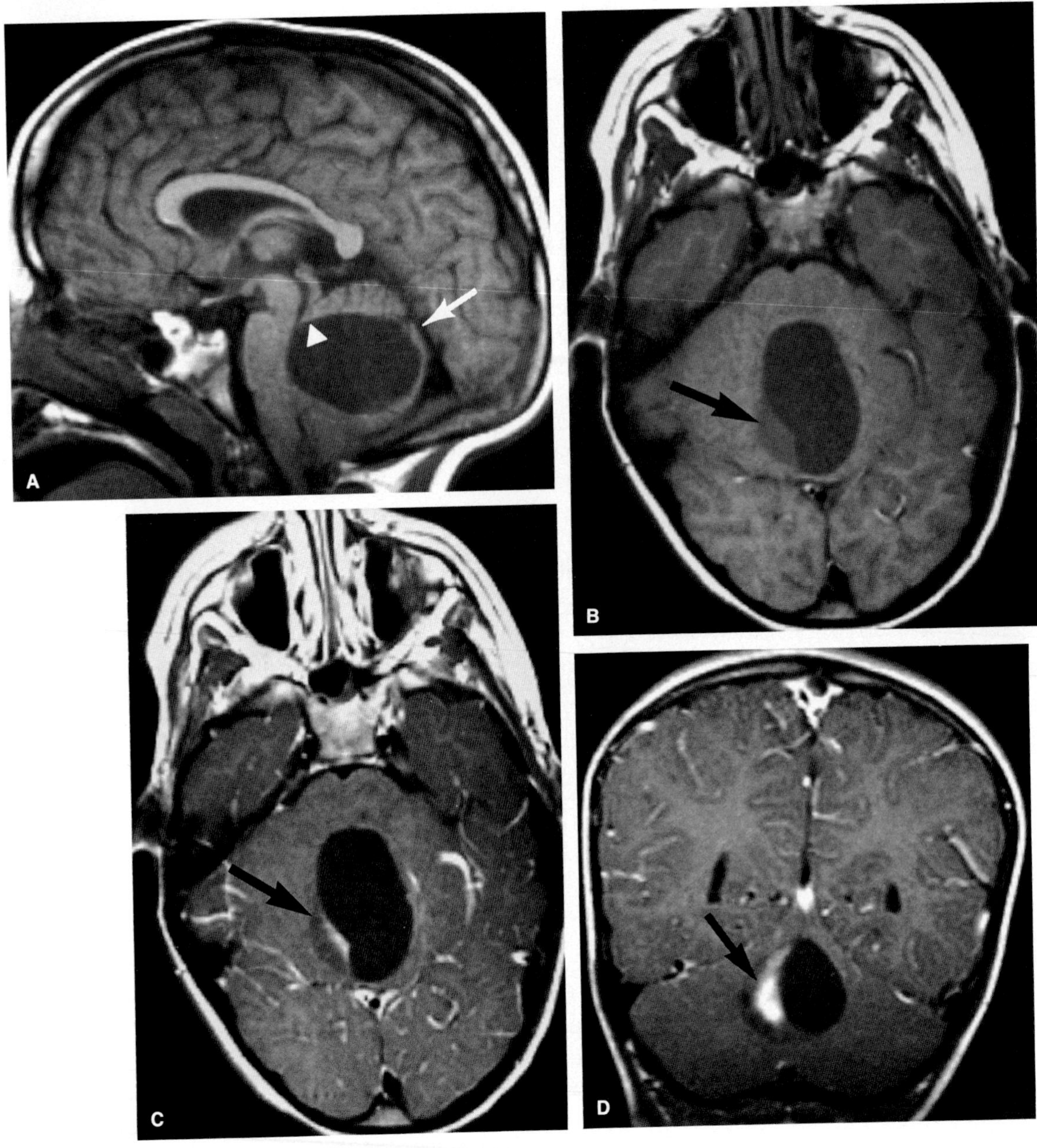

HISTORY

A 5-year-old with a 5-month history of vomiting and recent onset of headaches and ataxia

FINDINGS

(*A*) T1-weighted sagittal image demonstrates an oval, well-demarcated, 5 × 3.5 cm mass (*white arrow*) in the midline of the cerebellum. The mass displaces the brain stem and aqueduct of Sylvius (*white arrowhead*) anteriorly. (*B*) On the T1-weighted axial image, a nodular component (*black arrow*) with signal intensity isointense to brain is seen along the right lateral wall of the mass. The midline position of the tumor is confirmed. Postcontrast axial (*C*) and coronal (*D*) T1-weighted images demonstrate enhancement (*black arrow*) of the nodular component. (*E*) On the heavily T2-weighted axial image the signal intensity of the nodular component (*white arrow*) is greater than the adjacent gray matter. Most of the mass (*arrow*) has very high signal intensity on the T2-weighted image (*E*), corresponding to the area of very low signal intensity on the T1-weighted images. (*F*) T2-weighted axial image at a slightly lower level demonstrates almost complete obliteration of the fourth ventricle (*arrow*).

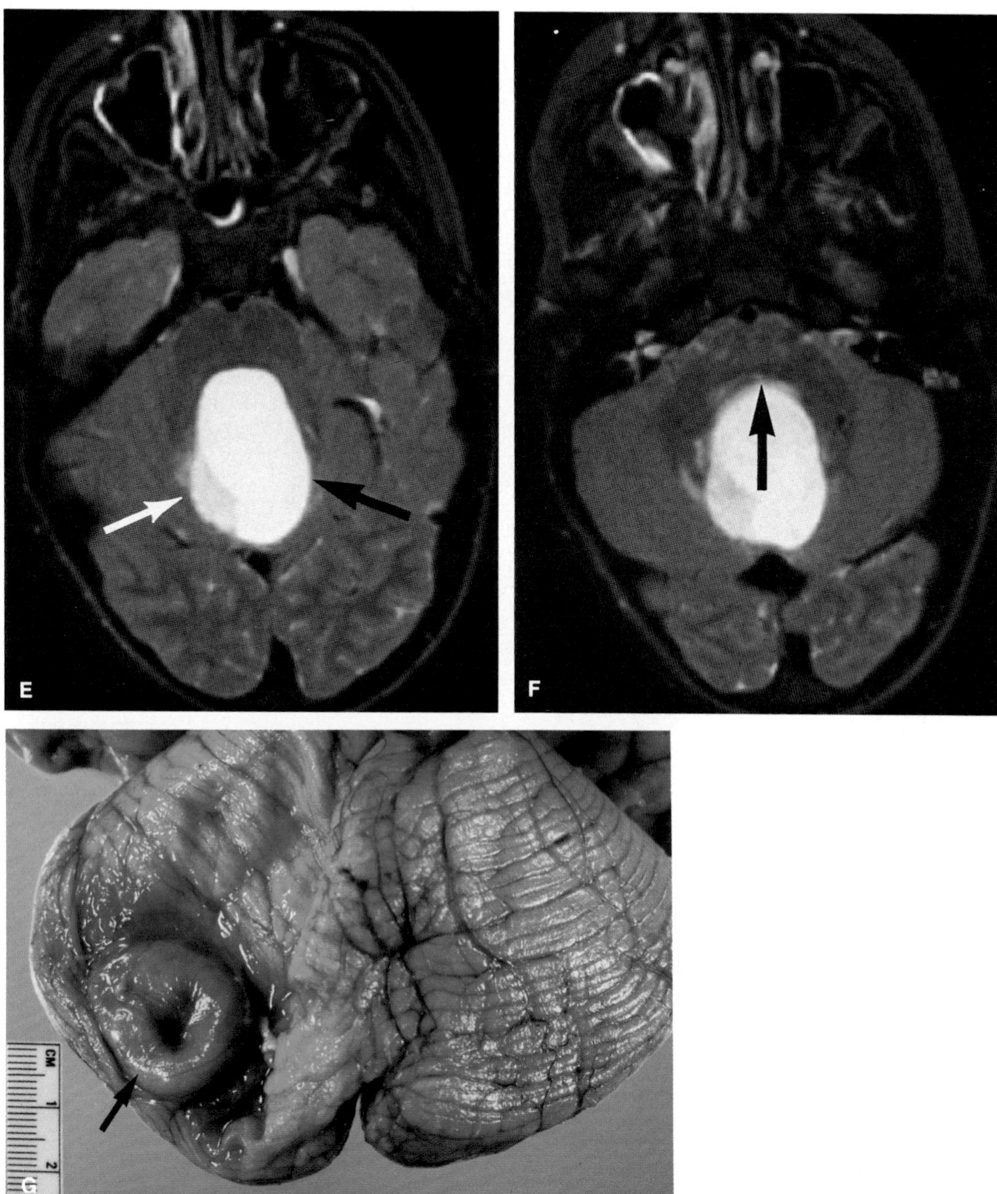

DIAGNOSIS

Cystic cerebellar astrocytoma

DISCUSSION

Cerebellar astrocytoma is the second most common posterior fossa neoplasm in childhood (slightly less common than primitive neuroectodermal tumor or medulloblastoma),[1] and constitutes 10% to 20% of all pediatric brain tumors. The peak incidence is in the first decade of life. Patients usually present with signs of increased intracranial pressure, such as headache, nausea and vomiting, or ataxia.

Most cerebellar astrocytomas are low-grade, slow-growing tumors, and are large at the time of diagnosis. Tumors may occur in the cerebellar hemisphere, the midline (vermis), or both. Hemispheric astrocytomas or those extending to the midline are cystic in 80% of cases, and midline astrocytomas are cystic in 50%. The small mural nodule is neoplastic tissue, which enhances after contrast infusion; the wall of the cyst consists of nonneoplastic cerebellar tissue, which does not enhance. For surgical planning, a cystic cerebellar astrocytoma must be differentiated from a solid astrocytoma with a necrotic center. The latter lesion may appear cystic but enhances along the entire periphery.

MR, with its multiplanar capabilities, is superior to CT for localization of posterior fossa tumors, especially with respect to the fourth ventricle. This case has typical signal intensity characteristics of a cystic astrocytoma, as described under Findings. The signal intensity of the cystic component is greater than CSF on all images because of the protein content of the cystic fluid.

Pitfalls in Image Interpretation

Differential diagnosis of a cystic posterior fossa lesion also includes hemangioblastoma, arachnoid cyst, Dandy-Walker malformation, cysticercosis, and mega cisterna magna. Medulloblastoma and ependymoma are rarely cystic.[2]

Pathologic Correlate

(*G*) Gross specimen demonstrates a cystic astrocytoma in the cerebellar hemisphere. The soft tissue component (*black arrow*) corresponds to a large neoplastic nodule. The large cystic component, which is partially decompressed, surrounds the soft tissue nodule and causes distortion of adjacent cerebellar tissue.

Clinical References

1. Gusnard D. Cerebellar neoplasms in children. Semin Roentgenol 1990;3:263–278.
2. Lee Y, Van Tassel P, Bruner JM. Juvenile pilocytic astrocytomas: CT and MR characteristics. AJNR 1989;10:363–370.

(G courtesy of Daron G. Davis, MD.)

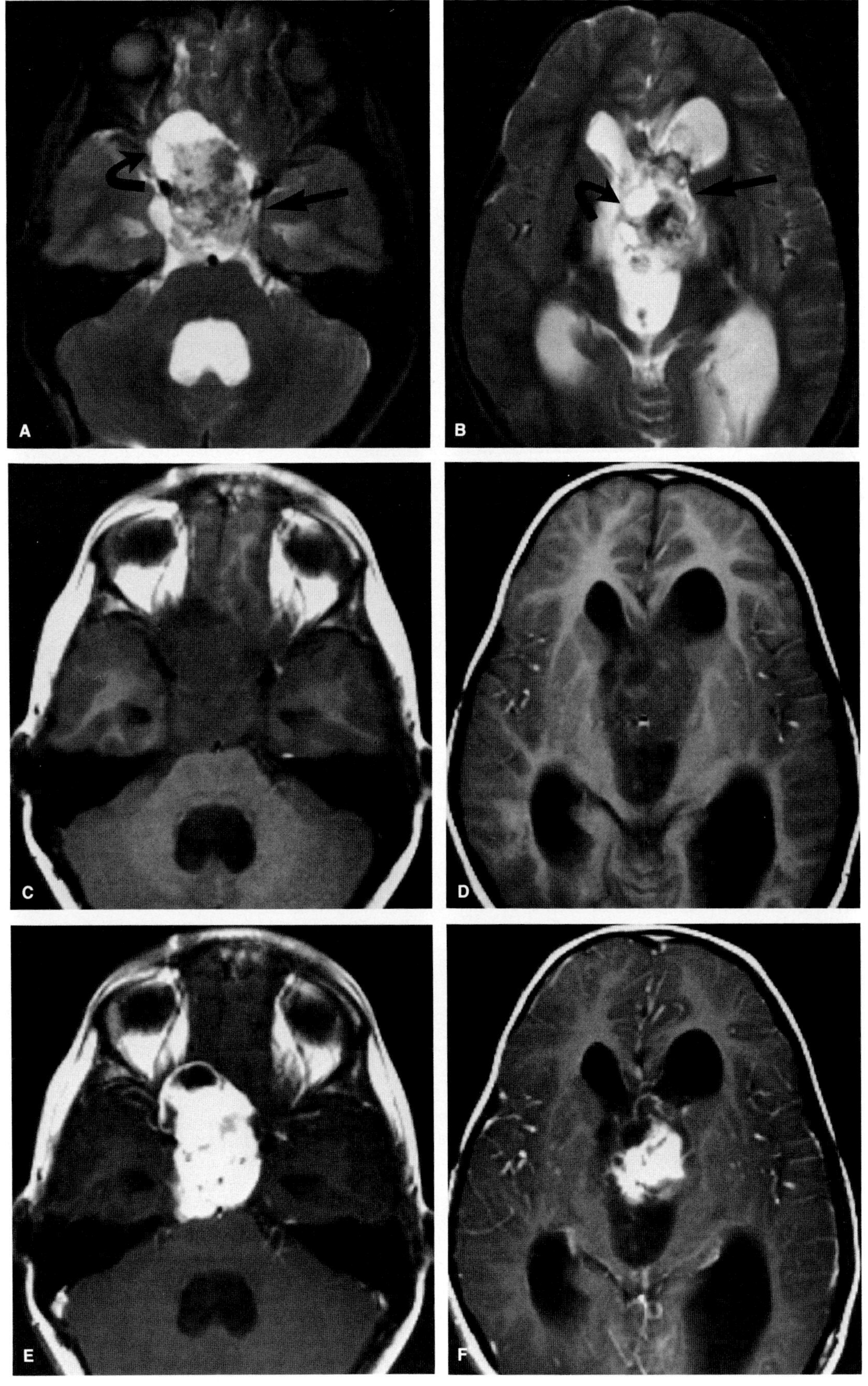
A
B
C
D
E
F

HISTORY

A child with hypothalamic dysfunction and visual problems

FINDINGS

T2-weighted (TE=90 msec) (*A and B*), precontrast T1-weighted (*C and D*), and postcontrast T1-weighted (*E and F*) scans at two levels are shown. On the axial T2-weighted images, a large heterogeneous midline mass (*arrows*) is seen, which on sagittal images (*not shown*) extended from the sella inferiorly to the lateral ventricles superiorly. The ventricular system is dilated, and the third ventricle is displaced posteriorly. Several cystic areas (*curved arrows in A and B*) can be identified within the mass. Precontrast T1-weighted scans (*C and D*) reveal the bulk of the mass to be slightly hypointense to brain, with heterogeneous but marked enhancement on the postcontrast images (*E and F*).

DIAGNOSIS

Juvenile pilocystic astrocytoma

DISCUSSION

Pilocystic astrocytomas are a distinctive histologic subtype of neoplasm. Two variants exist: an adult form, which can undergo anaplastic change, and a juvenile form, with a benign clinical course. In the juvenile type, tumor cells are elongated, thin, and tapering, with parallel formations characteristically sheathing blood vessels in a longitudinal manner. Areas remote from blood vessels are prone to microcystic degeneration.

Juvenile pilocystic astrocytomas occur in the second and third decades of life. These tumors commonly lie in the region of the third ventricle or midline in the cerebellum. They are typically well circumscribed, although those adjacent to the third ventricle may infiltrate the optic chiasm and tracts. On MR and CT, juvenile pilocystic astrocytomas appear sharply marginated, demonstrate marked contrast enhancement, and rarely have associated edema.[1] These lesions also tend to be round or oval, with cyst formation common.

In a study that examined treatment results in 36 patients with juvenile pilocystic astrocytoma, the overall survival rate was 83% at 10 years and 70% at 20 years after diagnosis. All patients who had complete tumor resection remained disease-free. Radiation therapy is recommended in patients with incomplete tumor resection.[2]

Pitfalls in Image Interpretation

The differential diagnosis for a lesion in the vicinity of the third ventricle in a child should include craniopharyngioma and germinoma. For a lesion in the posterior fossa, medulloblastoma and ependymoma should be considered.

Clinical References

1. Lee YY, Van Tassel P, Bruner JM, et al. Juvenile pilocystic astrocytomas: CT and MR characteristics. AJR 1989;152: 1263–1270.
2. Wallner KE, Gonzales MF, Edwards MS, et al. Treatment results of juvenile pilocystic astrocytoma. J Neurosurg 1988; 69:171–176.

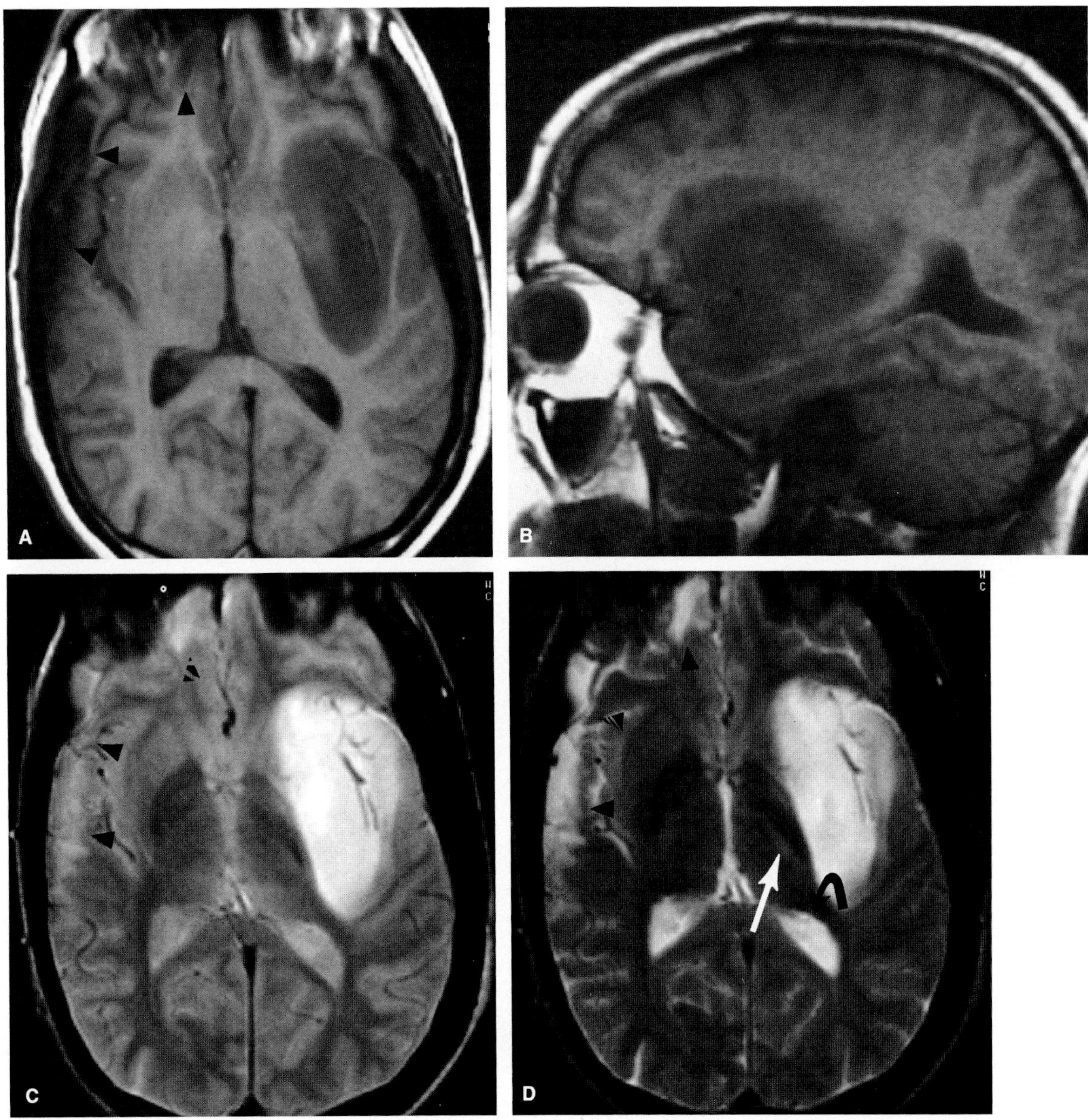

HISTORY

A 30-year-old with new onset of seizures

FINDINGS

(*A*) T1-weighted axial image, demonstrates a large, well-demarcated low-signal-intensity lesion in the left insular cortex and surrounding white matter. (*B*) On the T1-weighted sagittal image, the lesion is seen to extend into the superior left temporal lobe and into the white matter of the inferior left frontal lobe. On the intermediate (*C*) and heavily (*D*) T2-weighted images, the lesion has high signal intensity. There is no surrounding edema. The lesion is causing mass effect on the left globus pallidus (*white arrow in D*), and the trigone of the left lateral ventricle (*curved arrow in D*). There was no evidence for enhancement of the lesion after contrast infusion (*image not shown*). Note atrophy of the peripheral cortex of the anterior right temporal and right frontal lobes (*arrowheads in A, C, and D*), perhaps due to previous trauma.

DIAGNOSIS

Astrocytoma, grade II (of IV)

DISCUSSION

Gliomas are the most common type of primary brain neoplasm. Of the gliomas, glioblastoma multiforme (GBM) is the most common. Non-GBM, lower-grade (grades I and II) astrocytomas make up approximately 25% of supratentorial gliomas in adults. The peak incidence of low-grade astrocytomas is in the third through fifth decades, which is an earlier age range than for GBM. Patients present with seizures, focal neurologic deficits, or nonspecific signs of increased intracranial pressure such as headache, nausea, and vomiting. Low-grade astrocytomas have a better prognosis than GBM, and, in general, the younger the patient the longer the survival. Despite the relatively benign histologic characteristics of low-grade astrocytomas, the postoperative survival is usually only 3 to 10 years.[1]

Astrocytomas arise from glial cells in the white matter. Therefore, the most common locations are the frontal, temporal, and parietal lobes, reflecting the relative amount of white matter in these areas. Occipital astrocytomas are relatively rare. Cortical involvement is not uncommon with low-grade astrocytomas. The presence of tumor in the insular cortex in this case is typical.

Low-grade astrocytomas (see 1.3632) are usually well-defined, homogeneous, nonenhancing lesions with little mass effect and minimal surrounding vasogenic edema. MR is superior to CT in defining the borders of a low-grade astrocytoma. However, CT is better for detecting calcifications, which are present in about 25% of astrocytomas.

Pitfalls in Image Interpretation

When confined to a single vascular territory, a low-grade astrocytoma may have an appearance similar to that of an acute cerebral infarction, especially when there is cortical involvement.

Clinical References

1. Dean B, Drayer B, Bird C, et al. Gliomas: classification with MR imaging. Radiology 1990;174:411–415.

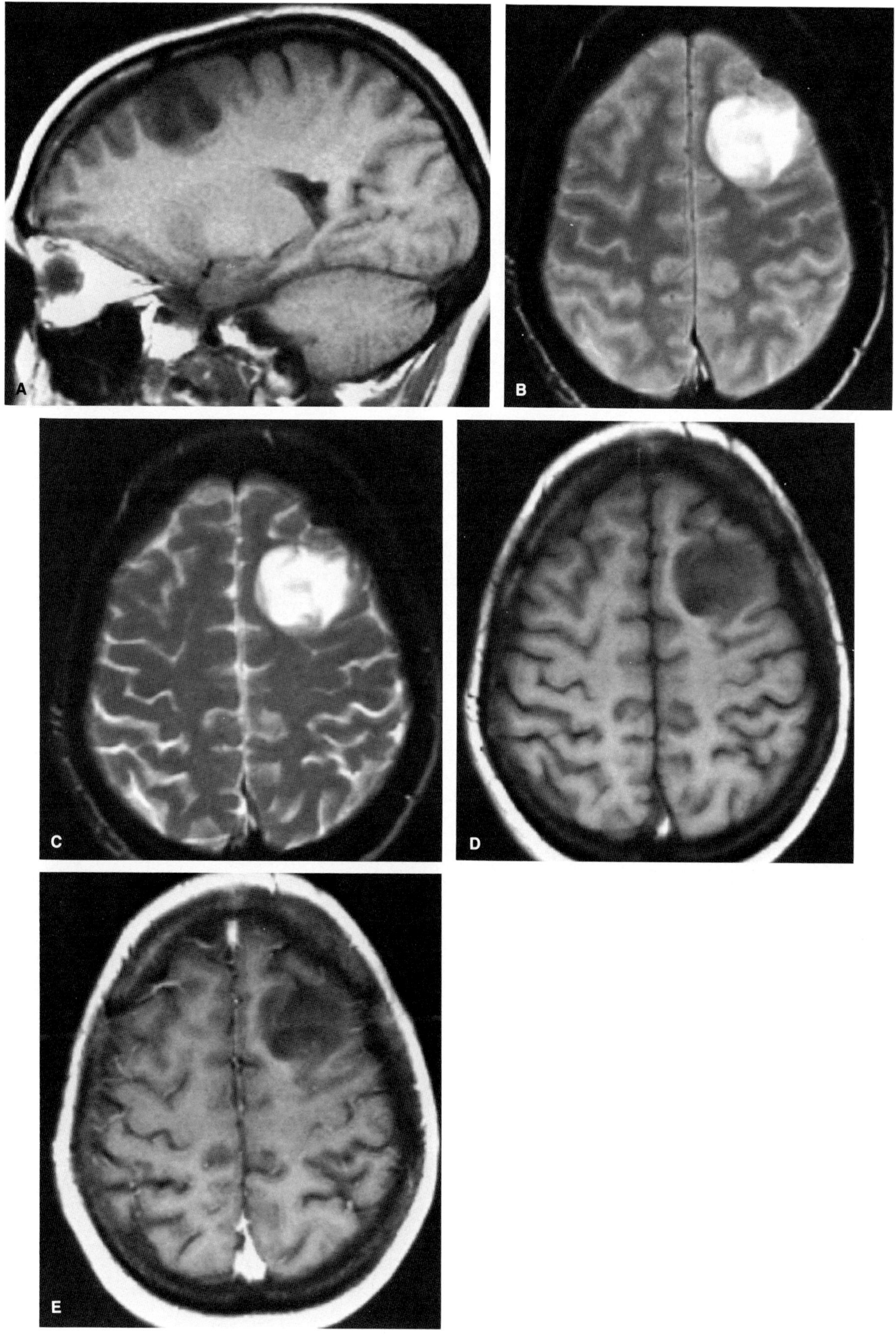
A
B
C
D
E

HISTORY

A 37-year-old woman with a 2-year history of seizures, progressive in severity

FINDINGS

A well-defined left frontal mass involving both gray and white matter, with prolonged T1 and T2 relaxation times (relative to gray matter), is identified on sagittal T1-weighted (*A*), axial T2-weighted (TE = 45,90 msec) (*B and C*), and axial precontrast T1-weighted (*D*) images. There is no associated vasogenic edema. The mass does not enhance postcontrast (*E*).

DIAGNOSIS

Astrocytoma, grade I to II (of IV)

DISCUSSION

On MR, low-grade astrocytomas are typically well-defined, homogeneous, with little mass effect or accompanying vasogenic edema, and do not enhance postcontrast.[1] The accuracy of MR classification of gliomas approaches that of neuropathologic diagnosis. Characteristics that should be assessed include lesion consistency (homogeneous versus heterogeneous), border definition, mass effect, hemosiderin (seen best on GRE scans), and vasogenic edema. Anaplastic astrocytomas on MR are less well defined and exhibit moderate mass effect, vasogenic edema, and heterogeneity. Glioblastomas are poorly defined, exhibiting greater mass effect, edema, and heterogeneity. Hemosiderin, seen most frequently with glioblastomas, aids in differentiation from an anaplastic astrocytoma. Necrosis (on histologic examination) is the hallmark of a glioblastoma.

Astrocytic tumors can be subdivided on the basis of cell type according to the 1979 World Health Organization classification into astrocytoma (protoplasmic, fibrillary, or gemistocytic), pilocystic astrocytoma, subependymal giant cell astrocytoma (seen in tuberous sclerosis), astroblastoma, and anaplastic (malignant) astrocytoma. The term *glioma* refers to a greater subset of lesions, in the strict sense referring to tumors composed of neuroglial cells, which include astrocytoma, ependymoma, oligodendroglioma, neuroastrocytoma, and medulloblastoma. Grading of tumors (by the degree of hypercellularity, pleomorphism, vascular proliferation, and presence or absence of necrosis) in the glioma group presents considerable problems, particularly when based on biopsy—with different portions of the lesion commonly displaying different histologic character. Furthermore, a lesion is not necessarily static cytologically, with temporal progression of tumor grade from highly differentiated to extreme anaplasia documented in many instances. Adding to possible confusion is the classification of astrocytomas by the Kernohan system into grades I to IV, as compared with three grades (I to III) by the National Brain Tumor Study Group[2]: astrocytoma, anaplastic astrocytoma, and glioblastoma multiforme. Significant prognostic value is associated with differentiation of an anaplastic astrocytoma from a glioblastoma multiforme, the latter tumor associated with more advanced age, shorter duration of preoperative symptoms, and shorter survival.

MR Technique

GRE scans can be used to improve visualization of hemosiderin, the presence of which favors the diagnosis of a glioblastoma as opposed to an anaplastic astrocytoma.

Clinical References

1. Dean BL, Drayer BP, Bird CR, et al. Gliomas: classification with MR imaging. Radiology 1990;174:411–415.
2. Burger PC, Vogel FS, Green SB, Strike TA. Glioblastoma multiforme and anaplastic astrocytoma: pathologic criteria and prognostic implications. Cancer 1985;56:1106–1111.

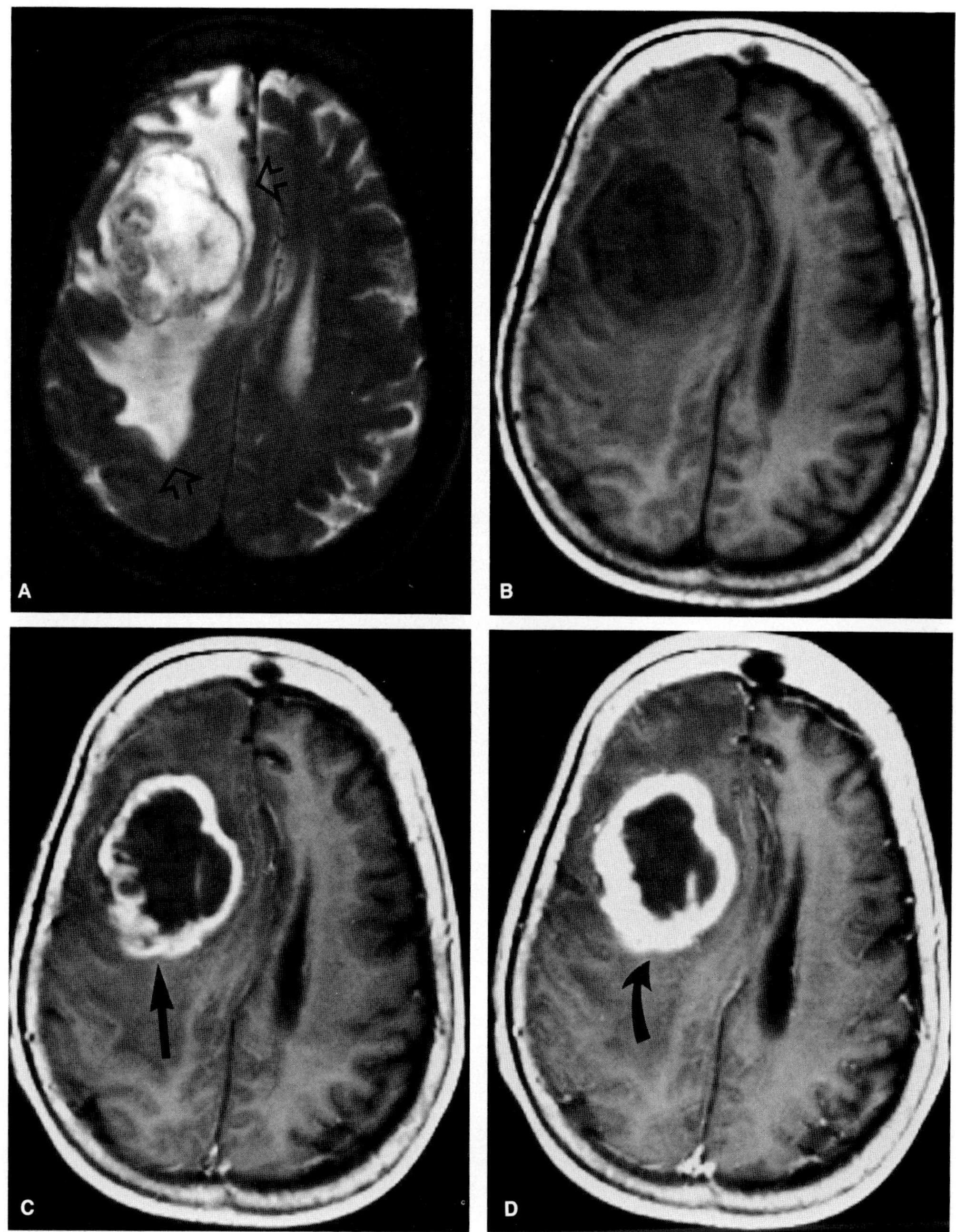

HISTORY

A 70-year-old woman with a 15-lb weight loss over 3 months, headache, fatigue, confusion, and a 10-day history of left arm and left leg weakness

FINDINGS

(*A*) Precontrast T2-weighted, (*B*) precontrast T1-weighted, (*C*) postcontrast T1-weighted (0.1 mmol/kg gadoteridol), and (*D*) high-dose postcontrast T1-weighted (0.3 mmol/kg gadoteridol) images are presented. Irregular rim enhancement (*arrow in C*) of a large right frontal lobe mass is noted postcontrast, with the enhancing rim both more intense and thicker at the high dose (*curved arrow in D*). Substantial surrounding abnormal hyperintensity (*open arrows in A*) on the T2-weighted image corresponds to cerebral edema.

DIAGNOSIS

Glioblastoma multiforme (GBM)

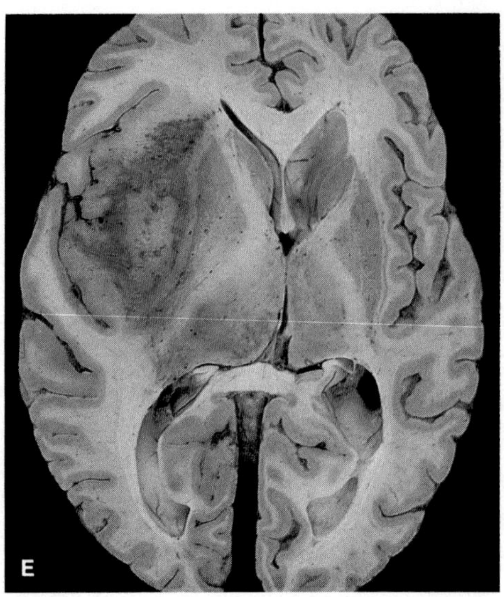

DISCUSSION

GBM is a highly malignant, widely infiltrative, astrocytic tumor that is typically located in the cerebral hemispheres. Multiple lobe involvement, ventricular rupture, and spread by way of the corpus callosum to the opposite hemisphere are not uncommon. This tumor is particularly resistant to radiation and chemotherapy. Gross total resection prolongs survival and improves quality of life.[1]

IV mannitol and dexamethasone can be given to brain tumor patients to control cerebral edema, with considerable temporary improvement in neurologic signs. Mannitol, an osmotic diuretic, acts to reduce brain water.

Characteristic MR imaging features for GBM include a thick irregular enhancing ring, central necrosis, and extensive peripheral white matter edema. The differential diagnosis includes metastatic disease and abscess.

MR Technique

Improved enhancement of intracranial lesions has been consistently demonstrated at high contrast dose (0.2 to 0.3 mmol/kg of a gadolinium chelate) in clinical trials, despite the potential for T2 shortening. Applications include improved lesion delineation in uncooperative patients, where motion artifact can markedly degrade both spatial and contrast resolution.

Pitfalls in Image Interpretation

In cerebral astrocytomas, tumor cells have been noted pathologically outside the region depicted as abnormal on CT (by contrast enhancement) and MR (by enhancement or by abnormalities on precontrast T1- and T2-weighted images).[2]

Pathologic Correlate

(*E*) Gross appearance of a glioblastoma involving the insula. A viable cellular zone (in which the blood–brain barrier is disrupted) surrounds the yellow necrotic center. Outside this rim, in "edematous" tissue, which actually constitutes the periphery of the tumor, small numbers of neoplastic astrocytes can be found. In this autopsy specimen, the ipsilateral thalamus is also involved by neoplastic cells.

Clinical References

1. Ammirati M, Vick N, Liao YL, et al. Effect of the extent of surgical resection on survival and quality of life in patients with supratentorial glioblastomas and anaplastic astrocytomas. Neurosurgery 1987;21:201–206.
2. Earnest F, Kelly PJ, Scheithauer BW, et al. Cerebral astrocytomas: histopathologic correlation of MR and CT contrast enhancement with stereotactic biopsy. Radiology 1988;166: 823–827.

(A to D from Runge VM, et al. J MRI 1992:2:9–18; E from Okazaki H, Scheithauer B. Slide atlas of neuropathology. New York, Gower Medical Publishing, 1988. By permission of Mayo Foundation.)

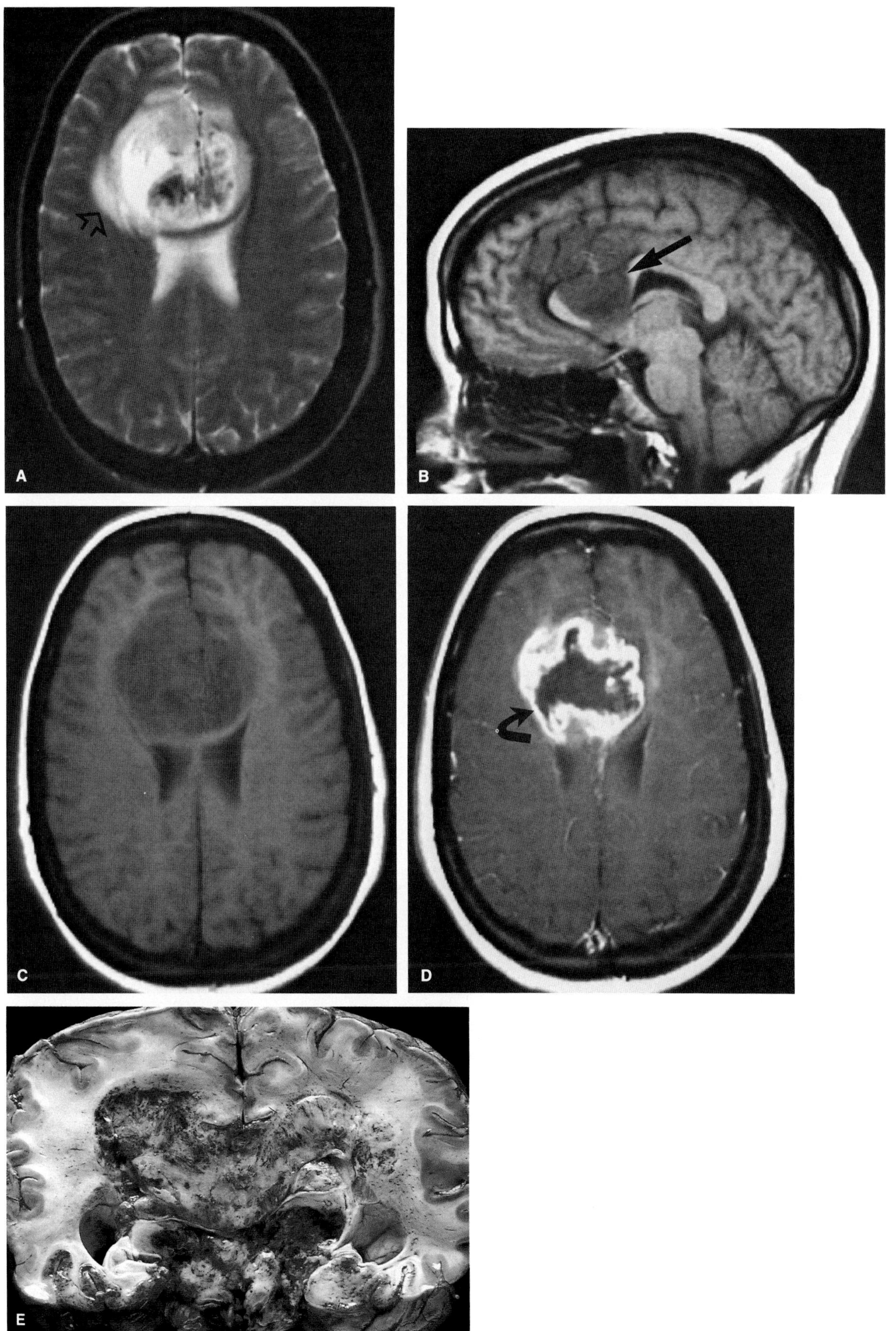
A
B
C
D
E

HISTORY

A 35-year-old woman with 1 month of persistent bitemporal headaches and recent onset of nausea and vomiting

FINDINGS

(*A*) T2-weighted (TE = 90 msec) image demonstrates a large midline lesion involving the frontal lobe and corpus callosum. There is a suggestion of cerebral edema (*open arrow*) immediately to the right of the lesion. (*B*) The sagittal T1-weighted image confirms involvement of the corpus callosum by the mass (*arrow*). Precontrast (*C*) and postcontrast (*D*) axial T1-weighted images demonstrate marked compression of the lateral ventricles, irregular ring enhancement, and central lesion necrosis (*curved arrow in D*).

DIAGNOSIS

Glioblastoma multiforme with involvement of the corpus callosum

DISCUSSION

MR is recommended over CT for the study of brain gliomas. Although MR does not allow a more specific diagnosis than CT, major advantages include superior depiction of tumor extent, cystic and necrotic change, and anatomic relationships.

Growth of glioblastomas occurs along white matter tracts, with spread across the corpus callosum producing a butterfly pattern.[1] With all brain tumors, symptoms are often due to increased intracranial pressure, which results in headaches, nausea, and vomiting, and at times leads to changes in mentation or loss of consciousness. These symptoms may be the result of obstruction to CSF flow, cerebral edema, tissue destruction or irritation, or traction or displacement of the brain.

Diagnosis was made in this patient by stereotaxic biopsy, which is recommended in particular for lesions that involve the septum-fornix-callosal region.[2]

Pitfalls in Image Interpretation

The differential diagnosis for a large ring-enhancing lesion includes neoplasia, infection, and multiple sclerosis. Principal involvement and destruction of white matter (and specifically the corpus callosum) in this case favors the diagnosis of a highly malignant neoplasm.

Pathologic Correlate

E demonstrates on pathologic section involvement of the splenium of the corpus callosum and white matter bilaterally by a butterfly glioblastoma. High-grade astrocytomas not infrequently grow into the contralateral hemisphere by way of the corpus callosum. Less commonly, these appear to originate in the midline with symmetric growth and extension into each hemisphere.

Clinical References

1. Price AC, Runge VM, Allen JH, et al. Primary glioma: diagnosis with magnetic resonance imaging. J Comput Assist Tomogr 1986;10:325–334.
2. Devaux B, Blond S, Roux FX, et al. Stereotaxic approach in extensive lesions of the septum–fornix–callosal region. Neurochirurgie 1988;34:315–322.

(E *from Okazaki H, Scheithauer B. Slide atlas of neuropathology. New York, Gower Medical Publishing, 1988. By permission of Mayo Foundation.)*

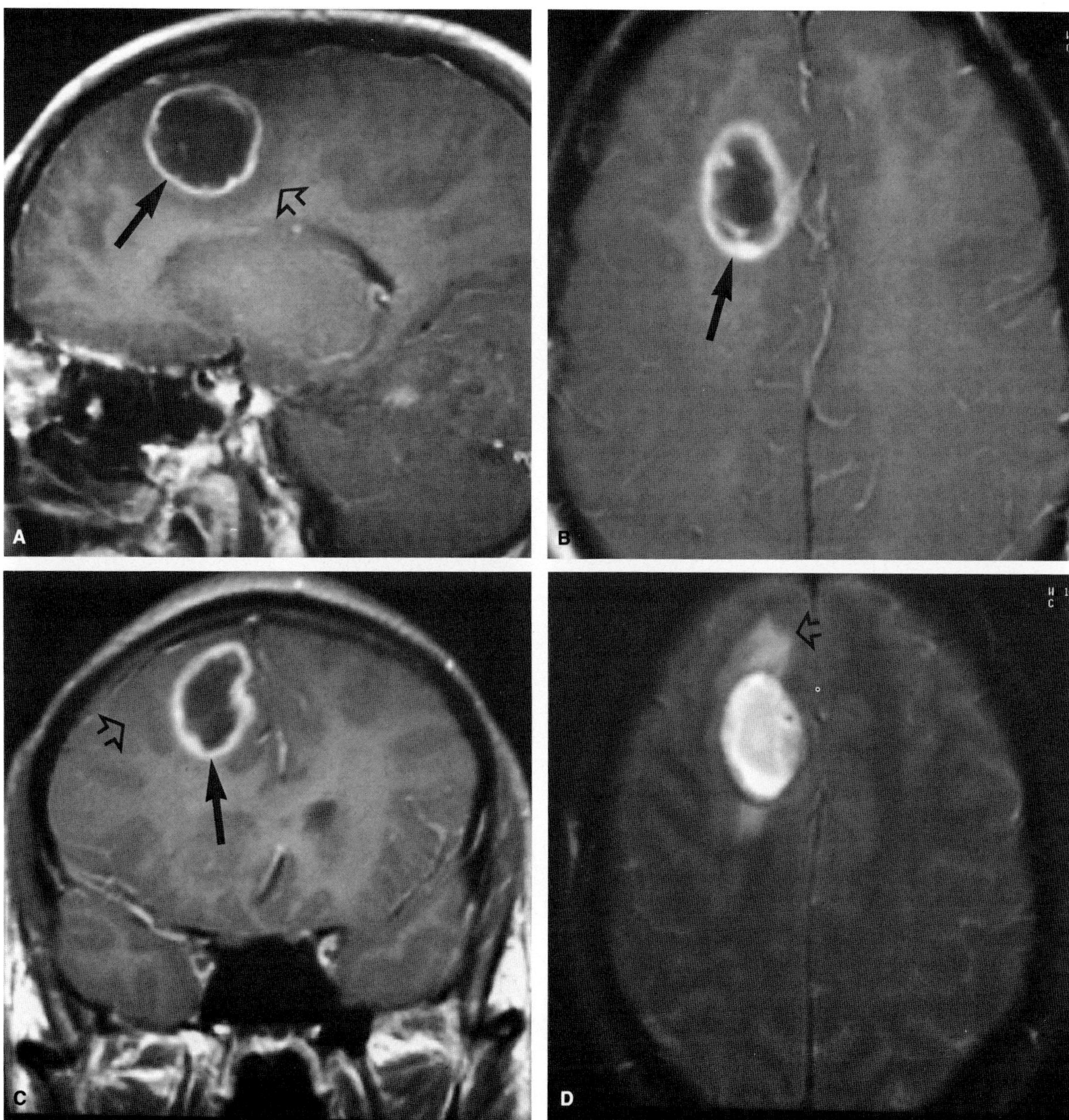

HISTORY

A 33-year-old patient with severe headaches for 4 weeks. After the initial MR (*A to E*), the lesion was excised completely, together with a 1-cm margin of normal brain. The second MR examination (*F to H*) is from 1 year later.

FINDINGS

On the initial MR examination, a single lesion with ring enhancement was identified. Following IV contrast administration, using a gadolinium chelate, T1-weighted images were acquired, first in the sagittal plane (*A*), followed by the axial plane (*B*), and then the coronal plane (*C*). The rim of enhancement (*arrows in A to C*) becomes thicker and more prominent on the delayed postcontrast images (*B and C*), a finding common in, but not specific for, neoplastic disease. (*D*) The axial T2-weighted image (TE = 90 msec), which is also postcontrast, demonstrates a prominent rim of hyperintensity that corresponds in position to the rim of enhancement seen on the T1-weighted images. Surrounding this rim, there is abnormal hyperintensity (*open arrow in D*) on the T2-weighted scan and hypointensity (*open arrows in A and C*) on the T1-weighted scans in the white matter in a pattern suggestive of edema. (*E*) At a lower anatomic level on the T2-weighted scan, abnormal hyperintensity can be

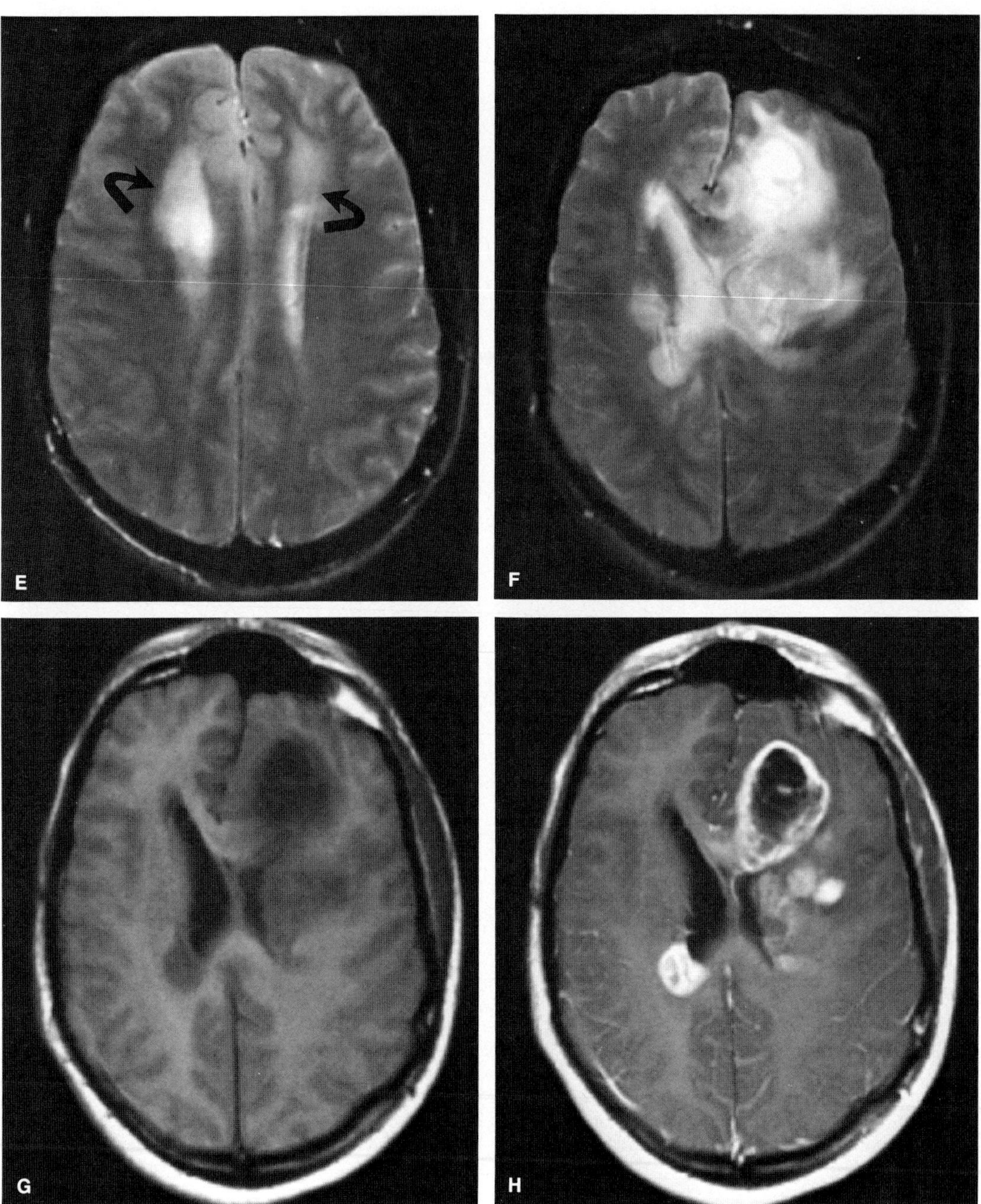

seen in the white matter bilaterally (*curved arrows*) adjacent to the more anterior portion of the lateral ventricles. On the MR 1 year later, there are multiple lesions bilaterally, with abnormal hyperintensity on the T2-weighted scan (*F*), hypointensity on the T1-weighted scan (*G*), and enhancement (*H*) after administration of a gadolinium chelate (using a dose of 0.1 mmol/kg). Additional enhancing lesions were also demonstrated at this time in the temporal lobes bilaterally and cerebellum (*images not shown*).

DIAGNOSIS

Multicentric glioblastoma

DISCUSSION

In the case presented, the pathologic diagnosis at the time of initial surgical resection was a mixed malignant glioma, with both astrocytic and oligodendroglial components. Conversion of an astrocytoma of low grade to an anaplastic astrocytoma and subsequently to a glioblastoma is not uncommon, although the exact incidence is unknown and timing in the individual patient is difficult to foretell. In tumor recurrences, an increase in the degree of malignancy has been observed in over 75% of cases. In the specific case examined, following complete surgical resection, the tumor recurred both with higher grade and in multiple areas. For astrocytomas in general,

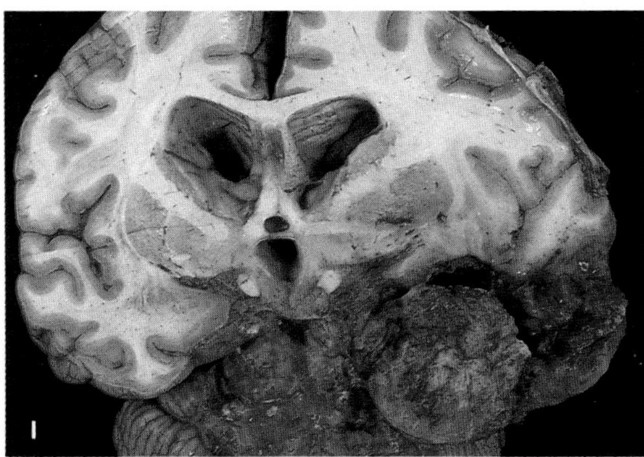

debulking (and likewise complete resection) and radiation therapy prolong survival.

Approximately 5% of patients with glioblastoma multiforme have multiple tumor foci. The lesions are termed synchronous if multiple on the first examination, and metachronous (as in the current clinical case) if multiple on examination months to years following documentation of the original glioma.[1] Postulated pathophysiologic mechanisms for the phenomenon of multiple lesions include simultaneous neoplastic transformation and seeding from a single lesion.

By definition, separate regions of tumor involvement in a *multicentric* glioblastoma do not demonstrate microscopic or macroscopic connection.[2] Demonstration of direct lesion continuity (microscopically or macroscopically), CSF spread, or local metastases characterize a *multifocal* glioblastoma.

MR Technique

T2-weighted images are not typically acquired postcontrast. Paramagnetic agents, however, decrease both T1 and T2, with a decrease in T1 (by itself) leading to increased signal intensity on SE images and a decrease in T2 (by itself) leading to decreased signal intensity. This results in positive contrast enhancement on T1-weighted scans, which are of course used routinely for the detection of IV contrast in current clinical practice. One might expect to see negative enhancement (with the lesion darker postcontrast) on T2-weighted scans. However, at the dosages employed and the selection of TE and TR typically used for T2-weighted images of the head, positive lesion enhancement is consistently seen on T2-weighted scans (*as in D*). Thus, in most cases, even on T2-weighted images, the T1 effect of the contrast agent predominates to cause positive lesion enhancement in head imaging.

Pitfalls in Image Interpretation

Differentiation of multicentric glioma from multiple metastases or abscesses is not possible by neuroradiologic evaluation.[3] Biopsy is suggested for diagnosis in patients without evidence of primary neoplastic disease or infection.

A pitfall in MR imaging is the tendency to equate contrast enhancement with tumor extent for glial lesions. Such a correlation is not supported by pathologic studies, with tumor cells demonstrated well beyond both the abnormality demonstrated on T2-weighted scans and by disruption of the blood–brain barrier (as delineated by postcontrast T1-weighted scans). Thus, the signal intensity abnormality adjacent to the left lateral ventricle on T2-weighted scans, which was observed on the first MR (*A to E*), could be due to additional tumor involvement at presentation in the left hemisphere. Preliminary results from contrast dose trials on MR in patients with high-grade astrocytomas suggest that greater tumor extension can be demonstrated after high-dose contrast administration, as compared with precontrast T2-weighted scans.

Pathologic Correlate

(*I*) Gross pathologic specimen of postoperative dissemination of a glioblastoma (in a different patient) is shown. There is local recurrence at the site of previous resection in the temporal lobe, as well as diffuse leptomeningeal seeding. The latter is particularly evident surrounding the brain stem and adjacent to the optic tracts.

Clinical References

1. Van Tassel P, Lee YY, Bruner JM. Synchronous and metachronous malignant gliomas: CT findings. AJNR 1988;9:725–732.
2. Prather JL, Long JM, van Heertum R, Hardman J. Multicentric and isolated multifocal glioblastoma multiforme simulating metastatic disease. Br J Radiol 1975;48:10–15.
3. Rao KC, Levine H, Itani A, et al. CT findings in multicentric glioblastoma: diagnostic-pathologic correlation. J Comput Assist Tomogr 1980;4:187–192.

(I from Okazaki H, Scheithauer B. Slide atlas of neuropathology. New York, Gower Medical Publishing, 1988. By permission of Mayo Foundation.)

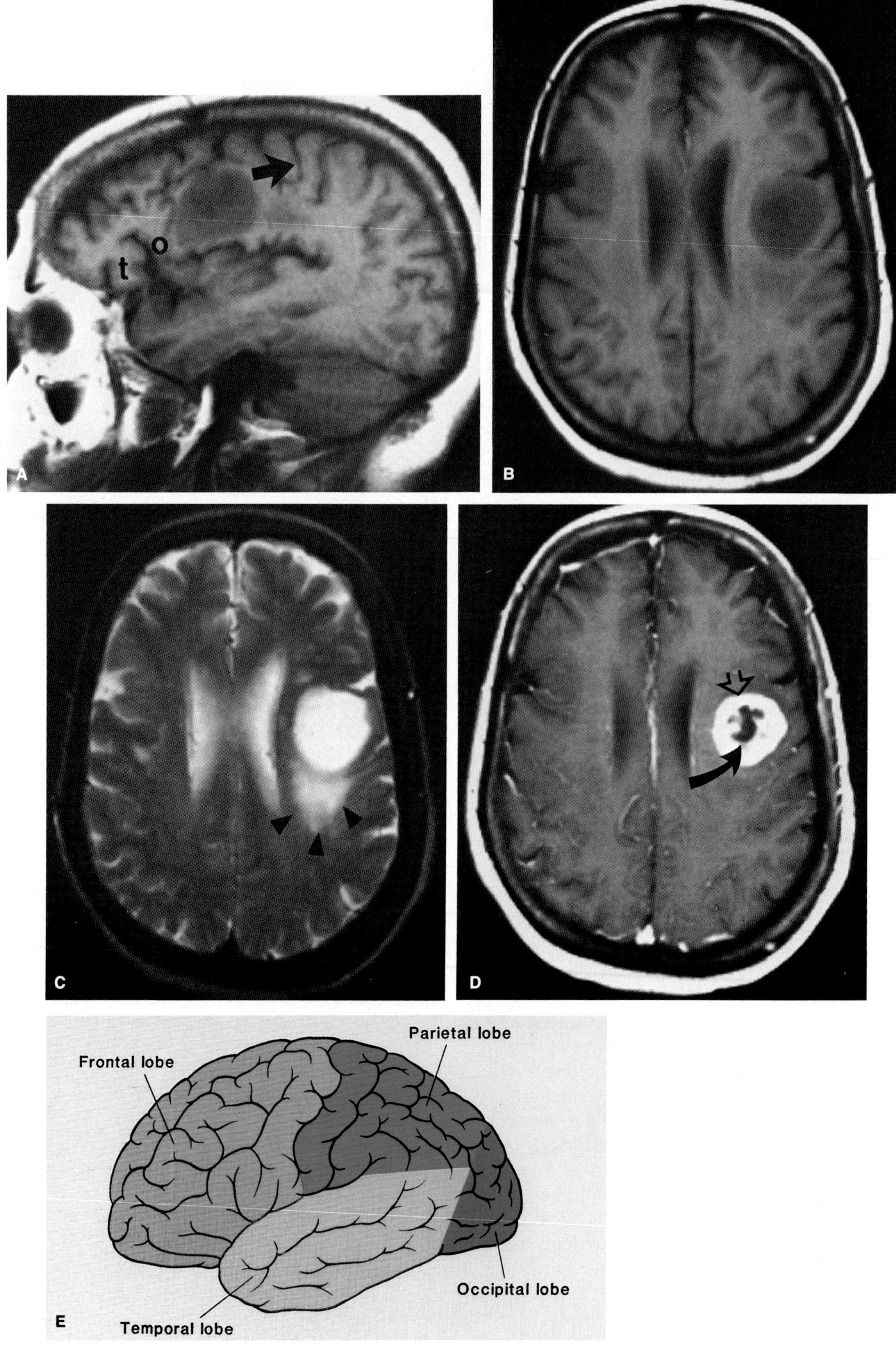
t
o
A
B
C
D
Parietal lobe
Frontal lobe
Occipital lobe
E
Temporal lobe

HISTORY

A 75-year-old woman with increasing difficulty in speaking

FINDINGS

Sagittal (*A*) and axial (*B*) precontrast T1-weighted images reveal a predominantly white matter mass measuring 3 × 3 × 3 cm. Identification of the central sulcus (*arrow in A*), as well as the pars triangularis (t) and pars opercularis (o) of the inferior frontal gyrus, places this mass in the frontal lobe. There is central necrosis, identified by the presence of lower signal intensity compared with viable tumor on the unenhanced T1-weighted image, higher signal intensity on the T2-weighted (TE=90 msec) image (*C*). On the postcontrast T1-weighted image (*D*), there is lack of central contrast enhancement (*curved arrow*). There is surrounding vasogenic edema (*arrowheads in C*), with thick irregular rim enhancement postcontrast (*open arrow in D*).

DIAGNOSIS

Glioblastoma multiforme, left frontal lobe

DISCUSSION

Typical features of a glioblastoma multiforme on MR demonstrated by this tumor include mass effect, the presence of vasogenic edema, and lesion heterogeneity, in particular, central necrosis. Cyst formation or necrosis, best assessed on postcontrast scans, has been shown statistically to be a positive predictor of higher tumor grade.[1] Contrast enhancement correlates with solid tumor neovascularity and endothelial proliferation.[2] Surgical resection may be limited in tumors of the frontal lobe by proximity to the motor speech area of Broca, typically located on the left (in right-handed individuals) in the inferior frontal gyrus. Ablation may result in loss of vocalization.

This patient was treated by primary excision and stereotactic placement of californium implants.

MR Technique

Tumor necrosis can be identified by use of heavily T1 (TR≤600/TE≤22) or T2 (TR≥2500/TE≥80) weighted images or by the administration of IV contrast, with the latter technique most efficacious.

Pitfalls in Image Interpretation

Caution should be exercised with localization of lesions on MR. (*E*) A sagittal examination aids in identification of the central sulcus, which serves to separate the frontal and parietal lobes. Axial CT images are tilted by about 25°, with MR images acquired without such tilt, complicating anatomic localization on transverse sections.

Clinical References

1. Dean BL, Drayer BP, Bird CR, et al. Gliomas: classification with MR imaging. Radiology 1990;174:411–415.
2. Ernest F, Kelly PJ, Scheithauer BW, et al. Cerebral astrocytomas: histopathologic correlation of MR and CT contrast enhancement with stereotactic biopsy. Radiology 1988; 166:823–827.

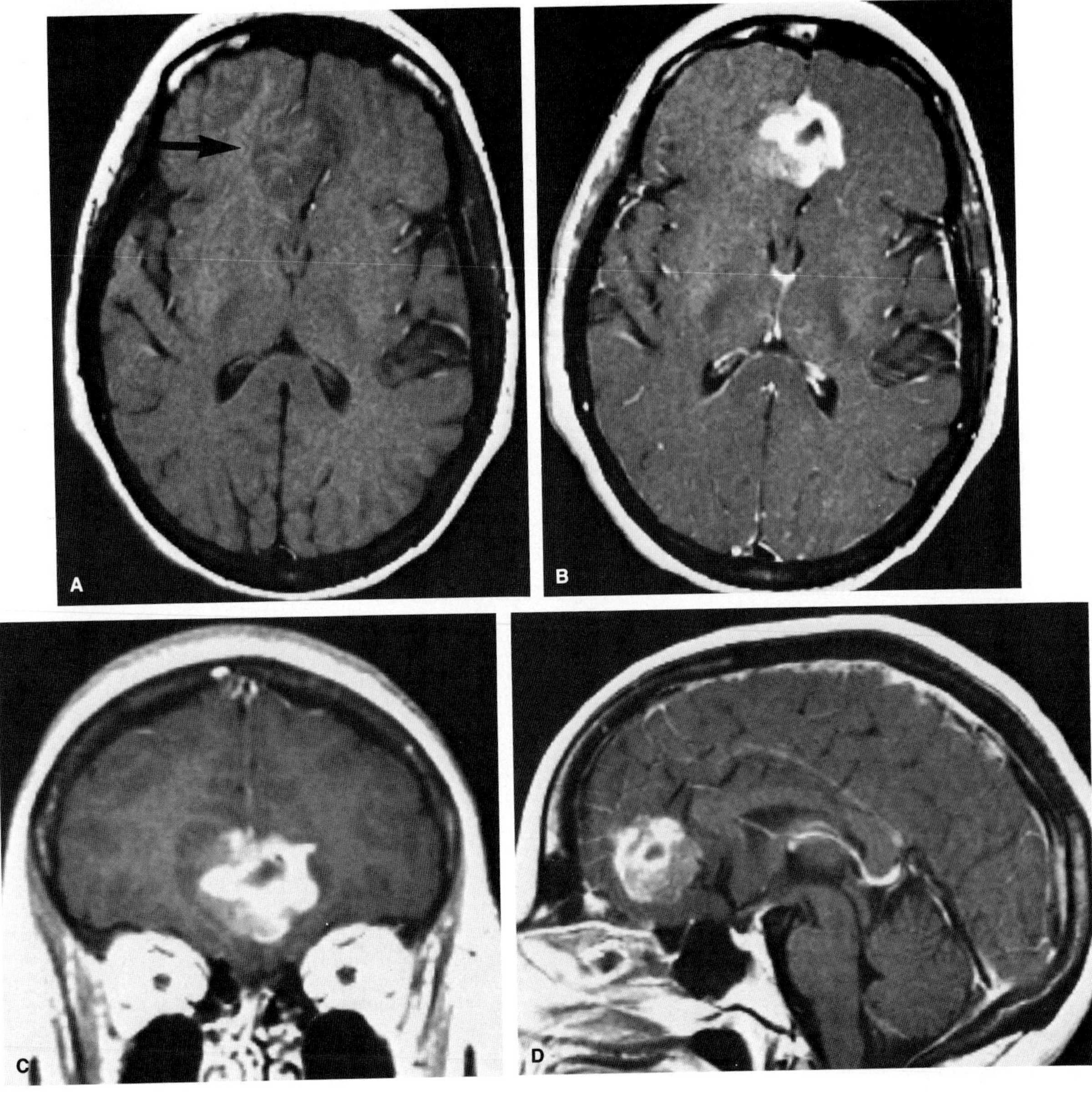

HISTORY

A 55-year-old woman who fell at work and lost consciousness

FINDINGS

(*A*) Precontrast axial T1-weighted image reveals an isointense midline frontal mass (*arrow*) anterior to the corpus callosum. This mass demonstrates irregular ringlike enhancement on axial (*B*), coronal (*C*), and sagittal (*D*) T1-weighted images postcontrast. The T2-weighted images showed a predominantly isointense mass (*images not shown*). Although the mass involves both frontal lobes, no MR characteristics are present to suggest that this is an extraaxial mass.

DIAGNOSIS

Glioblastoma multiforme

DISCUSSION

Glioblastomas are the most malignant of the primary neuralgia tumors, with a median survival of 6 months. They represent 15% to 20% of all intracranial tumors, and are the most common supratentorial neoplasm in the adult. These lesions show a 3:2 male predominance. The frontal lobe is the most common site of occurrence, followed by the temporal lobe.[1]

The differential diagnosis of a mass involving both hemispheres includes glioblastoma multiforme, lymphoma, sarcoidosis, and meningiosarcoma. Primary CNS lymphoma most often occurs as focal intracerebral masses, which are commonly multiple. These lesions are typically ill-defined with irregular borders. Classic locations include the deep gray matter structures, periventricular regions, and corpus callosum.[2] Sarcoidosis involves the meninges more often than the brain; brain involvement occurs most commonly by spread along the perivascular spaces. Although meningiosarcomas cannot be differentiated from their benign counterpart, poorly defined tumor margins, marked heterogeneity, and prominent edema are suggestive of a more aggressive tumor.

Clinical References

1. Russell DS, Rubinstein LJ. Pathology of tumors of the nervous system, 5th ed. Baltimore, Williams & Wilkins, 1989.
2. Atlas SW. Magnetic resonance imaging of the brain and spine. New York, Raven Press, 1991.

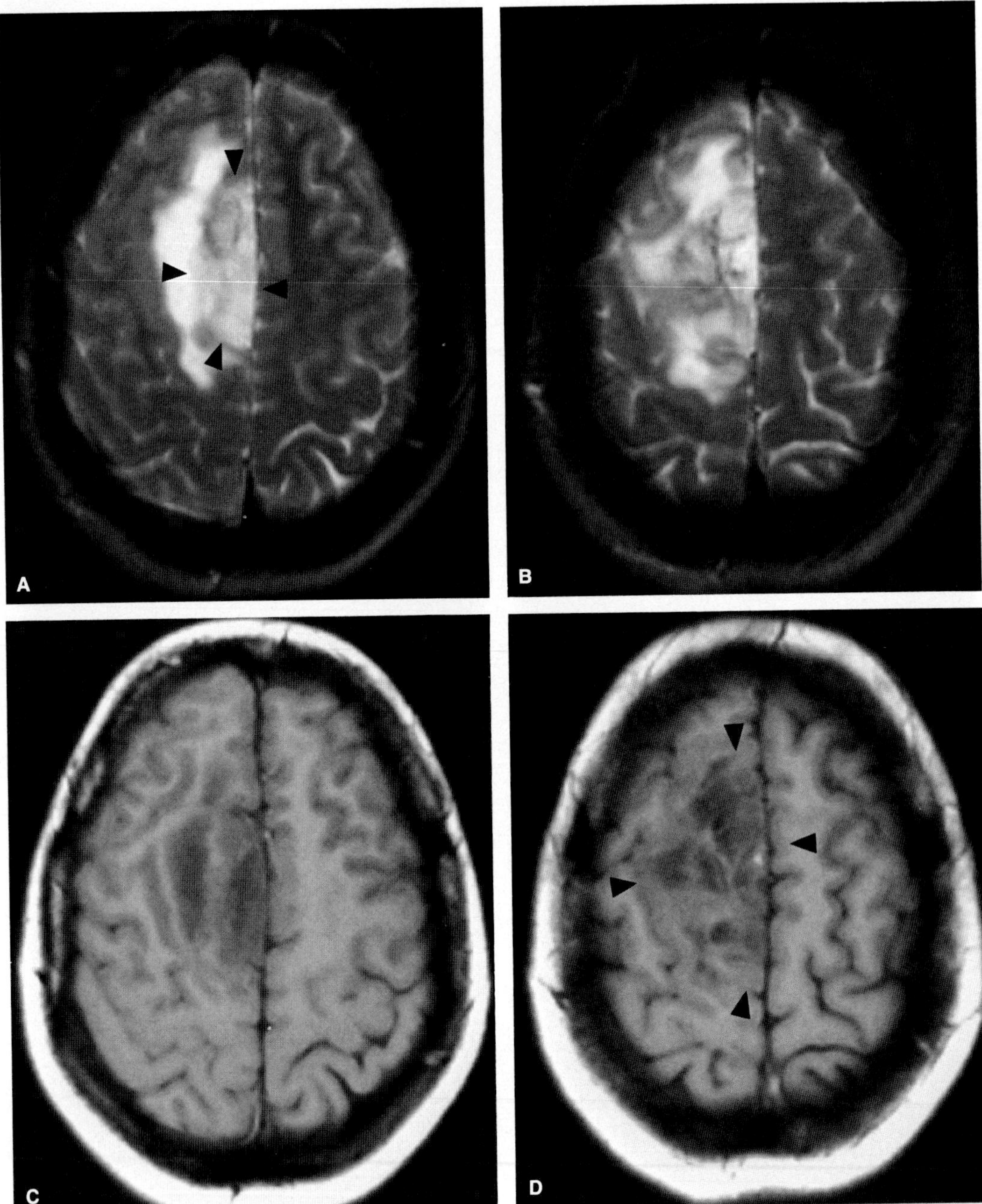

HISTORY

A 30-year-old woman with seizures involving her left side, accompanied by numbness and abnormal sensation of the face, arm, and leg on the left side

FINDINGS

(*A and B*) T2-weighted images demonstrate a moderately well defined, high-signal-intensity frontal lobe mass (*arrowheads* in *A*), with surrounding white matter edema. (*C to E*) Precontrast T1-weighted images reveal a heterogeneous mass (*arrowheads in D*), with punctate high signal intensity (*arrows in E*) medially, which is most likely due to the presence of calcification; these areas also demonstrate signal intensity compatible with fat on T2-weighted images (*not shown*). (*F*) Axial postcontrast image demonstrates enhancement in only one small region (*open arrow*), separate from the calcifications medially. (*G*) Postcontrast coronal T1-weighted scan reveals calvarial erosion (*curved arrow*). (*H*) On enhanced CT, the mass is low density with punctate calcifications.

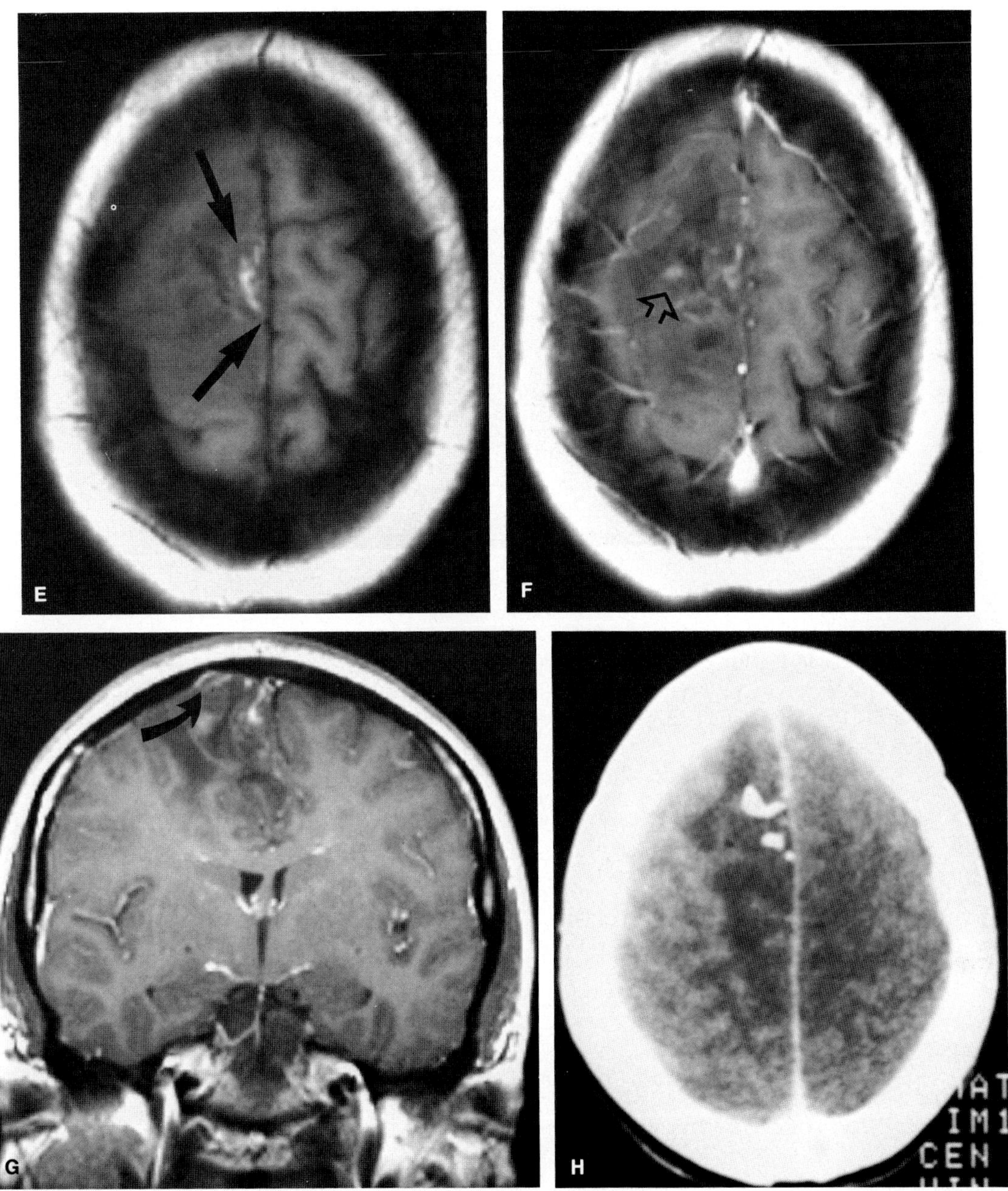

DIAGNOSIS

Mixed oligodendroglioma and astrocytoma

DISCUSSION

Oligoendrogliomas are relatively uncommon tumors, accounting for approximately 5% of intracranial gliomas.[1] These lesions often contain other glial elements, with 50% of mixed-cell type. Most occur in young adults and are located peripherally in the cerebral hemispheres (and in particular, the frontal lobe). Calvarial erosion may occur because of location and slow growth. Calcification, both nodular and linear, is extremely common. Hemorrhage and cystic formation are not infrequent. Enhancement is seen in about half the cases on CT, typically being mild and poorly defined. Lesions usually appear by imaging studies to be well defined, without significant edema.

Pathologically, oligodendrogliomas are infiltrating lesions,[2] with poorly defined borders (similar to low-grade astrocytomas). There is a wide range (low to high) of lesion grade, with little correlation to imaging findings.

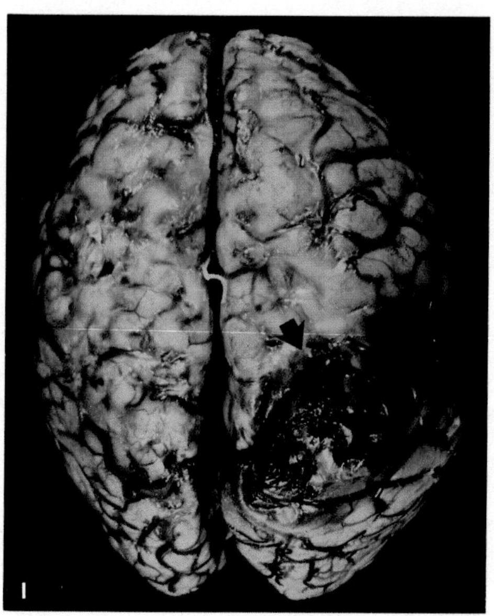

Treatment is by surgical excision and subsequent radiotherapy. Despite the typical history of long duration, survival after surgery is disproportionately short, with 10% to 30% 10-year survival rates.

Pitfalls in Image Interpretation

Intracranial calcification can appear as high signal intensity (explained in some cases by the presence of fat) on T1-weighted images and should be differentiated from hemorrhage.

Pathologic Correlate

I shows a large oligodendroglioma (*arrow*), which was followed for many years without treatment in a severely mentally retarded patient. Grossly, these tumors can appear well defined. Although they arise in white matter, there is a tendency for outward spread with infiltration of the cortex and obliteration of the gray–white matter junction.

Clinical References

1. Lee Y, Tassel PV. Intracranial oligodendrogliomas: imaging findings in 35 untreated cases. AJNR 1989;10:119–127.
2. Atlas SW. Adult supratentorial tumors. Semin Roentgenol 1990;25:130–154.

(I courtesy of Daron G. Davis, MD.)

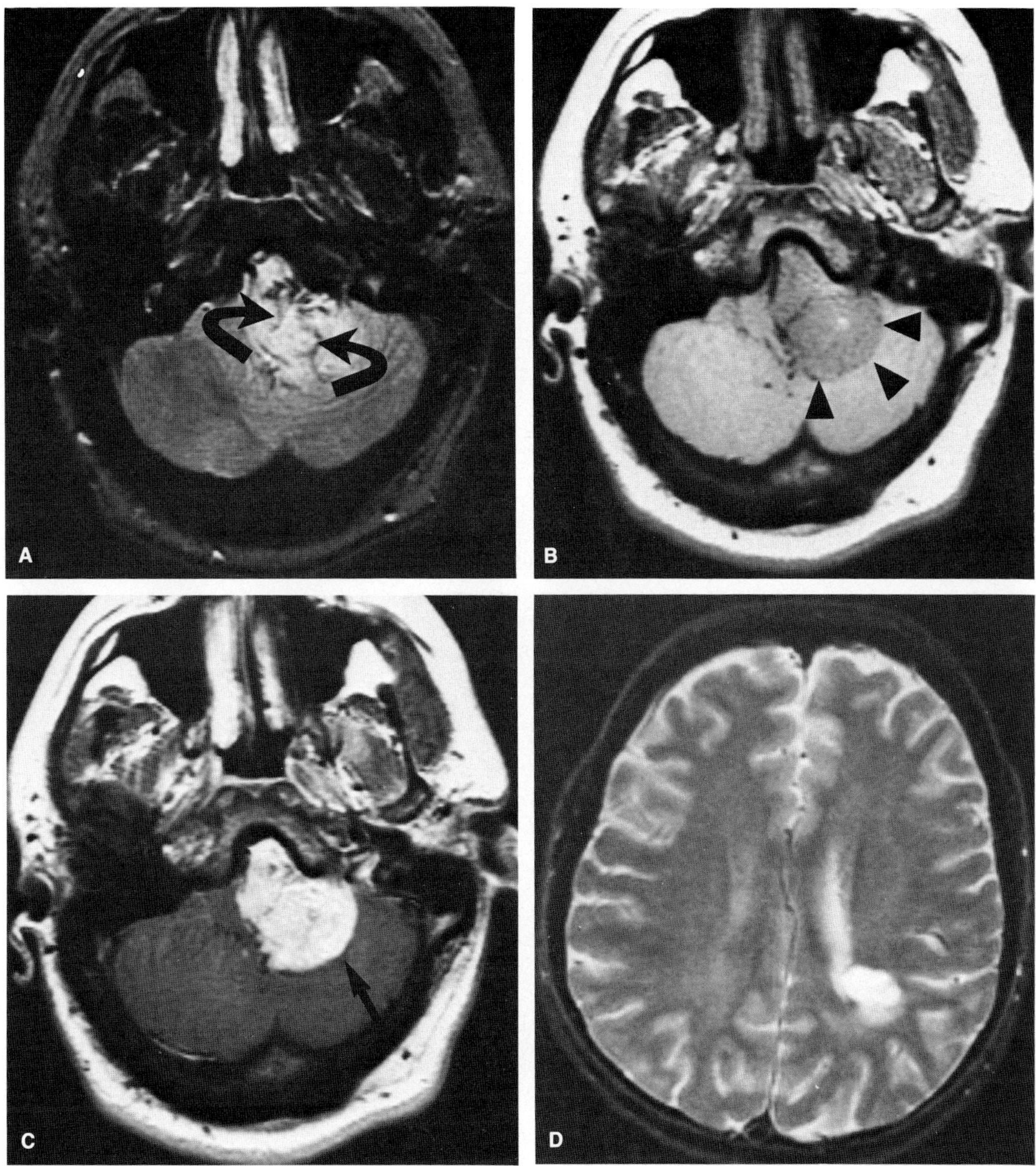

HISTORY

Two patients with the same tissue pathology, the first (patient 1) 32 years, and the second (patient 2) 40 years of age

FINDINGS

PATIENT 1: (*A*) Precontrast T2-weighted (TE = 80 msec) and precontrast (*B*) and postcontrast (*C*) T1-weighted axial images demonstrate an enhancing mass (*arrow in C*) with its epicenter in the left foramen of Luschka. There is marked distortion and displacement to the right of the medulla. There are large abnormal vessels (*curved arrows in A*) within the mass, best seen due to flow voids on the T2-weighted image. A faint rim of hypointensity (*arrowheads in B*) is noted on the precontrast T1-weighted image, suggesting an extraaxial location.

PATIENT 2: (*D*) Precontrast T2-weighted (TE = 80) and (*E and F*) postcontrast T1-weighted images reveal a mass contiguous with the left lateral ventricle. (*E and F*) The lesion is hyperintense on *D*, with both cystic and enhancing components.

DIAGNOSIS

Ependymoma

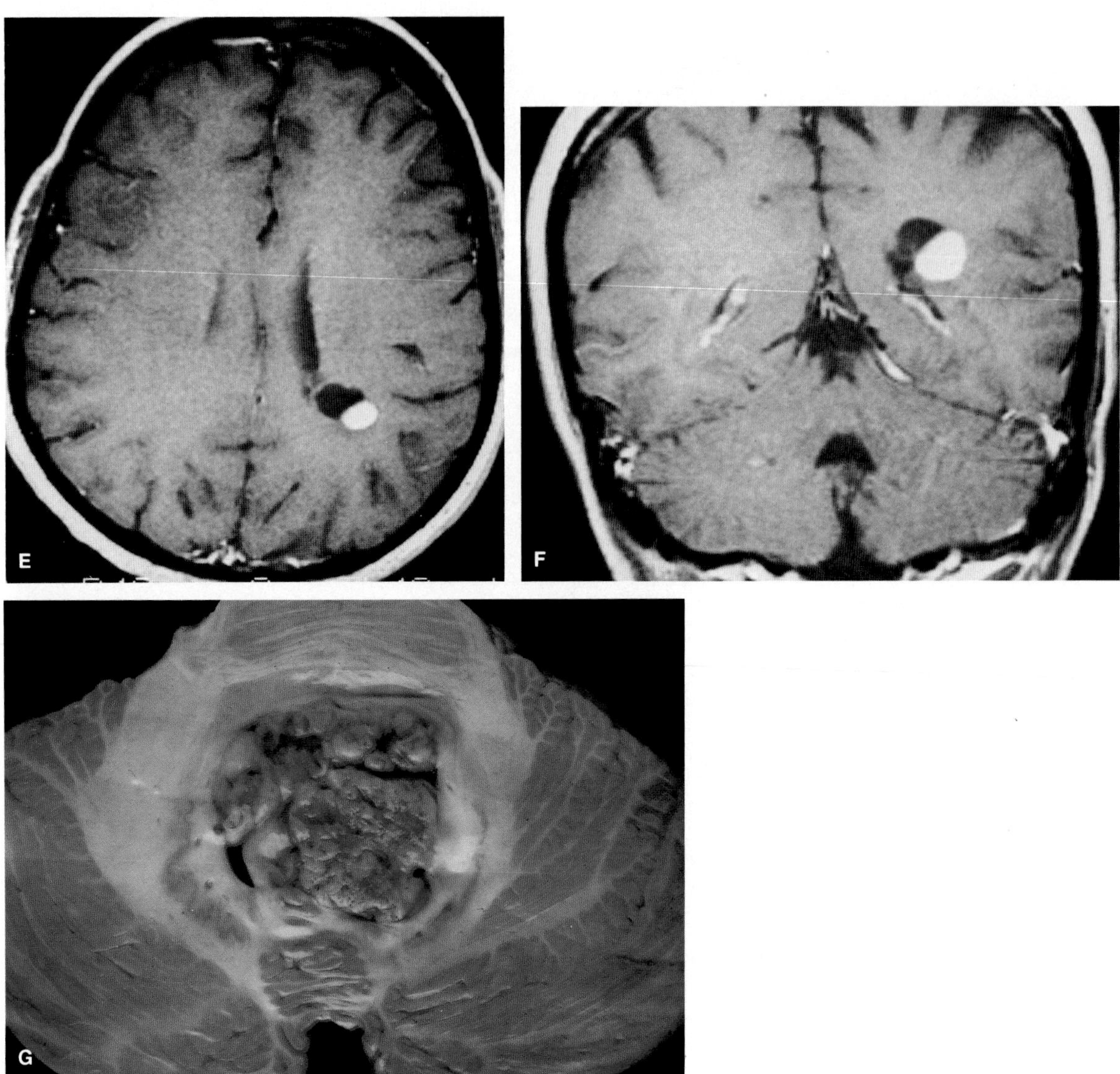

DISCUSSION

Ependymomas are rare tumors that can arise adjacent to any portion of the ventricular system, but most commonly the fourth ventricle. These lesions are generally slow growing and benign, but when intracranial represent a bad operative risk and thus poor prognosis. Ependymomas occur predominantly in children and adolescents.

On MR, differentiation of ependymomas from other gliomas cannot be achieved on the basis of signal intensity characteristics.[1] Lesion location and morphology may provide clues with respect to histologic diagnosis. The most common presentation is that of a solid heterogeneous mass arising in the fourth ventricle. The heterogeneity can be due to blood products, necrosis, or tumor vascularity. Tumor spread by way of CSF pathways is common. Supratentorial lesions are commonly periventricular in location with cystic components.

Pitfalls in Image Interpretation

The differential diagnosis for lesions involving the fourth ventricle includes ependymoma, glioma, cysticercosis, medulloblastoma, and epidermoid.[2] Although superior to CT, MR cannot provide an accurate histologic diagnosis for such lesions.

Pathologic Correlate

(*G*) Fresh pathologic section reveals a posterior fossa ependymoma, with typical lobulated appearance at the level of the fourth ventricle.

Clinical References

1. Spoto GP, Press GA, Hesselink JR, Solomon M. Intracranial ependymoma and subependymoma: MR manifestations. AJR 1990;154:837–845.
2. Barloon TJ, Yuh WT, Chiang FL, et al. Lesions involving the fourth ventricle evaluated by CT and MR: a comparative study. Magn Reson Imaging 1989;7:635–642.

(A to F courtesy of Mark Osborne, MD.; G from Okazaki H, Scheithauer B. Slide atlas of neuropathology. New York, Gower Medical Publishing, 1988. By permission of Mayo Foundation.)

1.3637-1

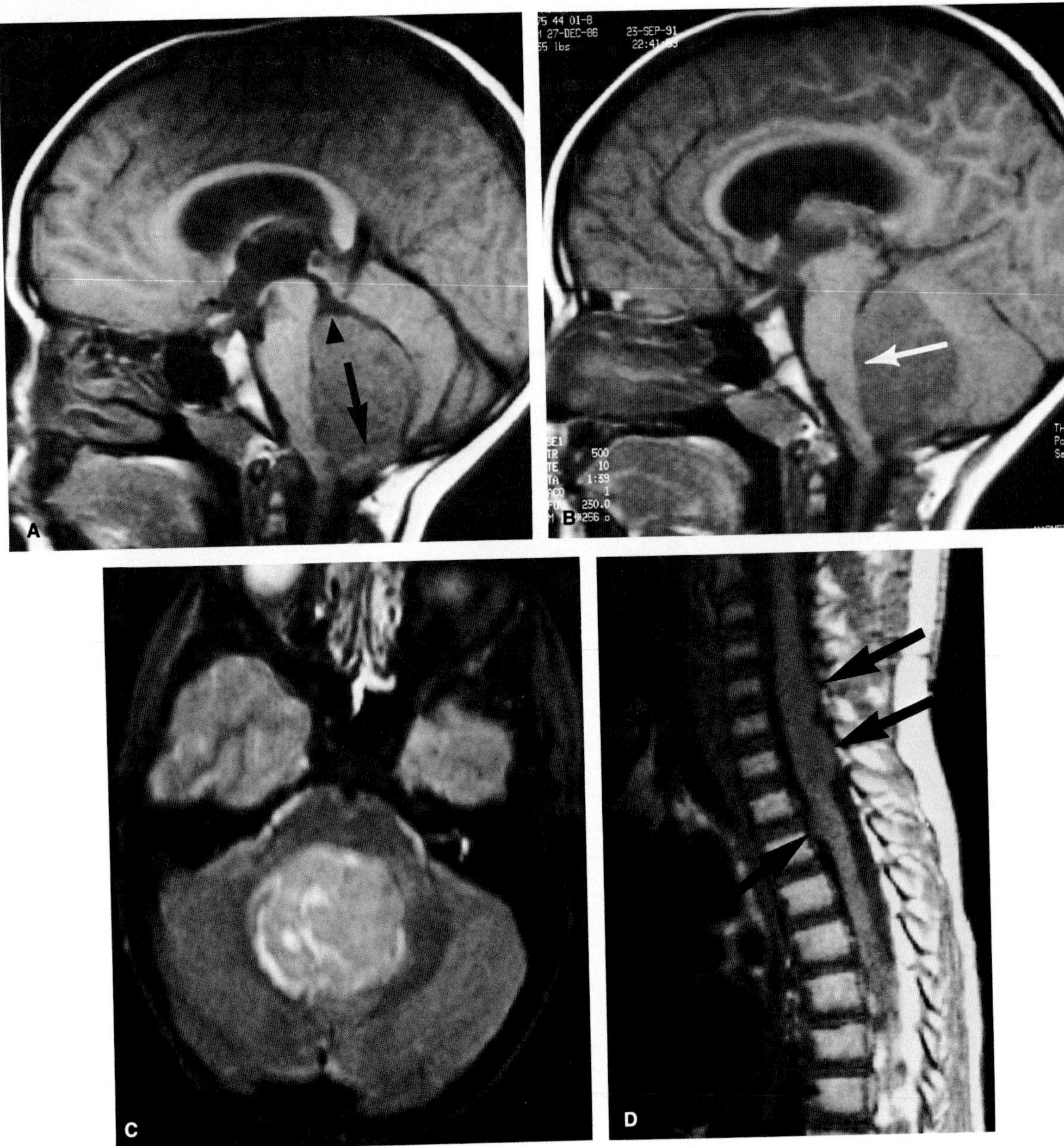

HISTORY

A 4-year-old with a 3-week history of headache and ataxia. There was papilledema on physical examination.

FINDINGS

(*A and B*) T1-weighted sagittal images at and just to the right of midline demonstrate a large mass extending from the anteroinferior cerebellum and filling the fourth ventricle. The brain stem (*white arrow in B*) is displaced anteriorly, and the inferior aspect of the aqueduct of Sylvius (*black arrowhead in A*) is widened. The mass is not clearly separable from the cerebellar tonsil (*black arrow in A*), which extends into and obliterates the foramen magnum. On *A* and *B,* the T1-weighted images, the signal intensity of the mass is similar to that of gray matter. (*C*) On the T2-weighted axial image, this midline mass has heterogeneous, though predominantly high, signal intensity. T1-weighted sagittal image (*D*) of the cervical and upper thoracic spine and T2-weighted sagittal image (*E*) of the lumbar and lower thoracic spine demonstrate multiple intradural, extramedullary masses (*black arrows in D; white arrows in E*), which have the same signal intensity as normal spinal cord.

DIAGNOSIS

Medulloblastoma with drop metastases

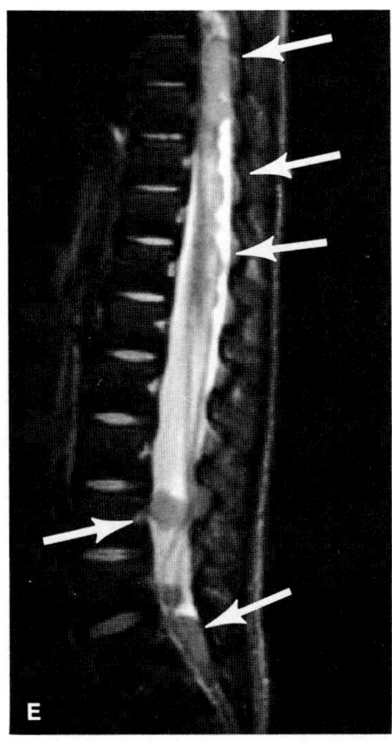

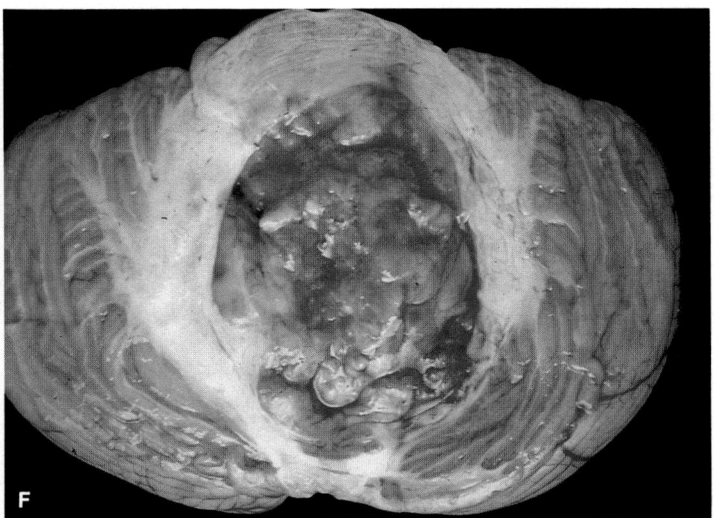

DISCUSSION

Medulloblastoma is a primitive neuroectodermal tumor (PNET) of the cerebellum,[1] and is the most common posterior fossa neoplasm in childhood.[2] About two thirds of patients with medulloblastoma present in the first decade of life, with a peak incidence between the ages of 5 and 9 years. However, up to one third of medulloblastomas occur in young adults, with a second late peak incidence between the ages of 20 and 24 years. These tumors grow rapidly, and patients usually present with nonspecific symptoms or signs of increased intracranial pressure (headache, nausea, vomiting, increasing head size) or of a posterior fossa mass (ataxia).[2]

Most medulloblastomas arise from the primitive neuroepithelial cells in the inferior medullary velum (roof of the fourth ventricle) and are located in the midline. These tumors typically encroach on or completely fill the fourth ventricle and extend inferiorly into the cisterna magna. The "classic" MR features of a midline mass with signal intensity equal to gray matter on both T1- and T2-weighted images, and intense homogeneous enhancement after contrast infusion are seen in just over half of cases. At least one "atypical" feature such as necrosis, a cystic component, calcification, or eccentric location is present in 47% of cases. Medulloblastomas in the cerebellar hemispheres are more common in the older age group.

Medulloblastomas are highly malignant, with dissemination into the subarachnoid cisterns and spinal cord ("drop metastases") common, as illustrated in the current case. These tumors are radiosensitive, however, and treatment with surgery and total craniospinal radiation has improved survival.[2]

Pitfalls in Image Interpretation

The differential diagnosis for a midline posterior fossa mass in a child includes ependymoma and astrocytoma. The most common primary CNS tumors to metastasize by way of the CSF spaces are medulloblastoma, ependymoma, pinealoma, choroid plexus papilloma, and glioblastoma multiforme.

Pathologic Correlate

(*F*) Gross pathologic specimen shows a large, irregular medulloblastoma in the midline, arising from the vermis and filling the fourth ventricle. Medulloblastomas, as might be anticipated from this specimen, commonly cause obstructive hydrocephalus.

Clinical References

1. Rorke L. The cerebellar medulloblastoma and its relationship to primitive neuroectodermal tumors. J Neuropathol Exp Neurol 1983;42:1–15.
2. Gusnard D. Cerebellar neoplasms in children. Semin Roentgenol 1990;25:263–278.

(F *from Okazaki H, Scheithauer B. Slide atlas of neuropathology. New York, Gower Medical Publishing, 1988. By permission of Mayo Foundation.)*

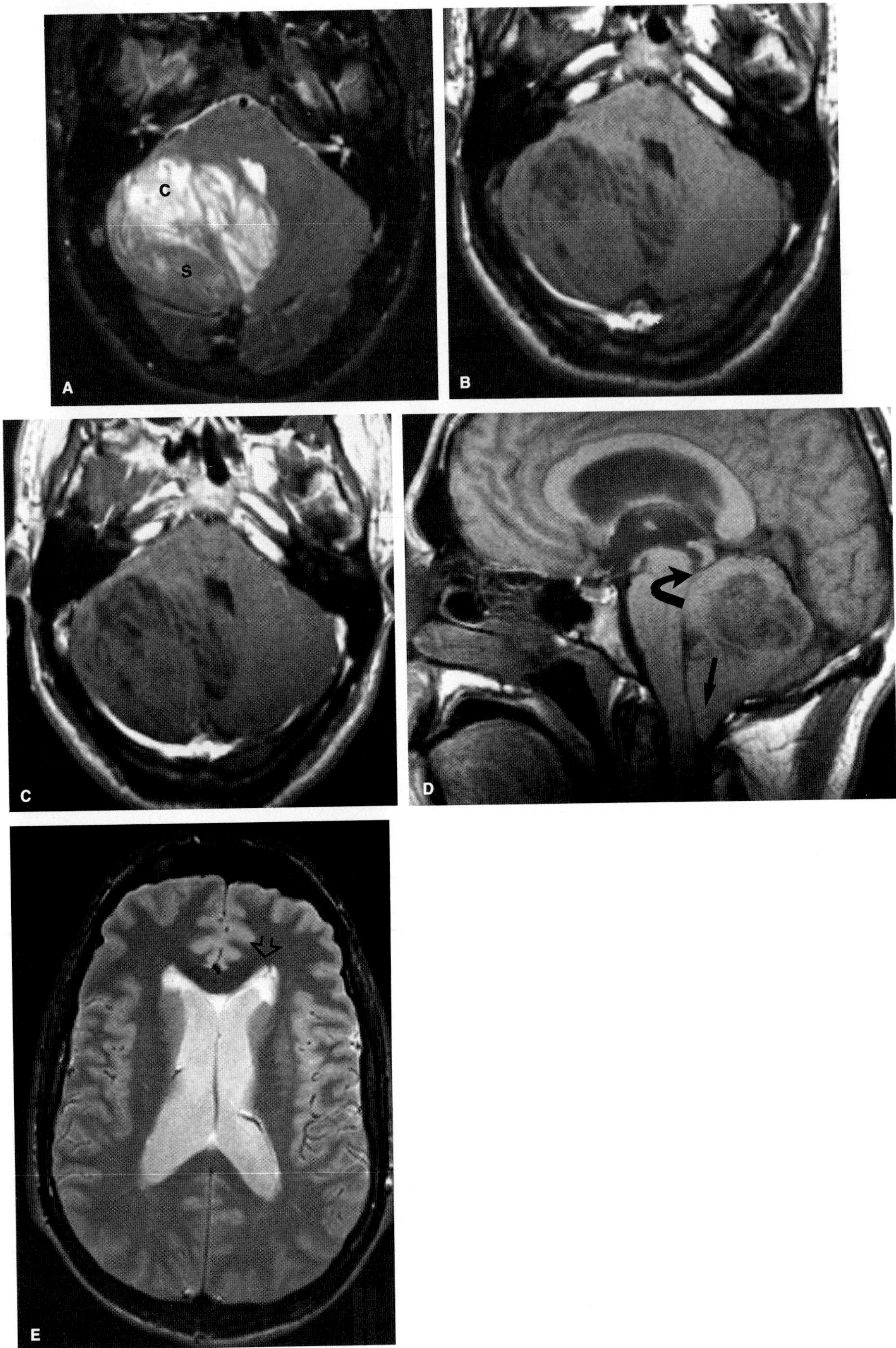

C
S
A
B
C
D
E

HISTORY

A 29-year-old man with a 1-week history of severe headache and papilledema

FINDINGS

T2-weighted (*A*), precontrast T1-weighted (*B*), and postcontrast T1-weighted (*C*) images depict a large right cerebellar mass, with solid (s) and cystic (c) components, which compresses the fourth ventricle and displays little contrast enhancement. (*D*) Precontrast sagittal T1-weighted image reveals compression of the distal aqueduct (*curved arrow*) and tonsillar herniation (*arrow*). (*E*) Axial T2-weighted image (TE = 45 msec) at the lateral ventricular level reveals that the compression has caused obstructive hydrocephalus with transependymal CSF flow (*open arrow*).

DIAGNOSIS

Gangliocytoma (ganglioneuroma)

DISCUSSION

Differentiated ganglion cell tumors of the CNS occupy a spectrum, which at one end consists of a tumor composed predominantly of mature atypical neurons (gangliocytoma) and, at the other, of a tumor with dominant glial elements (ganglioglioma). These two tumor types share common characteristics in terms of incidence, macroscopic features, and biologic behavior. The lesion may be cystic or solid, with about half demonstrating some contrast enhancement.[1] Patients typically present with long-standing symptoms; 80% of cases occur under the age of 30. The most frequent site is the temporal lobe, but no area of the CNS is exempt. Their slow growth and good demarcation from surrounding normal brain permit surgical resection in many cases—factors favoring a relatively good prognosis.

The mass in this patient was surgically excised.

MR Technique

Thin (3- to 4-mm) sections are required for detailed evaluation of the posterior fossa.

Pitfalls in Image Interpretation

Transependymal flow of CSF, due to obstructive hydrocephalus, should not be mistaken for frontal horn "capping," which may occur as a result of resorption of interstitial water or partial denuding of the ependyma. Ventricular enlargement and identification of extensive periventricular hyperintensity (not just at the frontal horns and atria) permit differentiation.

Clinical References

1. Castillo M, Davis PC, Takei Y, Hoffman JC. Intracranial ganglioglioma: MR, CT, and clinical findings in 18 patients. AJNR 1990;11:109–114.

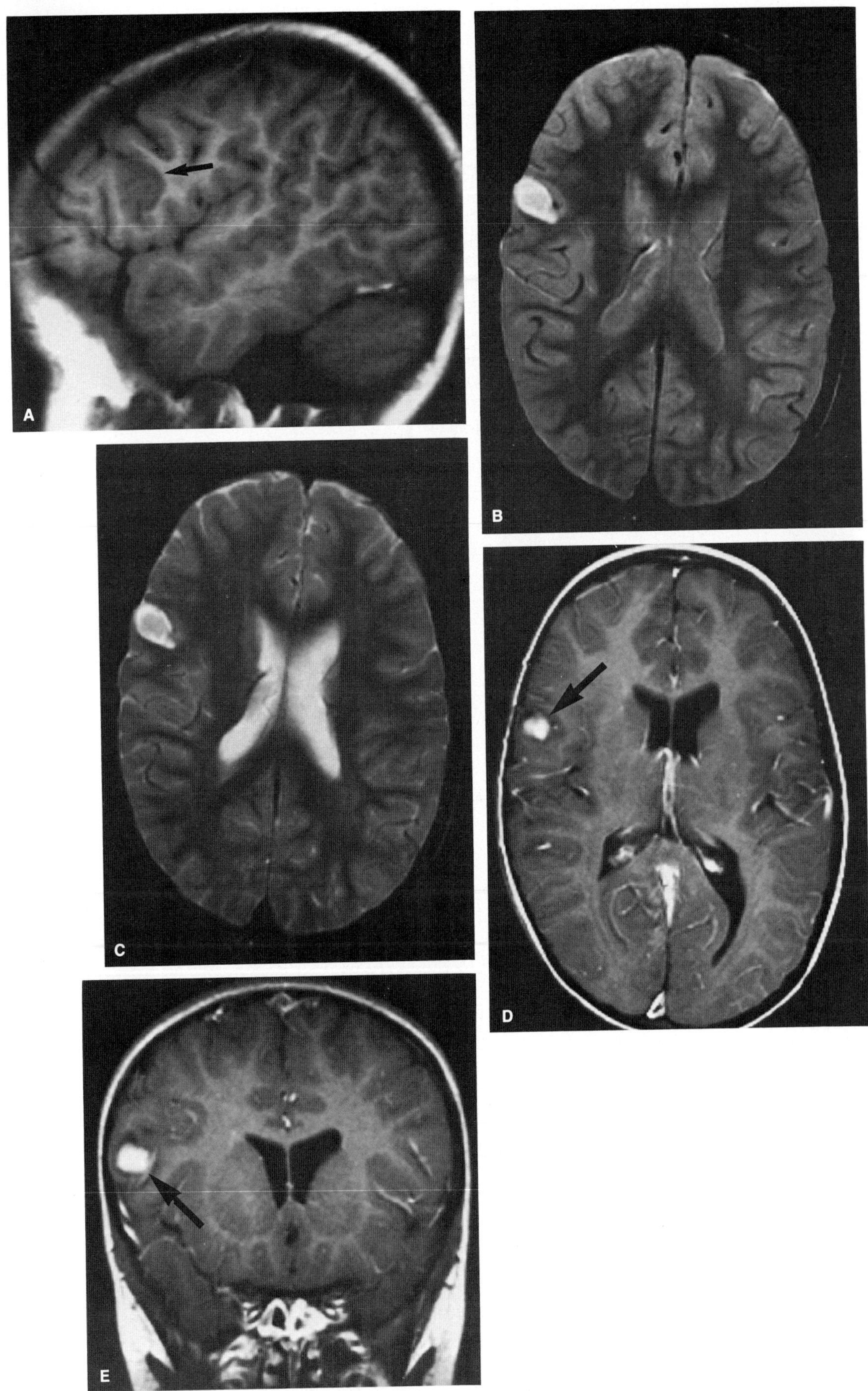
A
B
C
D
E

HISTORY

A 5-year-old child with new onset of seizures

FINDINGS

(*A*) The sagittal T1-weighted scout image reveals a small (less than 2 cm) low-signal-intensity mass (*arrow*) in the right frontal region. The lesion is of high signal intensity on both (*B*) intermediate (TE = 45 msec) and (*C*) heavily (TE = 90 msec) T2-weighted scans, appears well circumscribed, and is peripheral in location. Axial (*D*) and coronal (*E*) postcontrast T1-weighted scans reveal uniform lesion enhancement (*arrows*).

DIAGNOSIS

Polar spongioblastoma

DISCUSSION

True polar spongioblastoma is a rare type of PNET. The tumor cells are morphologically equivalent to migrating spongioblasts seen at 16 to 18 weeks of fetal development. The tumor is most common in the first and second decades of life, with preferential occurrence in the walls of the third or fourth ventricle.

The appearance of the lesion in this patient is not classic for either an astrocytoma or a PNET, raising the possibility of a less common histology. The well-defined nature of the lesion is not uncharacteristic of pediatric brain tumors. The marked enhancement, without definite evidence of surrounding edema, as well as lesion location (not in a vascular distribution), favors the diagnosis of neoplastic disease. Most PNETs, however, present as large, well-marginated, inhomogeneous masses and lie in the deep cerebral white matter.

Seizures, a frequent reason for clinical presentation, can be caused by many different disease entities, with the most likely cause varying with age and specific type. In the infant (0 to 2 years), the common causes of a seizure include perinatal ischemia, acute infection, metabolic disturbances, and congenital malformations. In children (2 to 12 years), causes include acute infection and trauma, although most cases are idiopathic. Febrile seizures, though also common, are characteristically short in duration and generalized rather than focal in nature. In adolescents (12 to 18 years) and young adults (18 to 35 years), trauma (which produces focal seizures) and drug or alcohol withdrawal (which produces generalized tonic-clonic seizures) are major causes. In this age group, focal seizures may also be due to an arteriovenous malformation. Between the ages of 30 and 50, brain tumors (of all types) become a common cause for seizures, and are present in up to 30% of patients with new onset. Above the age of 50, cerebrovascular disease dominates as the reason for seizures, which may be either focal or generalized in nature.

Clinical References

1. Figeroa RE, el Gammal T, Brooks BS, et al. MR findings on primitive neuroectodermal tumors. J Comput Assist Tomogr 1989;13:773–778.

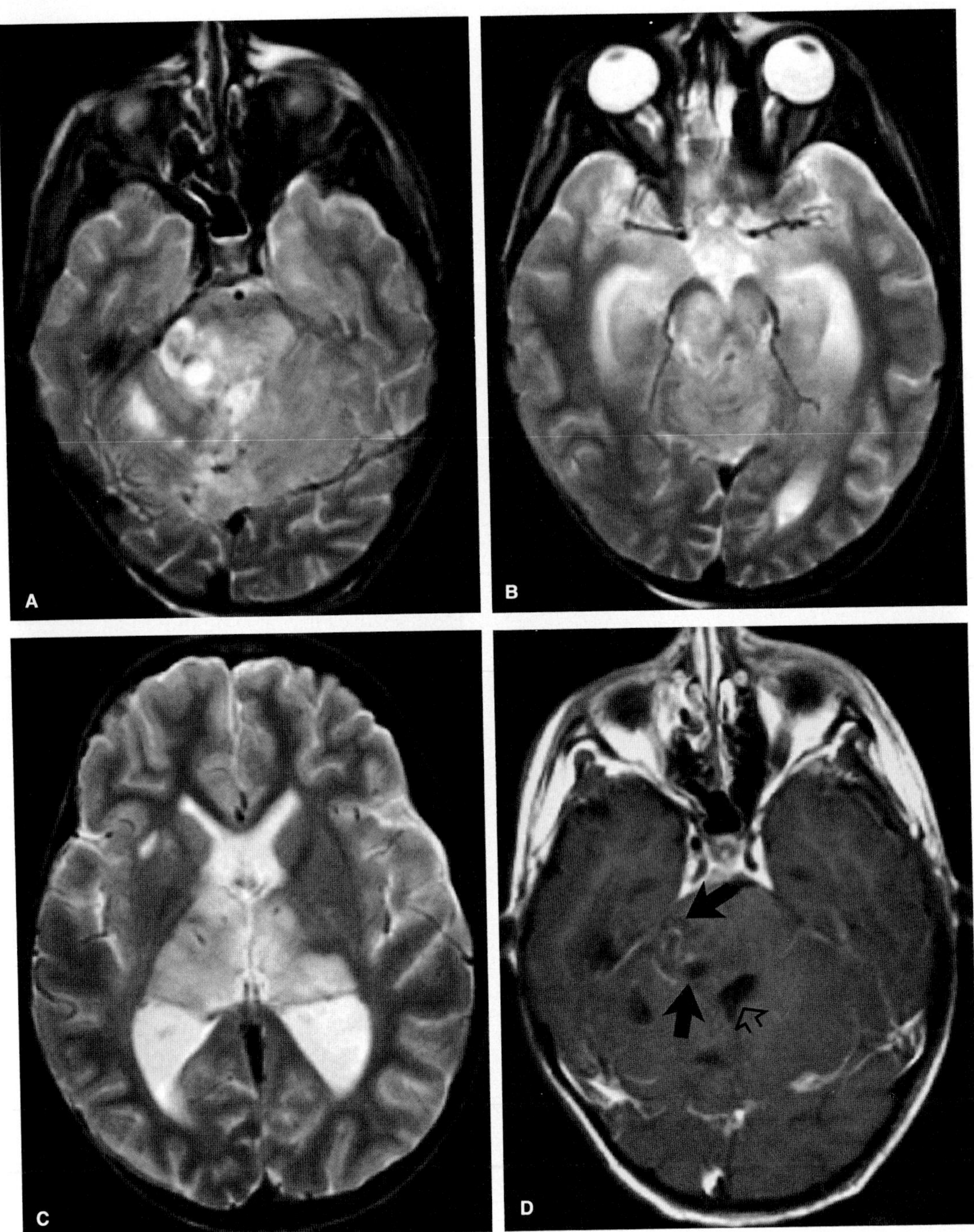

HISTORY

An 8-year-old patient with progressive headaches, worsening gait, and papilledema on ophthalmologic examination

FINDINGS

(*A to C*) T2-weighted images reveal a high-signal-intensity lesion that extends from the pons to the thalami. There is contiguous involvement of the rhombencephalon (hindbrain—medulla, pons, and cerebellum), mesencephalon (midbrain—cerebral peduncles, superior and inferior colliculi), and diencephalon (thalamus, hypothalamus). (*D to F*) Postcontrast T1-weighted images depict a predominantly nonenhancing mass, which expands the pons and right cerebral peduncle (*curved arrow in E*), with mass effect on the fourth ventricle (*open arrow in D*) and two small cystic foci (*arrows in D*).

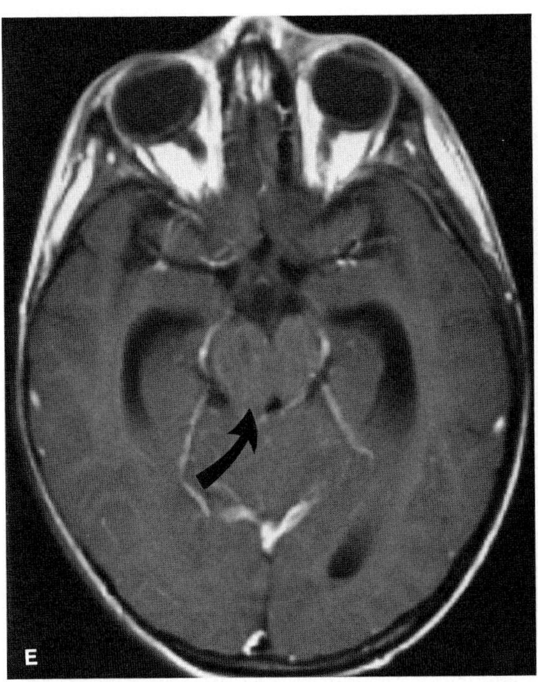

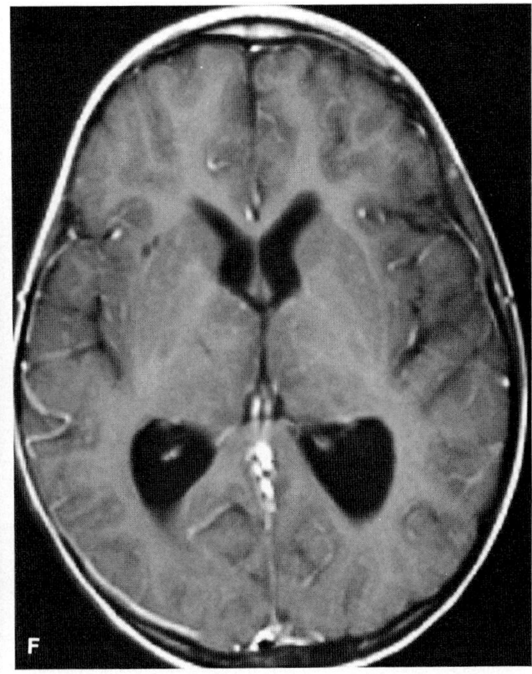

DIAGNOSIS

Primitive neuroectodermal tumor with astrocytomatous elements

DISCUSSION

The original biopsy in this patient revealed a low-grade astrocytoma. A second biopsy, performed at a later setting, showed predominantly primitive neuroectodermal elements. The lack of diagnostic concordance from biopsy to biopsy in this instance is due to the extremely small samples of tissue obtained. Small biopsies may be misleading, as in this instance, by not truly representing the complete pathologic spectrum of a tumor. It is well recognized that PNETs may be highly regionally variable in glial composition and degree of differentiation.

Recognition of the neuroectodermal elements in this tumor is important for patient management, given the propensity of PNETs for invasion locally, dissemination by way of the subarachnoid space, and metastases outside the CNS.[1] MR, of course, cannot provide histologic diagnosis but is invaluable for lesion detection and evaluation of the response to therapy.

Brain tumors constitute the second most common malignancy in childhood. In a recent large patient series, 45% of pediatric brain tumors were infratentorial in location and 55% supratentorial.[2] Astrocytomas were most common (30%), followed in incidence by neuroectodermal tumors (19%).

Clinical References

1. Figeroa RE, el Gammal T, Brooks BS, et al. MR findings on primitive neuroectodermal tumors. J Comput Assist Tomogr 1989;13:773–778.
2. Bonner K, Siegel KR. Pathology, treatment and management of posterior fossa brain tumors in children. J Neurosci Nurs 1988;20:84–93.

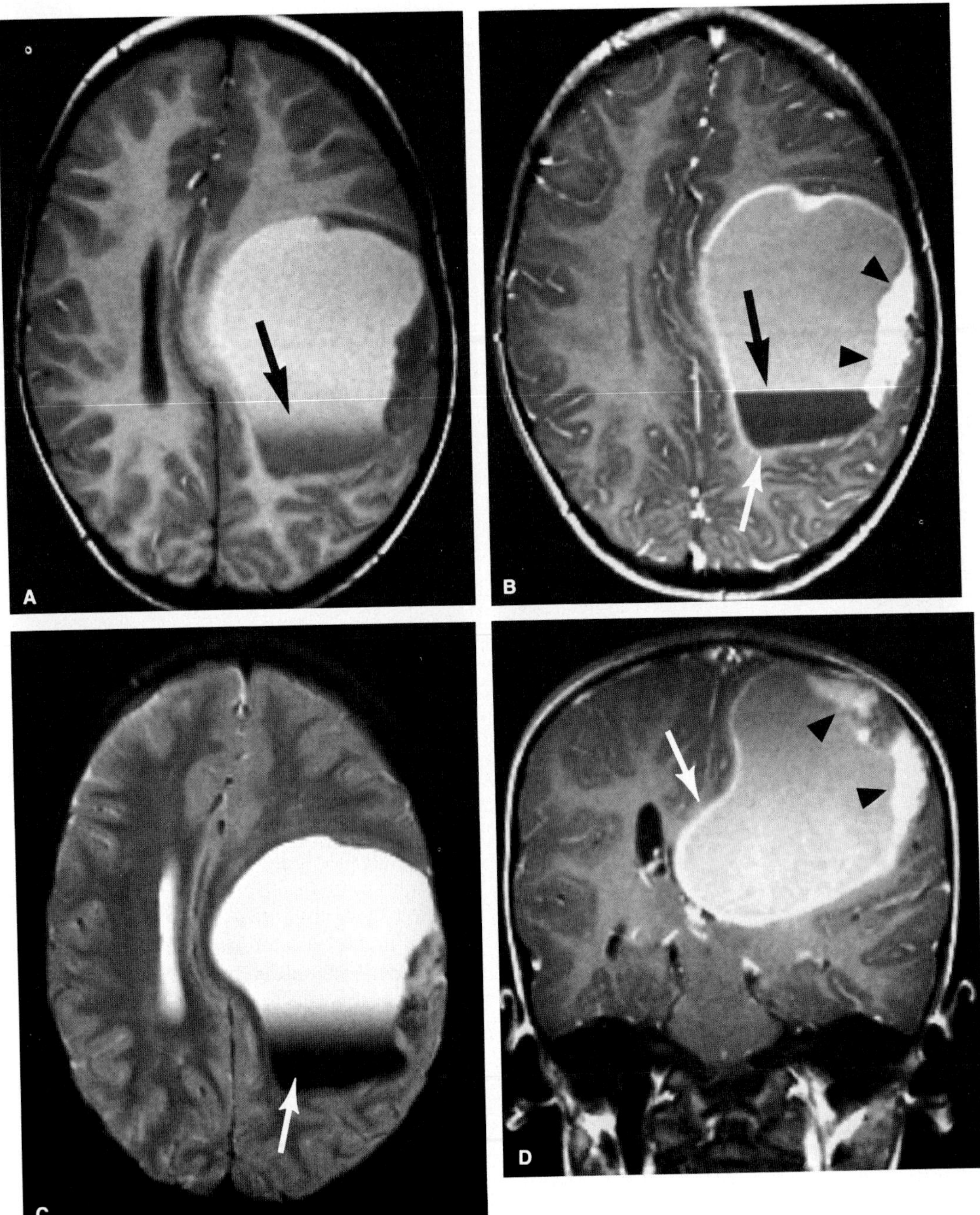

HISTORY

A 3-year-old patient with a 6-week history of right hemiparesis

FINDINGS

T1-weighted axial precontrast (*A*) and delayed postcontrast (*B*) images demonstrate a large, well-demarcated cystic mass within the left parietal and posterior frontal lobes. Within the cystic mass there is a fluid-fluid level (*black arrow*) representing separation of different hemoglobin degradation products. This fluid-fluid level is best defined on *B*, the delayed postcontrast scan. On T1-weighted (*B*) and T2-weighted (*C*) images the dependent layer (*white arrow*) has low signal intensity. The nondependent layer has high signal intensity on both *B* and *C*. Postcontrast T1-weighted axial (*B*) and coronal (*D*) images show enhancement of a soft tissue component (*black arrowheads in B and D*) along the lateral aspect of the mass, and enhancement of the entire rim. Subfalcine herniation (*white arrow in D*) of the mass and left-to-right shift of midline structures are best demonstrated on the coronal image (*D*). The body of the left lateral ventricle is completely obliterated by the mass effect.

DIAGNOSIS

Primitive neuroectodermal tumor

DISCUSSION

PNET is a term used for a rare group of CNS tumors composed of undifferentiated cells that resemble the germinal matrix of the embryonic neural tube.[1] When supratentorial, the nomenclature for these tumors is controversial, and *cerebral neuroblastoma* and *cerebral medulloblastoma* have often been used as synonyms for the currently preferred term, *PNET*.[2] PNET is usually detected in childhood or early adolescence, and patients present with headache, nausea, vomiting, increasing head size, papilledema, seizures, or neurologic deficit. These tumors are highly malignant and have a poor prognosis. Dissemination (seeding) along the CNS pathways is common.

Primitive neuroectodermal tumors are generally large, well-circumscribed masses[3] located most commonly in the frontal and parietal lobes. A cystic component is often the dominant feature, with enhancing soft tissue along the periphery of the tumor. Calcification (best seen on CT) and necrosis are also common. Hemorrhage into the cystic tumor is not uncommon and is often a presenting feature.[2] The MR appearance of the intracystic blood varies with time and often has distinct layers corresponding to different hemoglobin degradation products.

Pitfalls in Image Interpretation

The differential diagnosis for a large cystic supratentorial mass in childhood includes desmoplastic infantile ganglioglioma and astrocytoma.

Clinical References

1. Figueroa R, el Gammel T, Brooks B, et al. MR findings on primitive neuroectodermal tumors. J Comput Assist Tomogr 1989;13:773–778.
2. Hinshaw D, Ashwal S, Thompson J, Hasso AN. Neuroradiology of primitive neuroectodermal tumors. Neuroradiology 1983;25:87–92.
3. Chambers E, Turski P, Sobel D, et al. Radiologic characteristics of primary cerebral neuroblastomas. Radiology 1981; 139:101–104.

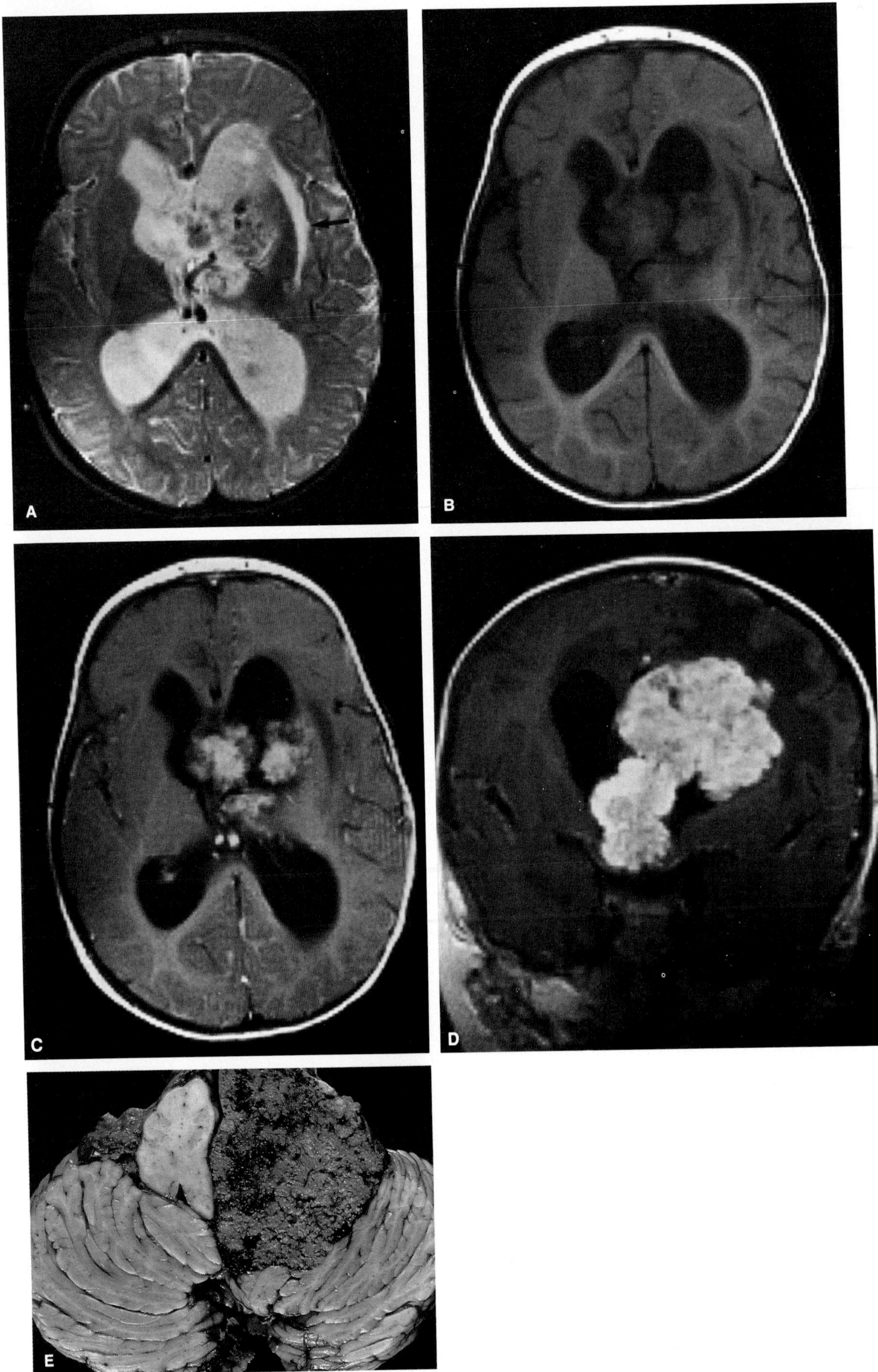
A
B
C
D
E

HISTORY

A young child who initially presented with obstructive hydrocephalus

FINDINGS

Precontrast T2-weighted (*A*) and T1-weighted (*B*) images reveal ventriculomegaly and a lobulated soft tissue mass lying principally within the left lateral ventricle. Edema, which was more extensive at a higher level, is seen tracking in the white matter of the external capsule (*arrow in A*). There are multiple large serpiginous signal voids, caused by the presence of large abnormal vessels, best seen on the T2-weighted scan. Intense lesion enhancement is noted on axial (*C*) and coronal (*D*) postcontrast T1-weighted images.

DIAGNOSIS

Choroid plexus papilloma

DISCUSSION

Choroid plexus papillomas are rare intracranial tumors, most commonly located in the lateral ventricles in children[1] and in the fourth ventricle in adults.[2] Intense, relatively homogeneous enhancement has been described on MR. These lesions are highly vascular and may demonstrate areas of signal void on precontrast scans because of blood flow in abnormal vessels. Calcification and hemorrhage have also been described. Malignant transformation is extremely unusual. Leptomeningeal seeding can occur, as well as communicating hydrocephalus, because of excessive production of CSF. Obstructive hydrocephalus can also be seen as a result of outlet obstruction and may be asymmetric in children. Treatment is by surgical resection.

MR Technique

Multiplanar imaging is important for surgical planning and postoperative follow-up, offering direct lesion visualization relative to normal anatomy and better definition of intraventricular location.[1] Contrast enhancement permits improved lesion identification, together with improved definition of lesion location and extent.[2]

Pitfalls in Image Interpretation

The most common lateral ventricular neoplasms are choroid plexus papilloma and meningioma.[3] The differential diagnosis should also include subependymoma, subependymal giant cell astrocytoma, metastasis, and lymphoma, although these lesions are less frequently encountered. With the exception of subependymoma, all demonstrate contrast enhancement. The MR and CT appearance of lateral ventricular tumors is not sufficiently specific to permit definitive tissue diagnosis.

Pathologic Correlate

(*E*) Pathologic section of a choroid plexus papilloma in the cerebellopontine angle. These tumors are typically well-demarcated, pedunculated, cauliflowerlike masses with delicate fronds resembling the appearance of normal choroid plexus.

Clinical References

1. Coates TL, Hinshaw DB, Peckman N, et al. Pediatric choroid plexus neoplasms: MR, CT, and pathologic correlation. Radiology 1989;173:81–88.
2. Girardot C, Boukobza M, Lamoureux JP, et al. Choroid plexus papillomas of the posterior fossa in adults: MR imaging and gadolinium enhancement: report of four cases and review of the literature. J Neuroradiol 1990;17:303–318.
3. Jelinek J, Smirniotopoulos JG, Parisi JE, Kanzer M. Lateral ventricular neoplasms of the brain: differential diagnosis based on clinical, CT, and MR findings. AJR 1990;155:365–372.

(A to D *from Runge VM. Clinical magnetic resonance imaging. Philadelphia, JB Lippincott, 1990;* E *from Okazaki H, Scheithauer B. Slide atlas of neuropathology. New York, Gower Medical Publishing, 1988. By permission of Mayo Foundation.)*

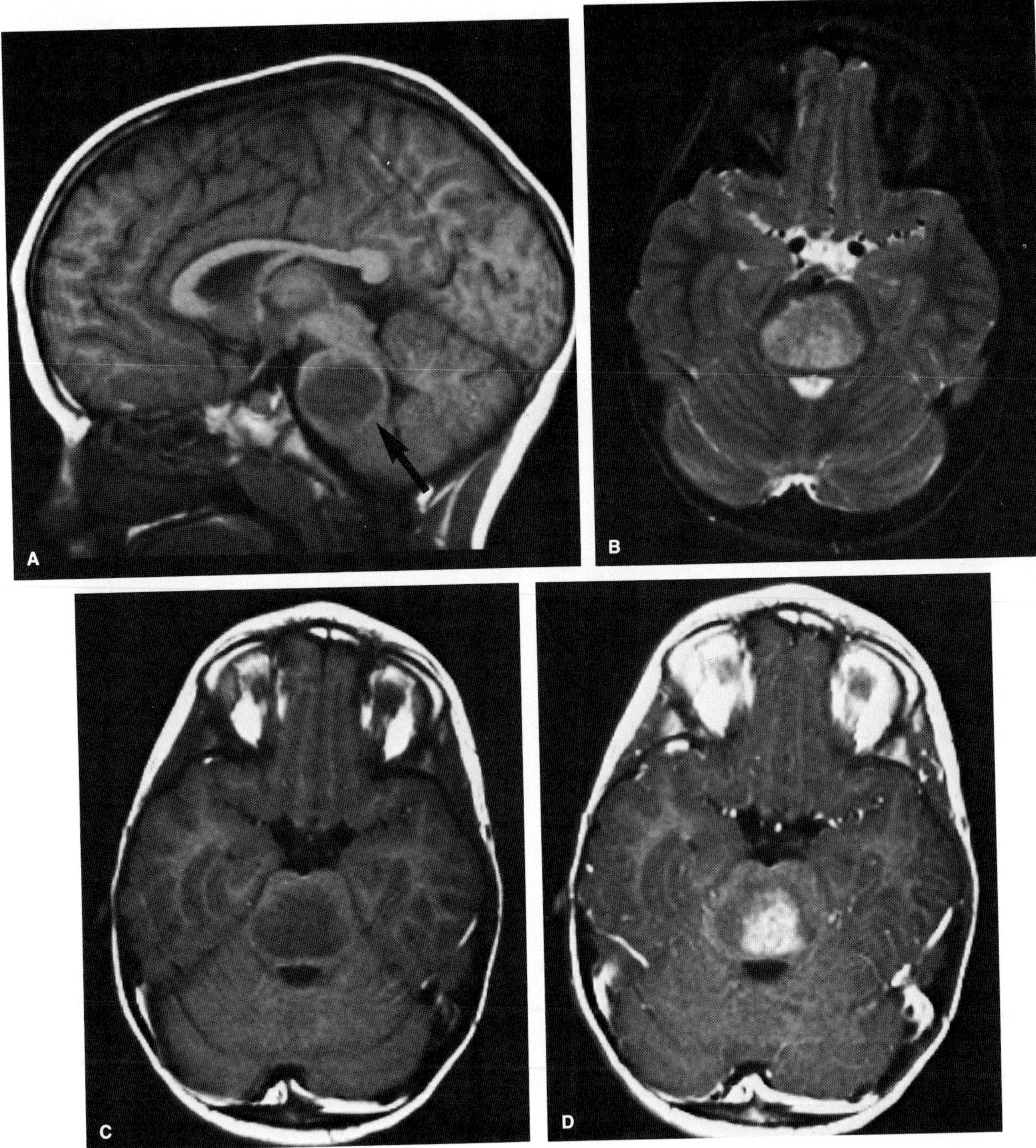

HISTORY

A 6-year-old patient with headaches for several weeks, ataxia for several days, and decreased hand-to-eye coordination

FINDINGS

(*A*) Midline sagittal T1-weighted image reveals a large low-signal-intensity mass (*arrow*) expanding the pons. (*B*) Inspection of the T2-weighted axial scan (TE = 90 msec) reveals the mass to occupy almost the entirety of the pons, leaving only a residual rim of normal tissue. Comparison of precontrast (*C*) and postcontrast (*D*) T1-weighted images discloses enhancement in a portion of the mass posteriorly. (*E*) Six weeks later, following radiation therapy to the brain stem, the T2-weighted image reveals enlargement of the mass. (*F*) Precontrast T1-weighted image now demonstrates hemorrhage (*curved arrow*) in the posterior portion of the mass. The enlargement of the lesion is at least in part due to the interval hemorrhage. The effects of radiation therapy can be noted on *F*, with mild enlargement of cortical sulci.

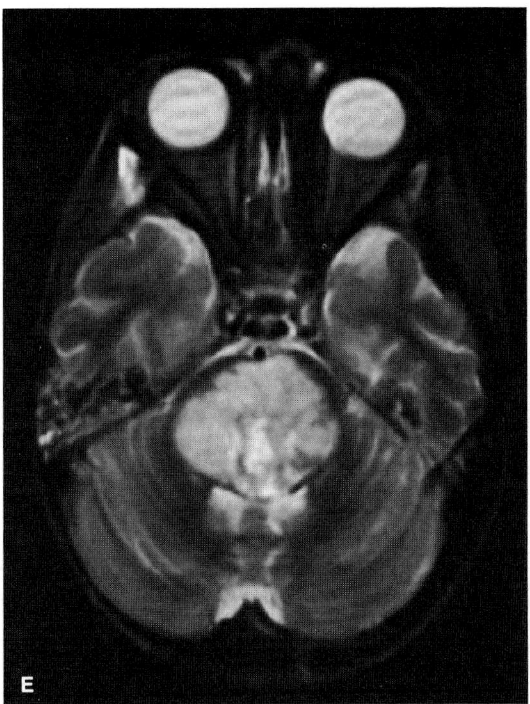

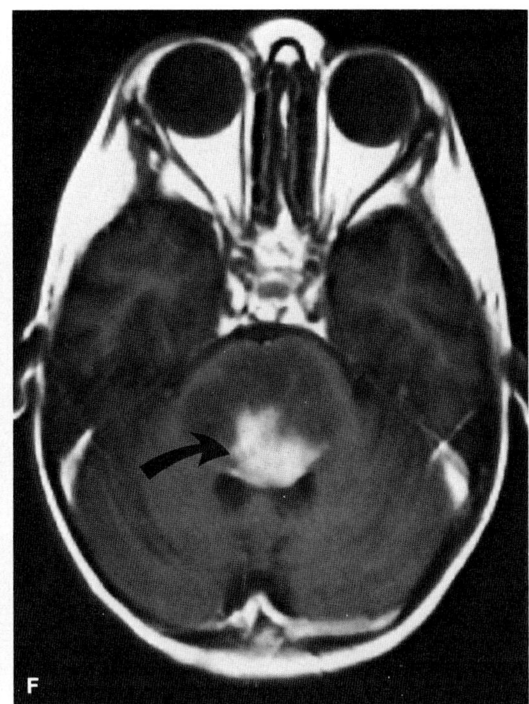

DIAGNOSIS

Brain stem (pontine) glioma

DISCUSSION

Brain stem gliomas tend to occur in childhood and adolescence. Histologically these lesions are pilocystic astrocytomas but share many features in common with fibrillary astrocytomas—in particular the tendency to undergo anaplastic change. Although lesions which involve the pons predominate, contiguous involvement of more than one division of the brain stem is extremely common, with high-grade lesions being more extensive. Exophytic extension, CSF seeding, and ventricular dilatation are common. Radiation therapy may produce a temporary improvement in clinical condition. In one series,[1] no patients with malignant lesions survived past 15 months, while those with low-grade lesions had a 50% 5-year survival.

MR is used both for diagnosis[2] and for monitoring therapeutic response, demonstrating tumor regression in response to radiation therapy, tumor progression before clinical deterioration, and cyst formation and hemorrhage, which may occur following treatment.[3]

MR Technique

MR is the modality of choice for examination of pediatric tumors and, in particular, those involving the brain stem and cerebellum.

Clinical References

1. Nishio S, Fukui M, Tateishi J. Brain stem gliomas: a clinicopathological analysis of 23 histologically proven cases. J Neurooncol 1988;6:245–250.
2. Hueftle MG, Hans JS, Kaufman B, Benson JE. MR imaging of brain stem gliomas. J Comput Assist Tomogr 1985;9:263–267.
3. Smith RR, Zimmerman RA, Packer RJ, et al. Pediatric brainstem glioma: post-radiation clinical and MR follow-up. Neuroradiology 1990;32:265–271.

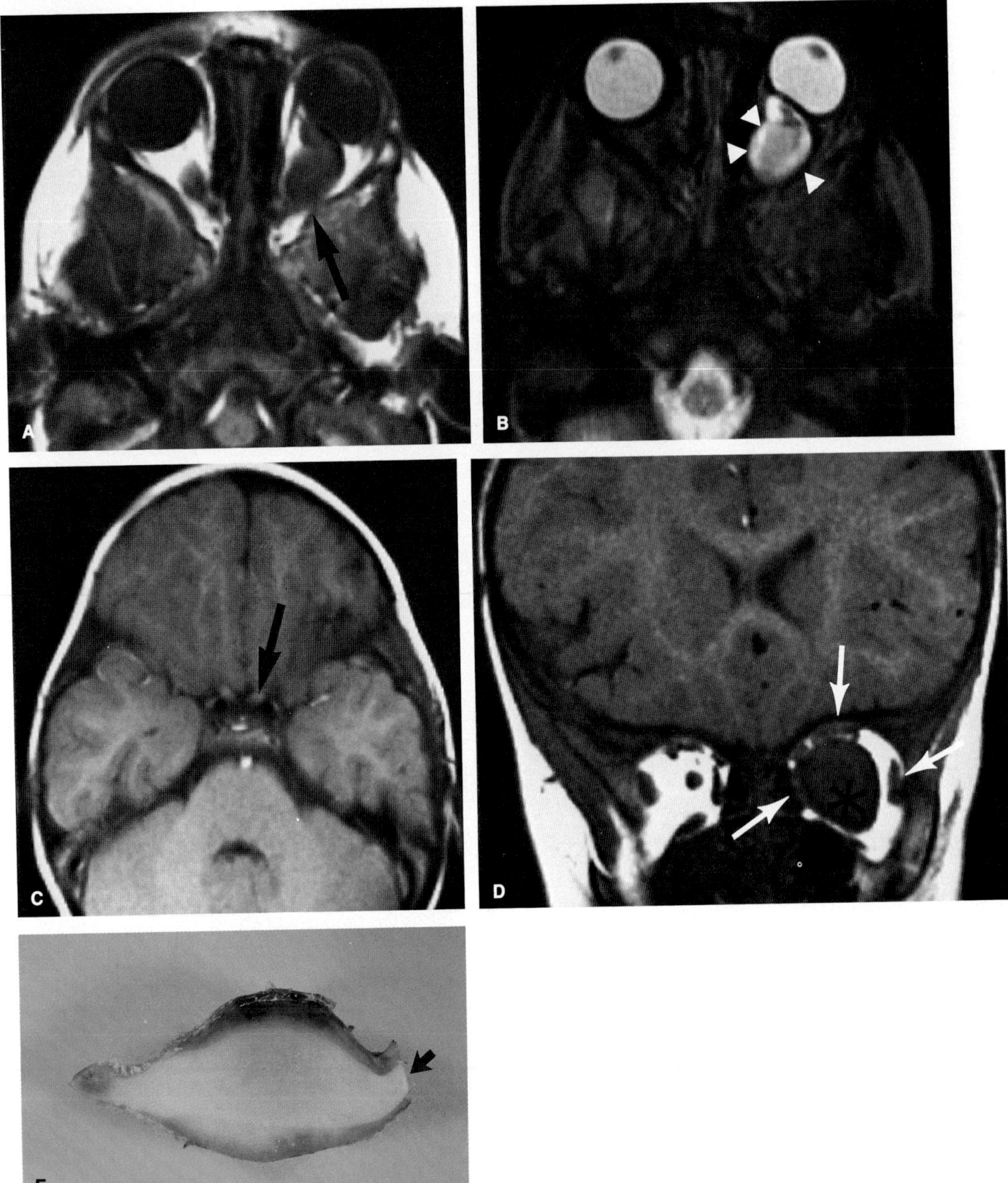
A
B
C
D
E

HISTORY

A 16-month-old with unilateral blindness and left proptosis

FINDINGS

(*A*) T1-weighted axial image demonstrates irregular fusiform enlargement of the intraorbital left optic nerve (*arrow*). (*B*) T2-weighted image shows high-signal-intensity CSF (*white arrowheads*) surrounding the abnormally enlarged nerve. (*C*) The posterior prechiasmal intracranial left optic nerve (*arrow*) is normal on a T1-weighted axial image at a higher level. (*D*) On the T1-weighted coronal image, the intraconal position of the enlarged optic nerve mass (*black asterisk*) and its relation to normal extraocular muscles (*white arrows*) are seen.

DIAGNOSIS

Optic nerve glioma

DISCUSSION

Optic nerve glioma is the most common cause of optic nerve enlargement. Seventy-five percent occur in the first decade of life, and the peak incidence is at 5 years of age. Patients present with visual disturbances and proptosis.[1] Optic nerve glioma is associated with neurofibromatosis type 1 in approximately 25% of cases.[2] In neurofibromatosis, optic nerve gliomas are often bilateral.

On MR, an optic nerve glioma is usually seen as a well-demarcated, fusiform enlargement of the optic nerve, with signal intensity similar to that of the normal optic nerve on T1-weighted images, and slightly high signal intensity on T2-weighted images. Extension posteriorly to involve the optic chiasm and optic tracts is well depicted on MR and indicates nonresectability.

Histologically, optic nerve glioma is a juvenile pilocystic astrocytoma, which is a low-grade neoplasm composed of distinctive, well-differentiated hairlike astrocytes, and characterized by a relatively benign clinical course.

Pitfalls in Image Interpretation

The differential diagnosis for optic nerve enlargement includes meningioma, inflammation (optic neuritis),[3] and leukemia or lymphoma. The differential diagnosis for an orbital mass in childhood includes rhabdomyosarcoma, hemangioma, lymphangioma, pseudotumor, lymphoma, abscess (often an extension of adjacent sinus disease), and dermoid cyst.

Pathologic Correlate

(*E*) Gross specimen from the same patient whose MR images are presented. There is fusiform enlargement of the midportion of the optic nerve itself, consistent with an optic nerve glioma. The posterior, prechiasmal portion (*arrow*) of the optic nerve is normal, confirming the findings on preoperative MR.

Clinical References

1. Alvord E, Lofton S. Gliomas of the optic nerve or chiasm. J Neurosurg 1988;68:85–98.
2. Borit A, Richardson E. The biological and clinical behaviour of pilocystic astrocytomas of the optic pathways. Brain 1982;105:161–187.
3. Holman R, Grimson B, Drayer B, et al. Magnetic resonance imaging of optic gliomas. Am J Opthalmol 1985;100:596–601.

(E *courtesy of Daron G. Davis, MD.)*

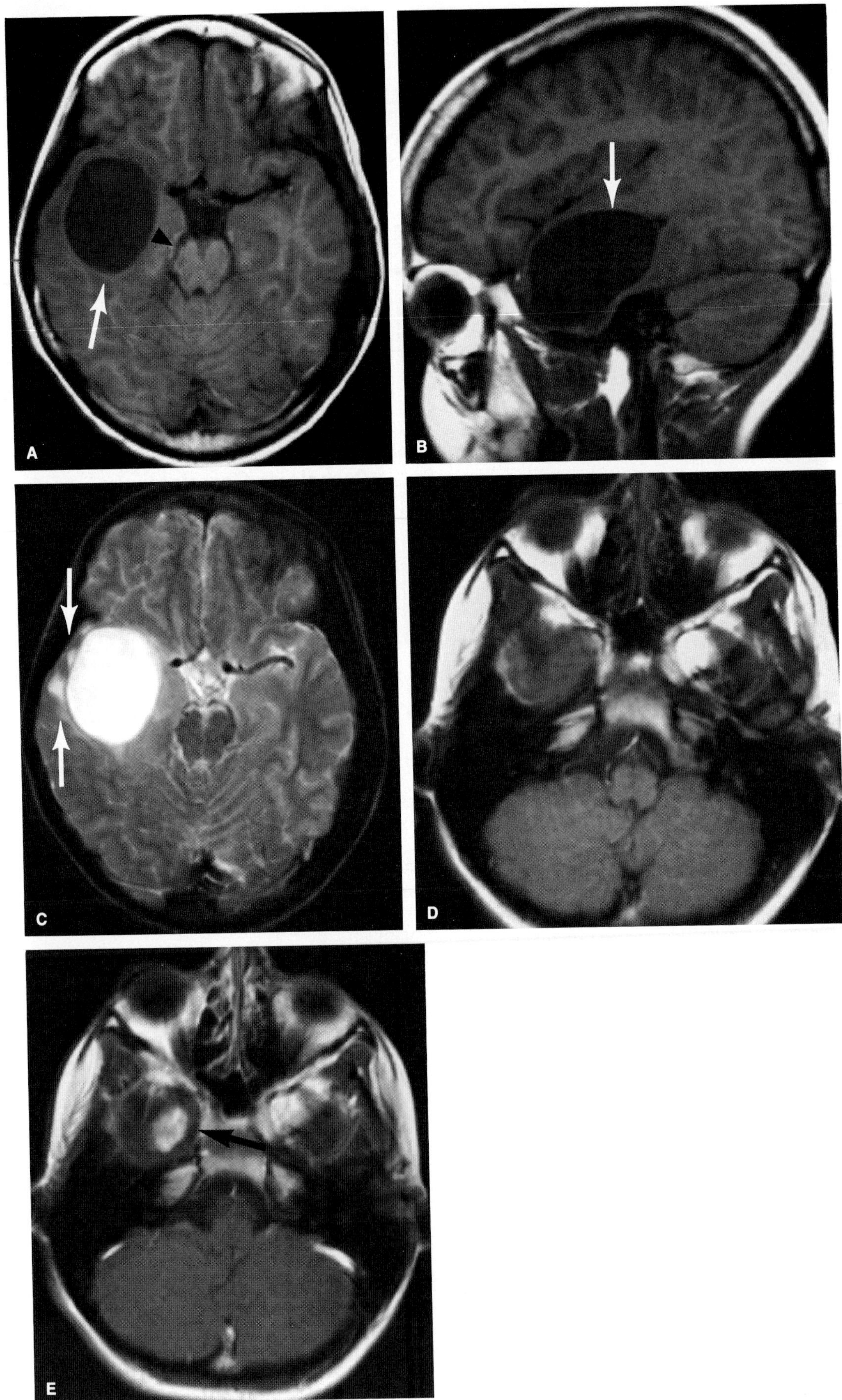
A
B
C
D
E

HISTORY

A 10-year-old with seizures

FINDINGS

T1-weighted axial (*A*) and sagittal (*B*) images demonstrate a large cystic mass (*white arrows in A and B*) in the anterior right temporal lobe. The tumor is causing mild mass effect on the brain stem (*arrowhead in A*). (*C*) T2-weighted axial image demonstrates a small amount of edema (*white arrows*) surrounding the lesion. The signal intensity of the cystic fluid is slightly higher than CSF on all images. Precontrast (*D*) and postcontrast (*E*) T1-weighted axial images at a more caudal position show a 1.5 × 1–cm enhancing soft-tissue nodule (*arrow in E*) along the inferior wall of the cyst.

DIAGNOSIS

Ganglioglioma

DISCUSSION

Gangliogliomas are rare primary brain neoplasms that contain both glial and neuronal elements. These tumors occur primarily in children and young adults, although the age range is from infancy through the eighth decade. The majority of ganglioglioma are supratentorial, and the most common site is the temporal lobe. However, they may also occur in the cerebellum, brain stem, spinal cord, and optic nerves.[1] Gangliogliomas are slow-growing, low-grade tumors that usually have relatively benign behavior and a good prognosis. Patients typically present with headaches or seizures.

About 60% of gangliogliomas are predominantly solid. The remaining 40% are predominantly cystic, and often consist of a large single cyst with a soft tissue nodule along the wall (mural nodule). Both cystic and solid gangliogliomas often contain calcifications, best seen with CT. On MR cystic gangliogliomas are well-circumscribed lesions with little or no associated edema. Solid gangliogliomas have less well defined tumor margins. The use of IV contrast material aids in tumor demarcation in those gangliogliomas which enhance.

Pitfalls in Image Interpretation

The differential diagnosis for a predominantly cystic supratentorial mass in a child or young adult includes juvenile pilocystic astrocytoma, primitive neuroectodermal tumor, and gangliocytoma. Gangliocytomas are composed of only neuronal elements and can be differentiated from gangliogliomas only histologically.

Clinical References

1. Castillo M, Davis P, Takel Y, et al. Intracranial ganglioglioma: MR, CT, and clinical findings in 18 patients. AJNR 1990;11:109–114.

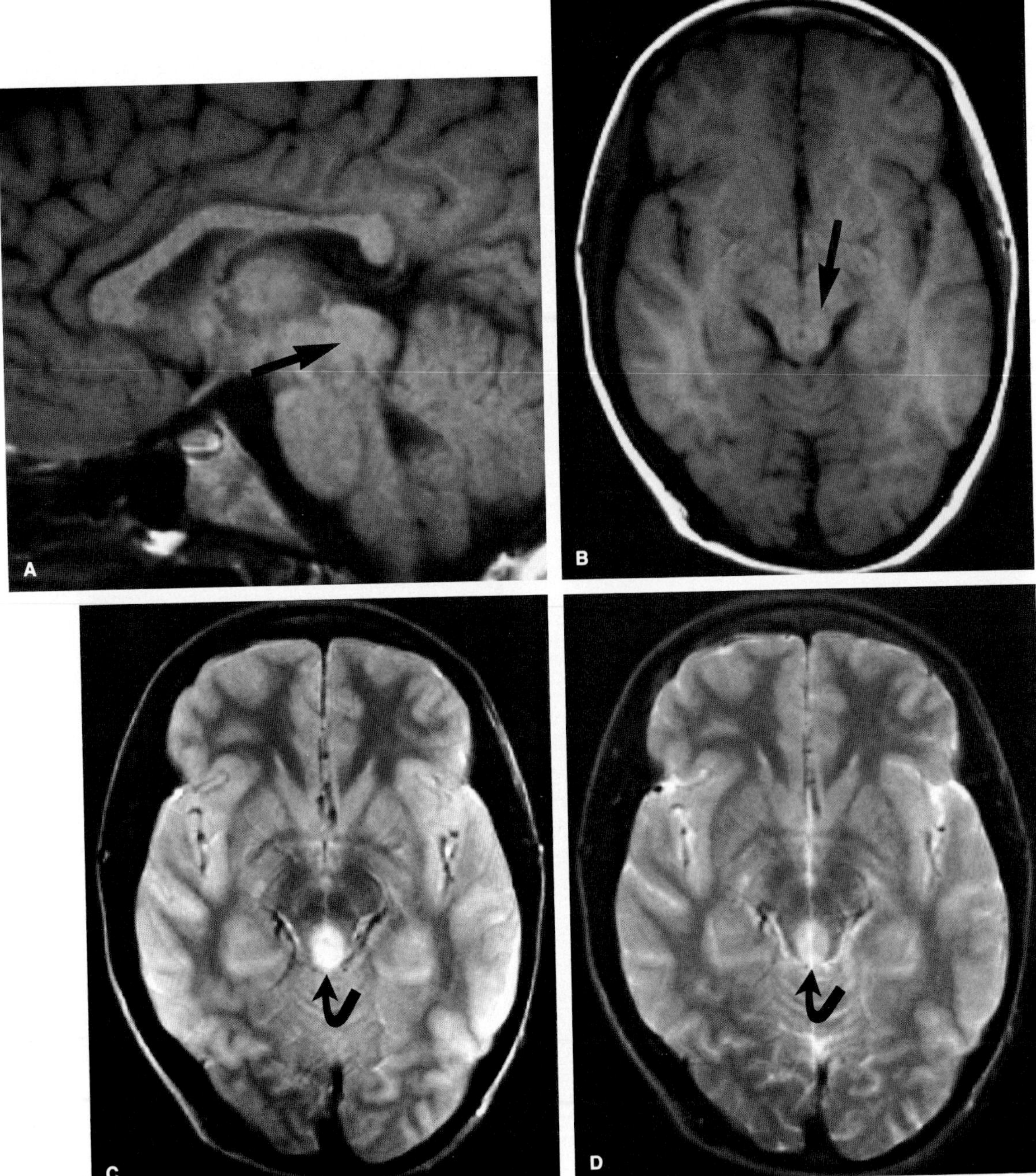
A
B
C
D

HISTORY

An adult who presented initially with papilledema and bifrontal headaches, findings suggestive of obstructive hydrocephalus

FINDINGS

Sagittal (*A*) and axial (*B*) T1-weighted images reveal bulbous enlargement of the tectum (*arrows in A and B*), with obliteration of the cerebral aqueduct anteriorly. The lateral and third ventricles are normal in size due to previous shunting. Intermediate (TE = 45 msec) (*C*) and heavily (TE = 90 msec) (*D*) T2-weighted images depict a tectal mass (*curved arrows in C and D*) with abnormal hyperintensity. The cerebral aqueduct, anterior to the mass, is compressed and not clearly visualized.

DIAGNOSIS

Tectal glioma

DISCUSSION

Aqueductal narrowing can be the result of stenosis, septum formation, gliosis, inflammatory conditions, and mass lesions.[1] Surprisingly, narrowing can also be the result, rather than the cause, of hydrocephalus. A high incidence of Chiari I malformation with nonneoplastic aqueductal stenosis has also been reported.

Tectal gliomas present as bulbous masses and may obstruct the aqueduct at any location along its length. These lesions typically exhibit prolonged T2 relaxation, which translates to high signal intensity on T2-weighted images. In benign aqueductal stenosis, thickening—but not bulbous enlargement—of the tectum is occasionally seen. A thin rim of periaqueductal hyperintensity, present in some patients, is presumed to represent gliosis or interstitial edema (from transependymal flow), although the possibility of an early presentation for neoplastic disease cannot be completely excluded.

MR Technique

The sagittal plane, in particular, is important for imaging of the cerebral aqueduct, providing depiction of both adjacent soft tissues and the entire length of this CSF pathway.

Pitfalls in Image Interpretation

Dilatation of the suprapineal recess in patients with proximal stenosis of the aqueduct (at the level of the superior colliculi) can produce shortening and thickening of the tectum, which should not be mistaken for tumor involvement. Ballooning of the aqueduct (and thinning of the tectum) in distal aqueductal stenosis can be confused with the appearance of an arachnoid cyst in the quadrigeminal plate cistern.

Clinical References

1. Barkovich AJ, Newton TH. MR of aqueductal stenosis: evidence of a broad spectrum of tectal distortion. AJNR 1989;10:471–476.

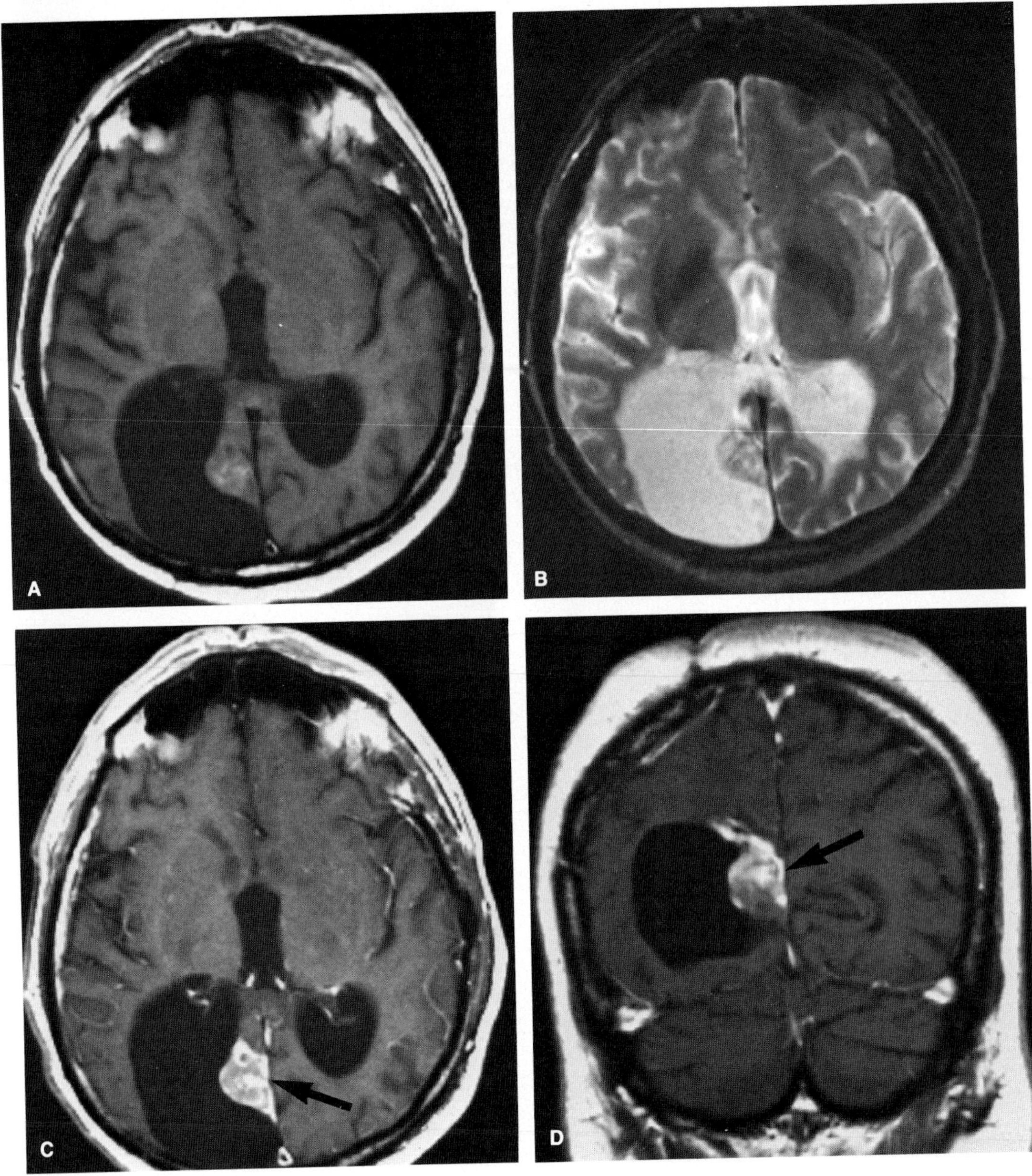

HISTORY

A 60-year-old patient with history of previous surgery for a glioma 4 years earlier

FINDINGS

A large postoperative porencephalic cavity is present in the right parietal lobe on the axial T1-weighted (*A*) and T2-weighted (*B*) images. Axial (*C*) and coronal (*D*) T1-weighted postcontrast images demonstrate a 2-cm enhancing nodular mass (*arrows in C and D*) along the medial aspect of the surgical defect.

DIAGNOSIS

Recurrent astrocytoma

DISCUSSION

Recurrent tumor usually enhances with administration of a gadolinium chelate, even if the preoperative original tumor did not.[1] Unfortunately, tumor recurrence cannot be reliably differentiated from radiation necrosis by conventional MR, and radiation necrosis and recurrent tumor can both be present. Necrosis from radiation usually occurs around the original tumor bed, whereas recurrent glioma is usually found in the immediate vicinity of the original lesion. Although radiation necrosis usually occurs more than 1 year after radiation treatment, it can occur sooner. Radiation therapy can result in disruption of the blood–brain barrier acutely (radiation encephalitis) and thus demonstrate enhancement with a gadolinium chelate.[2] MR perfusion techniques, currently available only on advanced instrumentation, can distinguish radiation necrosis from recurrent tumor by the measurement of cerebral blood volume. In current clinical practice, the diagnosis of recurrent tumor by MR depends on the detection of either new enhancement in or around the surgical bed, in comparison with the baseline postoperative study, or a focal mass lesion with anatomic distortion.

MR Technique

IV contrast is of great value in the diagnosis of recurrent tumor in the postoperative patient.

Pitfalls in Image Interpretation

The presence of abnormal contrast enhancement alone is insufficient to diagnose tumor recurrence postoperatively.

Clinical References

1. Atlas SW. Magnetic resonance imaging of the brain and spine. New York, Raven Press, 1991:246–248.
2. Burger PC. Malignant astrocytic neoplasms: classification, pathologic anatomy and response to treatment. Semin Oncol 1986;13:16.

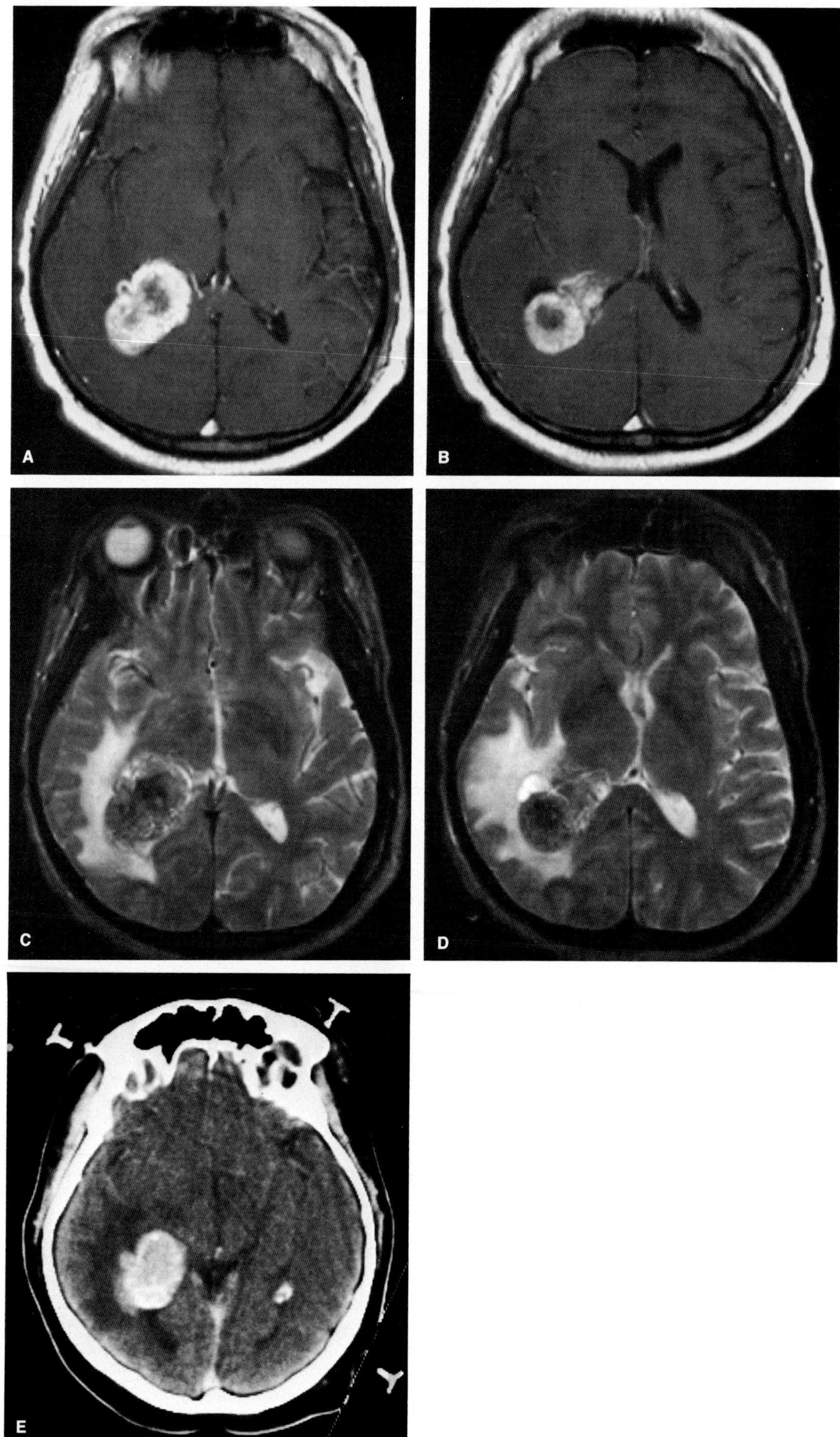
A
B
C
D
E

HISTORY

A 40-year-old man with headaches

FINDINGS

(*A and B*) Contiguous axial T1-weighted images demonstrate a 4-cm mass with predominant peripheral enhancement in or adjacent to the trigone of the right lateral ventricle. (*C and D*) On the corresponding axial T2-weighted images, the mass is of decreased signal intensity. Increased signal intensity, representing edema, is present surrounding this mass on the T2-weighted images. (*E*) CT image obtained without contrast administration depicts a densely calcified mass.

DIAGNOSIS

Intraventricular meningioma

DISCUSSION

Intraventricular meningiomas are rare tumors that usually arise in the atrium of the lateral ventricles. Less frequently they can arise in the foramen of Monro. They originate from arachnoid cells of the tela choroidea, extending through the choroidal fissure into the temporal horn of the lateral ventricles. Nests of meningeal cells may also be associated with the choroid plexus, giving rise to intraventricular meningiomas.[1]

Although only 1% of meningiomas are intraventricular in location, meningioma is the most common tumor of the atrium of the lateral ventricle in patients older than 30 years.[2] In this location, their arterial supply is usually from the anterior choroidal artery. There is an increased incidence of intraventricular meningiomas in patients with neurofibromatosis.

Pitfalls in Image Interpretation

Intraventricular meningiomas are frequently calcified. However, calcification is also seen in 50% of ependymomas and 25% to 80% of choroid plexus tumors. Thus, the presence of calcification does not narrow the differential diagnosis of an intraventricular tumor. The patient's age is, however, useful in differential diagnosis. Meningiomas have a peak incidence of 40 to 60 years. Ependymomas typically occur in children younger than 5 years, although there is a smaller peak in adults of 30 to 40 years. Seventy percent of ependymomas occur in the fourth ventricle. Most choroid plexus neoplasms occur in children younger than 5 years, and at least 80% occur in the atria of the lateral ventricles.

Clinical References

1. Jelinek J, Smirniotopoulos JG, Parisi JE, et al. Lateral ventricular neoplasms of the brain: differential diagnosis based on clinical, CT and MR findings. AJNR 1990;11:567–574.
2. Osborn AG. Handbook of neuroradiology. St Louis, Mosby–Year Book, 1991:219.

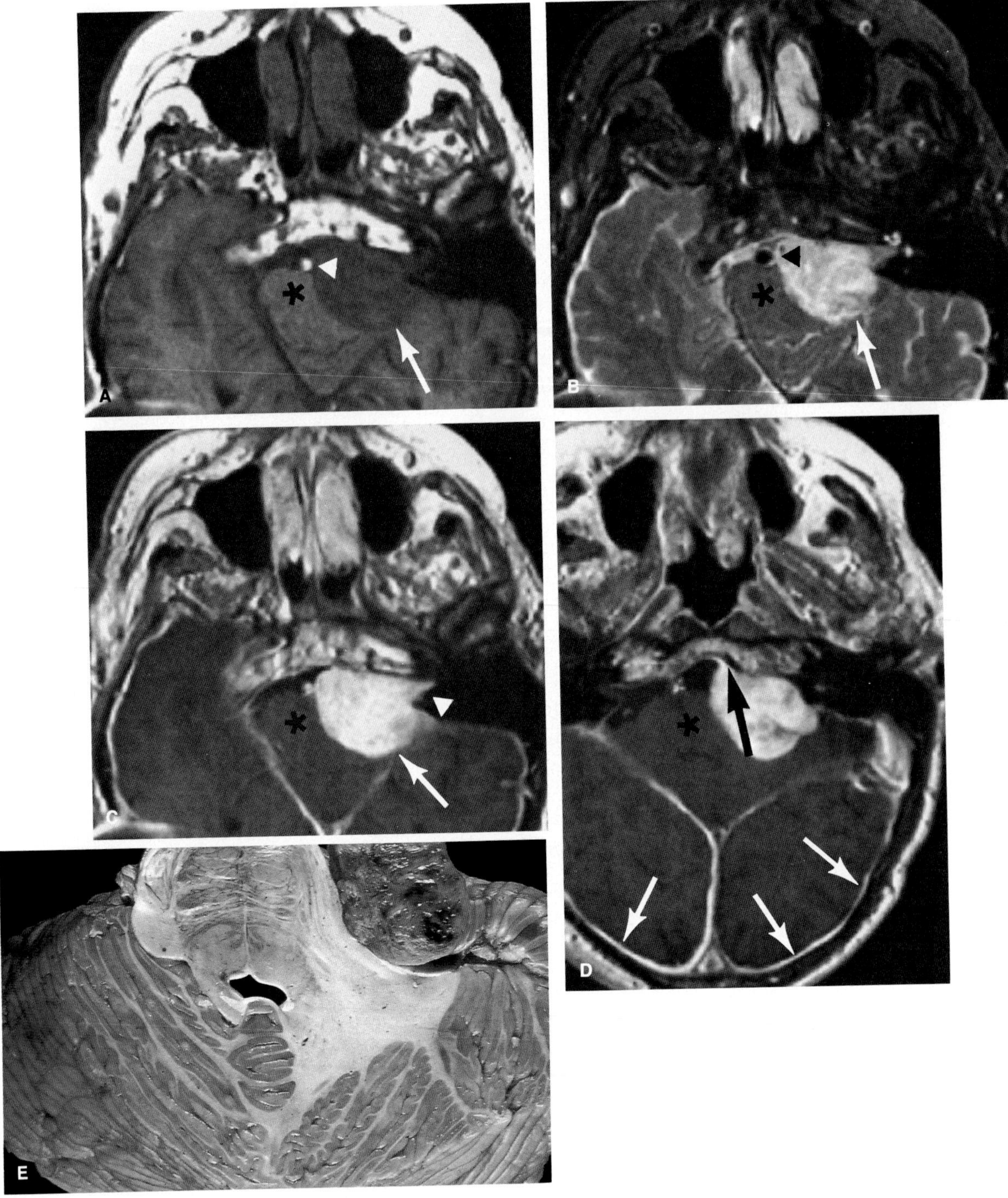

HISTORY

A 78-year-old with ataxia, headaches, left-sided hearing loss, and a history of previous intracranial surgery

FINDINGS

(*A*) Precontrast T1-weighted axial image demonstrates a 4 × 2.5 cm low-signal-intensity mass (*white arrow*) in the left cerebellopontine angle (CPA). (*B*) On the heavily T2-weighted axial image the mass (*white arrow*) has high signal intensity. (*C*) Postcontrast T1-weighted axial image shows intense homogeneous enhancement (*white arrow*) of the lesion. Extension of the mass into the left internal auditory canal (IAC) (*white arrowhead*) is clearly seen. (*D*) Postcontrast T1-weighted axial image at a lower level demonstrates an enhancing dural "tail" (*arrow*). The mass compresses the brain stem (*asterisks in A through D*), and displaces the basilar artery (*arrowheads in A and B*) to the right. The dura (*white arrows in D*) enhances diffusely after contrast infusion, a finding which may persist indefinitely following intracranial surgery.

DIAGNOSIS

Acoustic neuroma

DISCUSSION

Acoustic neuromas are benign Schwann cell tumors that arise at the neuroglial–Schwann cell junction of the vestibular division of the eighth cranial nerve. The majority of acoustic neuromas have both an intracanalicular and an extracanalicular component, and are centered at the porus acusticus of the internal auditory canal. Although usually unilateral, acoustic neuromas can be bilateral, typically in association with neurofibromatosis type 2.

Acoustic neuroma is the most common extraaxial CPA tumor, accounting for 80% of neoplasms at this site. The age at presentation is usually between 35 and 60 years. Symptoms usually include unilateral sensorineural hearing loss and tinnitus. Tumors with a large extracanalicular component have a mass effect on the brain stem, and may cause ataxia, vertigo, headache, and diminished corneal reflexes.

The extracanalicular portion of an acoustic neuroma is usually round, as opposed to a more plaquelike configuration typical for a meningioma, from which it must be differentiated. An acoustic neuroma also causes enlargement of the porus acusticus, and extends into the IAC, both of which are rare with meningioma. Enlargement of the IAC and canal asymmetry are best seen on T2-weighted images, with high-signal-intensity CSF outlining the osseous margin of the IAC. An acoustic neuroma typically is hypointense to isointense on T1-weighted images, and isointense to hyperintense on T2-weighted images compared with the pons,[1] although the high signal intensity of CSF may obscure a small tumor on T2-weighted images. After contrast infusion, there is intense enhancement, greater than for any other intracranial tumor.[2] Enhancement is usually homogeneous, and a heterogeneous appearance on precontrast or postcontrast T1-weighted images suggests necrosis, hemorrhage, or calcification.[2] An enhancing dural "tail" can be seen in both meningioma and acoustic neuroma.[3]

MR Technique

Postcontrast images are essential for demonstrating the exact dimensions and intracanalicular extension of an acoustic neuroma.

Pitfalls in Image Interpretation

The differential diagnosis for a CPA tumor includes meningioma, epidermoid, fifth nerve schwannoma, seventh nerve schwannoma, ninth and tenth nerve schwannoma, glomus jugulare tumor, arachnoid cyst, basilar artery aneurysm, exophytic brain stem glioma,[1] and chordoma.

Pathologic Correlate

(*E*) Freshly cut gross specimen shows a large acoustic neuroma in the CPA, compressing the brain stem and adjacent cerebellum. Acoustic neuromas, like all schwannomas, displace rather than incorporate the affected nerve, which sometimes allows for surgical salvage of the nerve.

Clinical References

1. Press G, Hesselink J. MR imaging of cerebellopontine angle and internal auditory canal lesions at 1.5T. AJR 1988; 150:1371–1381.
2. Jackler R, Shapiro M, Dillon W, et al. Gadolinium-DTPA enhanced magnetic resonance imaging in acoustic neuroma diagnosis and management. Otolaryngol Head Neck Surg 1990;102:670–677.
3. Kutcher T, Brown D, Maurer P, et al. Dural tail adjacent to acoustic neuroma: MR features. J Comput Assist Tomogr 1991;15:669–670.

(E *from Okazaki H, Scheithauer B. Slide atlas of neuropathology. New York, Gower Medical Publishing, 1988. By permission of Mayo Foundation.*)

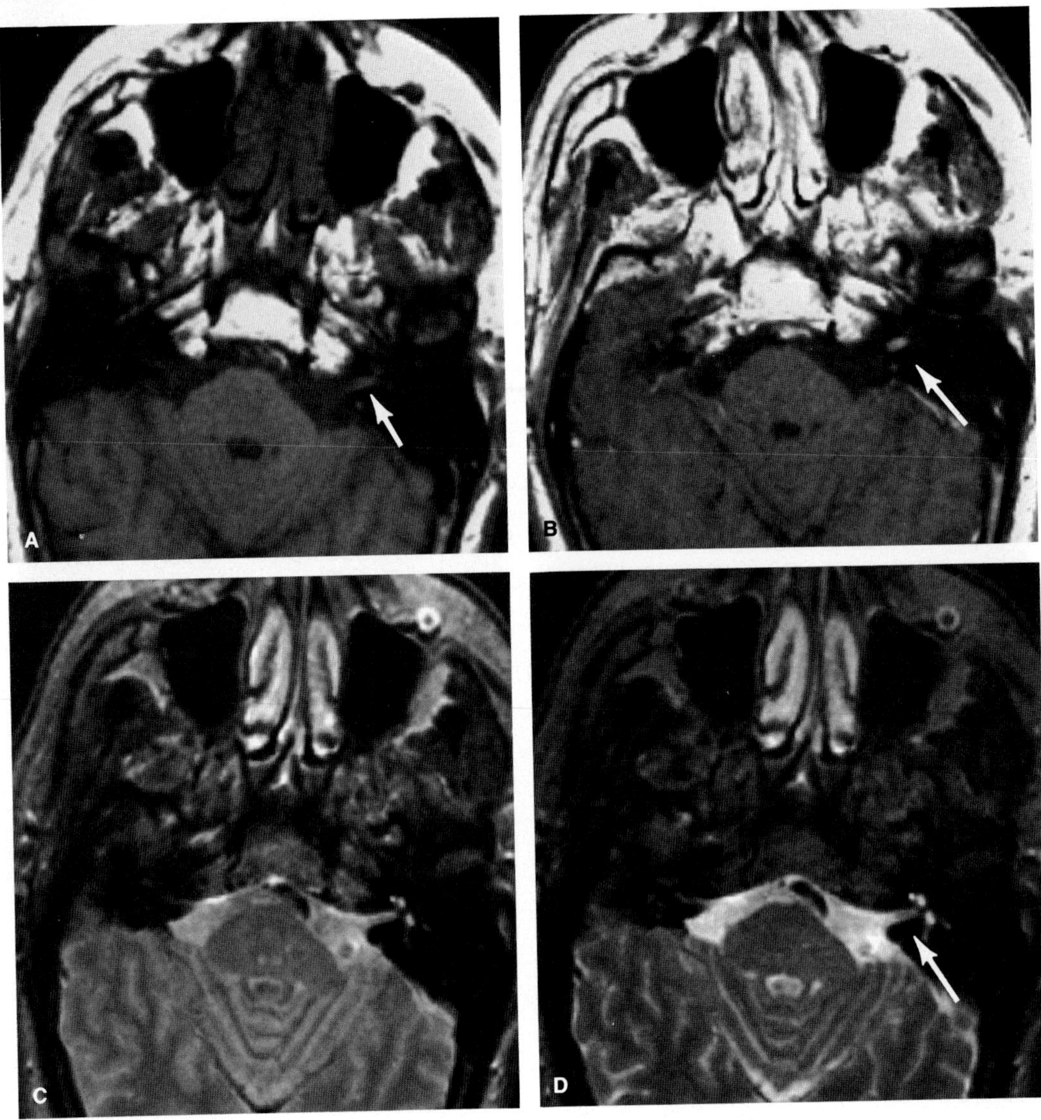

HISTORY

A 62-year-old with tinnitus and left-sided sensorineural hearing loss

FINDINGS

(*A*) T1-weighted axial image through the left internal auditory canal (IAC) demonstrates a small focal area (*white arrow*) with mildly increased signal intensity compared with the remainder of the seventh and eighth cranial nerve complex. (*B*) Postcontrast T1-weighted axial image shows intense enhancement of the lesion (*white arrow*), which measures 4 × 7 mm. (*C*) An abnormality is not definitely seen on the intermediate T2-weighted image. (*D*) On the heavily T2-weighted axial image the lesion (*white arrow*) is isointense to gray matter, and displaces high-signal-intensity CSF.

DIAGNOSIS

Intracanalicular acoustic neuroma

DISCUSSION

Nearly all acoustic neuromas have some intracanalicular component. Up to 35% are purely intracanalicular.[1] MR has replaced CT as the imaging modality of choice for diagnosis of small intracanalicular acoustic neuromas.[2] Mild expansion of the IAC, best seen on T2-weighted images, and obscuration of the margins of the seventh and eighth nerves, best seen on T1-weighted images, may be present. However, localized enhancement after contrast infusion within the IAC is often the only finding on MR. Up to 20% of intracanalicular acoustic neuromas less than 1 cm in diameter would be missed without contrast infusion.[3]

The seventh and eighth cranial nerves, both of which lie in the IAC, normally do not enhance after IV contrast infusion. Although an acoustic neuroma is the most common cause of enhancement within the IAC, other entities may also enhance. A facial nerve (seventh cranial nerve) neuroma mimics acoustic neuroma on MR. Inflammation of the vestibulocochlear nerve, without evidence of tumor at surgical exploration, can demonstrate enhancement on MR.[2] Enhancement of the entire facial nerve from the IAC to the stylomastoid foramen has been documented in Bell's palsy.[3] Postoperatively, enhancement may be caused by residual tumor, granulation tissue (scar), or nerve inflammation.[3]

MR Technique

Postinfusion T1-weighted images must be obtained to rule in or out the presence of a small intracanalicular acoustic neuroma. MR without contrast enhancement can produce both false-negative and false-positive results.

Clinical References

1. Press G, Hesselink J. MR imaging of cerebellopontine angle and internal auditory canal lesions at 1.5T. AJR 1988; 150:1371–1381.
2. Han M, Jabour B, Andrews J, et al. Nonneoplastic enhancing lesions mimicking intracanalicular acoustic neuroma on gadolinium-enhanced MR images. Radiology 1991;179:795–796.
3. Jackler R, Shapiro M, Dillon W, et al. Gadolinium-DTPA enhanced magnetic resonance imaging in acoustic neuroma: diagnosis and management. Otolaryngol Head Neck Surg 1990;102:670–677.

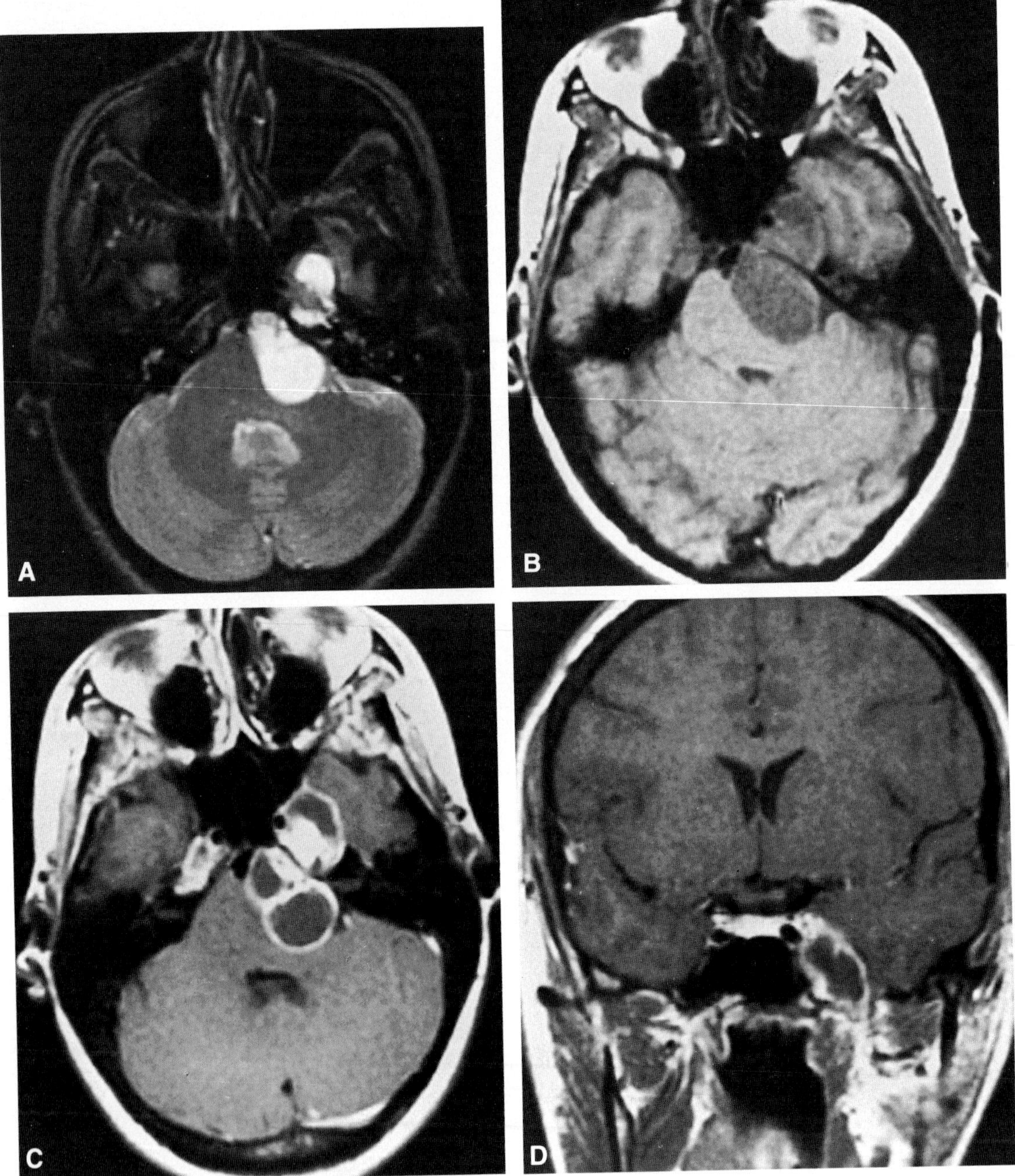

HISTORY

Facial pain and numbness

FINDINGS

(*A*) T2-weighted scan demonstrates a predominantly hyperintense parasellar mass with extension into both the middle and posterior cranial fossae. Marked compression of the pons by the mass is clearly seen on the precontrast T2-weighted (*A*) and T1-weighted (*B*) scans. (*C*) Following IV contrast administration, there is heterogeneous enhancement, with both solid and cystic components identified. The mass also appears to involve the cavernous sinus. (*D*) Coronal postcontrast T1-weighted scan reveals extension of the mass into the foramen ovale, along the normal course of the mandibular nerve (V3). The coronal scan also demonstrates atrophy, on the side of involvement, of the masseter, lateral pterygoid, and medial pterygoid muscles.

DIAGNOSIS

Trigeminal schwannoma

DISCUSSION

Schwannomas account for about 8% of all primary intracranial tumors, with 80% to 90% of these lesions occurring in the cerebellopontine angle and originating from the acoustic nerve (eighth cranial nerve). The trigeminal nerve (cranial nerve V) is the next most common site of involvement by a solitary tumor. Primary lesions of other nerves, such as the vagus and glossopharyngeal, and multiplicity of involvement generally points to von Recklinghausen's disease (neurofibromatosis).

Trigeminal tumors most commonly arise from the gasserian ganglion and remain confined to the middle cranial fossa. When large, there can be erosion of the petrous bone. In a minority of patients, the lesion extends into both the middle and posterior fossae, as illustrated by the current case. In this instance, the tumor is usually hourglass or dumbbell in shape, with constriction between the two major tumor masses at the petrous apex where the trigeminal nerve penetrates the dura.

The trigeminal nerve is the chief sensory nerve for the face (giving rise to the ophthalmic, maxillary, and mandibular nerves) and the motor nerve for mastication. Facial pain is a common presenting feature in patients with trigeminal schwannoma. There may also be atrophy of the muscles of mastication (masseter, temporalis, medial pterygoid, and lateral pterygoid). With regard to surgical removal, adherence of the tumor to the brain stem or lateral wall of the cavernous sinus can preclude total resection. Postoperatively, permanent loss of trigeminal nerve function is common.[1]

The superior soft-tissue detail and absence of artifacts from the skull base make MR markedly superior to CT for diagnosis and anatomic depiction of trigeminal schwannomas.[2] In particular, tumor extension into Meckel's cave, the orbit, or infratemporal fossa is more clearly shown by MR.

Pitfalls in Image Interpretation

The differential diagnosis in this case is limited to lesions which can involve the cavernous sinus and demonstrate perineural extent. Several head and neck tumors,[3] including squamous cell and adenoid cystic carcinoma, can track along nerves; however, the degree of intracranial involvement seen would be unusual. Of possible intracranial lesions, both lymphoma and meningioma should be considered. The absence of tumor extension along the dura makes the diagnosis of a meningioma less likely.

Nerves which run through the cavernous sinus include the oculomotor (III), trochlear (IV), abducens (VI), ophthalmic (V1), and maxillary (V2).

Clinical References

1. McCormick PC, Bello JA, Post KD. Trigeminal schwannoma: surgical series of 14 cases with review of the literature. J Neurosurg 1988;69:850–860.
2. Saito A, Nakazawa T, Matsuda M, Handa J. Comparison of computed tomographic scanning and magnetic resonance imaging in the diagnosis of trigeminal schwannoma: report of four cases. Neurol Med Chir (Tokyo) 1989;29:1101–1106.
3. Laine FJ, Braun IF, Jensen ME, et al. Perineural tumor extension through the foramen ovale: evaluation with MR imaging. Radiology 1990;174:65–71.

(A *to* D *from Runge VM. Magnetic resonance imaging: clinical principles. Philadelphia, JB Lippincott, 1992.*)

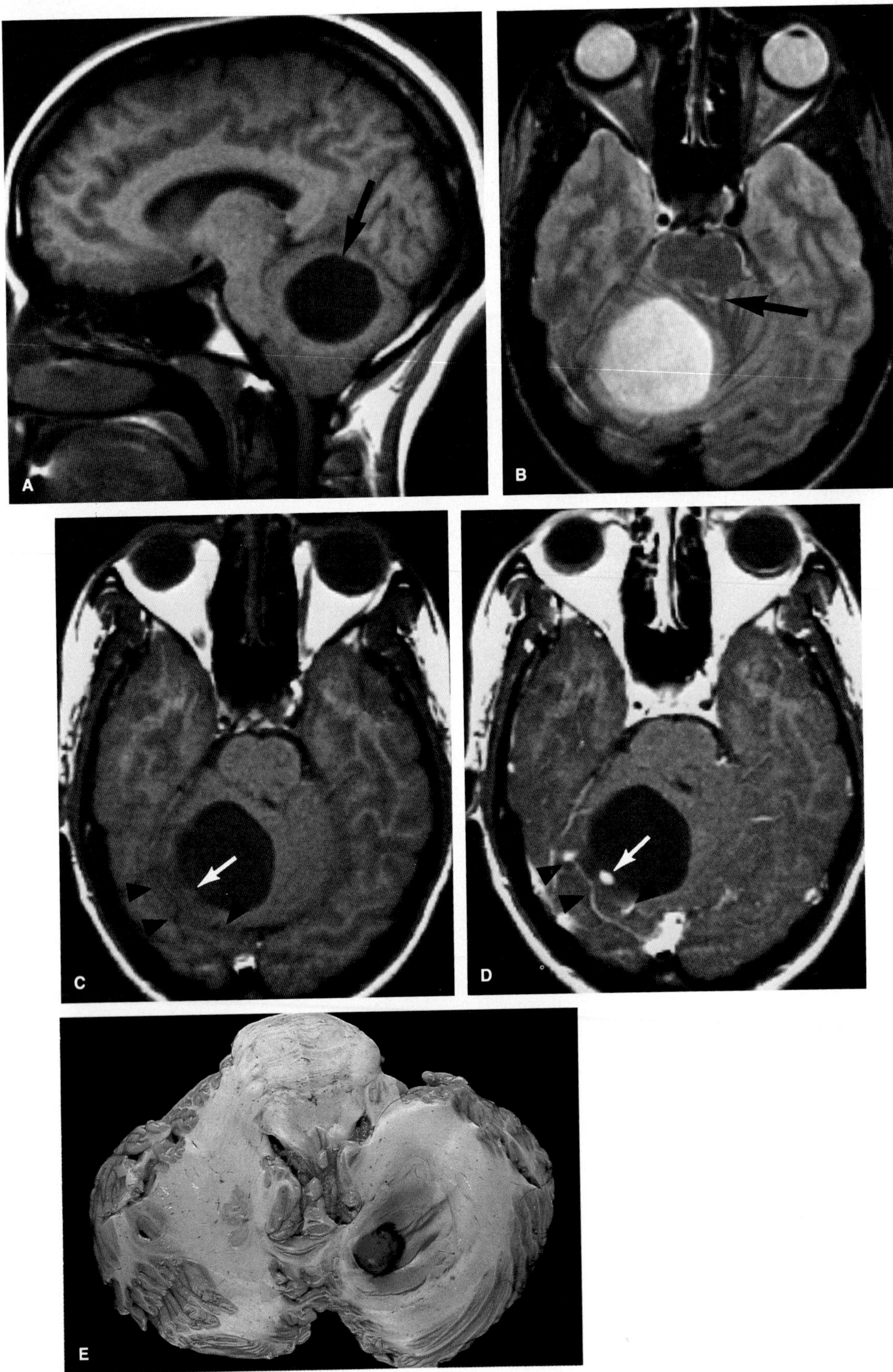
A
B
C
D
E

HISTORY

A 30-year-old with a 2-year history of intermittent throbbing headaches

FINDINGS

(*A*) T1-weighted sagittal image, 7 mm to the right of midline, demonstrates a well-marginated, low-signal-intensity mass (*arrow*) in the cerebellum, measuring 3 cm in diameter. (*B*) On the intermediate T2-weighted axial image the mass has high signal intensity, and compresses the fourth ventricle (*arrow*). (*C*) Precontrast T1-weighted axial image demonstrates a soft tissue nodule (*white arrow*) along the posterolateral wall of the mass, and several serpiginous flow voids (*arrowheads*), which may be abnormal tumor vessels or simply prominent normal tentorial vessels. (*D*) Postcontrast T1-weighted axial image shows enhancement of both the mural nodule (*white arrow*) and the adjacent blood vessels (*arrowheads*).

DIAGNOSIS

Hemangioblastoma

DISCUSSION

Hemangioblastoma is a rare benign tumor of the CNS composed of embryonic vascular elements. These tumors are usually solitary and the cerebellum is the most common site of occurrence, followed by the cervical spinal cord, and the medulla. Hemangioblastoma is the most common primary cerebellar neoplasm found in adults, and the average age at detection is 33 years. Headache, papilledema, and ataxia are common clinical features.

Hemangioblastomas may occur sporadically (80%) or as part of the von Hippel–Lindau syndrome, an inherited autosomal dominant neurocutaneous disorder which also may include retinal angiomas (50% of cases), renal cell carcinoma (25% to 38%), pheochromocytoma (over 10%), and cysts of the kidneys, pancreas, liver, and epididymis.[1] Patients with von Hippel–Lindau syndrome typically have multiple CNS hemangioblastomas, which may be detected in childhood.

Most hemangioblastomas are sharply marginated cystic masses with a peripheral mural nodule. The signal intensity of the cystic fluid is slightly greater than that of CSF on both T1- and T2-weighted images because of greater protein content. The mural nodule (tumor nidus) is hypointense to isointense on T1-weighted images, and slightly hyperintense on T2-weighted images, relative to gray matter, and enhances after contrast infusion.[2] The mural nodule always abuts the pia mater, from which the tumor receives its vascular supply.[3] Abnormal tumor vessels may be present, appearing as serpiginous signal voids within, and at the periphery of, the mass.

Less commonly (33% of cases), hemangioblastomas are solid masses. These lesions are also usually sharply marginated, enhance after contrast infusion, and have abnormal vascularity. Solid hemangioblastomas are usually small, averaging about 1 cm in diameter.

MR Technique

The difference in signal intensity between the cyst fluid and CSF is best seen on intermediate T2-weighted images.

Pitfalls in Image Interpretation

Differential diagnosis for a cystic cerebellar mass in an adult includes metastasis, astrocytoma, and abscess. However, the association of a peripheral cyst with a mural nodule supplied by enlarged vessels is virtually pathognomonic for hemangioblastoma.[3]

Pathologic Correlate

(*E*) A fixed, stained gross cerebellar specimen from a different patient demonstrates a discrete hemangioblastoma nodule, and surrounding gliotic parenchyma. The tumor in a hemangioblastoma is limited to the mural nodule; the cyst wall is composed of gliotic cerebellar tissue, and is not neoplastic.

Clinical References

1. Sato Y, Waziri M, Smith W, et al. Hippel–Lindau disease: MR imaging. Radiology 1988;166:241–246.
2. Anson J, Glick R, Crowell R. Use of gadolinium-enhanced magnetic resonance imaging in the diagnosis and management of posterior fossa hemangioblastomas. Surg Neurol 1991;35:300–304.
3. Lee S, Sanches J, Mark A, et al. Posterior fossa hemangioblastomas: MR imaging. Radiology 1989;171:463–468.

(E from Okazaki H, Scheithauer B. Slide atlas of neuropathology. New York, Gower Medical Publishing, 1988. By permission of Mayo Foundation.)

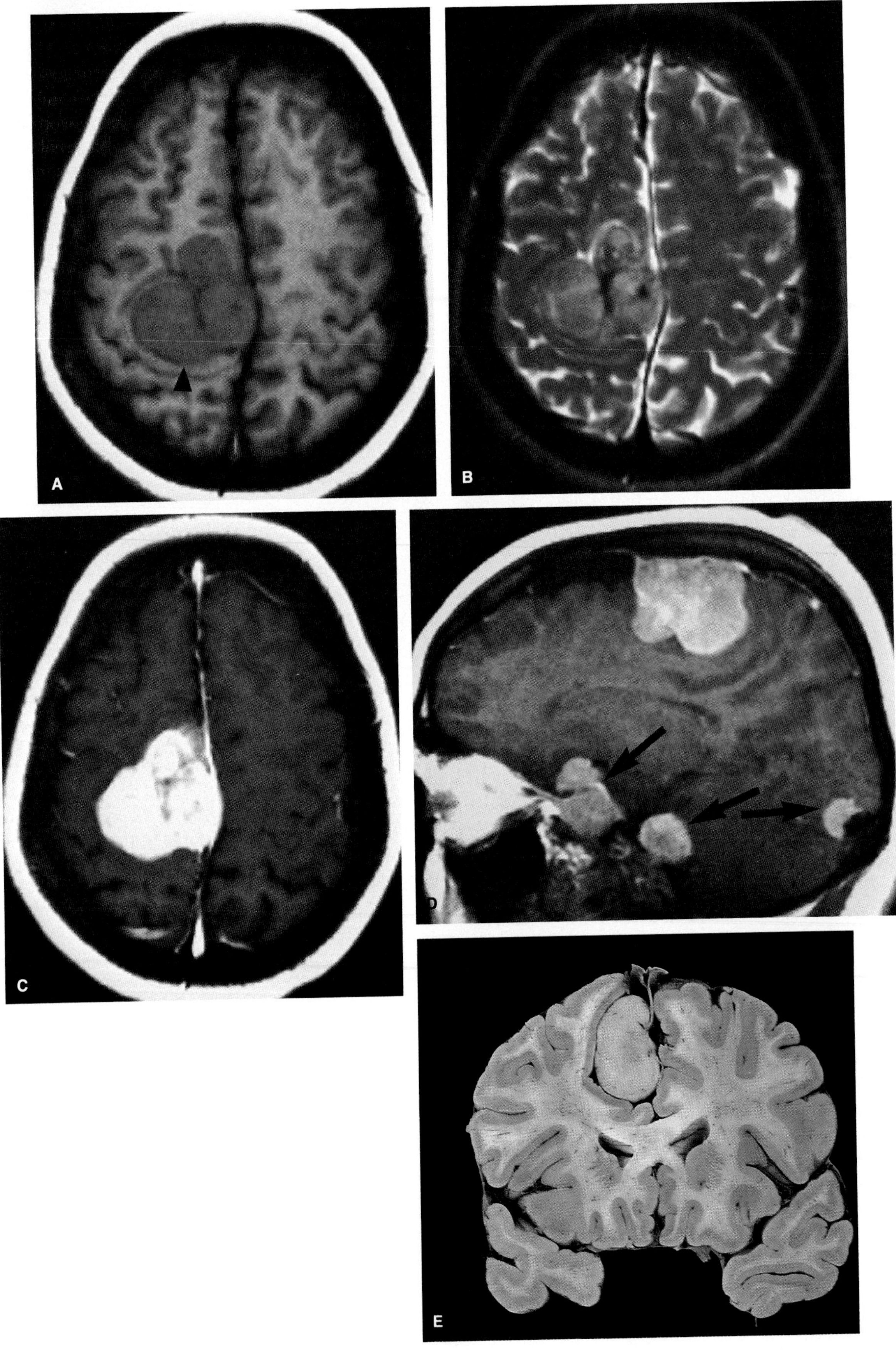
A
B
C
D
E

HISTORY

A 48-year-old woman with a change in mental status

FINDINGS

Axial T1-weighted (*A*) and T2-weighted (*B*) images precontrast reveal a large extraaxial predominantly isointense mass (*arrowhead in A*) directly adjacent to the falx in the right frontal lobe. This mass demonstrates homogenous enhancement on axial (*C*) and sagittal (*D*) T1-weighted images after contrast administration. Several other enhancing extraaxial masses (*arrows in D*) are identified in this patient with neurofibromatosis type 2.

DIAGNOSIS

Falx meningioma

DISCUSSION

Meningiomas account for about 15% of all intracranial tumors in adults. They are multiple in 6% to 8% of cases. They have a peak age incidence in the fifth decade of life and are twice as common in women than in men.[1]

The hallmark of these tumors is their extraaxial location. Extraaxial tumors typically cause displacement of adjacent brain tissue, and are broad based along a bony or dural surface. Meningiomas usually demonstrate prolonged T1 and T2 relaxation times, although the degree of T1 and T2 prolongation is not as great as that seen with most intraaxial tumors.

Meningiomas are commonly of homogeneous signal intensity on MR imaging.[2] Factors producing tumor inhomogeneity include calcification, vascularity, and necrotic or cystic change. The incidence of necrosis and cystic degeneration of meningiomas is approximately 14%. On MR these areas are of decreased signal intensity on T1-weighted images, and increased signal intensity on T2-weighted images (cystic components closely parallel the signal intensity of water).

The incidence of edema associated with meningiomas is variable. Some tumors have extensive edema, while others have only minimal or no edema. There is no correlation between tumor size and the amount of edema.

MR Technique

Multiplanar imaging is useful in differentiating whether a mass is intraaxial or extraaxial.

Pathologic Correlate

(*E*) On gross coronal section, an intermediate-size meningioma is seen arising along the falx, displacing the ipsilateral cerebral hemisphere and compressing the body of the lateral ventricle. Mass effect on vital structures is a frequent reason for clinical presentation of a patient with a meningioma.

Clinical References

1. Bird CR, Hasso AN, LeBeau DJ. Meningiomas and skull base neoplasms. Top Magn Reson Imag 1989;1:52–68.
2. Schubeus P, Schorner W, Henkes H, et al. Intracranial meningiomas: comparison of plain and contrast-enhanced examinations in CT and MRI. Neuroradiology 1990;32:12–18.

(E *from Okazaki H, Scheithauer B. Slide atlas of neuropathology. New York, Gower Medical Publishing, 1988. By permission of Mayo Foundation.)*

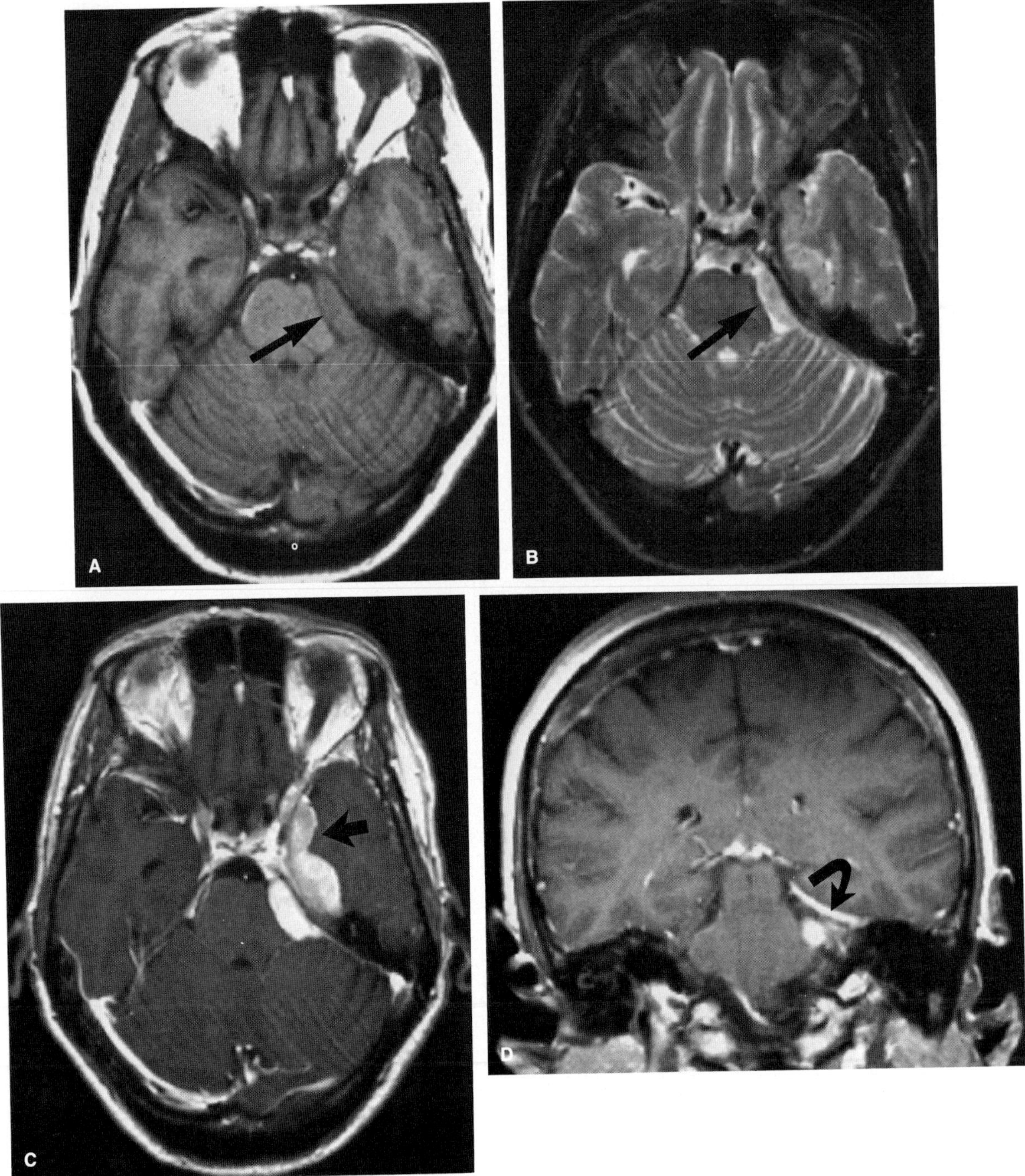

HISTORY

A 65-year-old woman with headaches

FINDINGS

(*A*) Precontrast axial T1-weighted image reveals an isointense mass (*arrow*) in the left cerebellopontine angle. (*B*) On the axial T2-weighted image, the mass (*arrow*) is of increased signal intensity. (*C*) Homogeneous enhancement is demonstrated on the postcontrast axial T1-weighted image. The mass extends anteriorly along the left sphenoid wing (*arrow*). (*D*) Postcontrast coronal T1-weighted image demonstrates an enhancing dural "tail" (*curved arrow*). (*E*) Digital subtraction angiography demonstrates a tumor blush (*arrowheads*) and an enlarged artery of Bernasconi-Cassinari (*black arrow*) arising from the lateral tentorial branch of the meningohypophyseal trunk.

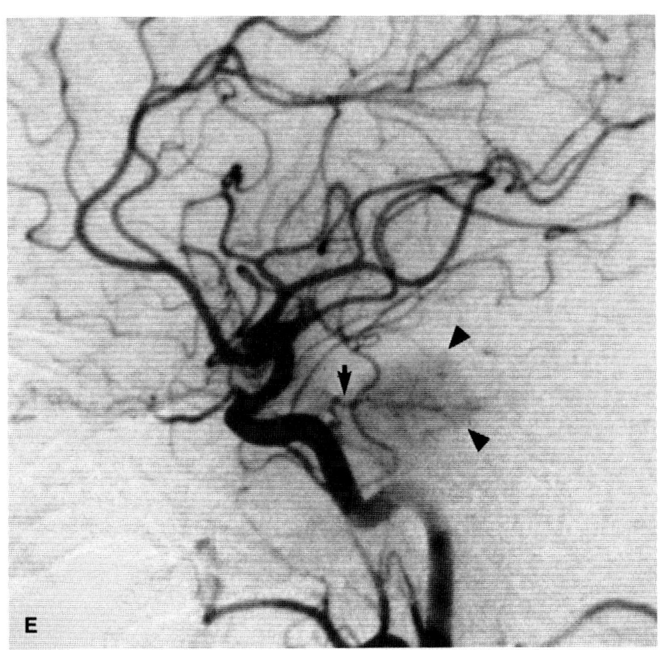

DIAGNOSIS

Meningioma

DISCUSSION

Meningiomas are the most common benign intracranial neoplasm, and the most common extraaxial adult tumor. They are more common in women than in men, and most frequently occur from the ages of 40 to 70 years.[1] These lesions are commonly broad based along a dural or bony surface, producing imaging findings characteristic of an extraaxial mass. The most common tumor of the cerebellopontine angle is the acoustic neuroma, followed by meningioma.

The value of MR enhanced with a gadolinium chelate for extraaxial masses has been well documented. Meningiomas are commonly isointense on T1- and T2-weighted images, and demonstrate intense homogeneous enhancement postcontrast due to the lack of a blood–brain barrier. The dural "tail" sign (*curved arrow in C*) has been reported to be suggestive of meningiomas but not specific.[2] This is a linear-enhanced meningeal thickening or "tail" extending away from the tumor along the dural surface, seen in about 60% of cases.[3] It has also been reported in patients with lymphoma, chloroma, sarcoidosis[4] and acoustic neuroma.[5] Meningiomas are often highly vascular and demonstrate a tumor blush on x-ray angiography.

MR Technique

IV contrast is useful in detecting small extraaxial masses, the full extent of the lesion, and a dural tail.

Pitfalls in Image Interpretation

An acoustic neuroma, schwannoma, or neurofibroma are other extraaxial masses that may be confused with a meningioma. The dural tail sign is suggestive of but not specific for meningioma.

Clinical References

1. Elster AD, Venkata VR, Gilbert TH, et al. Meningiomas: MR and histopathologic features. Radiology 1989;170:857–862.
2. Tolumaru A, Toshihiro O, Tsuneyoshi E, et al. Prominent meningeal enhancement adjacent to meningioma on Gd-DTPA-enhanced MR images: histopathologic correlation. Radiology 1990;175:431–433.
3. Goldsher D, Litt AW, Pinto RS, et al. Dural "tail" associated with meningiomas on Gd-DTPA-enhanced MR images: characteristics, differential diagnostic value, and possible implications for treatment. Radiology 1990;176:447–450.
4. Tien RD, Yang PJ, Chu PK. "Dural tail sign"—a specific MR sign for meningioma? J Comput Assist Tomogr 1991;15:64–66.
5. Kutcher TJ, Brown DC, Maurer PK, et al. Dural tail adjacent to acoustic neuroma. J Comput Assist Tomogr 1991;15:669–670.

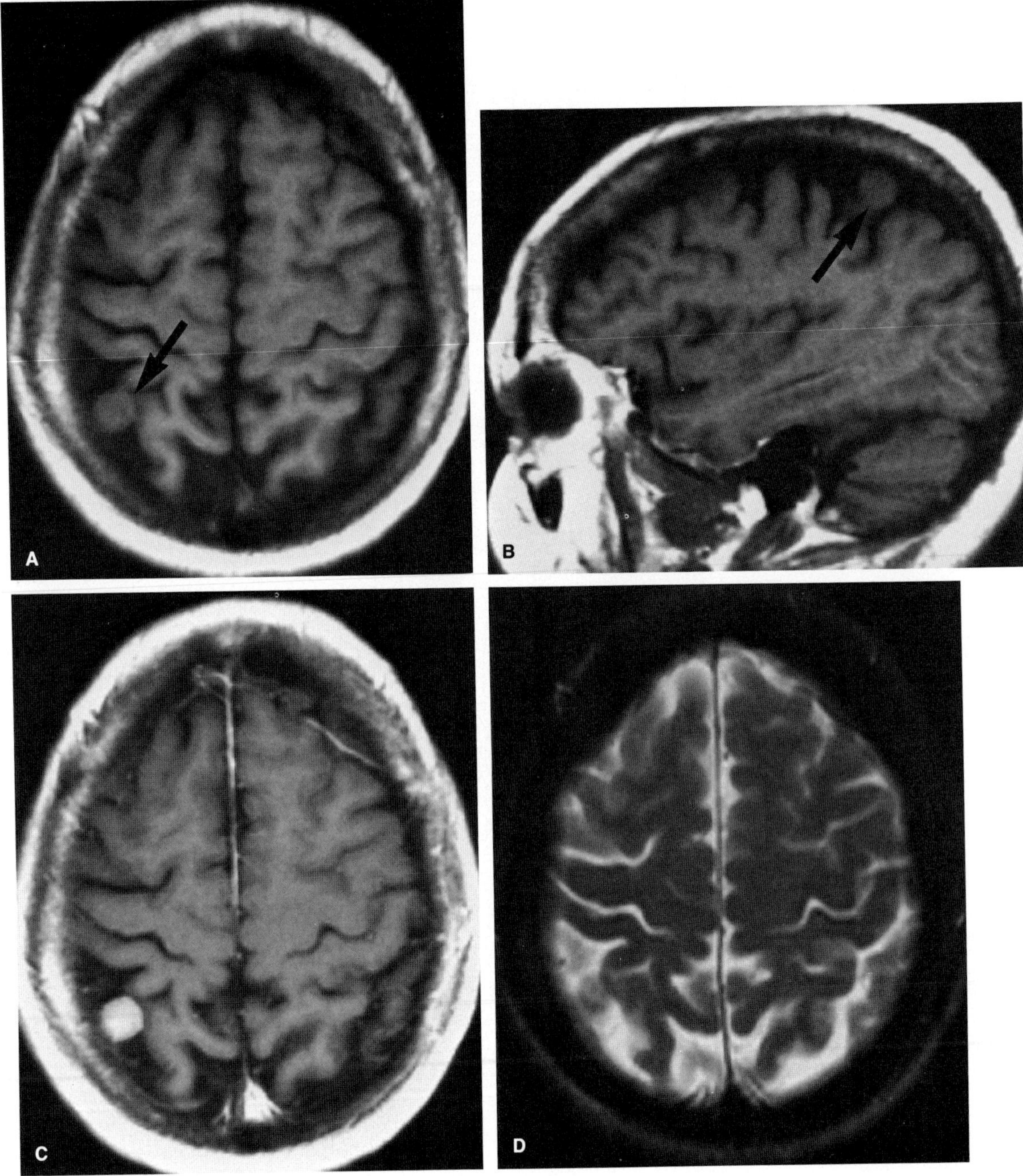

HISTORY

A 62-year-old woman with a single episode of loss of consciousness 1 month previously

FINDINGS

Axial (*A*) and sagittal (*B*) T1-weighted images demonstrate a 1.8-cm isointense extraaxial mass (*arrows in A and B*) over the convexity of the right posterior frontal/anterior parietal lobe. (*C*) On the axial T1-weighted image postcontrast this extraaxial mass demonstrates intense homogeneous contrast enhancement. (*D*) The lesion is difficult to identify on the corresponding axial T2-weighted image.

DIAGNOSIS

Convexity meningioma

DISCUSSION

The incidence of meningiomas in postmortem series is 1% to 2%. The largest number of meningiomas is found in patients over 80 years of age. Incidental meningiomas are rare in patients younger than 30 years. The male/female ratio is approximately 1:3. Most incidental meningiomas are less than 1 cm in diameter. Multiple incidental meningiomas not associated with neurofibromatosis are seen in about 8% of cases.[1]

The annual growth rate of meningiomas has been reported to range from 0.5% to 21%, with a median growth rate of 3.6%. Tumor growth rate is not related to patient age.[2]

Clinical References

1. Nakasu S, Hirano A, Shimura T, et al. Incidental meningiomas in autopsy study. Surg Neurol 1987;27:319–322.
2. Firsching RP, Fischer A, Peters R, et al. Growth rate of incidental meningiomas. J Neurosurg 1990;73:545–547.

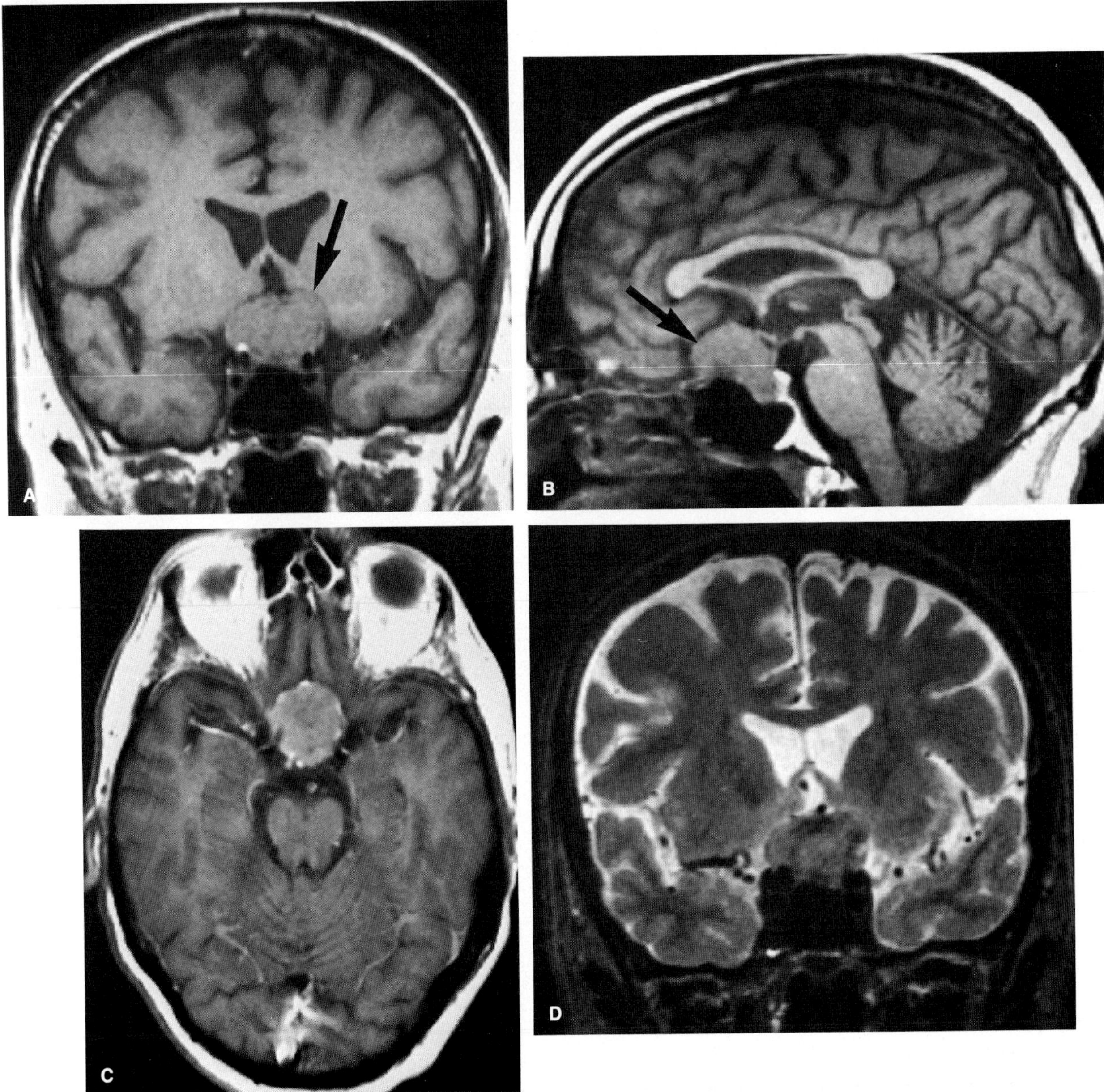

HISTORY

A 62-year-old man with severe headaches, hypersensitive smell, and vision loss in the left eye

FINDINGS

On coronal (*A*) and sagittal (*B*) T1-weighted images a 2-cm isointense mass (*arrows in A and B*) is identified in the suprasellar cistern. (*C*) The lesion demonstrates homogeneous enhancement on the axial T1-weighted image postcontrast. (*D*) On the coronal T2-weighted image, the mass is predominantly isointense to cerebral tissue.

DIAGNOSIS

Suprasellar meningioma

DISCUSSION

Suprasellar meningiomas most commonly arise from the tuberculum or diaphragma sellae, and can result in visual field defects secondary to compression of the optic chiasm. Meningiomas arising from the greater wing of the sphenoid or the planum spheniodale can also extend into the suprasellar region.[1]

Common locations of meningiomas include the parasagittal region, cortical convexity, sphenoid wing, parasellar region, olfactory groove, tentorium cerebelli, petrous ridge, cerebellopontine angle, and foramen magnum. They are more frequent in the anterior cranium than the posterior fossa. Although meningiomas are usually benign, they can locally invade venous sinuses or the skull.[2]

Bony changes in the skull include hyperostosis and invasion. En plaque meningiomas are particularly prone to these changes.

The histopathologic classification of meningiomas subdivides benign meningiomas into four basic subtypes: fibroblastic, transitional, syncytial, and angioblastic. Mixed types are also recognized.[3]

Pitfalls in Image Interpretation

The differential diagnosis of a suprasellar mass includes pituitary macroadenoma, meningioma, craniopharyngioma, optic nerve glioma, aneurysm, metastasis, chordoma, hypothalamic glioma, and infundibular tumor.

Clinical References

1. Johnsen DE, Woodruff WW, Allen IS, et al. MR imaging of the sellar and juxtasellar regions. Radiographics 1991; 11:727–758.
2. Bird CR, Hasso AN, LeBeau DJ. Meningiomas and skull base neoplasms. Top Magn Reson Imaging 1989;1:52–68.
3. Elster AD, Challa VR, Gilbert TH, et al. Meningiomas: MR and histopathologic features. Radiology 1989;170:857–862.

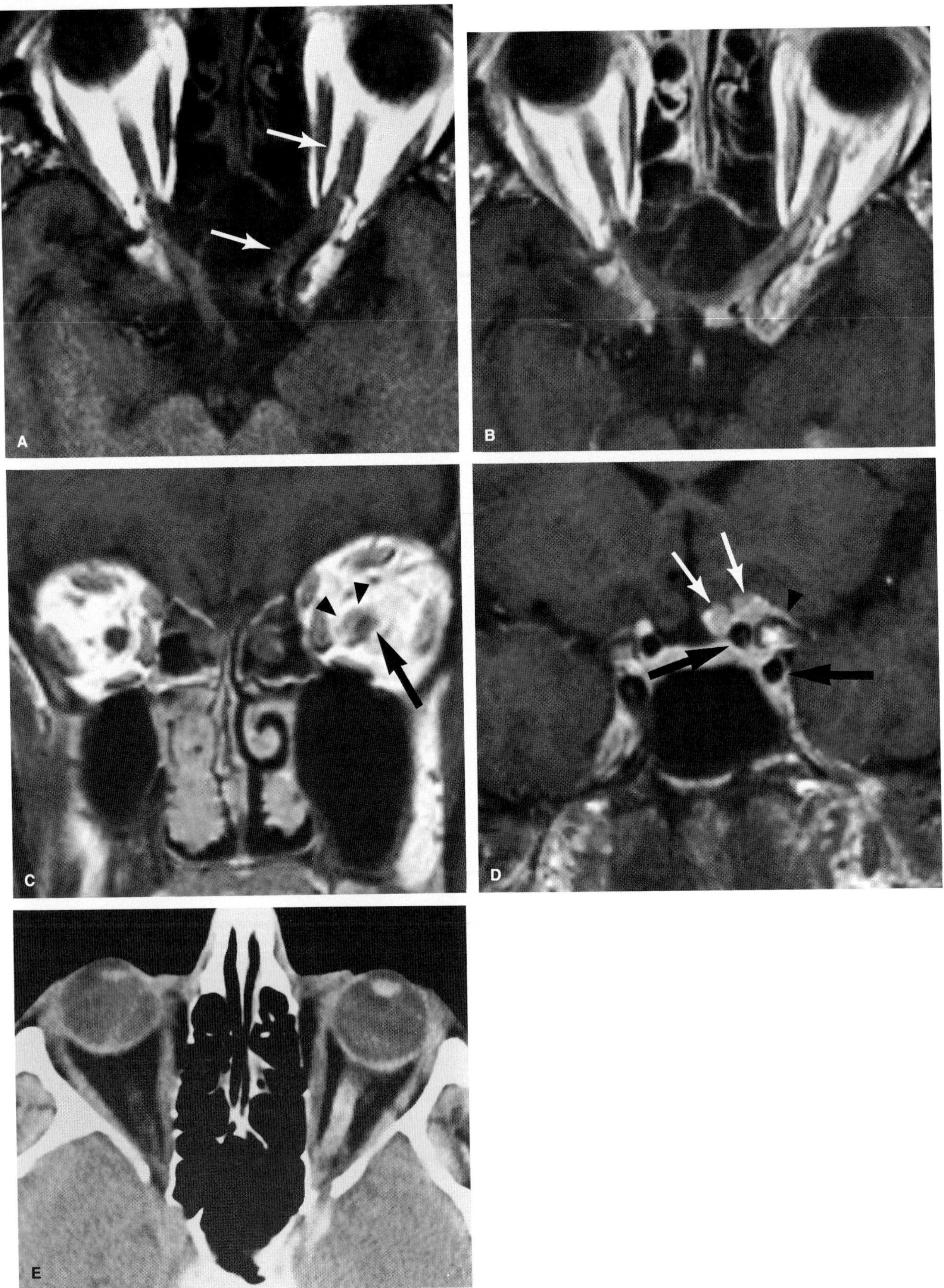
A
B
C
D
E

HISTORY

A 45-year-old with loss of vision in the left eye

FINDINGS

(*A*) T1-weighted axial image demonstrates slight enlargement of the intraorbital and intracranial portions of the left optic nerve (*white arrows*). (*B*) The postcontrast T1-weighted axial image shows enhancement along the periphery of the nerve. (*C*) On the postcontrast T1-weighted coronal image through the midportion of the orbit the left optic nerve (*arrow*) is surrounded by enhancing soft tissue (*arrowheads*). (*D*) The postcontrast T1-weighted coronal image just anterior to the optic chiasm demonstrates abnormal enhancing soft tissue (*white arrows*) along the floor of the anterior cranial fossa, adjacent to the inferior left frontal lobe and the left internal carotid artery (*arrows*). The enhancing tumor has a thin "dural tail" (*arrowhead*) extending laterally. (*E*) The left optic nerve has high density throughout its length on the noncontrast orbital CT, consistent with calcification.

DIAGNOSIS

Perioptic meningioma

DISCUSSION

Perioptic meningiomas arise from the optic nerve sheath, and represent the most common type of orbital meningioma. Perioptic meningiomas account for about 33% of all tumors of the optic nerve and sheath, and 5% of all primary orbital tumors. Most perioptic meningiomas occur in the third to fifth decades, and there is a decidedly female predominance, with about 80% of these tumors occurring in women. Patients present with visual loss and proptosis.[1]

On MR, perioptic meningiomas are isointense to muscle on T1-weighted images, and isointense to fat on T2-weighted images.[2] The signal intensity may vary, however, probably because of the presence of calcification, which is common. Most perioptic meningiomas show mild enhancement of the intraorbital tumor and intense enhancement of the intracranial component after contrast infusion.[3] However, the classically described perineural enhancement or "tram-track" sign is nonspecific, and is not pathognomonic for perioptic meningioma. CT remains superior to MR for detection of calcification, but MR is better for defining the intracanalicular and posterior extent of these lesions.[1]

MR Technique

Small-diameter surface coils provide greater S/N and are useful for evaluation of superficial eye lesions or intraorbital lesions. However, the gain in S/N with small-diameter coils is reduced as the distance from the coil increases. The orbital apex and optic chiasm may not be optimally imaged with a surface coil. Therefore, it is recommended that a standard head coil be used for imaging of lesions, such as perioptic meningiomas, that may have intracranial extension.[2] Sagittal oblique images along the axis of the optic nerve depict well the intracranial extension of such lesions through the optic canal or superior orbital fissure.

Pitfalls in Image Interpretation

The differential diagnosis for a mass involving the optic nerve or sheath includes optic nerve glioma, optic nerve hemangioblastoma, neurofibroma, leukemia, lymphoma, metastases, pseudotumor, granulomatous disease, and hematoma. Optic nerve gliomas are usually found in children, with 90% occurring before the age of 20, as opposed to perioptic meningiomas, which usually occur in adults.

Clinical References

1. Atlas S. Magnetic resonance imaging of the orbit: current status. Magn Reson Q 1989;5:39–96.
2. Atlas S, Bilanuik L, Zimmerman R, et al. Orbit: initial experience with surface coil spin-echo MR imaging at 1.5 T. Radiology 1987;164:501–509.
3. Zimmerman C, Schatz N, Glaser J. Magnetic resonance imaging of optic nerve meningiomas: enhancement with gadolinium-DTPA. Ophthalmology 1990;97:585–591.

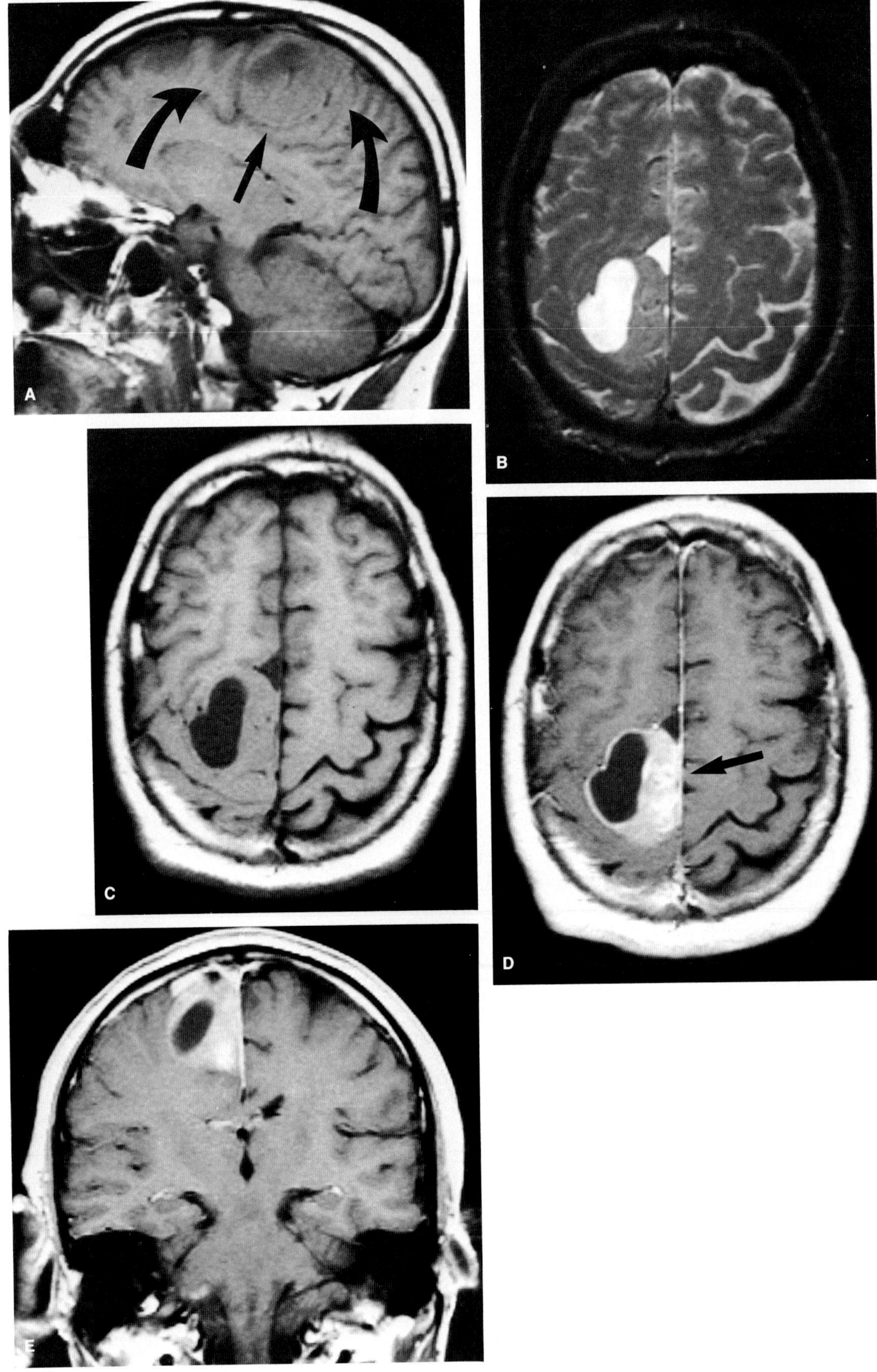
A
B
C
D
E

HISTORY

A 68-year-old patient with a mass on CT

FINDINGS

(*A*) Sagittal T1-weighted scout image identifies a mass (*arrow*) just to the right of midline, which appears to displace surrounding gyri (*curved arrows*) and thus to be extraaxial in nature. Axial precontrast T2-weighted (TE = 80 msec) (*B*) precontrast T1-weighted (*C*) and postcontrast T1-weighted (*D*) images demonstrate the mass to lie adjacent to the falx, with cystic and solid components, and intense enhancement (*arrow in D*). (*E*) Mass effect on the right lateral ventricle is best appreciated on the coronal postcontrast T1-weighted image.

DIAGNOSIS

Hemangiopericytoma

DISCUSSION

Three histologically similar vascular neoplasms, namely hemangioblastomas, angioblastic meningiomas, and hemangiopericytomas, are thought to arise from embryonic vascular elements (angioblasts). Hemangioblastomas are confined to the posterior fossa and do not demonstrate a dural attachment. Angioblastic meningiomas are characterized by high cellularity and rapid growth. The numerous vascular spaces within the tumor are considered to be derived from the tumor cells themselves, not the supporting stroma, and thus are the basis of their distinction from other types of meningiomas. Five percent of tumors involving the meninges are hemangiopericytomas, an extremely vascular neoplasm with high cellularity and numerous mitoses, reflecting its malignant nature. A peak in age incidence between the fourth and sixth decades has been reported. This aggressive neoplasm has a high rate of recurrence, with systemic metastases described in 20% of cases. At surgery, because of its location and tendency to compress underlying brain, it is often mistaken for a meningioma.[1] Because of tumor vascularity, marked enhancement of a hemangiopericytoma should be expected on MR after administration of a gadolinium chelate.[2]

Clinical References

1. Kruse F Jr. Hemangiopericytoma of the meninges (angioblastic meningioma of Cushing and Eisenhardt): clinicopathologic aspects and follow-up studies in 8 cases. Neurology 1961;11:771–777.
2. Parizel PM, Degryse HR, Gheuens J, et al. Gadolinium DOTA enhanced MR imaging of intracranial lesions. J Comput Assist Tomogr 1989;13:378–385.

(A through E courtesy of Mark Osborne, MD.)

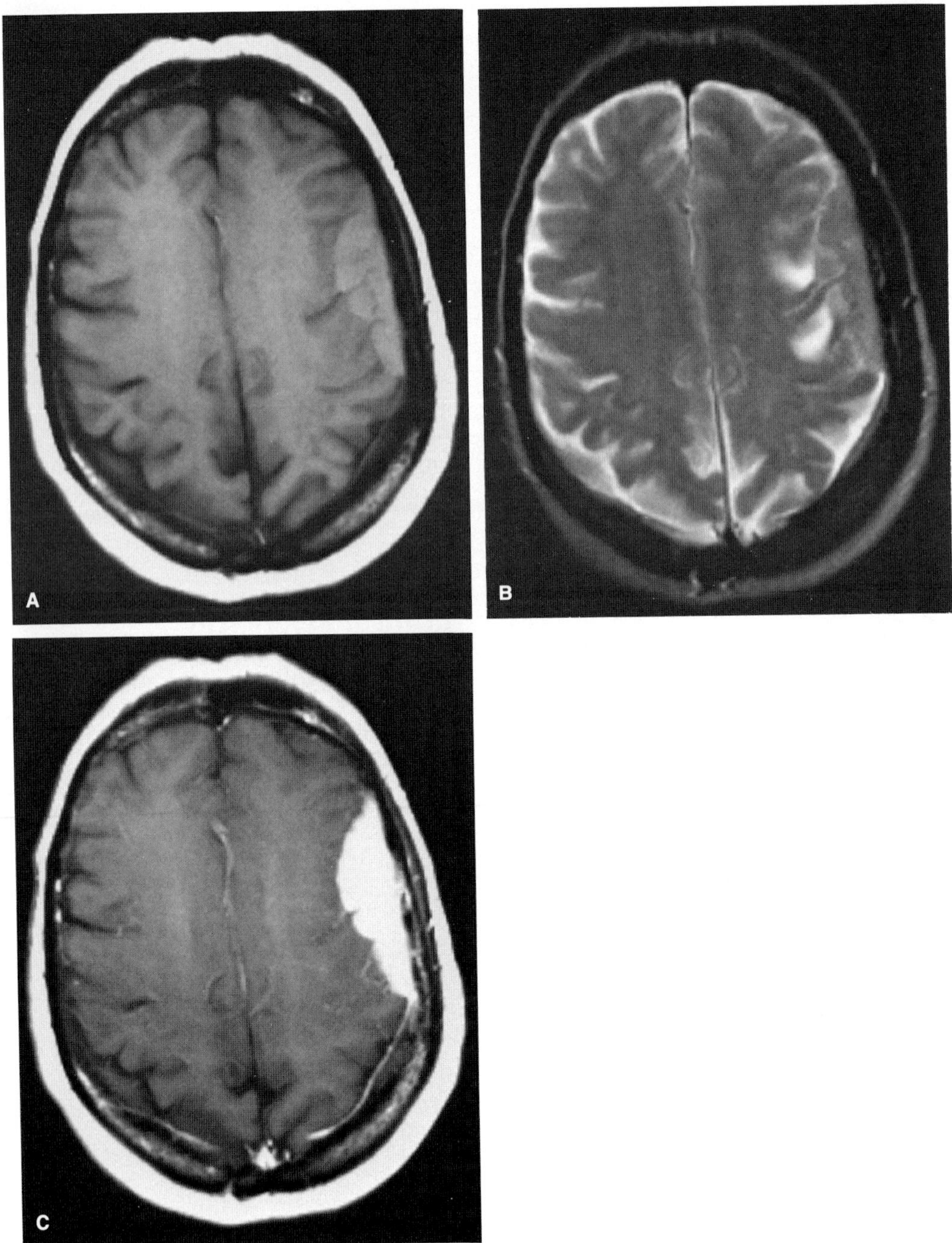

HISTORY

A 60-year-old woman with headaches

FINDINGS

A soft-tissue–intensity extraaxial, dural-based mass is identified along the left frontal and parietal lobes on axial T1-weighted (*A*) and T2-weighted (*B*) images. Minimal edema is present adjacent to this mass on the T2-weighted image. (*C*) The mass demonstrates intense, homogeneous enhancement after administration of a gadolinium chelate on the postcontrast axial T1-weighted image.

DIAGNOSIS

En plaque meningioma

DISCUSSION

En plaque meningiomas are meningiomas that are only slightly raised above the dura mater and grow along the planes of the leptomeninges. The most common location is along the sphenoid ridge or over the convexity (frequently in the vicinity of the coronal suture).

These tumors can be difficult to detect on both CT and MR (the latter when used without contrast media). The administration of a gadolinium chelate increases the sensitivity of MR in the diagnosis of all meningiomas. En plaque meningiomas can be especially difficult to diagnose on CT either with or without contrast because of the high attenuation of the adjacent bony calvarium. They are prone to invade adjacent bone and it is not uncommon to see marked hyperostosis of the adjacent bone, particularly along the skull base.[1] This hyperostosis can be associated with increased blood flow to the meninges and diploic space. The amount of hyperostosis is often out of proportion to the size of the underlying intracranial meningioma. The hyperostosis of adjacent bony structures can produce symptoms secondary to the mass effect from the bony hyperostosis. When the hyperostosis occurs along the sphenoid ridge, it can be confused with fibrous dysplasia. Associated cerebral vasogenic edema is relatively uncommon when compared with globoid meningiomas.[2]

The visualization of a tumor stain or encasement of vessels by these tumors is uncommon, although an enlarged middle meningeal artery is sometimes observed.

MR Technique

En plaque meningiomas are difficult to detect on MR without administration of a gadolinium chelate.

Pitfalls in Image Interpretation

Dural-based metastases can have a similar appearance to en plaque meningiomas.

Clinical References

1. Russell DS, Rubinstein LJ. Pathology of tumours of the nervous system. Baltimore, Williams & Wilkins, 1989:461.
2. Kim KS, Rogers LF, Globlatt D. CT features of hyperostosing meningioma en plaque. AJR 1987;149:1017–1023.

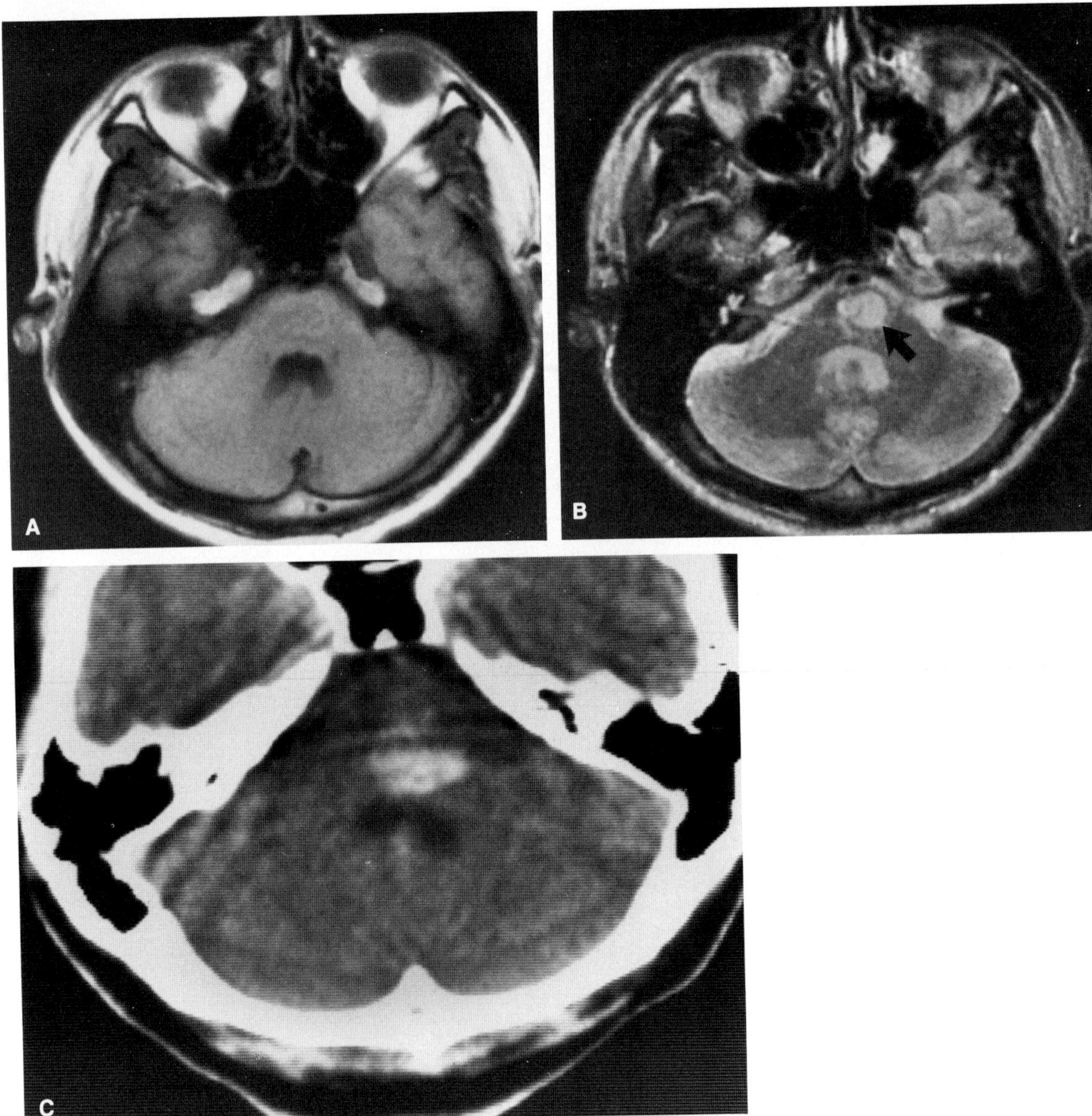

HISTORY

A 26-year-old with acute onset of quadriparesis

FINDINGS

(*A*) No definite abnormality is seen on the T1-weighted axial image obtained at 0.35 T. (*B*) The corresponding T2-weighted axial image, also obtained at 0.35 T, demonstrates a high-signal-intensity lesion in the pons (*arrow*). (*C*) A noninfused CT acquired 5 days later shows hyperdensity in the posterior pons, consistent with hemorrhage. (*D and E*) MR was repeated, 9 days after the initial MR, at 1 T. T1-weighted axial image (*D*) now shows a lesion in the pons (*white arrow*) that is predominantly high signal intensity, with a center that is isointense to the surrounding brain. (*E*) On the T2-weighted axial image the lesion has high signal intensity anteriorly (*white arrow*) and low signal intensity posteriorly (*curved open arrow*).

DIAGNOSIS

Hyperacute hematoma (oxyhemoglobin)

DISCUSSION

Intracranial intraparenchymal hemorrhage undergoes complex changes in signal intensity on MR that are influenced by several intrinsic and extrinsic factors.[1] The major intrinsic factor is the time at which the brain is imaged after development of the hematoma. The extrinsic factors are the pulse sequences used and the field strength of the magnet.[1]

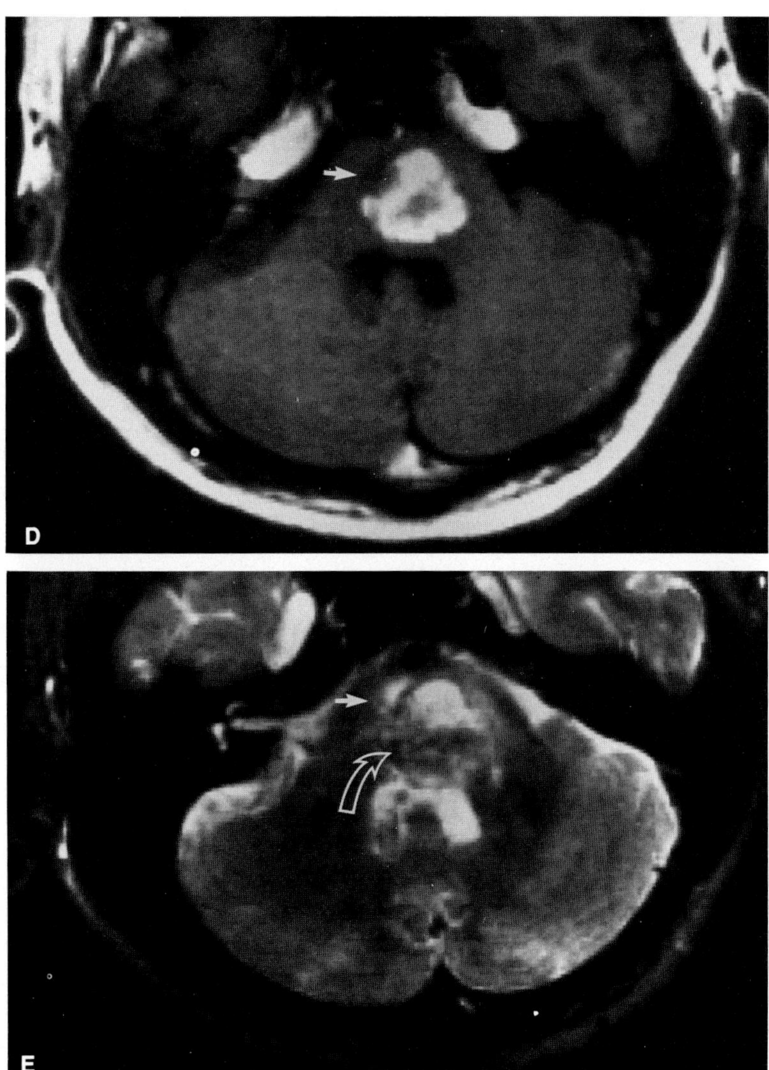

Hyperacute hemorrhage has been defined as that occurring between 0 and 12 hours of age.[1] Hyperacute intraparenchymal intracranial hemorrhage is isointense or slightly hypointense relative to brain on T1-weighted images, independent of field strength. A hyperacute hematoma is hyperintense relative to brain on T2-weighted images at both mid and high field strengths.[1] The appearance of hyperacute hematomas reflects the signal intensity of nonflowing blood, which is a proteinaceous fluid with higher water content than brain parenchyma.

In the hyperacute stage, hemoglobin remains oxygenated (oxyhemoglobin). The subsequent appearance of low signal intensity within a hematoma on T2-weighted images, reflecting deoxyhemoglobin (acute hematoma), depends on field strength. Hypointensity on T2-weighted images develops sooner and is more pronounced at high field strength (1.5 T) than at mid (0.5 to 1 T) or low (0.35 T or less) field strength.

Deoxyhemoglobin breaks down to methemoglobin, which has high signal intensity on T1-weighted images, as seen on images *D* and *E* obtained 9 days postictus. The signal intensity of intracellular methemoglobin is low on T2-weighted images. After cell lysis, extracellular methemoglobin has high signal intensity on T2-weighted images.[2] Thus, the hematoma in the pons seen on scan *E* is composed of intracellular methemoglobin in the dependent posterior pons, and extracellular methemoglobin in the anterior pons, with a small amount of residual deoxyhemoglobin centrally.

MR Technique

Hemorrhage consistently has low signal intensity on T2-weighted GRE scans, regardless of age or field strength. Therefore, GRE pulse sequences can be helpful in characterizing lesions as hemorrhagic before the development of hyperintensity on T1-weighted images and hypointensity on T2-weighted images.[1]

Pitfalls in Image Interpretation

The signal intensity characteristics of hyperacute hemorrhage are nonspecific. The differential diagnosis for a lesion that is isointense on T1-weighted images and hyperintense on T2-weighted images includes infarct, tumor, and demyelination.

Clinical References

1. Weingarten K, Zimmerman R, Deo-Narine V, et al. MR imaging of acute intracranial hemorrhage: findings on sequential spin-echo and gradient-echo images in a dog model. AJNR 1991;12:457–467.
2. Gomori J, Grossman R, Hackney D, et al. Variable appearances of subacute intracranial hematomas on high-field spin-echo MR. AJNR 1987;8:1019–1026.

*(*A *to* E *from Runge VM. Clinical magnetic resonance imaging. Philadelphia, JB Lippincott, 1990.)*

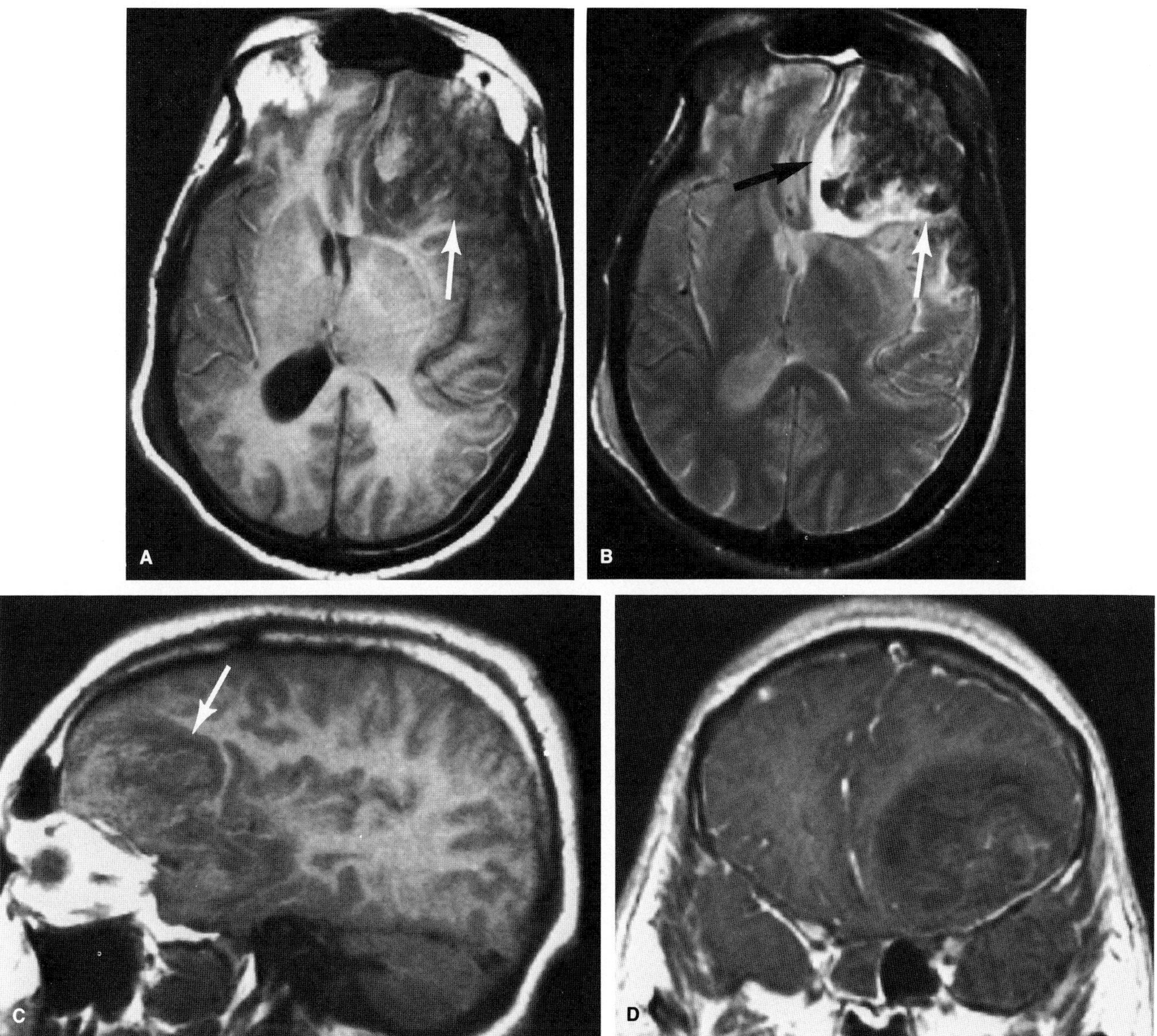

HISTORY

A 30-year-old man who fell off a barn the previous day

FINDINGS

(*A to C*) A large round lesion (*white arrow*) of predominantly decreased signal intensity is identified in the left frontal lobe on axial T1-weighted (*A*) and T2-weighted (*B*) images. Increased signal intensity (*black arrow in B*), representing edema, is present surrounding the lesion. Extension of the mass to the left temporal lobe is seen on precontrast sagittal (*C*) and postcontrast coronal (*D*) T1-weighted images.

DIAGNOSIS

Acute hematoma (deoxyhemoglobin)

DISCUSSION

Intracranial hematomas have a variable appearance on high-field-strength MR. There are five classic stages (oxygenated blood, deoxygenated blood, intracellular methemoglobin, hemolysis to extracellular methemoglobin, and protein resorption leading to hemosiderin) of intracranial hematomas, which are associated with characteristic signal intensity patterns at 1.5 T.[1]

1—Hyperacute hematomas (oxyhemoglobin) are slightly hypointense on T1-weighted images and hyperintense on T2-weighted images.

2—Acute hematomas (intracellular deoxyhemoglobin) are isointense to gray matter on T1-weighted images, and of marked decreased signal intensity on T2-weighted images.

3—Early subacute hematomas (intracellular methemoglobin) are hyperintense on T1-weighted images and hypointense on T2-weighted images.

4—Late subacute hematomas (extracellular methemoglobin) form secondary to cell lysis and are hyperintense on T1- and T2-weighted sequences.

5—Chronic hematomas (hemosiderin or ferritin) are slightly hypointense on T1-weighted sequences and markedly hypointense on T2-weighted sequences.

Often hematomas do not display one of the above characteristic patterns on MR. This can be secondary to dilutional effects on extracellular methemoglobin, a combination of intracellular methemoglobin and deoxyhemoglobin, or different degrees of lysis of intracellular methemoglobin.[2]

Clinical References

1. Brooks RA, Di Chiro G, Patromas N. MR imaging of cerebral hematomas at different field strengths: theory and applications. J Comput Assist Tomogr 1989;13:194–206.
2. Gomori JM, Grossman RI, Hackney DB, et al. Variable appearances of subacute intracranial hematomas on high-field spin-echo MR. AJNR 1987;8:1019–1026.

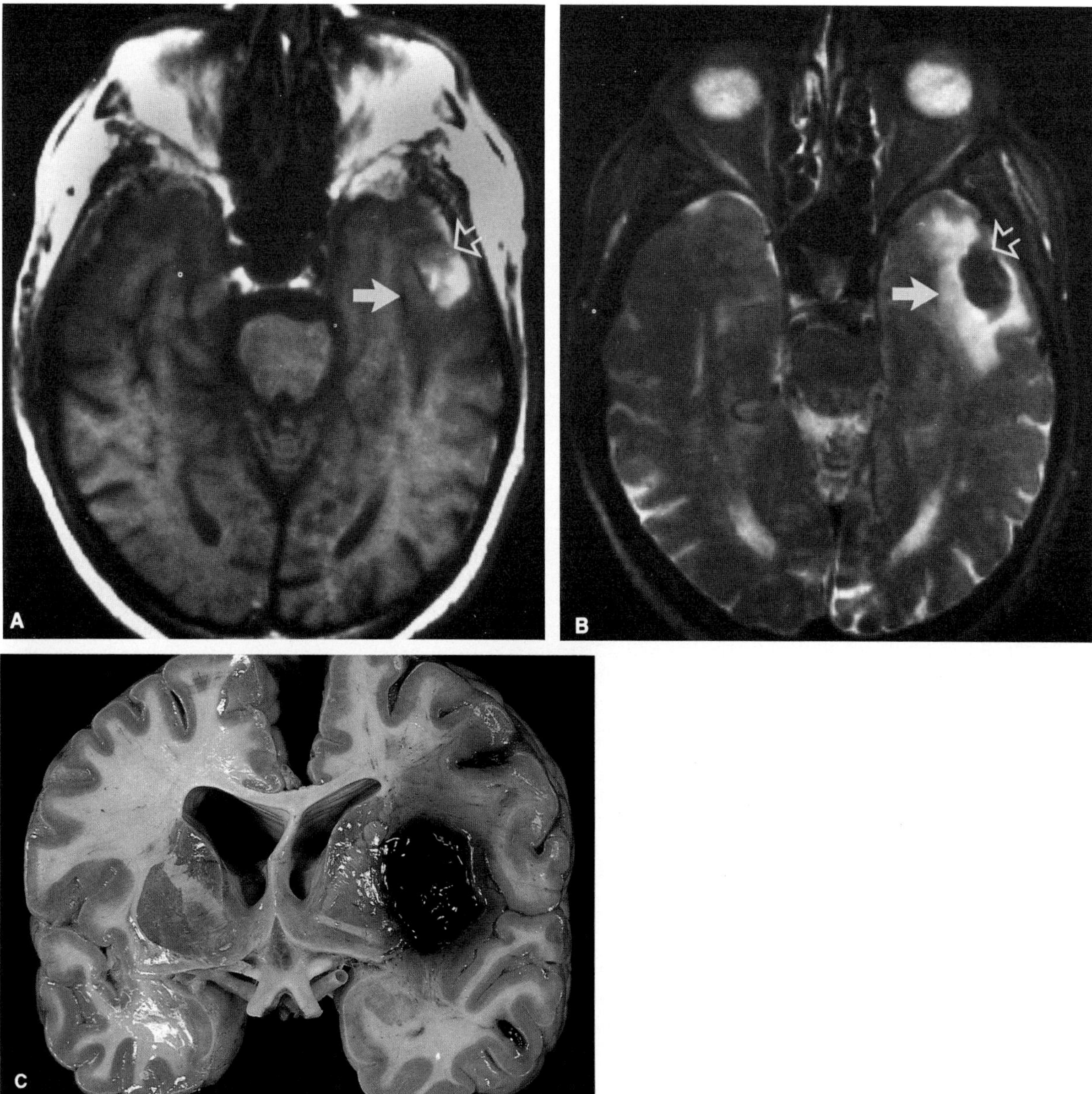

HISTORY

A 71-year-old man

FINDINGS

(*A*) Axial T1-weighted image shows an irregular mass (*open arrow*) of increased signal intensity in the left temporal lobe. (*B*) On the axial T2-weighted image this mass (*open arrow*) is hypointense. Edema surrounding the mass is identified primarily on the basis of the T2-weighted scan with increased signal intensity (*arrow in B*), although there is corresponding mild hypointensity (*arrow in A*) on the T1-weighted scan.

DIAGNOSIS

Early subacute hematoma (intracellular methemoglobin)

DISCUSSION

Intracellular methemoglobin is of high signal intensity on T1-weighted images and decreased signal intensity on T2-weighted images at high field strength. Intracellular methemoglobin results in significant shortening of T1 and T2 relaxation times. Intracellular methemoglobin demonstrates two properties termed *selective T2 relaxation enhancement* and *proton–electron dipole–dipole proton relaxation enhancement*.

Selective T2 relaxation enhancement results from dephasing of water molecules secondary to the inhomogeneous distribution of a paramagnetic substance. The presence of paramagnetic forms of hemoglobin (deoxyhemoglobin and methemoglobin) within red blood cells results in inhomogeneous susceptibility effects which result in signal loss on T2-weighted images. Hemolysis of red blood cells eliminates the inhomogeneous susceptibility effect of the methemoglobin and thus the signal loss. The cause of this signal loss is due to a susceptibility effect and not to direct T2 shortening, as the term implies. Extracellular methemoglobin is of increased signal intensity on T1- and T2-weighted images.

Methemoglobin has five unpaired electrons. The presence of unpaired electrons causes large fluctuations in the local magnetic field which enhance relaxation of protons: this property is called *proton–electron dipole–dipole proton relaxation enhancement.* This interaction depends on the ability of water protons to approach within 3 angstroms of the unpaired electron. This results in a more efficient energy transfer, and the end result is shortening of the T1 and T2 relaxation times. The unpaired electrons of deoxyhemoglobin and hemosiderin are inaccessible to water molecules and this interaction cannot occur. Proton–electron dipole–dipole proton relaxation enhancement causes the hyperintensity of methemoglobin on T1-weighted images.[1,2]

Methemoglobin is usually seen initially at the periphery of a hematoma and later throughout the hematoma.

Pitfalls in Image Interpretation

The signal intensity of hematomas varies depending on magnetic field strength. Selective T2 relaxation enhancement increases as the square of the magnetic field. The proton–electron dipole–dipole proton relaxation enhancement of methemoglobin is not affected by field strength.

Pathologic Correlate

(*C*) Coronal section of an unfixed brain demonstrates a moderate-size left putamen hemorrhage (without rupture into the lateral ventricle). Pathologically, a zone of tissue necrosis is seen around a resolving hematoma.

Clinical References

1. Brooks RA, Di Chiro G, Patronas N. MR imaging of cerebral hematomas at different field strengths: theory and applications. J Comput Assist Tomogr 1989;13:194–206.
2. Gomori JM, Grossman RI, Hackney DB, et al. Variable appearances of subacute intracranial hematomas on high-field spin-echo MR. AJNR 1987;8:1019–1026.

*(*A *and* B *from Runge VM. Clinical magnetic resonance imaging. Philadelphia, JB Lippincott, 1990;* C *from Okazaki H, Scheithauer B. Slide atlas of neuropathology. New York, Gower Medical Publishing, 1988. By permission of Mayo Foundation.)*

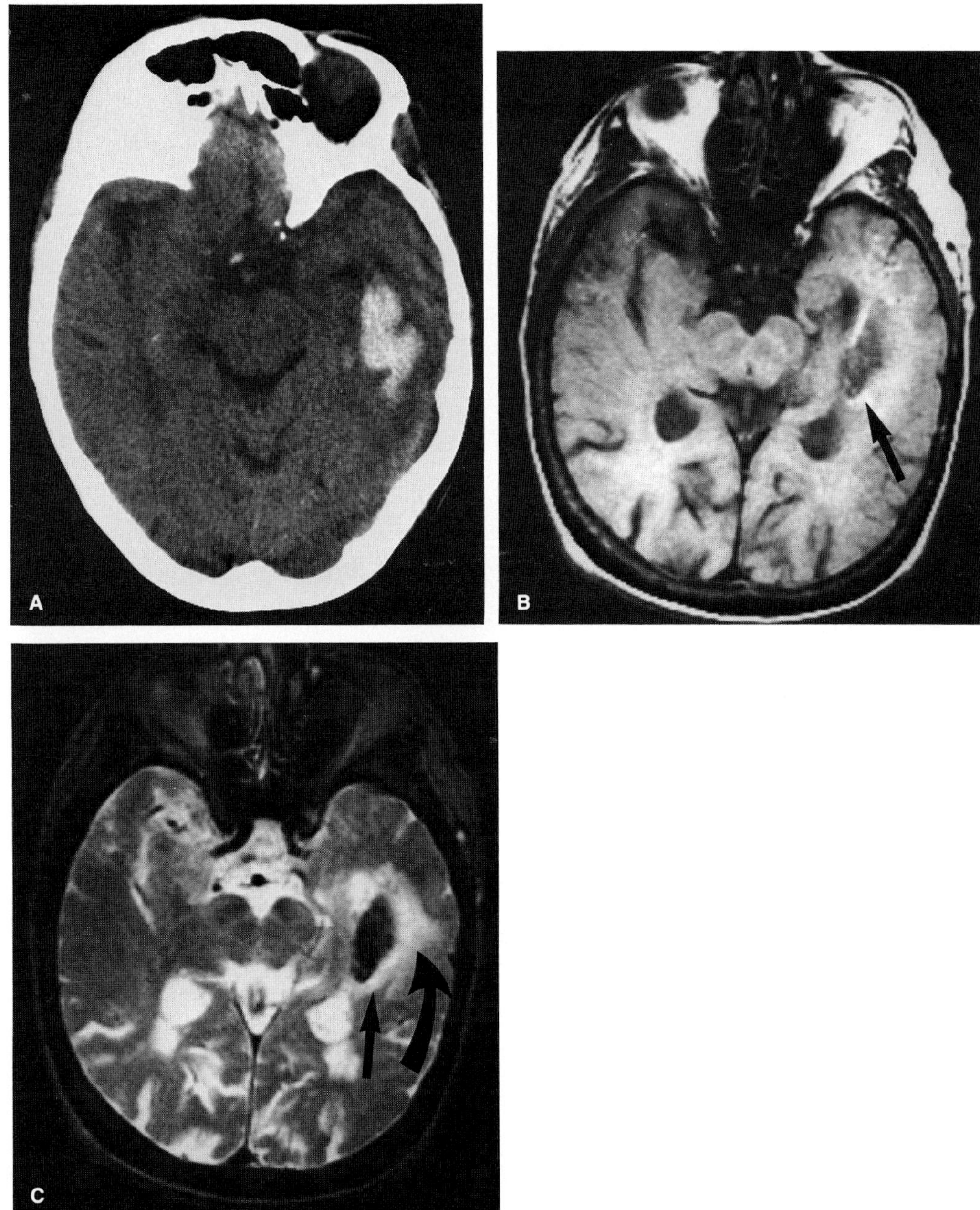

HISTORY

An 85-year-old with abrupt onset of confusion

FINDINGS

(*A*) Unenhanced x-ray CT reveals a high attenuation mass in the left temporal lobe, with a suggestion of surrounding hypodensity. An MR examination was obtained 4 days later using a 1.5-T magnet. At this time, the mass (*arrows in B and C*) is mildly hypointense on T1-weighted (*B*) and markedly hypointense on T2-weighted (*C*) images. Abnormal hyperintensity (*curved arrow in C*), consistent with edema, can also be identified surrounding the mass on the T2-weighted scan. MR imaging was repeated 45 days following presentation. At this latter date, the majority of the mass (*arrows in D and E*) is hyperintense on both T1-weighted (*D*) and T2-weighted (*E*) scans. A peripheral rim of marked hypointensity (*open arrow in E*) is also noted on the T2-weighted scan, consistent with hemosiderin or ferritin deposition. The surrounding cerebral edema resolved by the time of the second examination.

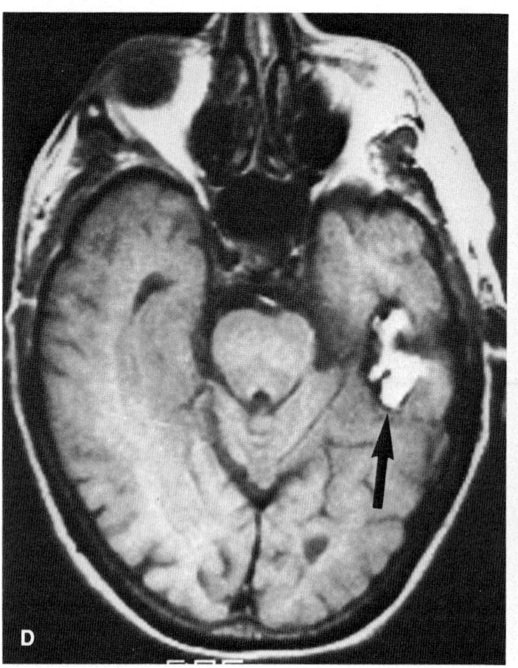

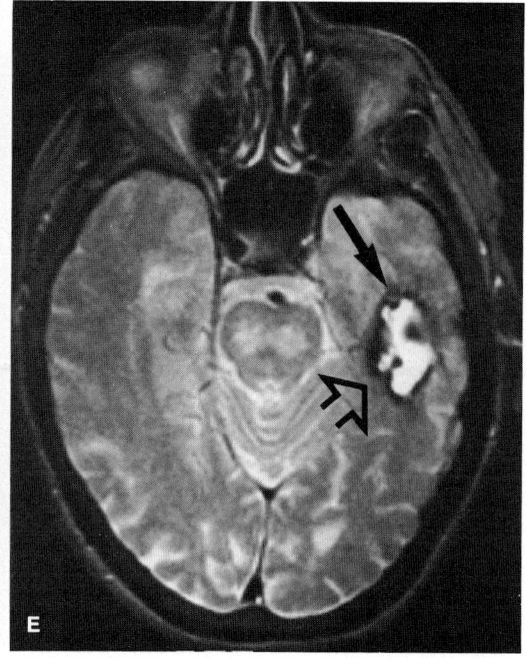

DIAGNOSIS

Acute hematoma (deoxyhemoglobin), with temporal evolution to late subacute hematoma (extracellular methemoglobin)

DISCUSSION

Intracranial hemorrhagic lesions can have a different appearance depending on the field strength at which MR is performed.[1,2] On both low-field and high-field imaging, subacute intracranial hematomas are hyperintense on T1-weighted images as a result of the presence of methemoglobin. On high-field T2-weighted images, the appearance is variable, with undiluted intracellular methemoglobin being markedly hypointense, undiluted free (extracellular) methemoglobin being isointense to slightly hypointense, and dilute free methemoglobin being hyperintense. However, at low field (less than 1 T), the T2* or susceptibility effect of blood products is not well appreciated. Thus, subacute hematomas at low field appear hyperintense on T2-weighted, as well as T1-weighted, images.

The ultimate long-term appearance of intracranial bleeding depends on whether resorption of the central fluid collection occurs. If the fluid is resorbed, only a hemosiderin cleft is left, which can be seen only at high field. If no fluid resorption occurs, a fluid collection which appears bright on all pulse sequences, due to the presence of extracellular methemoglobin, is seen regardless of field strength. A surrounding hemosiderin rim is also present, but of course visible (as marked hypointensity) only at high field.

Pitfalls in Image Interpretation

Early subacute hematomas may be difficult to differentiate from melanotic melanoma metastases. In both entities, the lesion can present with hyperintensity on T1-weighted images, surrounded by cerebral edema.

On first glance, intracranial fat could be confused with a chronic subacute hematoma. However, differentiation in this case is easily achieved by attention to chemical shift artifact or by repeat imaging with fat suppression or chemical shift techniques.

Clinical References

1. Gomori JM, Grossman RI, Hackney DB, et al. Variable appearances of subacute intracranial hematomas on high-field spin-echo MR. AJR 1988;150:171–178.
2. Dooms GC, Uske A, Brant-Zawadzki M, et al. Spin-echo MR imaging of intracranial hemorrhage. Neuroradiology 1986; 28:132–138.

(A *through* E *courtesy of Clifford Wolf, MD.)*

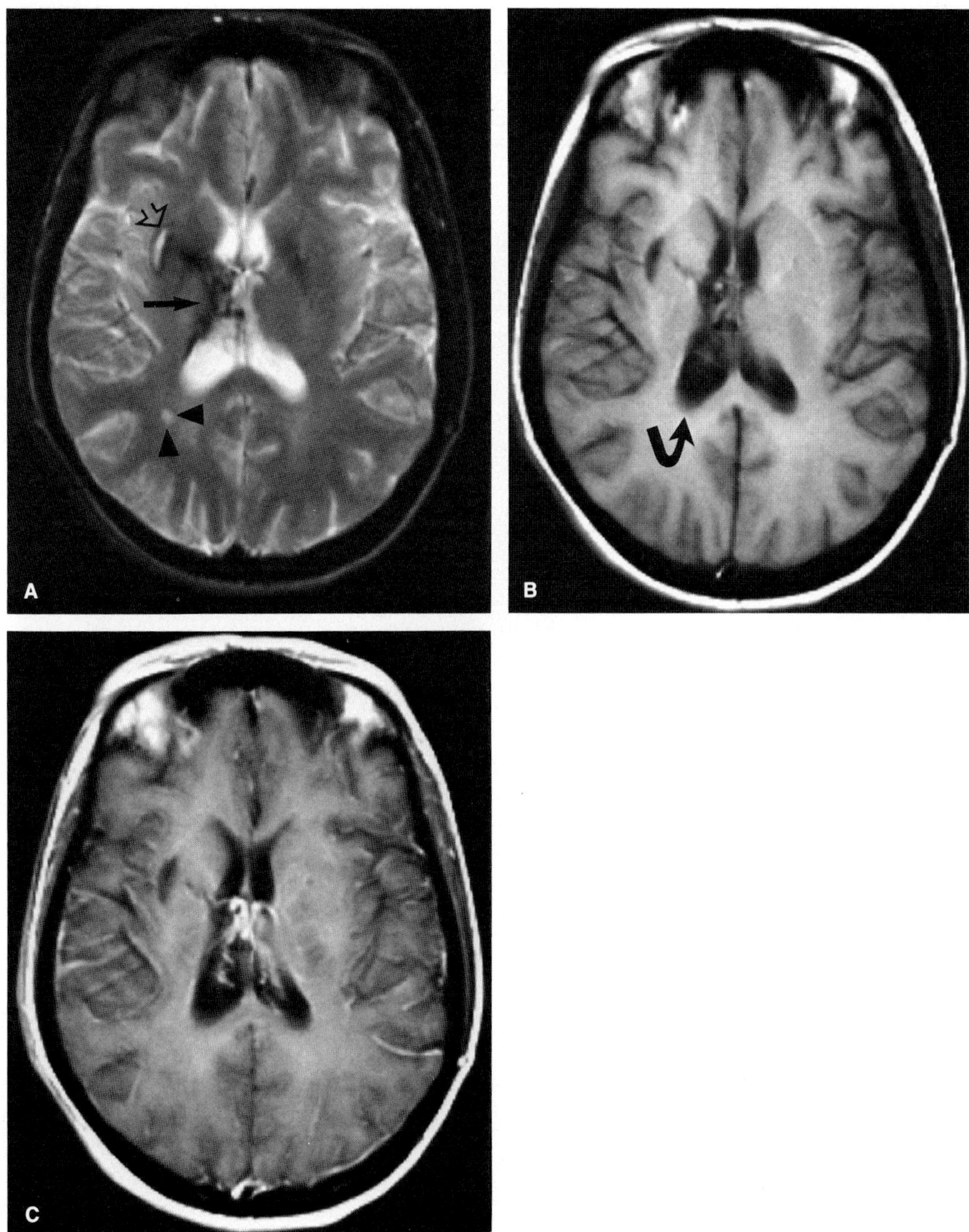

HISTORY

A 30-year-old woman with chronic headaches, hospitalized 18 months before the current examination with severe headaches, nausea, and vomiting. In the emergency department (during the prior hospital admission), she became obtunded and had a seizure. CT revealed blood within the right thalamus and third ventricle. By the time of discharge, there had been partial resolution of the patient's left hemiparesis

FINDINGS

Precontrast T2-weighted (TE=90 msec) (*A*) and T1-weighted (*B*) SE images reveal abnormal iron deposition (*arrow in A*) in the right thalamus (extending to the border of the lateral ventricle), slight ex vacuo dilatation of the atrium of the right lateral ventricle (*curved arrow in B*), and a cystic lesion (*open arrow in A*), surrounded by iron staining in either the external capsule or putamen on the right. The latter abnormality could represent

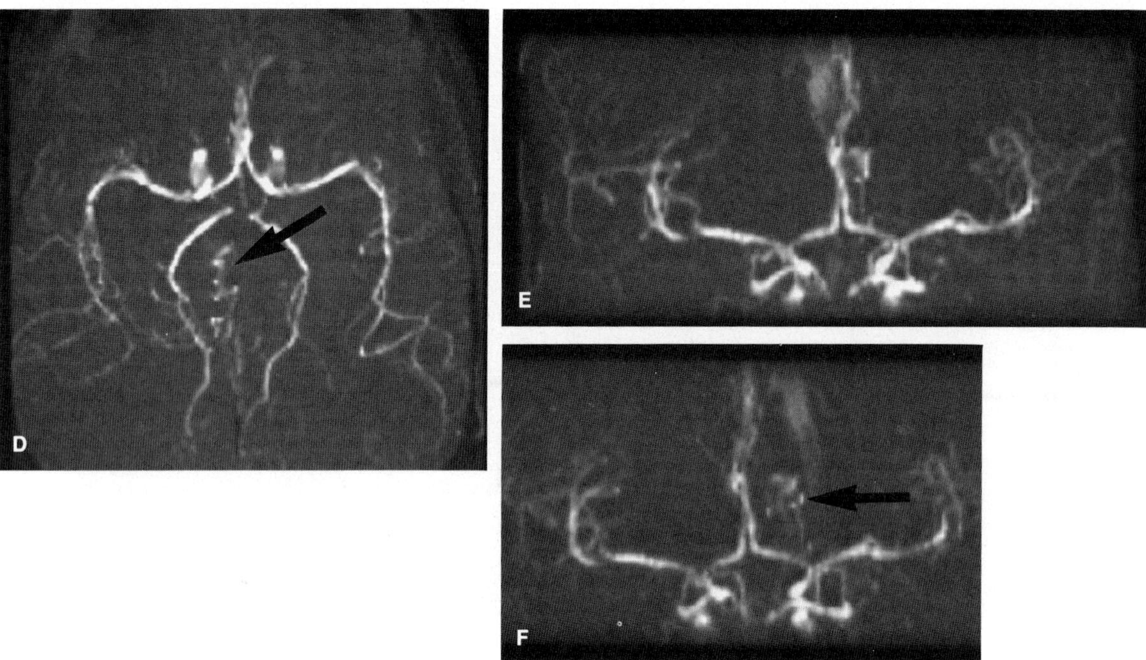

either the residual of cerebral hemorrhage or a large lacunar infarct. Incidental note is made of a nonspecific ischemic or gliotic focus (*arrowheads in A*) adjacent to the atrium of the right lateral ventricle. (*C*) The postcontrast T1-weighted SE image reveals no abnormal enhancement. MRA was performed precontrast using 3D TOF technique, with 2D image reconstruction by maximum intensity projection (MIP) in the craniocaudal (*D*), anteroposterior (AP) (*E*), and oblique AP (*F*) directions. An abnormal tangle of vessels (*arrows in D and F*), seen to the right of midline and superior to the posterior cerebral artery, is noted only on MRA. Although this is well depicted in *D,* vessel overlap obscures visualization in the straight AP view (*E*). The slight obliquity of the projection displayed in *F* improves lesion identification on the AP view.

DIAGNOSIS

Thalamic arteriovenous malformation (AVM) with residual from prior intraparenchymal hemorrhage

DISCUSSION

The case presented illustrates the ability of MRA to diagnose an AVM (documented by conventional x-ray angiography) not seen on conventional MR images. Prior hemorrhage has resulted in partial ablation of the lesion and abnormal iron deposition in brain parenchyma. MR is superior to both CT and contrast angiography for demonstration of the precise anatomic relation between an AVM (its nidus, arterial feeders, and draining veins) and surrounding brain parenchyma.[1] MR is also superior to CT for demonstration of associated parenchymal abnormalities and subacute and chronic hemorrhage.

Vascular malformations of the brain stem are a common cause of spontaneous hemorrhage in normotensive young adults.[2] Before the advent of MR, these malformations often went undetected. MR provides for both diagnosis and accurate localization. Characteristic MR findings include multiple hemorrhages of varying age and surrounding abnormal iron deposition.

From biochemical and histochemical studies,[3] both ferritin and hemosiderin are known to be present late in resolution of a cerebral hematoma. The MR signal changes (low intensity on T2-weighted scans at high field strength) correlate more closely in distribution to that of abnormal ferritin deposition. The central fluid component in certain instances can be completely resorbed, leaving only a ferritin or hemosiderin cleft.

Cerebral angiography (*not shown*), performed both during the prior hospitalization and concurrent with the present examination, demonstrated an abnormal cluster of enlarged arteries and draining veins in the right thalamus and along the right lateral ventricular wall, consistent with an AVM. The major arterial supply was by way of the right posteromedial choroidal artery with minor contributions from the right medial lenticulostriate and thalamoperforate arteries. Venous drainage was principally by way of the right internal cerebral vein. The patient was not an operable candidate because of the deep location of the lesion. She was referred for gamma knife stereotactic radiation therapy.

MR Technique

MRA can reveal significant arterial and venous abnormalities that would otherwise go undetected on conventional SE images. When an arteriovenous abnormality is suspected clinically, or due to abnormal iron deposition, MRA is mandated.

Pitfalls in Image Interpretation

Cerebral hemorrhage, specifically methemoglobin, can be confused for abnormal vasculature on MR TOF angiography. Blood in this stage of evolution can appear bright (high intensity) on the GRE sequences used in MR TOF angiography and thus be visualized on the final image obtained using MIP reconstruction. Careful comparison of routine SE images and the MR angiogram avoids misdiagnosis.

Clinical References

1. Smith HJ, Strother CM, Kikuchi Y, et al. MR imaging in the management of supratentorial intracranial AVMs. AJR 1988; 150:1143–1153.
2. Kashiwagi S, van Loveren HR, Tew JM Jr, et al. Diagnosis and treatment of vascular brainstem malformations. J Neurosurg 1990;72:27–34.
3. Thulborn KR, Sorensen AG, Kowall NW, et al. The role of ferritin and hemosiderin in the MR appearance of cerebral hemorrhage: a histopathologic biochemical study in rats. AJR 1990;154:1053–1059.

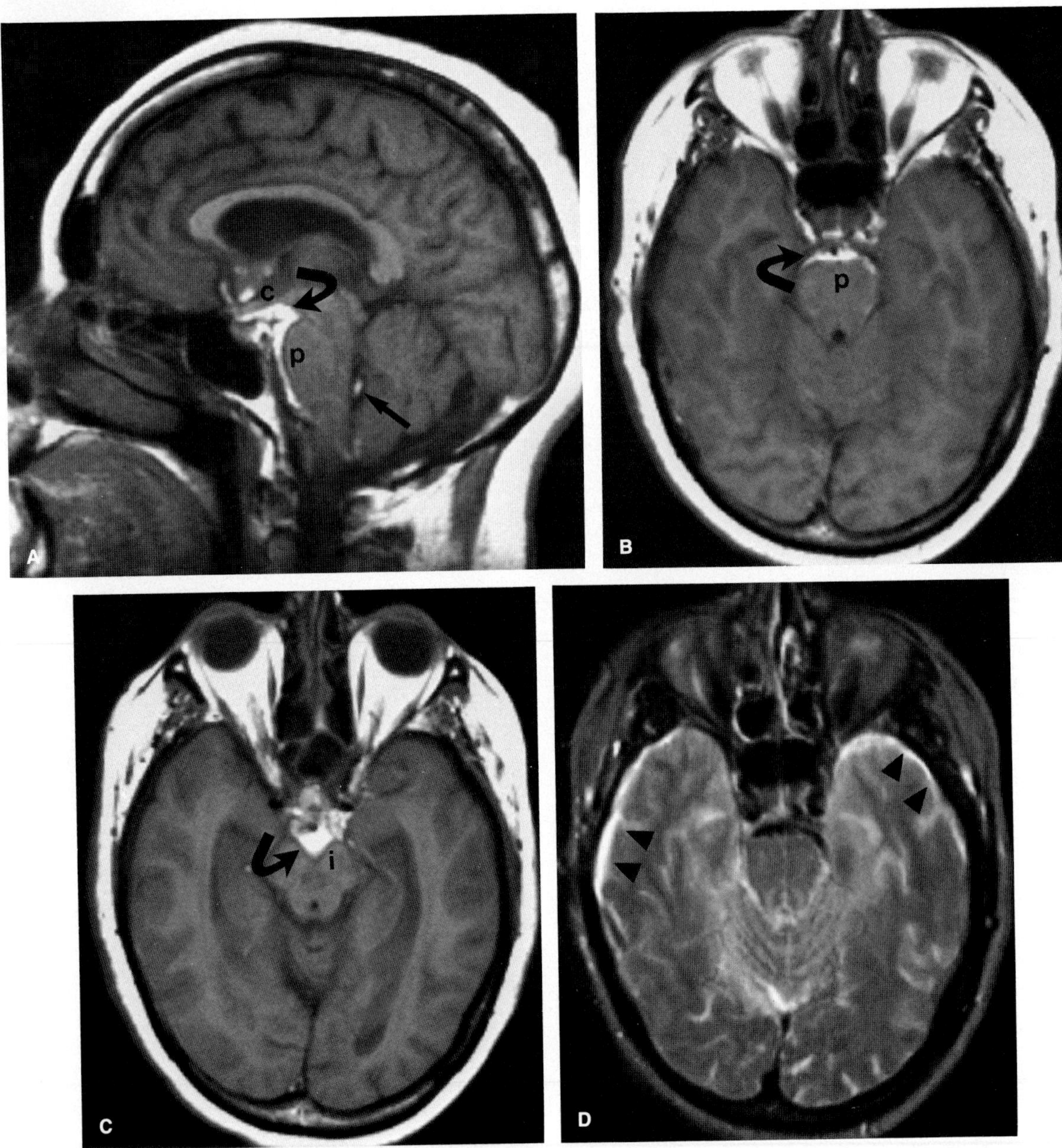

HISTORY

A 67-year-old hypertensive patient with "the worst headache of her life," accompanied by nausea and vomiting, 4 days before the current examination. The pain did not abate.

FINDINGS

(*A to C*) Sagittal and axial T1-weighted images reveal abnormal, hyperintense soft tissue (*curved arrows*), representing methemoglobin in clotted blood, in the pontine (p), interpeduncular (i), and chiasmatic cisterns (c). Clotted blood can also be identified in the fourth ventricle (*arrow in A*). (*D and E*) On the T2-weighted images (TE = 90 msec), these areas are of predominantly low signal intensity, indicating that the methemoglobin is intracellular in location. Clotted blood can be recognized prospectively in the occipital horns (*open arrows in E*) only on the T2-weighted image. This appearance, with abnormal low signal intensity on the T2-weighted scan and isointensity (relative to CSF) on the T1-weighted scan, is due to deoxyhemoglobin. The prepontine clot appears more extensive on the T2-weighted image, which depicts both deoxyhemoglobin and intracellular methemoglobin as abnormal hypointensity. An abnormal extraaxial fluid collection with extremely high signal intensity (greater than CSF), corresponding to subarachnoid blood, is noted on both T2-weighted images adjacent to the temporal lobes (*arrowheads in D and E*). (*F*) CT, performed 2 days before MR, reveals hemorrhage in the chiasmatic

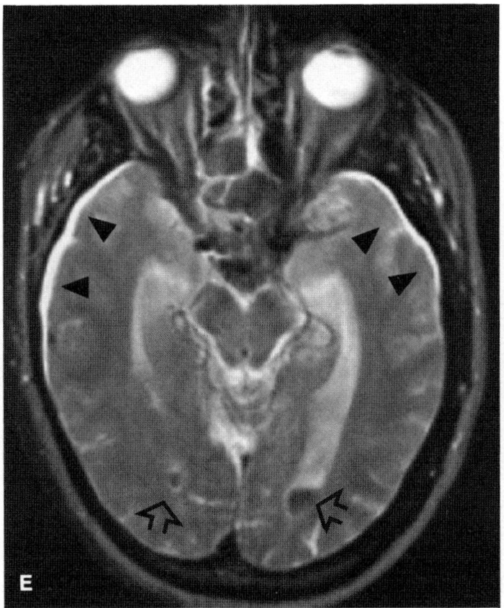

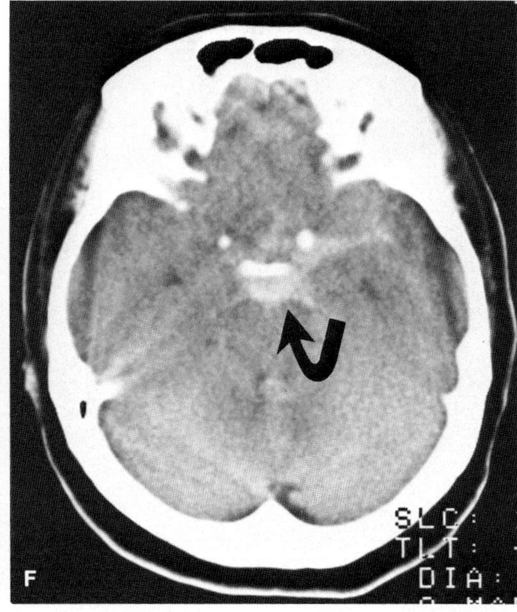

cistern (*curved arrow*) and fourth ventricle (*not illustrated*). No abnormal extraaxial fluid collection or blood within the lateral ventricles was noted on CT. Cerebral angiography (*not illustrated*) was normal.

DIAGNOSIS

Subarachnoid hemorrhage (subacute)

DISCUSSION

Deoxyhemoglobin is well visualized, because of its hypointensity on T2-weighted scans, by high field MR. When hemorrhage occurs in the subarachnoid space (as opposed to within the brain parenchyma), high oxygen tension may prevent conversion of oxyhemoglobin to deoxyhemoglobin. Thus, some authors have hypothesized that acute diffuse subarachnoid hemorrhage might be missed by MR, although blood clots (within which the conversion to deoxyhemoglobin does occur) would be visualized.[1] The use of CT instead of MR in subarachnoid hemorrhage has thus been debated, with the previous article strongly advocating CT. However, CT images can give negative results in patients with subarachnoid hemorrhage, as a result of either the presence of only a small amount of extravasated blood or a delay in time between hemorrhage and imaging. Subsequent clinical research[2] has demonstrated MR to be slightly superior to CT for detection of acute (0 to 24 hours) subarachnoid blood and markedly superior for detection of subacute (4 to 16 days) subarachnoid blood. Because of T1 shortening, acute subarachnoid hemorrhage is well visualized by MR on T2 weighted-scans as abnormal hyperintensity. In high-risk neonates,[3] MR has also been shown to be superior to CT and ultrasonography for the evaluation of extracerebral hemorrhage.

A very small number of patients with ruptured brain aneurysms (the presence of which was suspected in the current case) have a normal angiogram because of local hemorrhage or spasm causing nonfilling. In such cases, a second cerebral angiogram performed at a later date may reveal the lesion. If the original angiogram is technically adequate and there is no vasospasm, repeat angiography is seldom justified.

Pitfalls in Image Interpretation

On T2-weighted images, acute subarachnoid hemorrhage is "brighter" or higher in signal intensity than normal CSF. However, if T2-weighted images are filmed with a "narrow" window level, this contrast difference may not be evident. Careful film photography is required for all MR examinations in order not to obscure valuable clinical information.

Clinical References

1. Barkovich AJ, Atlas SW. Magnetic resonance imaging of intracranial hemorrhage. Radiol Clin North Am 1988;26:801–820.
2. Satoh S, Kadoya S. Magnetic resonance imaging of subarachnoid hemorrhage. Neuroradiology 1988;30:361–366.
3. Keeney SE, Adcock EW, McArdle CB. Prospective observations of 100 high-risk neonates by high-field (1.5 tesla) magnetic resonance imaging of the central nervous system. I. Intraventricular and extracerebral lesions. Pediatrics 1991;87:421–430.

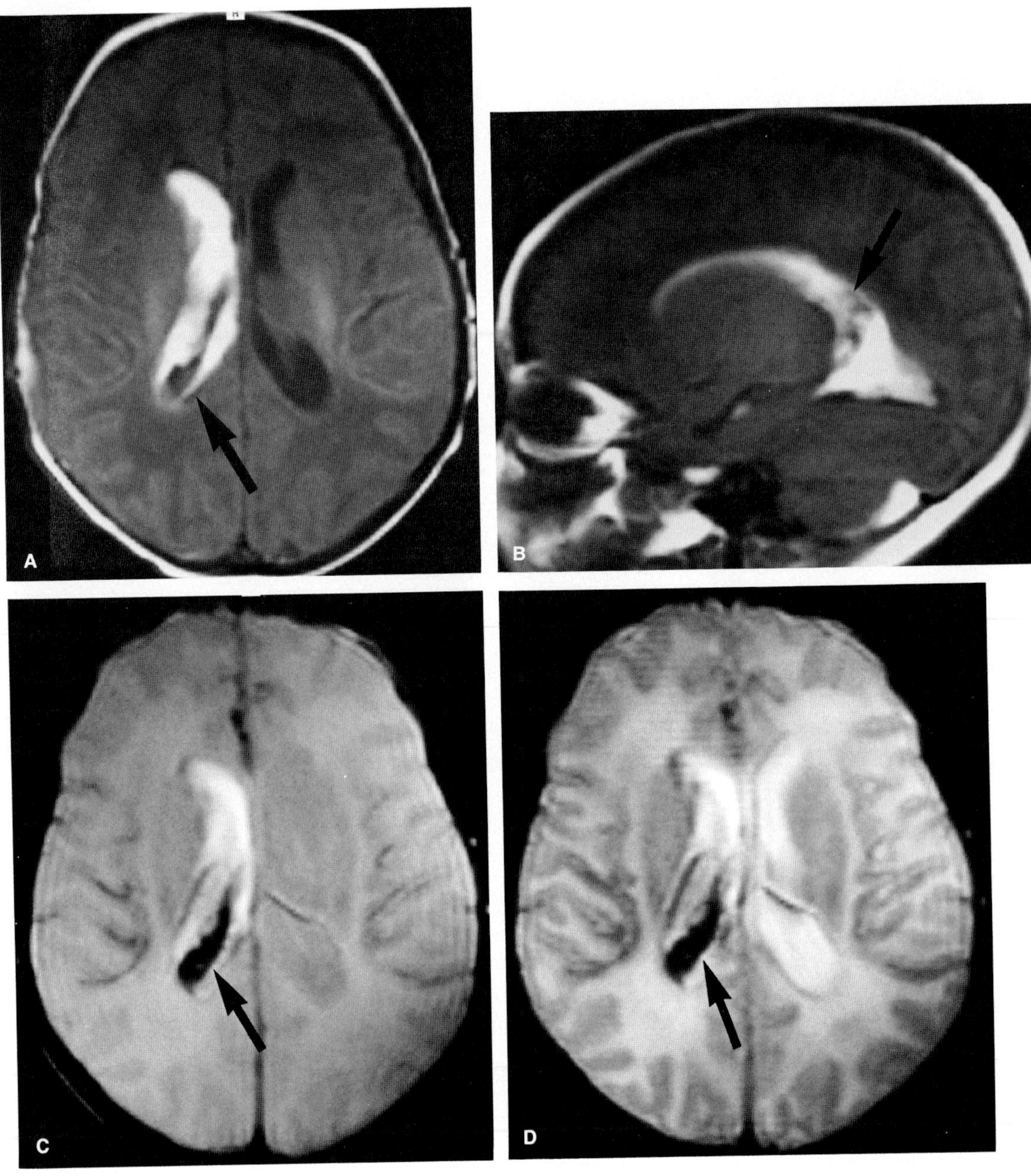

HISTORY

A 2-week-old, full-term infant with seizures. On the second day of life, the patient had an episode of apnea and cyanosis.

FINDINGS

T1-weighted axial (*A*) and sagittal (*B*) images demonstrate high signal intensity representing blood (extracellular methemoglobin) filling the frontal horn, body, atrium, and occipital horn of the right lateral ventricle. The blood has high signal intensity on the intermediate T2-weighted axial image (*C*), much higher than CSF, which is isointense to gray matter. (*D*) The blood is obscured by high-signal-intensity CSF on the heavily T2-weighted image. A portion of the clot (*black arrows in A to D*) has low signal intensity on all pulse sequences. (*E*) The maximum intensity projection (MIP) image obtained from a 3D TOF MRA demonstrates the clotted blood within the ventricle, in addition to flowing blood in the arterial system. (*F and G*) The raw images from the 3D MRA reveal that much of the ventricular cast is of high signal intensity, and thus reconstructed as a "vascular structure" on the MIP image.

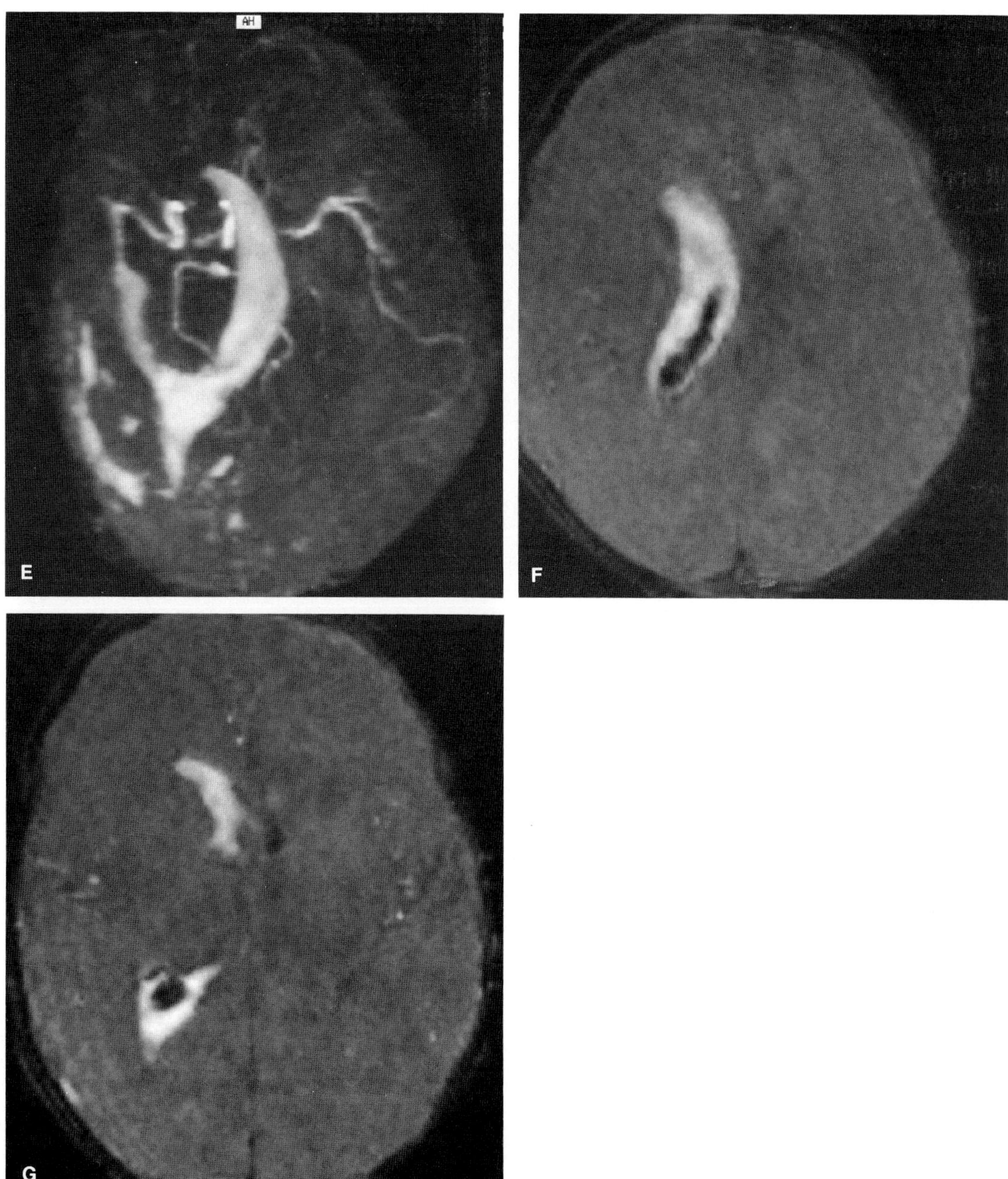

DIAGNOSIS

Intraventricular hemorrhage

DISCUSSION

Intraventricular hemorrhage (IVH) in newborn infants is most often the result of rupture of the ependyma caused by expansion of a subependymal germinal matrix bleed. The germinal matrix is a highly vascular, highly cellular, fragile growth zone of the developing fetal brain in the subependyma of the lateral ventricles. It is most prominent in the region of the caudate nucleus, the caudothalamic groove, and along the lateral walls of the ventricular bodies.[1] The germinal matrix decreases in size with increasing fetal age, usually with complete involution by 34 gestational weeks. Thus, most infants with germinal matrix hemorrhage (GMH) are born prematurely, at less than 32 weeks' gestation, and weigh less than 1500 g. IVH in premature and full-term infants can also be caused by hemorrhage into the choroid plexus.[2] Hypoxia, metabolic acidosis, and loss of autoregulation contribute to the development of GMH and IVH.

There are four grades of germinal matrix hemorrhage. The higher the grade, the worse the prognosis.

Grade I: Confined to the subependyma.
Grade II: Extends from the subependyma into a nondilated ventricle (IVH).
Grade III: IVH with ventricular dilatation.
Grade IV: IVH with associated parenchymal hemorrhage.

The MR appearance of intraventricular hemorrhage depends on its age. Extracellular methemoglobin (subacute hemorrhage) has high signal intensity on both T1- and T2-weighted images.

MR Technique

Extracellular methemoglobin has a very short T1 and long T2. As a result, it can have a high signal intensity on 3D TOF MRA despite the fact that it is stationary and nonflowing.

Pitfalls in Image Interpretation

Intraventricular extracellular methemoglobin can be obscured by the high signal intensity of CSF on heavily T2-weighted images.[3]

Clinical References

1. Nakamura Y, Okudera T, Fukuda S, et al. Germinal matrix hemorrhage of venous origin in preterm neonates. Hum Pathol 1990;21:1059–1062.
2. Leech R, Kohnen P. Subependymal and intraventricular hemorrhages in the newborn. Am J Pathol 1974;77:465–476.
3. McArdle C, Richardson C, Hayden C, et al. Abnormalities of the neonatal brain: MR imaging. Part I. Intracranial hemorrhage. Radiology 1987;163:387–394.

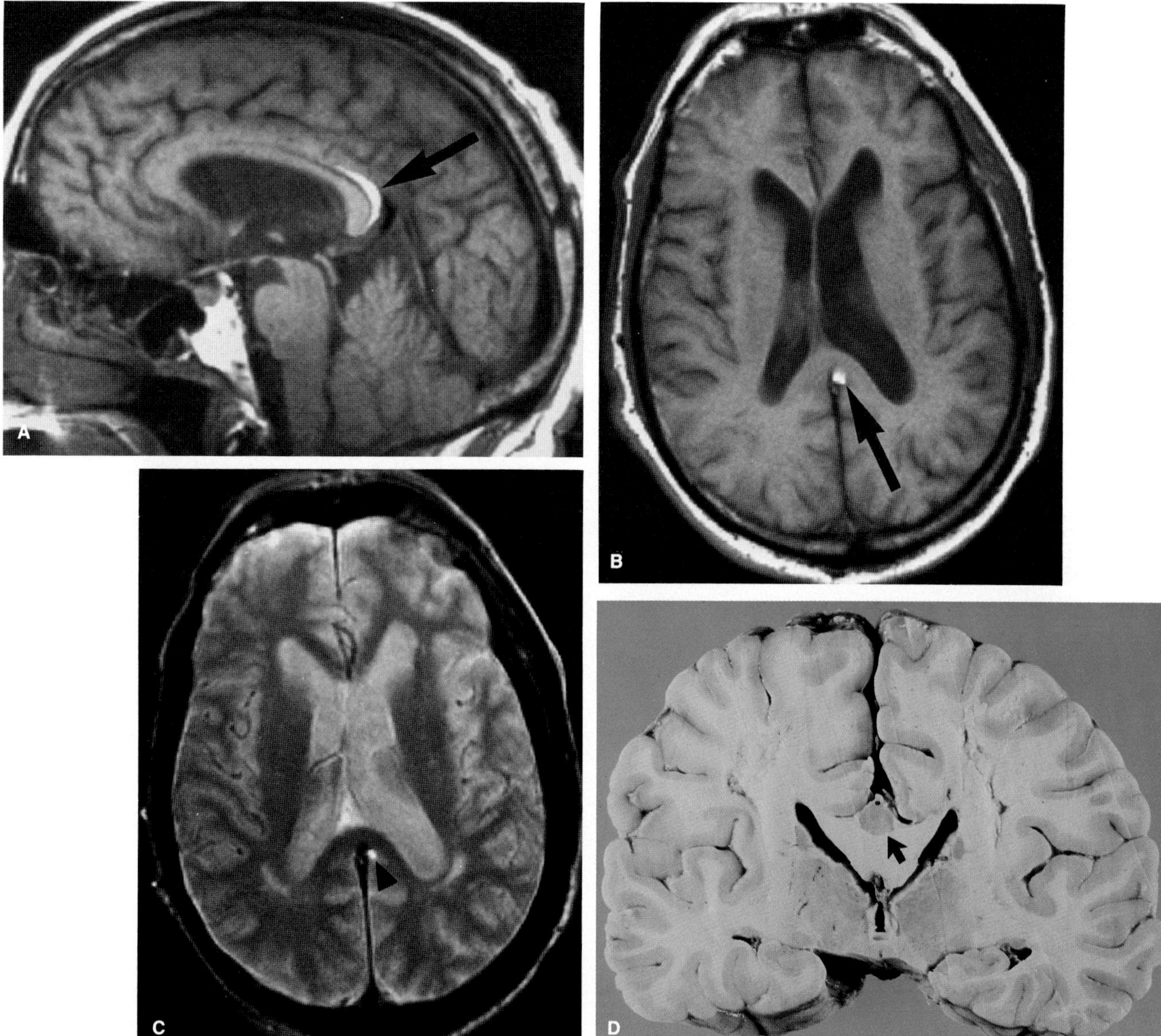

HISTORY

A 73-year-old patient with multiple myeloma, being evaluated for possible brain metastases

FINDINGS

Sagittal (*A*) and axial (*B*) T1-weighted images reveal a curvilinear lesion (*arrow*) of increased signal intensity adjacent to the splenium of the corpus callosum. (*C*) On the axial T2-weighted image the lesion (*arrowhead*) is identified to the left of the vein of Galen. On the T2-weighted image, the abnormal high signal intensity associated with this lesion appears displaced laterally as compared with the T1-weighted images, raising the question of chemical shift artifact. No abnormal contrast enhancement was noted (*images not shown*).

DIAGNOSIS

Interhemispheric lipoma

DISCUSSION

Intracranial lipomas are uncommon lesions, and tend to occur in specific, characteristic locations within the brain. They occur most frequently in the interhemispheric region, with the remainder occurring in the quadrigeminal, superior cerebellar, suprasellar, interpeduncular, cerebellopontine angle, and sylvian cisterns. In 55% of cases, they are associated with brain malformations. Intracranial nerves and vessels course through these masses rather than being displaced by them. Intracranial lipomas are generally asymptomatic and require no therapy.

The current theory is that intracranial lipomas are congenital malformations (not hamartomas or true neoplasms) that result from persistence and maldifferentiation of the meninx primitiva during the development of the subarachnoid cisterns. The meninx primitiva is a mesenchymal derivative of the neural crest. Normally, the meninx is resorbed as its extracellular space expands to create the subarachonid cisterns.[1]

Corpus callosal lipomas are associated with agenesis of the corpus callosum in about half of cases. They most frequently involve the genu of the corpus callosum, and are not uncommonly associated with frontal bone defects. Calcification is commonly noted on pathologic examination.

Lipomas demonstrate hyperintensity on T1-weighted images, and show progressive diminution of signal intensity (characteristic of fat) with increasing T2 weighting. Lipomas do not demonstrate enhancement with a gadolinium chelate. Because of their characteristic MR appearance, lipomas are seldom confused with other midline tumors.

Pitfalls in Image Interpretation

Colloid cysts are midline lesions that may have increased signal intensity on T1-weighted images and should not be confused with a lipoma.

Pathologic Correlate

(*D*) A lipoma (*black arrow*) is seen in a superior pericallosal location on gross brain coronal section at the level of the anterior horns of the lateral ventricles.

Clinical References

1. Truwit CL, Barkowich JA. Pathogenesis of intracranial lipoma: an MR study in 42 patients. AJNR 1990;11:665–674.

(D *courtesy of Daron G. Davis, MD.*)

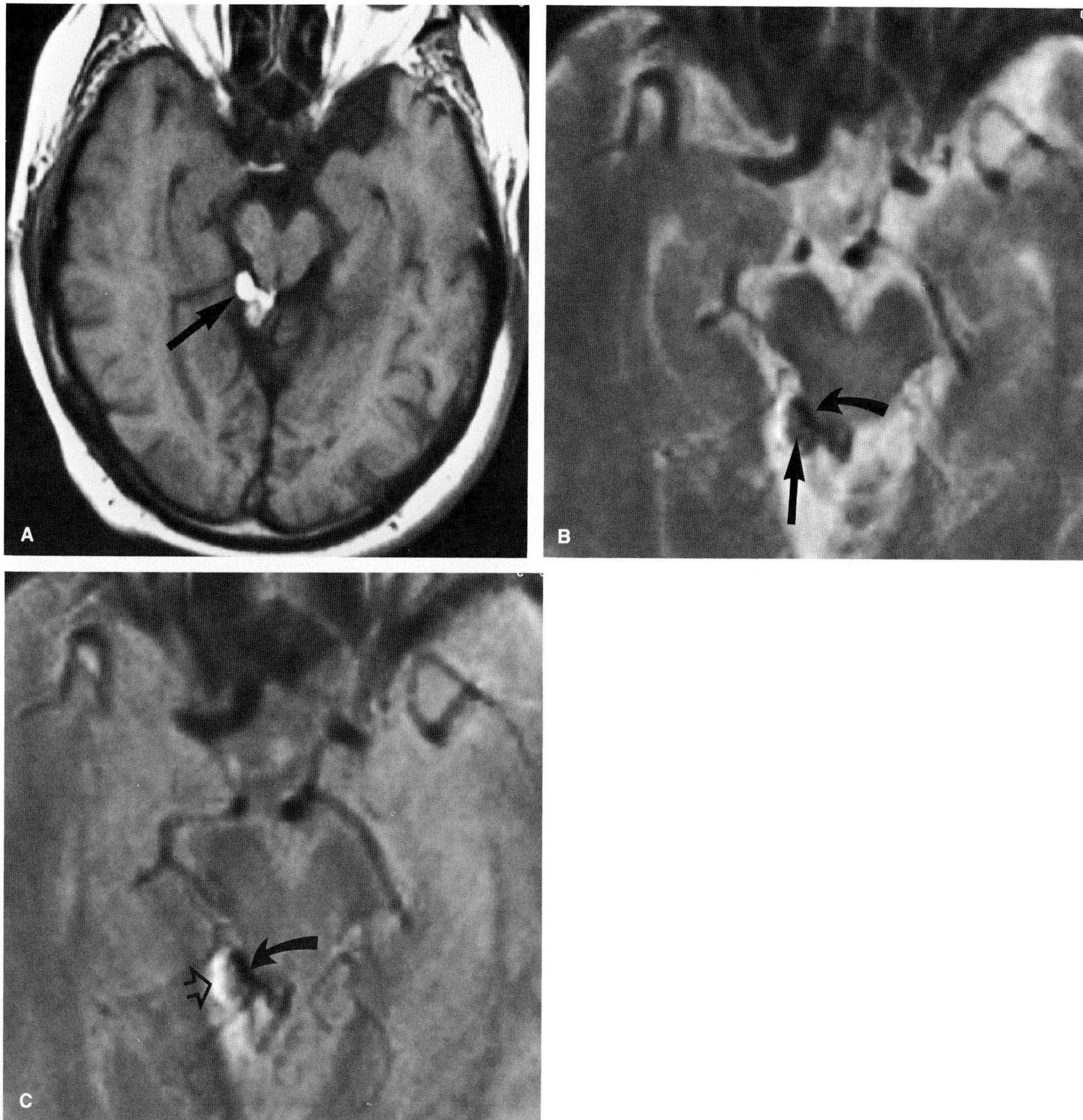

HISTORY

Noncontributory

FINDINGS

(*A*) Axial T1-weighted scan depicts abnormal hyperintensity (*arrow*) in the ambient cistern. (*B*) On a magnified view, at the same anatomic level, the T2-weighted (TE = 90 msec) image shows the lesion (*arrow*) appearing predominantly of intermediate signal intensity, although a dark line (*curved arrow*) can be noted along one border. (*C*) The magnified view from the first echo (TE = 45 msec) of the T2-weighted scan reveals artifactual hyperintensity (*open arrow*) on the right side of the lesion and hypointensity (*curved arrow*) on the left due to chemical shift in the frequency encoding direction.

DIAGNOSIS

Ambient cistern lipoma

DISCUSSION

As previously described, intracranial lipomas are rare developmental lesions and usually asymptomatic. The second most common location for an intracranial lipoma, as illustrated in this case, is the quadrigeminal plate or superior cerebellar cistern (also referred to as the ambient cistern), accounting for 25% of cases.[1] The most common location (45%) is interhemispheric. Less common sites include suprasellar or interpeduncular (14%), cerebellopontine angle (9%), and sylvian fissure (5%). Obstructive hydrocephalus, requiring CSF shunting, is a rare reported complication.[2]

The presence of chemical shift artifact, at the boundary between a lipoma and surrounding soft tissue or CSF, can be used to confirm the diagnosis of a fatty lesion on MR. This permits ready differentiation from other abnormalities that can have high signal intensity on T1-weighted scans (such as a hematoma). Chemical shift artifacts are seen only in the frequency encoding axis, with the magnitude of effect dependent on field strength and imaging bandwidth.[3]

Pitfalls in Image Interpretation

Although falx calcification per se is rarely visualized on MR, falx ossification is commonly seen, particularly in the elderly population. The marrow within such an ossification demonstrates signal characteristics similar to fat, with high signal intensity on T1-weighted images, surrounded by low-signal-intensity cortical bone. This appearance should not be confused with an interhemispheric lipoma, which is much less common.[4]

Clinical References

1. Truwit CL, Barkovich AJ. Pathogenesis of intracranial lipoma: an MR study in 42 patients. AJR 1990;155:855–864.
2. Maiuri F, Cirillo S, Simonetti I, et al. Intracranial lipomas: diagnostic and therapeutic considerations. J Neurosurg Sci 1988;32:161–167.
3. Smith AS, Weinstein MA, Hurst GC, et al. Intracranial chemical-shift artifacts on MR images of the brain: observations and relation to sampling bandwidth. AJR 1990;154:1275–1283.
4. Lee DH, Larson TC, Norman D. Falx ossification: MR visualization. Can Assoc Radiol J 1988;39:260–262.

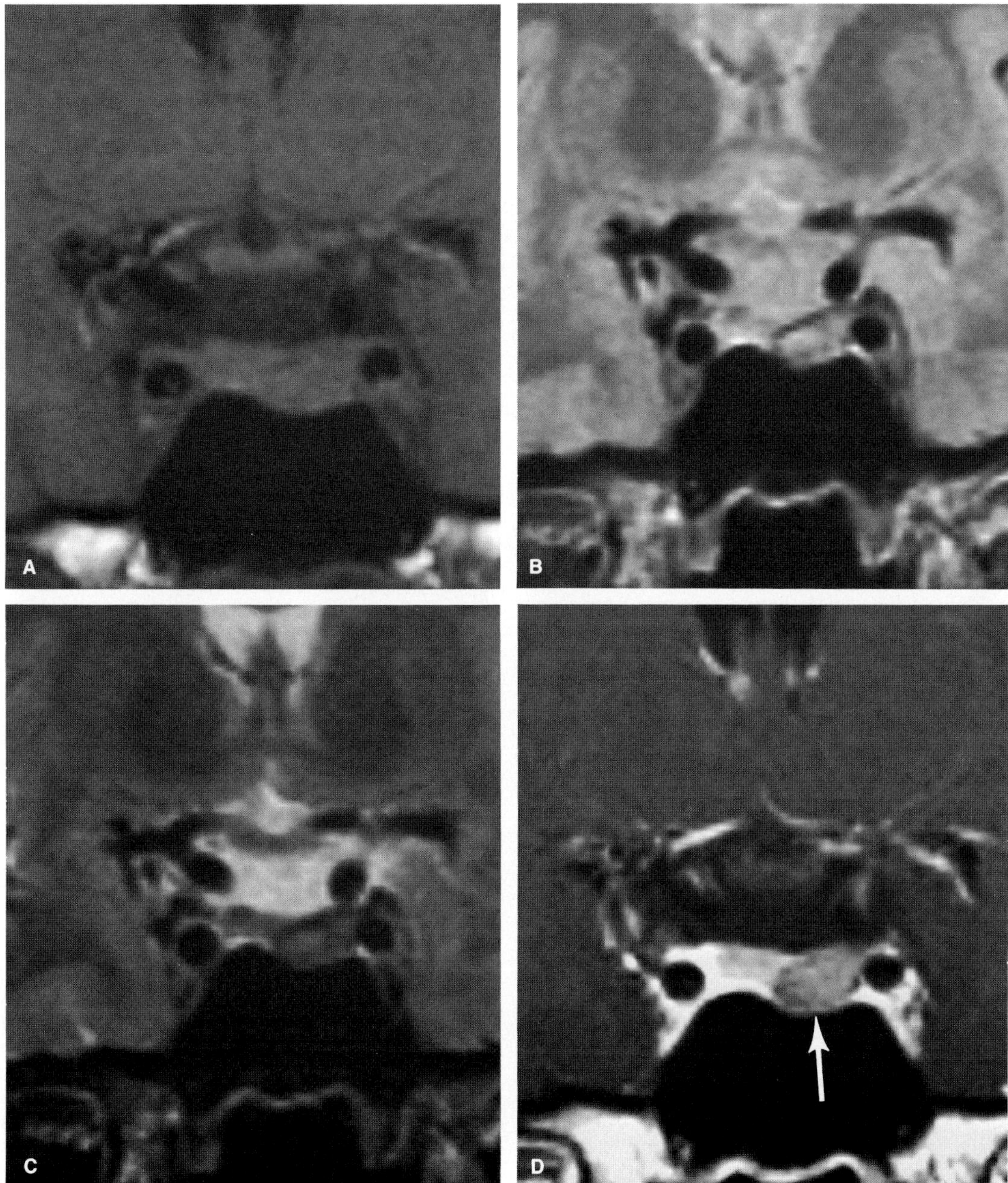

HISTORY

A 28-year-old woman with irregular menses, galactorrhea, and a prolactin level of 135 μg/L

FINDINGS

(*A*) A thin-section (3-mm) coronal T1-weighted image shows slight asymmetry of the pituitary gland and sellar floor, raising the question of a space occupying mass on the left. There is slight inhomogeneity in signal intensity of the pituitary on both intermediate (TR/TE = 3000/45) (*B*) and heavily (TR/TE = 3000/90) (*C*) T2-weighted images, also acquired with a 3-mm slice thickness. (*D*) The immediate postcontrast (0.1 mmol/kg) coronal T1-weighted image reveals a large left-sided pituitary microadenoma (*arrow*), with greater enhancement of the pituitary and cavernous sinus as compared with the lesion itself.

DIAGNOSIS

Pituitary microadenoma (prolactinoma)

DISCUSSION

After IV contrast administration, there is immediate prominent enhancement of the normal infundibulum, anterior pituitary, and cavernous sinus.[1] Maximum enhancement occurs within 1 to 2 minutes of injection, followed by a gradual decrease in signal enhancement. Conversely, pituitary adenomas (both microadenomas and macroadenomas) demonstrate a later peak of enhancement with slower washout.[2] Thus, dynamic scans or early postcontrast conventional thin-section SE imaging can be used to improve differentiation between the normal gland and a pituitary adenoma. Use of this diagnostic approach improves not only detection of pituitary microadenomas but also identification of the displaced pituitary gland with large macroadenomas.

In a study of 11 patients with surgical confirmation in all cases, a microadenoma was detected in 3 patients only after contrast enhancement.[1] Tumor delineation was improved by contrast administration in an additional two cases. One false-positive examination and one false-negative examination (the latter despite the use of both precontrast and postcontrast imaging) were also reported. Delayed postcontrast scans (obtained at 30 minutes after injection) were of no additional benefit.

MR is considerably more sensitive (approximately twofold) than CT for detection of pituitary microadenomas,[3] a conclusion strongly supported by the scientific literature, although isolated reports exist with positive CT and false-negative MR. The two modalities equally demonstrate infundibular displacement, sellar floor abnormality, and focal gland convexity. Thin-section T2-weighted imaging at high field (with good S/N) can be used to detect some microadenomas that are not well demonstrated on the precontrast T1-weighted examination alone.

Prolactinomas are the most common secretory pituitary lesion, with 90% of patients being women. Presenting symptoms include irregular menses, amenorrhea, and galactorrhea. A serum prolactin level above 300 μg/L is diagnostic, with levels above 100 μg/L in a nonpregnant patient typically due to an adenoma. Dopamine agonist drugs, such as bromocriptine, are effective in lowering prolactin levels. When indicated, bromocriptine is the therapy of choice for patients with a prolactin-secreting microadenoma.

MR Technique

Immediate postcontrast coronal T1-weighted imaging is the most sensitive MR technique for detection of intrasellar lesions.[1] A complete examination should consist of thin-section (less than or equal to 3 mm) precontrast sagittal and coronal T1-weighted, coronal T2-weighted, and postcontrast coronal T1-weighted scans. A small field-of-view (20 to 25 cm) is also mandatory for high in-plane spatial resolution. Successful pituitary imaging for microadenomas can only be performed at this time at high field (1 to 1.5 T), where sufficient S/N is available.

Pitfalls in Image Interpretation

MR has not been proved to be either 100% sensitive or 100% accurate for demonstration of pituitary microadenomas. The differential diagnosis for an intrasellar lesion includes a Rathke's cleft cyst, a midline embryonic remnant that is usually small and asymptomatic.

Clinical References

1. Newton DR, Dillon WP, Norman D, et al. Gd-DTPA-enhanced MR imaging of pituitary adenomas. AJNR 1989; 10:949–954.
2. Miki Y, Matsuo M, Nishizawa S, et al. Pituitary adenomas and normal pituitary tissue: enhancement patterns on gadopentetate-enhanced MR imaging. Radiology 1990;177:35–38.
3. Kulkarni MV, Lee KF, McArdle CB, et al. 1.5-T MR imaging of pituitary microadenomas: technical considerations and CT correlation. AJNR 1988;9:5–11.

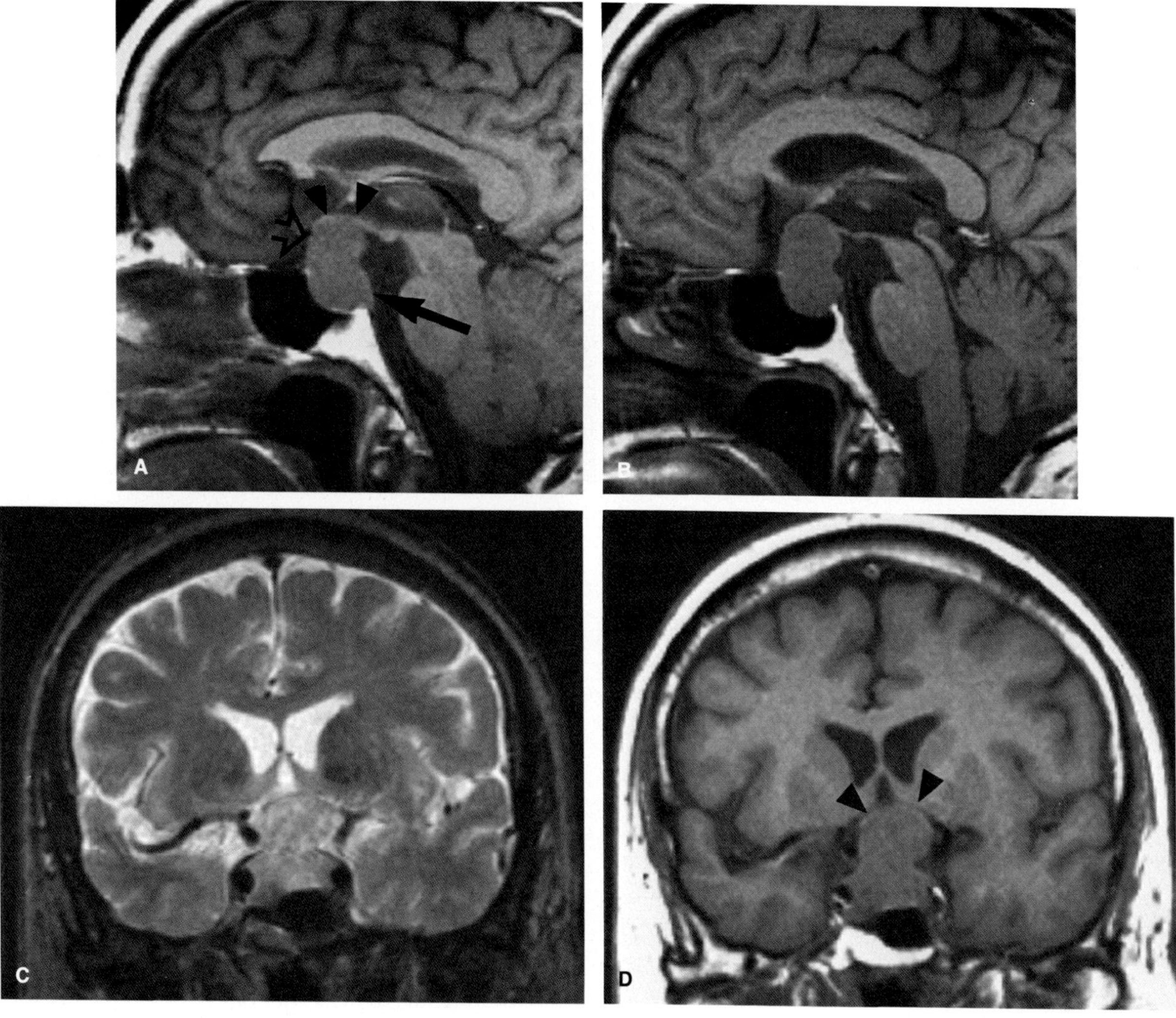

HISTORY

A 75-year-old patient with adrenal insufficiency and decreased peripheral vision

FINDINGS

Precontrast sagittal T1-weighted (*A and B*), coronal T2-weighted (*C*), coronal T1-weighted (*D*), and postcontrast coronal T1-weighted (*E*) images are presented. The slice thickness was 3 mm for all images. A large soft tissue mass (*arrow in A*) is noted expanding the sella with suprasellar extent (*open arrow in A*). The optic chiasm (*arrowheads in A and D*) is compressed and splayed by the mass. The lesion is isointense with brain on both T1- and T2-weighted images precontrast and displays fairly uniform enhancement (increasing its conspicuity) following IV administration of a gadolinium chelate.

DIAGNOSIS

Pituitary macroadenoma

DISCUSSION

MR is superior to CT for identification of infundibular and focal diaphragma sellae abnormalities, cavernous sinus invasion, and optic chiasm compression.[1] On this basis, MR has become the technique of choice for study of patients in whom a pituitary macroadenoma is suspected.

Tumors that are large at the time of diagnosis are frequently nonsecretory and present with pressure symptoms, in particular hypopituitarism and visual loss. The optic chiasm lies superior and anterior to the pituitary gland, with the most common visual field defect in a patient with a pituitary macroadenoma being bitemporal hemianopsia. Macroadenomas are defined as lesions

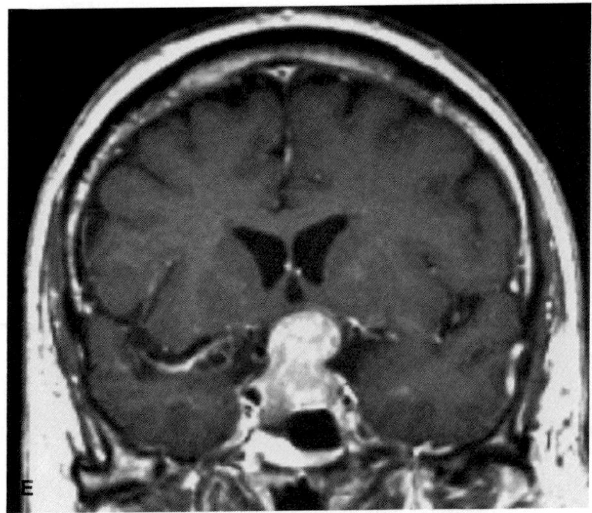

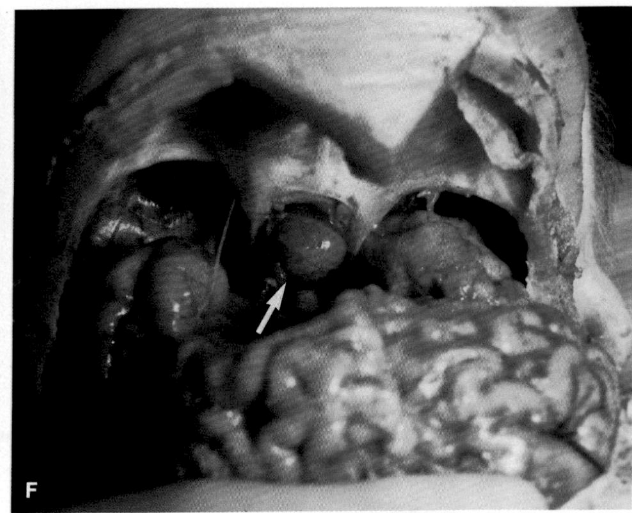

greater than 10 mm in diameter. Approximately 25% of pituitary adenomas that come to surgery are nonsecretory.

The patient in this case underwent transsphenoidal resection of the lesion without complication.

MR Technique

The imaging protocol for the sella region should include thin-section (2 to 3 mm) precontrast and postcontrast sagittal and coronal images, providing tumor localization and margin definition.

Pathologic Correlate

(*F*) Gross specimen (viewed from above with the frontal lobes retracted) shows a small macroadenoma (*white arrow*) seen extending into the suprasellar cistern. Suprasellar extension is always preceded by expansion of the sella, with the tumor often being dumbbell-shaped as a result of constriction by the diaphragma sellae and circle of Willis. The direction of expansion is usually midline, with the lesion confined by a capsule formed of the leptomeninges.

Clinical References

1. Davis PC, Hoffman JC, Spencer T, et al. MR imaging of pituitary adenoma: CT, clinical, and surgical correlation. AJR 1987;148:797–802.

(F *courtesy of Daron G. Davis, MD.*)

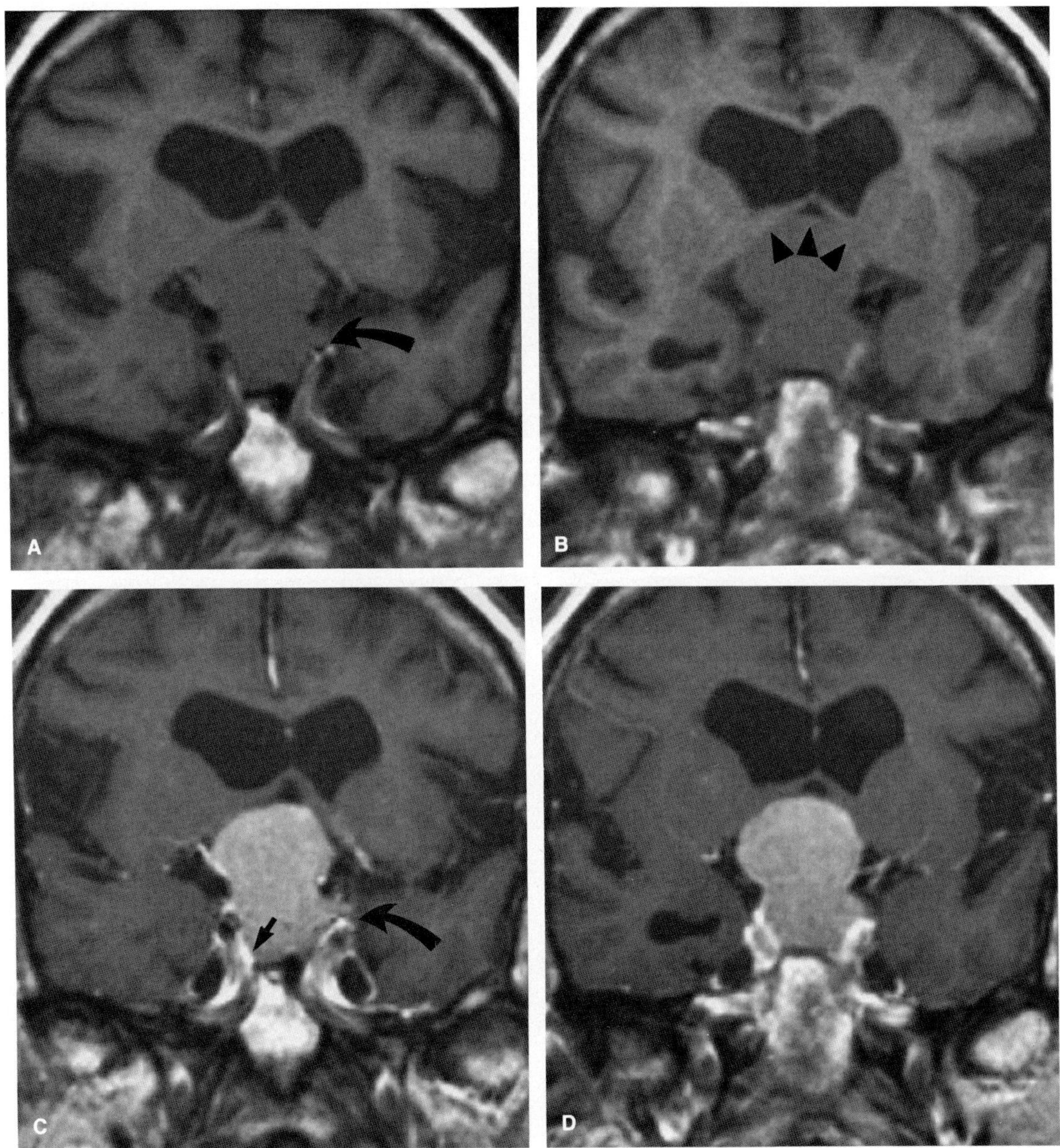

HISTORY

A 72-year-old with decreased visual acuity and loss of lateral visual fields

FINDINGS

(*A to D*) The preoperative MR sequence demonstrates a large pituitary mass with suprasellar extension. The lesion is isointense to gray matter on precontrast T1-weighted scans (*A and B*), with homogeneous enhancement postcontrast (*C and D*). The optic chiasm (*arrowheads in B*) is markedly thinned, and appears draped over the mass, an observation best made on the precontrast scans. There is apparent invasion of the left cavernous sinus by the mass (*curved arrow in A*), with partial encasement of the left cavernous carotid noted on the precontrast scans. This finding is confirmed postcontrast, with differential enhancement of venous blood (*small arrow in C*) and neoplastic tissue (*curved arrow in C*), the former being more intense.

(*E to J*) On the first postoperative scan (*E* and *F*—precontrast T1; *G* and *H*—postcontrast T1; *I* and *J*—precontrast T2 with TE = 90 msec), residual tumor is noted anteriorly (*arrows in E and G*), although the bulk of the tumor has been successfully resected. Residual tumor (*curved arrows in F and H*) can also be seen within the left cavernous sinus. Abnormal hyperintensity (*open arrow in F*) is seen within the sella on the T1-weighted examination, representing the fat graft placed at surgery. The optic chiasm (*arrow in F*) has returned to a more

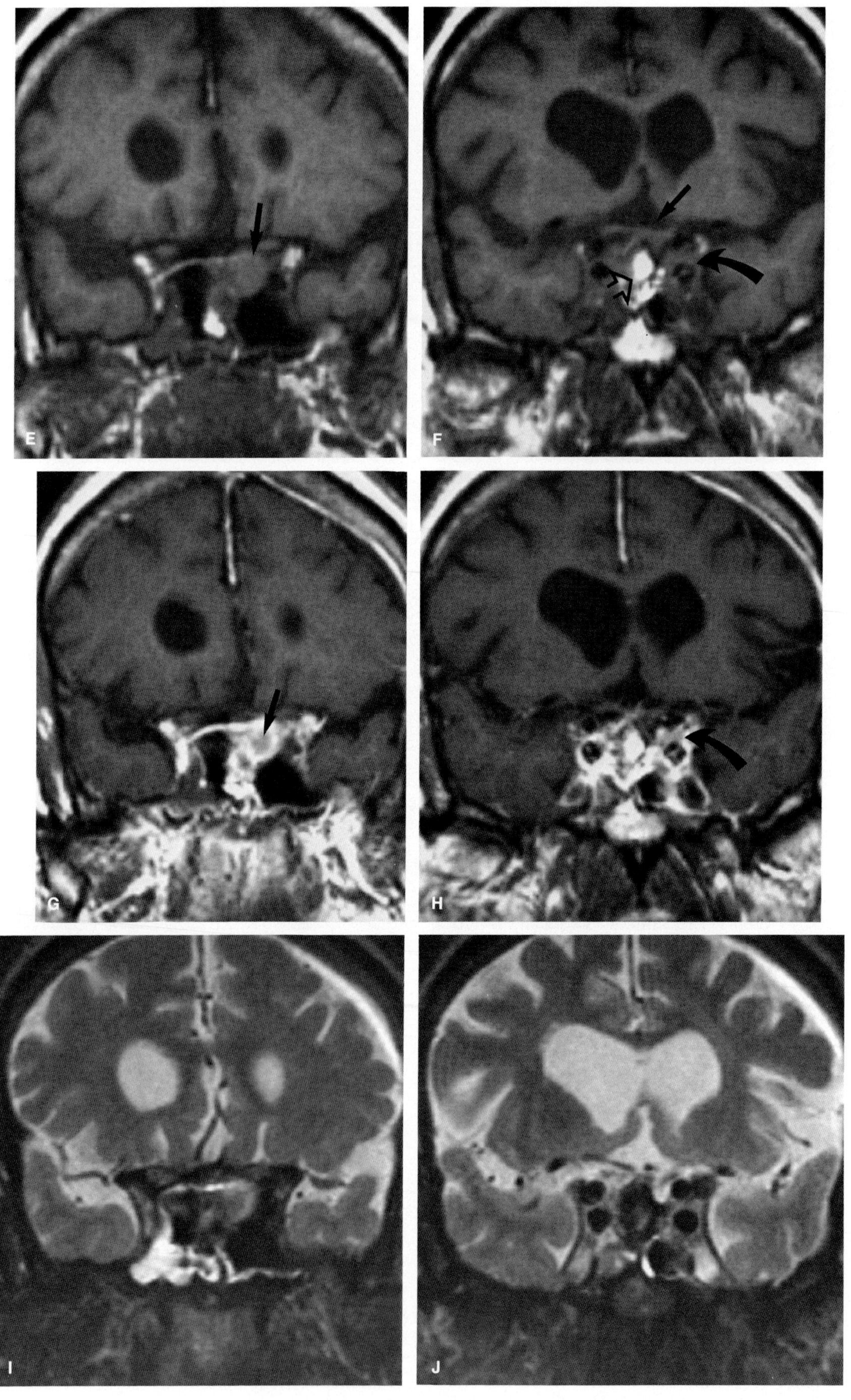
E
F
G
H
I
J

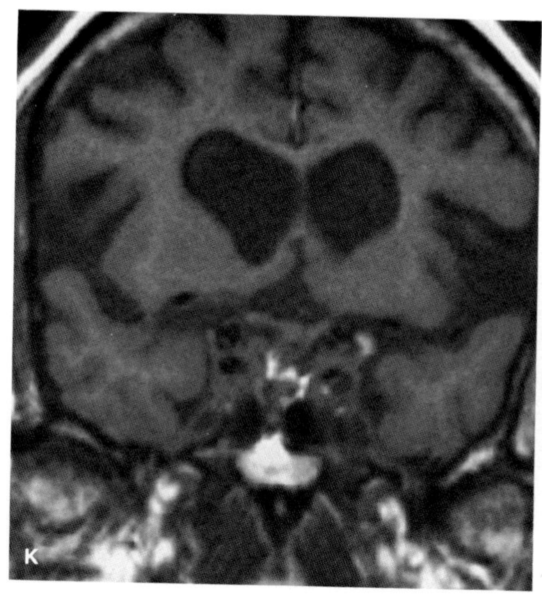

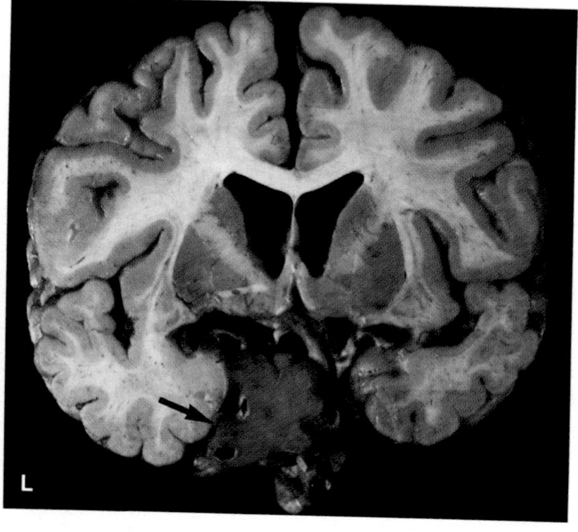

normal position and configuration. The T2-weighted examination (*I and J*) is of high quality but adds little information. (*K*) By the time of the second postoperative examination 6 months later, little remains of the fat graft placed at surgery.

DIAGNOSIS

Pituitary macroadenoma with cavernous sinus invasion, preoperative and postoperative appearances

DISCUSSION

MR is the preferred modality, as compared with CT, for the evaluation of pituitary macroadenomas.[1] The superiority of MR is greatest in the demonstration of tumor relation to the carotids and optic chiasm, cavernous sinus invasion, and tumoral hemorrhage.

Cavernous sinus invasion by a pituitary macroadenoma is not uncommon. On unenhanced MR, the medial wall of the cavernous sinus cannot be consistently identified, with unilateral carotid artery encasement being the only reliable sign of sinus invasion.[2] However, contrast administration facilitates depiction of cavernous sinus invasion as a result of differential enhancement between tumor and venous blood.[3]

Pituitary apoplexy (*not illustrated*) is caused by sudden infarction, either bland or hemorrhagic in nature, within a normal gland or a pituitary tumor. With sudden enlargement of the pituitary, compression of adjacent structures occurs, producing characteristic signs and symptoms. MR is more sensitive than CT for detection of subacute hemorrhage (occurring greater than 12 hours after onset of symptoms) within the pituitary gland.[4] Intratumoral hemorrhage can also be seen unaccompanied by clinical evidence of apoplexy.

Large pituitary adenomas that secrete prolactin are likely to benefit from medical therapy. Bromocriptine, a dopamine agonist, can be used to induce shrinkage, which is typically complete after 8 weeks of therapy. For lesions with low prolactin levels, surgery is advised for decompression (particularly if vision is impaired) and histologic diagnosis.[5]

In the postoperative case, MR has also been shown to be superior to CT. MR can identify residual tumor tissue, permits differentiation of surgical packing from adenomatous tissue, and better delineates abnormalities of the infundibulum, diaphragma sellae, and chiasm.[6]

MR Technique

IV contrast enhancement is recommended for improved delineation of a pituitary macroadenoma from surrounding structures, and in particular for improved definition of cavernous sinus invasion.

Pitfalls in Image Interpretation

An intrasellar meningioma can simulate a pituitary macroadenoma. Nonvisualization of the diaphragma sellae and elevated prolactin levels do not exclude a nonpituitary neoplasm.[7]

Pathologic Correlate

(*L*) A large macroadenoma with invasion of the cavernous sinus (*black arrow*) is seen on this gross coronal specimen. Lateral encroachment on the cavernous sinus is more common than suprasellar extension. In this instance, the dural capsule of the gland is often breached. There can be pressure on the cranial nerves within the cavernous sinus, which may be either encased or stretched by the lesion.

Clinical References

1. Lundin P, Bergstrom K, Thuomas KA, et al. Comparison of MR imaging and CT in pituitary macroadenomas. Acta Radiol 1991;32:189–196.
2. Johnsen DE, Woodruff WW, Allen IS, et al. MR imaging of the sellar and juxtasellar regions. Radiographics 1991; 11:727–758.
3. Nakamura T, Schorner W, Bittner RC, Felix R. The value of paramagnetic contrast agent gadolinium-DTPA in the diagnosis of pituitary adenomas. Neuroradiology 1988;30:481–486.
4. Onesti ST, Wisniewski T, Post KD. Clinical versus subclinical pituitary apoplexy: presentation, surgical management, and outcome in 21 patients. Neurosurgery 1990;26:980–986.
5. Bevan JS. Interpreting prolactin levels: implications for the management of large pituitary lesions. Br J Neurosurg 1991;5:3–6.
6. Candrina R, Gasparotti R, Galli G, et al. Comparison between computed tomography and magnetic resonance imaging in the postoperative evaluation of acromegalic patients. Rec Prog Med 1991;82:509–513.
7. Michael AS, Paige ML. MR imaging of intrasellar meningiomas simulating pituitary adenomas. J Comput Assist Tomogr 1988;12:944–946.

(L courtesy of Daron G. Davis, MD.)

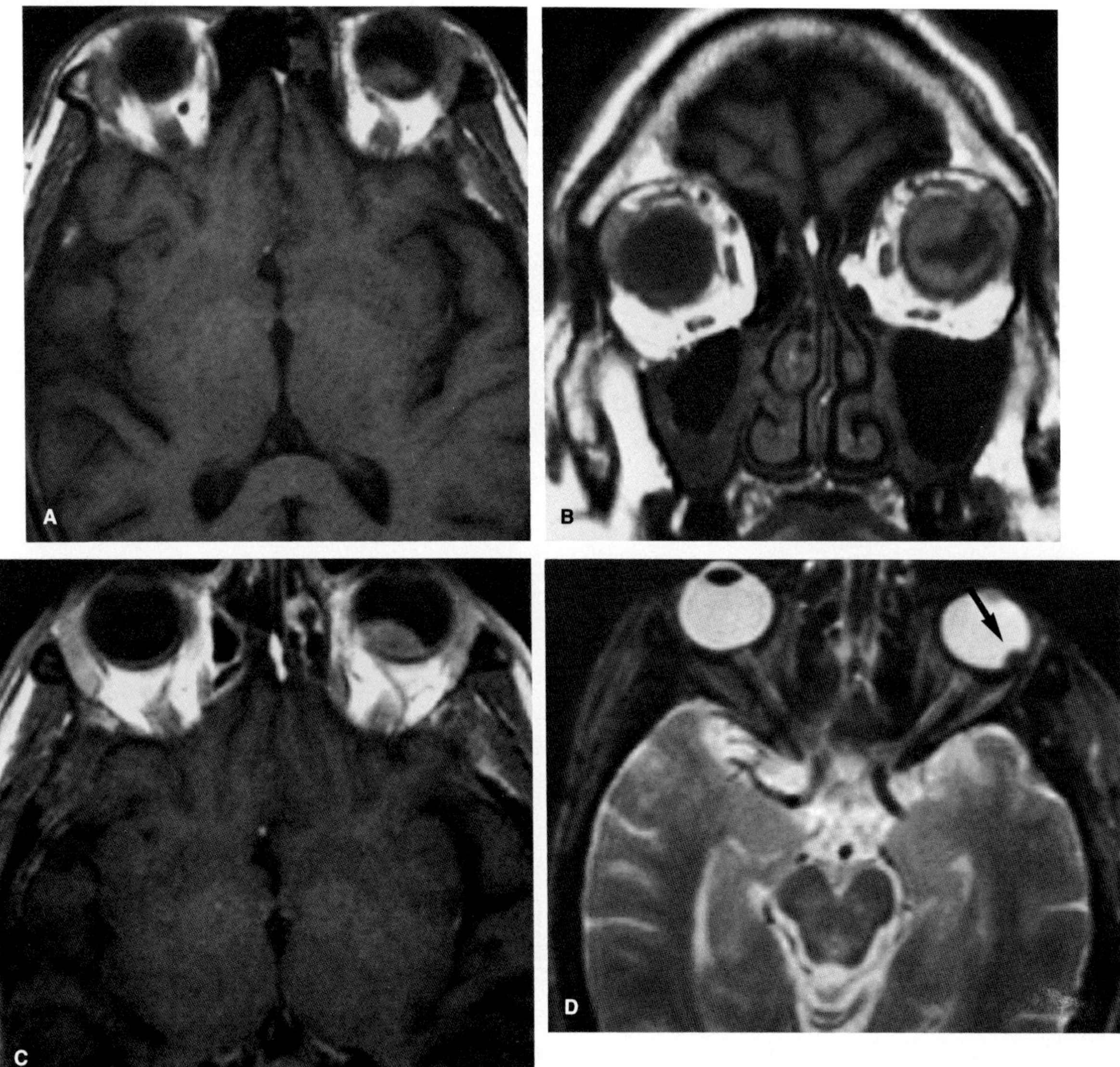

HISTORY

Patient with a 4-week history of decreased visual acuity in the left eye

FINDINGS

T1-weighted axial (*A*) and coronal (*B*) images demonstrate a soft tissue mass within the posterior left globe. The mass is contiguous with the retina, and does not extend beyond the globe. The signal intensity of the lesion on T1-weighted images is greater than gray matter and much greater than the surrounding vitreous. (*C*) The mass enhances homogeneously on the postcontrast T1-weighted axial image. (*D*) The T2-weighted axial image in a different patient shows a smaller, similar lesion (*black arrow*) that has very low signal intensity compared with the adjacent vitreous.

DIAGNOSIS

Ocular melanoma

DISCUSSION

Uveal tract (choroid, ciliary body, iris) melanoma is the most common primary intraocular neoplasm in adults. The peak age incidence is around 50 years. Ocular melanoma is uncommon in children. Ocular melanoma is

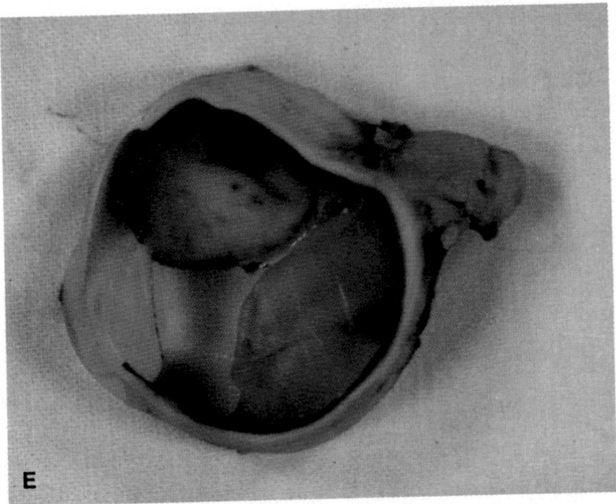

almost always unilateral and patients present with decreased visual acuity or pain. Associated retinal detachment is common.

Ocular tumors are usually initially diagnosed by ophthalmoscopy. Although it is highly sensitive, ophthalmoscopy is often nonspecific and cannot distinguish melanoma from retinal detachment or from other neoplasms. The main role of MR in intraocular masses is to characterize pathology and to determine the extent of tumor.

Melanotic melanomas have a characteristic signal-intensity pattern on MR, which is attributed to the paramagnetic properties of stable free-radicals within melanin.[1] These tumors are markedly hyperintense on T1-weighted images, and markedly hypointense on T2-weighted images relative to the normal vitreous.[2] Subretinal fluid associated with a retinal detachment has very high signal intensity on T2-weighted images and is readily distinguished from melanoma, allowing for accurate measurement of tumor size.[2]

Pitfalls in Image Interpretation

The only intraocular tumors that may have the same signal-intensity characteristics as melanotic melanoma are the choroidal nevus, which also contains melanin, and retinoblastoma.[2] Retinoblastoma occurs mainly in children, and contains calcification on CT in nearly all cases. Amelanotic melanoma has a nonspecific signal-intensity pattern and cannot be differentiated from other ocular neoplasms, such as metastases.

Pathologic Correlate

(*E*) Sagittal gross section shows two large ocular melanomas with associated retinal detachment. Ocular melanomas occur most commonly in the choroid, which is a highly vascular tissue located between the retina and the sclera.

Clinical References

1. Gomori J, Grossman R, Shields J, et al. Choroidal melanomas: correlation of NMR spectroscopy and MR imaging. Radiology 1986;158:443–445.
2. Peyster R, Augsburger J, Shields J, et al. Intraocular tumors: evaluation with MR imaging. Radiology 1988;168:773–779.

(E courtesy of Daron G. Davis, MD.)

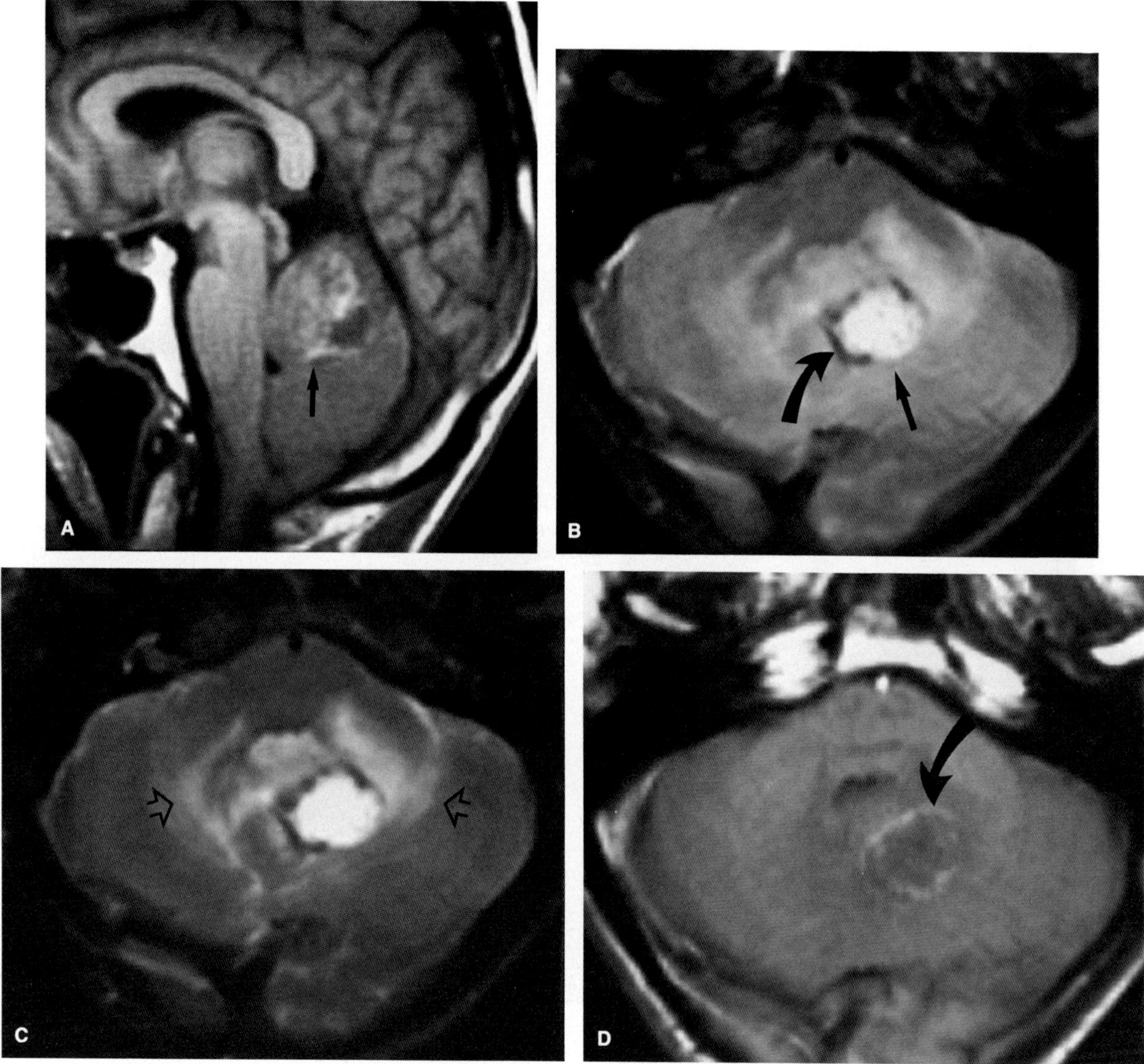

HISTORY

A 49-year-old patient with excision of a bulky tumor in the right axilla 3 months before the current examination. Presenting symptoms at this time include nausea, vomiting, weight loss, and general fatigue.

FINDINGS

(*A*) The midline sagittal T1-weighted image reveals a mass (*arrow*) with mixed low and high signal intensity in the superior cerebellum. On intermediate (*B*) and heavily (*C*) T2-weighted images the lesion (*arrow in B*) is principally hyperintense, with an incomplete rim of hypointensity (*curved arrow in B*) and extensive edema with high signal intensity (*open arrows in C*) in the white matter of both cerebellar hemispheres. (*D*) The precontrast T1-weighted axial examination reveals effacement of the fourth ventricle and a faint rim of hyperintensity (*curved arrow in D*) partially surrounding the mass. Inhomogeneous lesion enhancement is noted on postcontrast axial (*E*) and coronal (*F*) T1-weighted images. Extension of the lesion to the tentorium is seen on the coronal image. A second small enhancing nodule was noted in the left temporal lobe (*images not shown*).

DIAGNOSIS

Metastatic melanoma

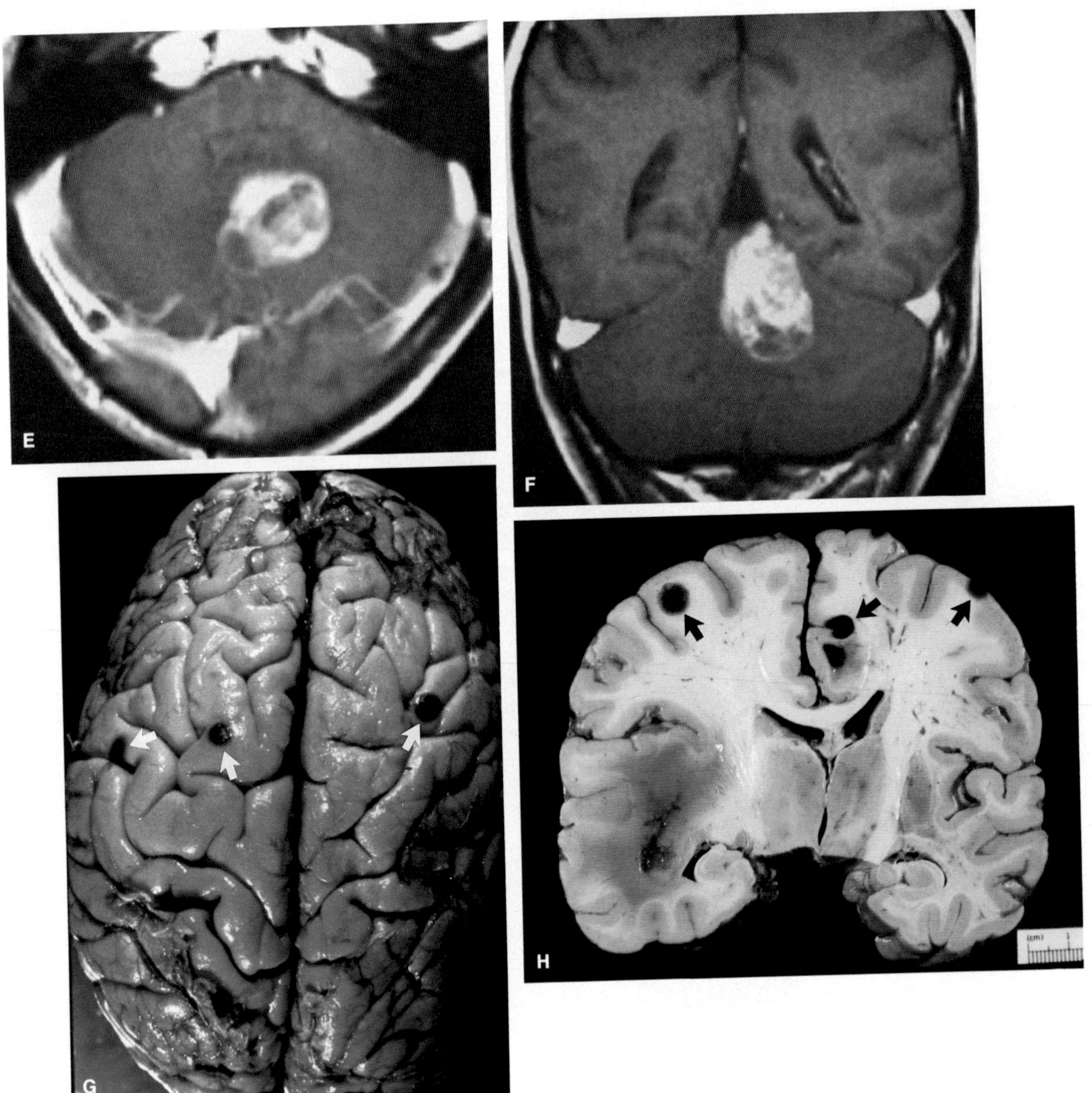

DISCUSSION

In metastatic brain deposits due to melanoma, either melanin or hemorrhage (or both) may be present. Both could potentially influence the observed signal intensity of the lesion on MR. It has been reported, on the basis of limited histologic data, that nonhemorrhagic melanotic melanoma has a distinctive (but not unique) MR appearance, with marked hyperintensity on T1-weighted images resulting from the paramagnetic effect of melanin.[1,2] Hemorrhagic melanoma metastases have a variable appearance on T1- and T2-weighted images, depending on the blood products which are present.[2]

For the present case, there are no specific differentiating features with respect to pathologic diagnosis, other than the evidence for hemorrhage. The rim of high signal intensity on the T1-weighted examination likely represents methemoglobin, whereas the low-signal-intensity rim on the T2-weighted images may represent deoxyhemoglobin, intracellular methemoglobin, or hemosiderin (and ferritin). The rim seen in *D* does not correspond exactly to that on the T2-weighted images.

The posterior fossa mass in this patient was surgically resected and the temporal lobe lesion treated by stereotactic radiation (gamma knife). Despite the predominantly intermediate signal intensity on precontrast T1-weighted scans, microscopic examination of the tumor revealed melanin pigment. The patient died 2 months later of disseminated systemic disease.

Pitfalls in Image Interpretation

In addition to melanoma, many other metastatic tumors can show evidence of hemorrhage, including commonly renal cell carcinoma, bronchogenic carcinoma, thyroid carcinoma, and choriocarcinoma.

Pathologic Correlate

Whole brain (*G*) and coronal autopsy specimens (*H*) reveal multiple brain metastases (*arrows*) from melanoma. Melanoma typically produces lesions that are both pigmented and grossly hemorrhagic. In certain instances, melanin may be absent or sparse. Metastases in general appear sharply marginated at surgery.

Clinical References

1. Uozumi A, Saegusa T, Ohsato K, Yamaura A. Computed tomography and magnetic resonance imaging of nonhemorrhagic, metastatic melanoma of the brain—case report. Neurol Med Chir (Tokyo) 1990;30:143–146.
2. Atlas SW, Grossman RI, Gomori JM, et al. MR imaging of intracranial metastatic melanoma. J Comput Assist Tomogr 1987;11:577–582.

(*G and* H *courtesy of Daron G. Davis, MD.*)

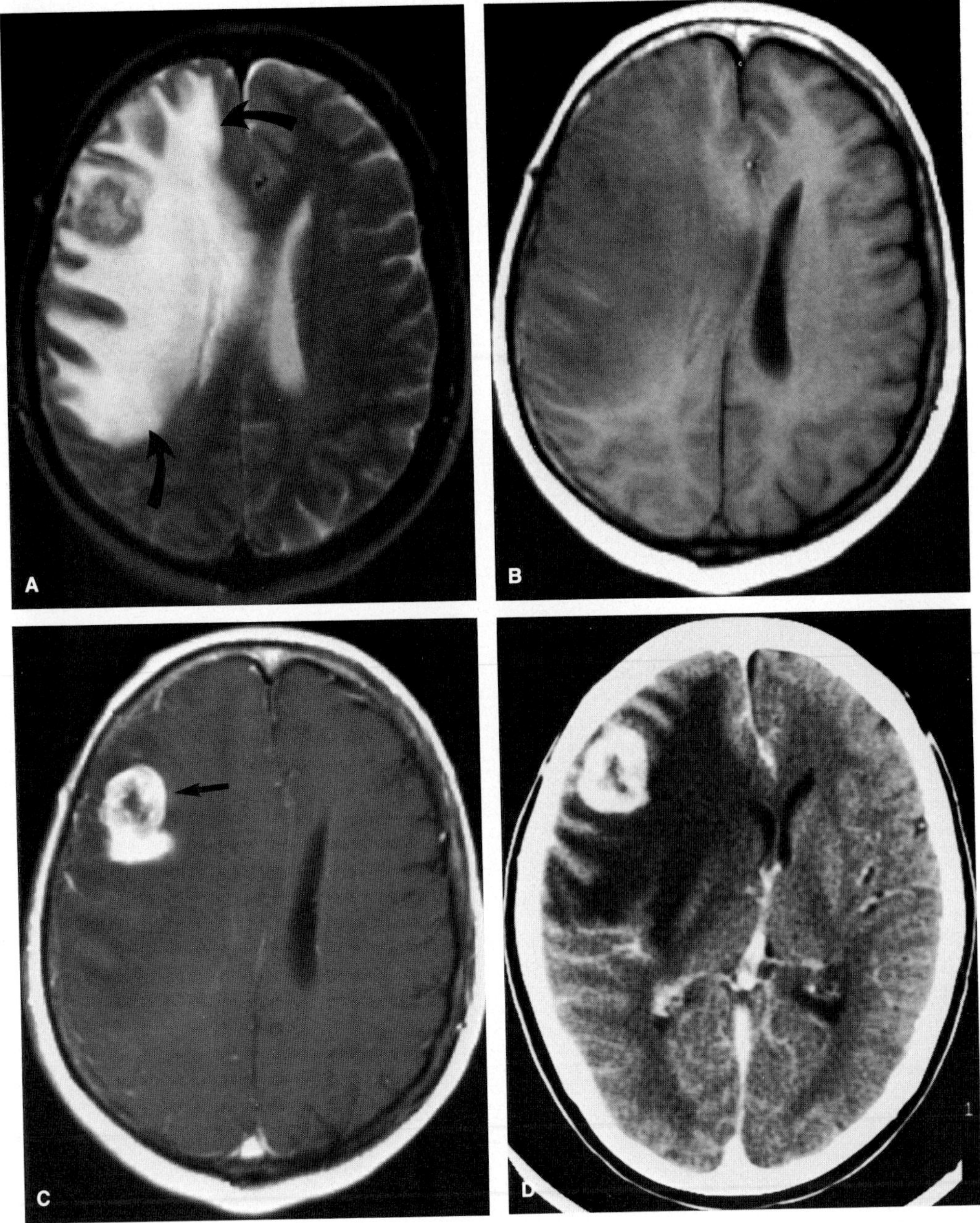

HISTORY

A 64-year-old woman with a 2-week history of right frontal headaches, new onset of left face, arm, and leg weakness, and a history of smoking

FINDINGS

Precontrast T2-weighted (*A*) and T1-weighted (*B*) images and a postcontrast T1-weighted image (*C*) are presented for interpretation. A 2 × 2 cm ring enhancing right frontal lobe brain mass (*arrow in C*) is noted with significant associated edema (*curved arrows in A*), compression of the right lateral ventricle, and shift of the midline structures. The lesion and surrounding edema are also well depicted by enhanced CT (*D*). (*E*) Chest radiograph reveals a large left-upper-lobe mass.

DIAGNOSIS

Metastatic large cell lung carcinoma

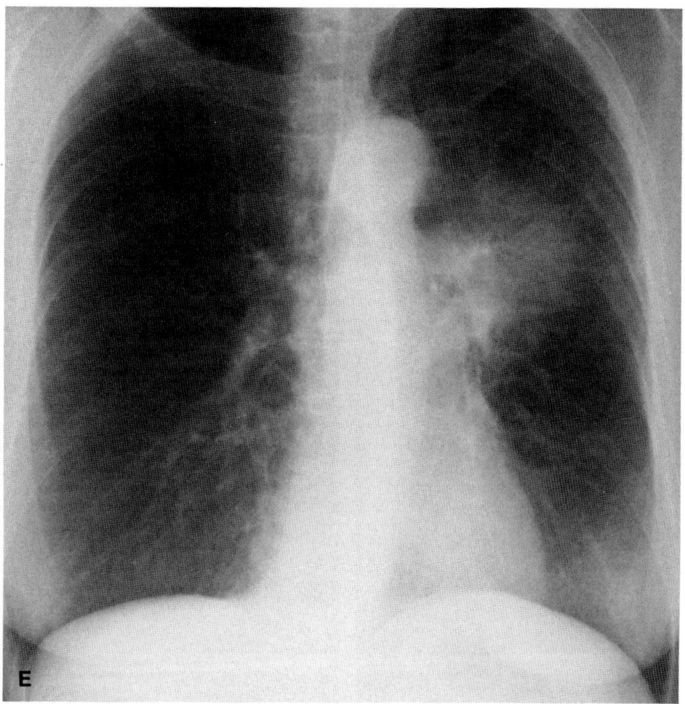

DISCUSSION

The location of this lesion at the gray–white matter junction, as well as the large amount of associated cerebral edema, favors the diagnosis of a metastasis, although a primary brain tumor must be considered. Clinical trials have shown that surgical resection combined with radiotherapy for single brain metastases, as compared with radiotherapy alone, leads to longer survival, fewer brain recurrences, and a better quality of life.[1]

In the United States, lung cancer is responsible for more deaths (both men and women) than any other type of cancer. The incidence of disease continues to rise in women. The cure rate is low, with most patients presenting with advanced disease. The four major histopathologic types, in decreasing order of incidence in the United States, are squamous cell, adenocarcinoma, large cell, and small cell. There is a strong association of lung cancer with cigarette smoking,[2] with 93% of cancers seen in smokers in one large study. Large cell cancer typically is peripheral in origin (unlike the present case) and presents as a large bulky lung mass. Clinically, as with adenocarcinoma, there is early preferential metastasis to the central nervous system.

MR Technique

T2-weighted images, as in this case, often provide for differentiation of neoplastic tissue from surrounding normal brain and edema. Contrast enhancement, however, can improve the depiction of lesion necrosis, in addition to increasing the conspicuity of the lesion itself.

Clinical References

1. Patchell RA, Tibbs PA, Walsh JW, et al. A randomized trial of surgery in the treatment of single metastases to the brain. N Engl J Med 1990;323:132–133.
2. Hammond EC, Horn D. Smoking and death rates—report on forty-four months of follow-up of 187,783 men. JAMA 1984;251:2840–2853.

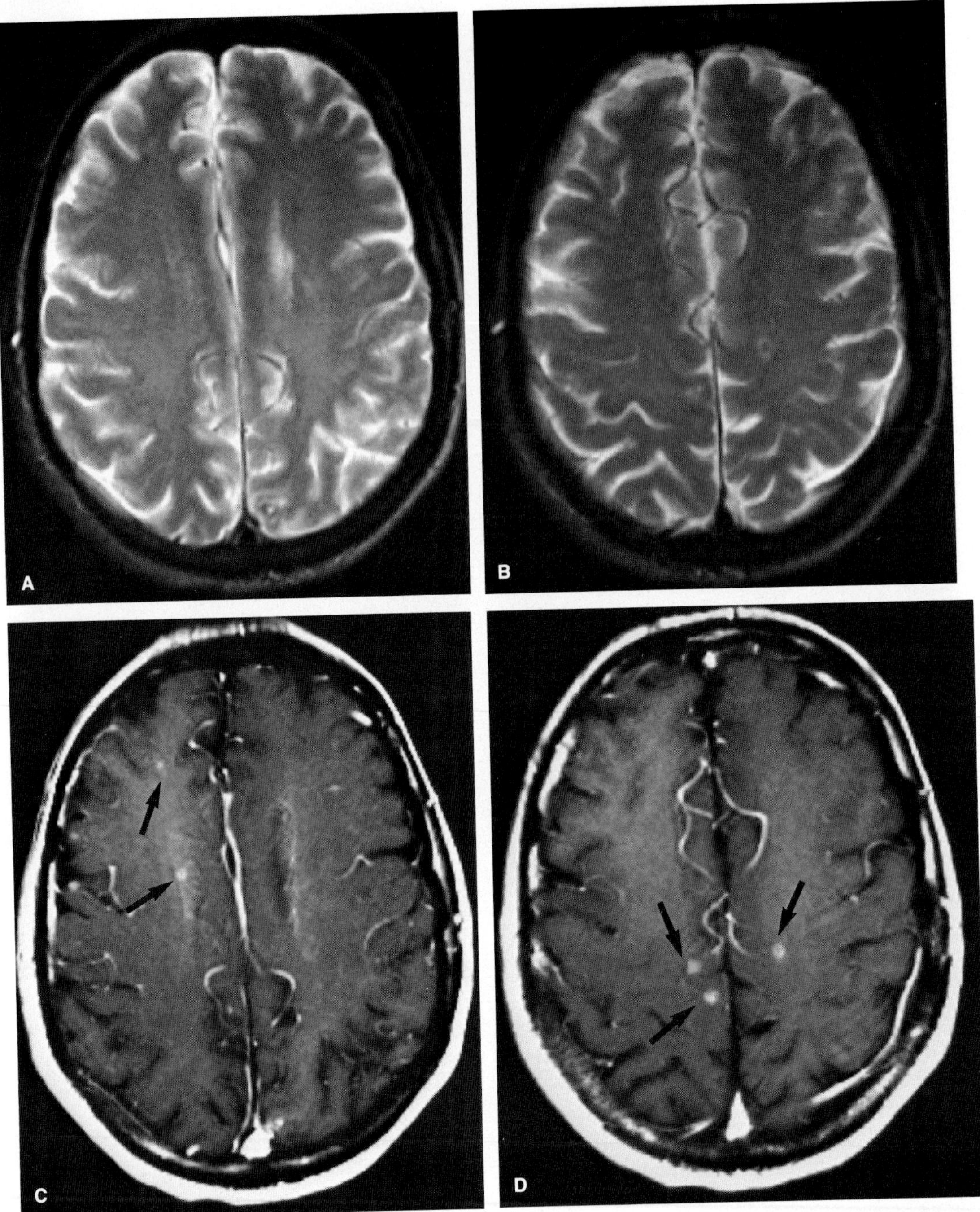

HISTORY

A 64-year-old man with transient dizziness, blurred vision, blurred speech, and right extremity weakness 1 month ago. The history is positive for smoking (80 pack-years), with a 20-lb weight loss in the previous 6 months. Chest CT reveals a right upper lobe mass with hilar and mediastinal adenopathy.

FINDINGS

(*A and B*) T2-weighted images at two anatomic levels reveal no gross abnormality, in particular no definite evidence for metastatic disease. The corresponding precontrast T1-weighted scans were normal (*images not shown*). (*C and D*) Postcontrast, on T1-weighted scans, at least five discrete enhancing lesions (*arrows in C and D*)

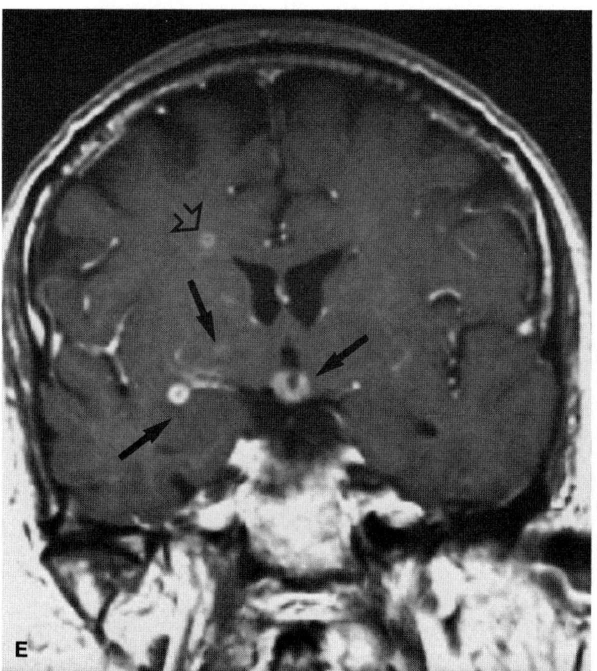

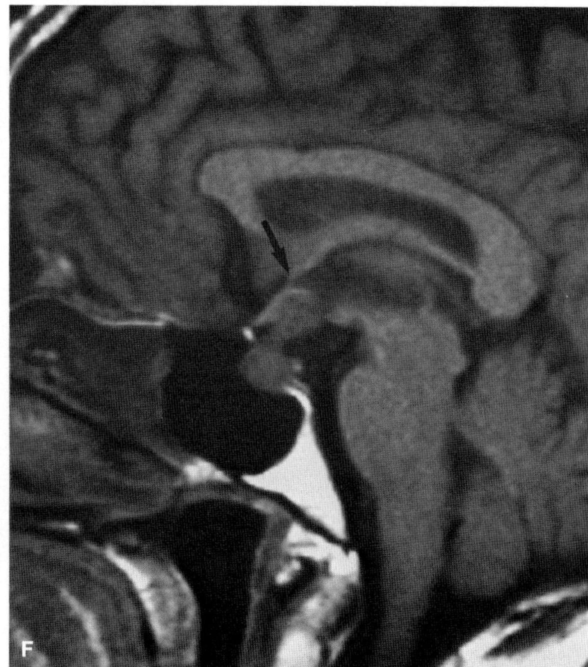

can be identified. In retrospect, a questionable abnormality can be identified on the T2-weighted scan (at the higher level), which corresponds in position to the solitary left-sided lesion. (*E*) A postcontrast coronal T1-weighted scan confirms the presence of the one lesion immediately above the right lateral ventricle (*open arrow*) and identifies three additional lesions (*arrows*), including involvement of the tuber cinereum and adjacent pituitary infundibulum. (*F*) A precontrast sagittal T1-weighted image reveals an abnormal soft tissue mass (*arrow*) in the latter location.

DIAGNOSIS

Metastatic adenocarcinoma of the lung (diagnosed only postcontrast)

DISCUSSION

On review of the entire head examination (all sections, in retrospect), T2-weighted images revealed six questionable white matter abnormalities, one of which is illustrated. Of these, three proved to represent edema associated with metastatic lesions and three were chronic ischemic foci. The T2-weighted scan was considered suspicious, but not diagnostic, for metastatic disease. The presence of such lesions in the brain was confirmed, of course, on the postcontrast T1-weighted scan. Bronchoscopy in this patient revealed adenocarcinoma. Bony metastatic disease, although asymptomatic at present, was confirmed by radionuclide scan. Palliative radiotherapy to the brain and chest was prescribed.

It has been shown in clinical trials that small metastatic tumor nodules may go undetected on unenhanced brain MR. At least one metastatic focus was uncovered postcontrast, which went undetected precontrast, in six of seven patients with multiple metastases in one early investigation.[1] Metastases that can be missed on unenhanced MR include small nodules without associated cerebral edema, lesions adjacent to CSF-containing spaces, and small foci lying within the edema elicited by a larger adjacent lesion.

MR Technique

IV contrast enhancement (with a gadolinium chelate) must be employed for identification of certain metastatic lesions.[2] The edema elicited in many cases is not sufficient to allow recognition of metastatic disease on precontrast scans alone.

Clinical References

1. Russell EJ, Geremia GK, Johnson CE, et al. Multiple cerebral metastases: detectability with Gd-DTPA–enhanced MR imaging. Radiology 1987;165:609–617.
2. Hosten N, Schorner W, Schubeus P, Felix R. MRT of brain metastases. 1. What is the place of screening with T2-weighted sequences? ROFO 1990;153:321–326.

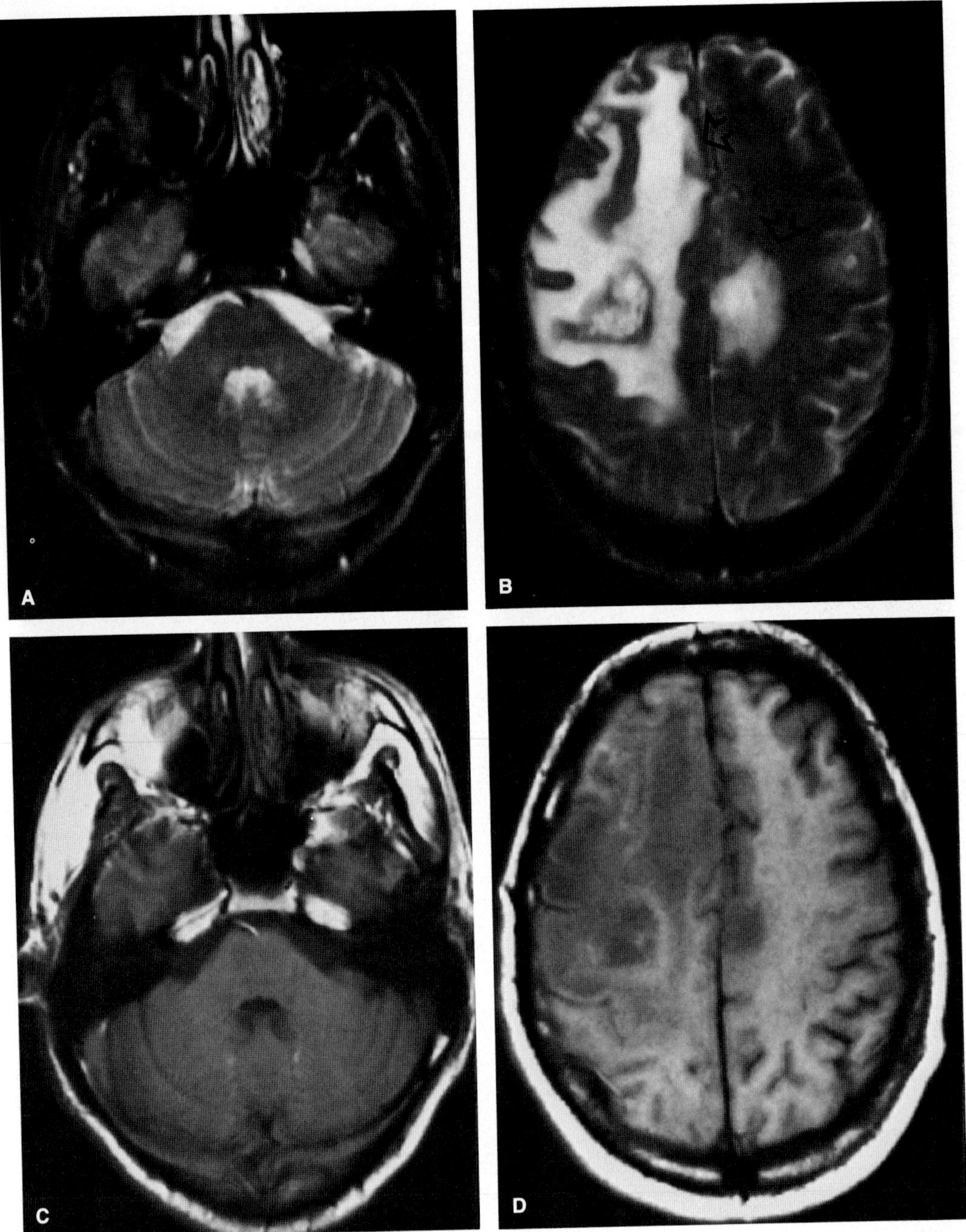

HISTORY

A 43-year-old man with a 2-month history of a 20-lb weight loss, headache, nausea, and left neck, arm, and hand pain. Chest CT scan reveals partial atelectasis of the right middle lobe with nonvisualization of the bronchus, raising the question of an endobronchial lesion. Bronchoscopy is positive for malignant cells.

FINDINGS

T2-weighted precontrast (*A and B*), T1-weighted precontrast (*C and D*), T1-weighted postcontrast (0.1 mmol/kg gadoteridol) (*E and F*), and high-dose T1-weighted postcontrast (0.3 mmol/kg gadoteridol) (*G and H*) images at two anatomic levels are presented. In the posterior fossa, a single enhancing lesion (*arrow in G*) is seen

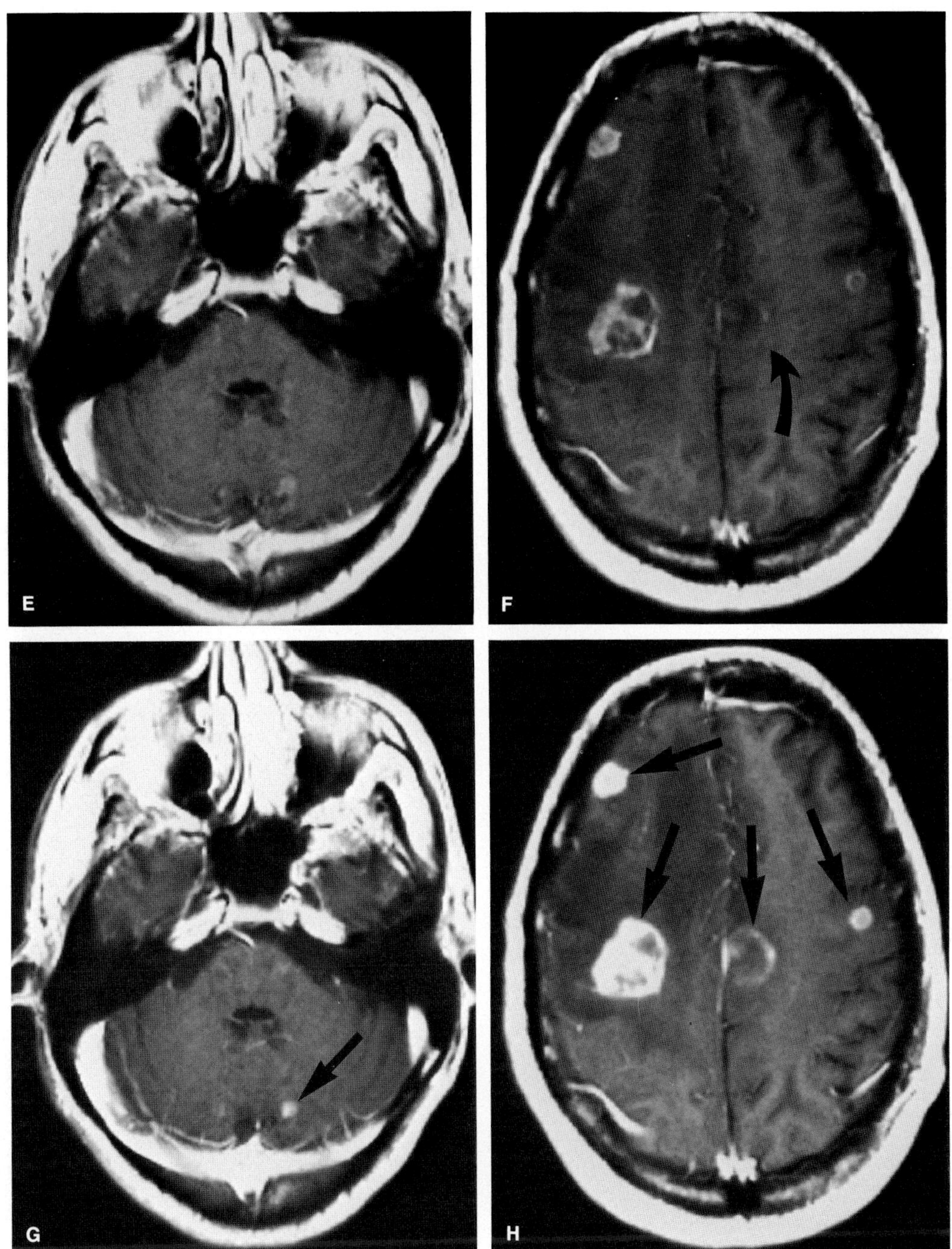

only on the high-dose postcontrast examination. In retrospect, this lesion demonstrates faint enhancement on the 0.1-mmol/kg postcontrast scans, with a questionable increase in signal intensity on the precontrast T2-weighted scans (*A and B*). Above the ventricular level, there is substantial cerebral edema (*open arrows in B*) recognized as abnormal hyperintensity on the T2-weighted images. Delineation of the four metastatic lesions (*arrows in H*) at this level is greatest on the high-dose scans. At 0.1 mmol/kg, the degree of contrast enhancement for each lesion is less, with that of the lesion (*curved arrow in F*) bordering the falx quite subtle. (*G and H*) The abnormal blood–brain barrier associated with this lesion is well demonstrated by contrast enhancement at high dose.

DIAGNOSIS

Metastatic non–small cell lung carcinoma (improved detection at high contrast dose)

DISCUSSION

High-dose (greater than 0.1 mmol/kg) intravenous gadolinium chelate administration provides superior lesion enhancement and detection of additional lesions, compared with standard-dose (0.1 mmol/kg), in metastatic brain disease.[1,2] The ability to precisely identify the number and location of brain metastases is key for therapeutic decision making. Treatment options include surgery, radiation therapy, and chemotherapy. Prolonged survival has been demonstrated with two treatment regimens: resection of single lesions (combined with radiotherapy) and high-dose focal radiation therapy (gamma surgery).

MR Technique

Some metastatic brain lesions will be missed on enhanced MR using 0.1 mmol/kg IV of a gadolinium chelate. Higher doses (0.2 to 0.3 mmol/kg) reveal lesions not seen at 0.1 mmol/kg and improve reader certainty for diagnosis of other lesions.

Pitfalls in Image Interpretation

Arterial and venous pulsation artifacts are more prominent on postcontrast studies and should not be mistaken for enhancing pathology. In the case presented, thin-section imaging was used to confirm the presence of a metastatic lesion in the left cerebellum. Alternatively, the phase encoding axis can be switched, which changes the direction of propagation of motion-related artifacts.

Clinical References

1. Yuh WT, Fisher DJ, Engelken JD, et al. MR evaluation of CNS tumors: dose comparison study with gadopentetate dimeglumine and gadoteridol. Radiology 1991;180:485–491.
2. Runge VM, Kirsch JE, Burke V, et al. High dose gadoteridol in MR imaging of intracranial neoplasms. J Magn Reson Imaging 1992;2:9–18.

(A *through* H *from Runge VM, Kirsch JE, Burke V, et al. High dose gadoteridol in MR imaging of intracranial neoplasms. J Magn Reson Imaging 1992;2:9–18.)*

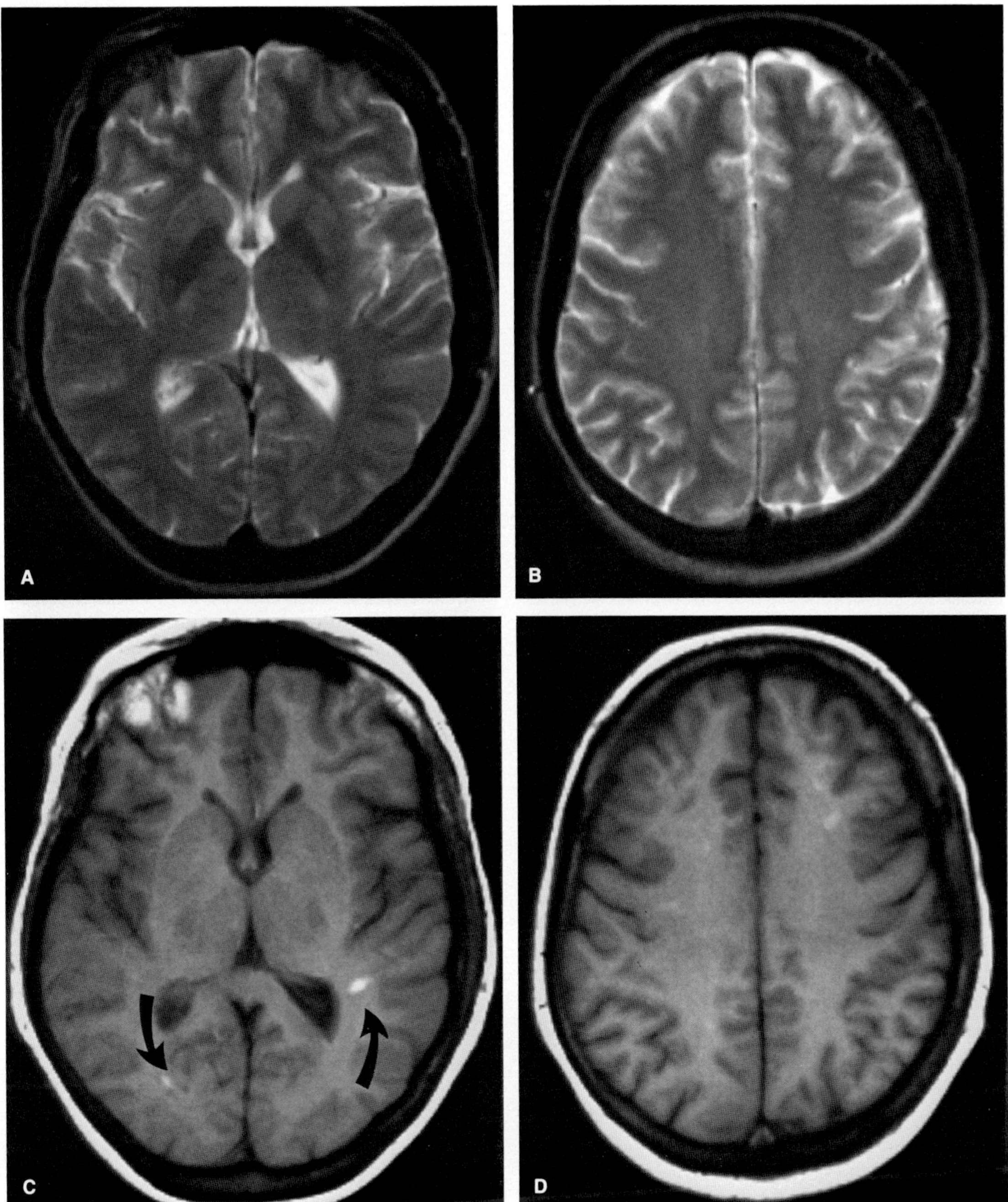

HISTORY

A 46-year-old woman, 2 years after mastectomy for breast cancer. Radionuclide scans confirm bony metastatic disease.

FINDINGS

(*A and B*) No abnormalities were noted on the T2-weighted images, with two representative axial sections (TE = 90 msec) illustrated. (*C and D*) On the corresponding precontrast T1-weighted sections, two small, abnormal high-signal-intensity foci are identified (*curved arrows in C*). (*E and F*) T1-weighted images following IV contrast administration reveal multiple enhancing foci (*arrows in F*), in addition to the two lesions previously identified (*arrows in E*). In retrospect, each appears slightly hyperintense to brain on the precontrast T1-weighted scan. On contrast-enhanced CT (*not shown*), only a single abnormal enhancing focus was seen, adjacent to the left frontal horn.

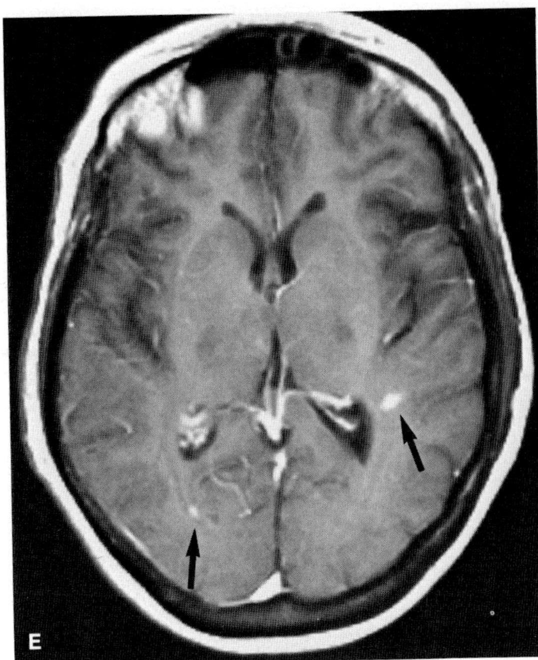

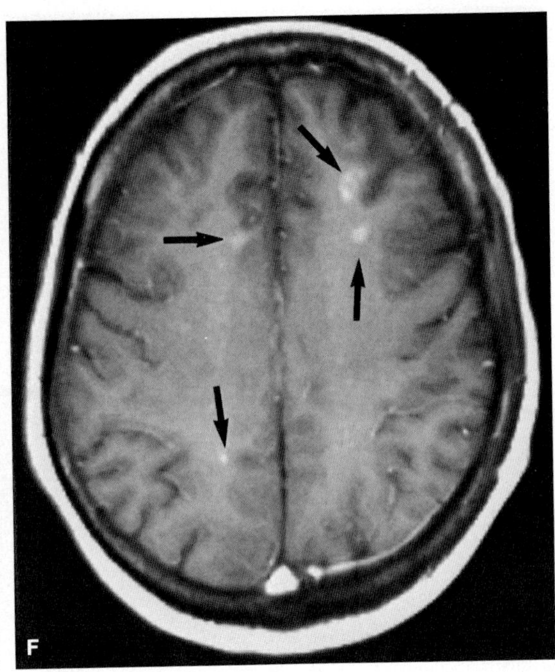

DIAGNOSIS

Metastatic breast carcinoma (hemorrhagic)

DISCUSSION

MR with contrast enhancement, using a dose of 0.1 mmol/kg IV of a gadolinium chelate, has been shown to be superior to double-dose delayed CT for lesion detection in metastatic brain disease.[1] Comparison of immediate and delayed postcontrast T1-weighted scans has not demonstrated the delayed scans to be of significant additional value for lesion detection.[2]

Hemorrhage within intracranial neoplasms can be hypointense, isointense, or hyperintense relative to brain on T1-weighted sequences, depending on the stage of hemoglobin degradation.[3] High signal intensity from blood products on T1-weighted scans is caused by the presence of methemoglobin. Metastases from melanoma, choriocarcinoma, lung (oat cell), kidney, colon, and thyroid demonstrate a propensity for hemorrhage.

MR Technique

Precontrast T1-weighted scans are required to differentiate between hemorrhage and contrast enhancement.

Pitfalls in Image Interpretation

T2-weighted scans are not sufficient to rule out metastatic brain disease.

Clinical References

1. Davis PC, Hudgins PA, Peterman SB, Hoffman JC. Diagnosis of cerebral metastases: double-dose delayed CT vs contrast-enhanced MR imaging. AJNR 1991;12:293–300.
2. Sze G, Milano E, Johnson C, Heier L. Detection of brain metastases: comparison of contrast-enhanced MR with unenhanced MR and enhanced CT. AJNR 1990;11:785–791.
3. Destian S, Sze G, Krol G, et al. MR imaging of hemorrhagic intracranial neoplasms. AJR 1989;152:137–144.

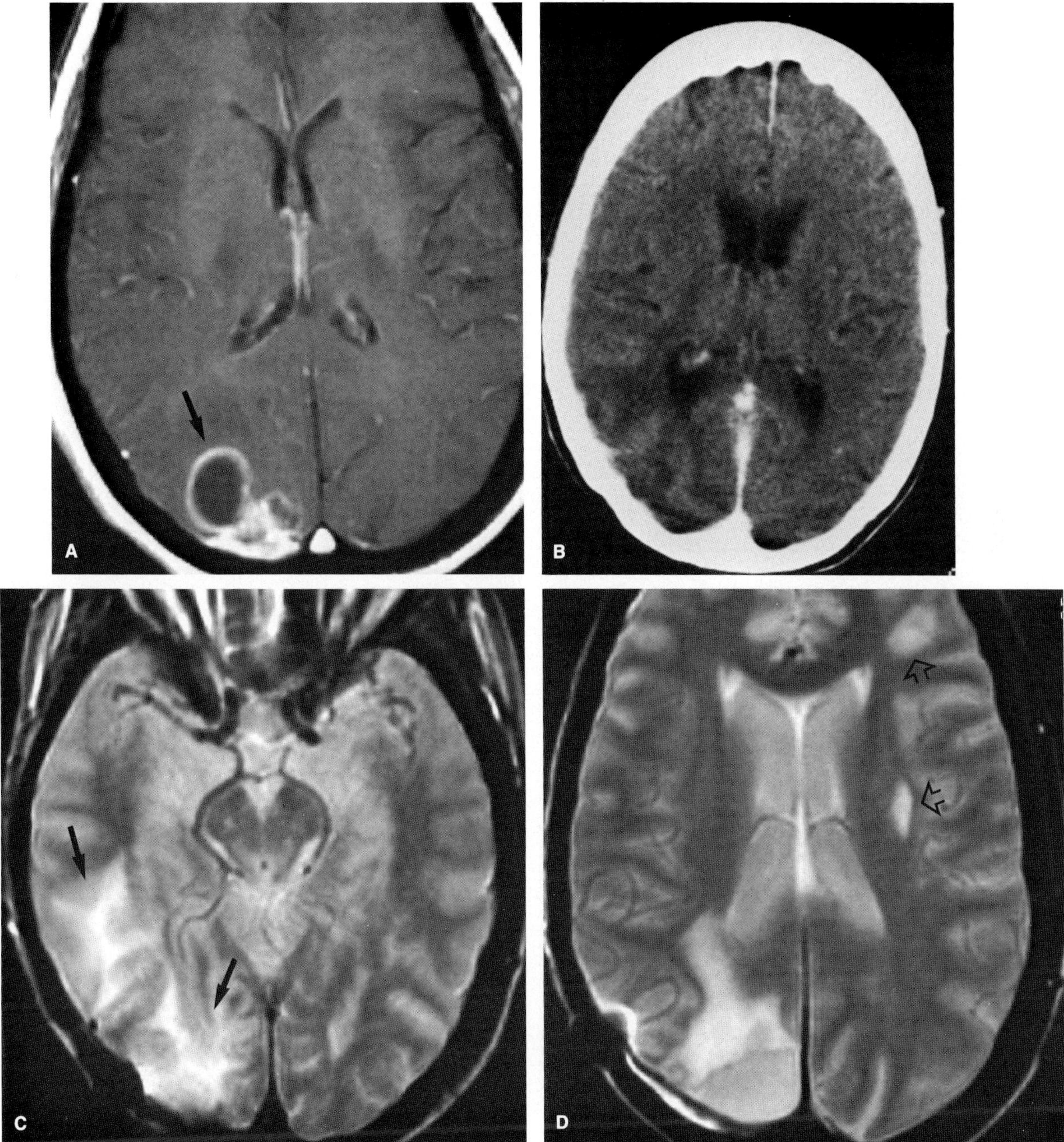

HISTORY

A 65-year-old woman diagnosed with breast carcinoma and treated by modified radical mastectomy 4 years before the current hospital admission. One year ago, she presented with a seizure. MR (*A*) documented a single right occipital brain metastasis which was surgically excised. Two lung nodules were also noted, for which the patient received chemotherapy. Presenting problems at the current time include poor appetite, 40-lb weight loss, and neurologic symptoms.

FINDINGS

(*A*) A single postcontrast T1-weighted image is presented from the patient's original hospital admission. A large right occipital metastasis (*arrow*), with a cystic nonenhancing component and involvement of brain immediately adjacent to the leptomeninges, is noted. The lesion was treated by surgical resection followed by whole-brain irradiation (5000 rad). The patient was readmitted 1 year later because of increasing problems with balance and positional vertigo. CT with and without IV contrast

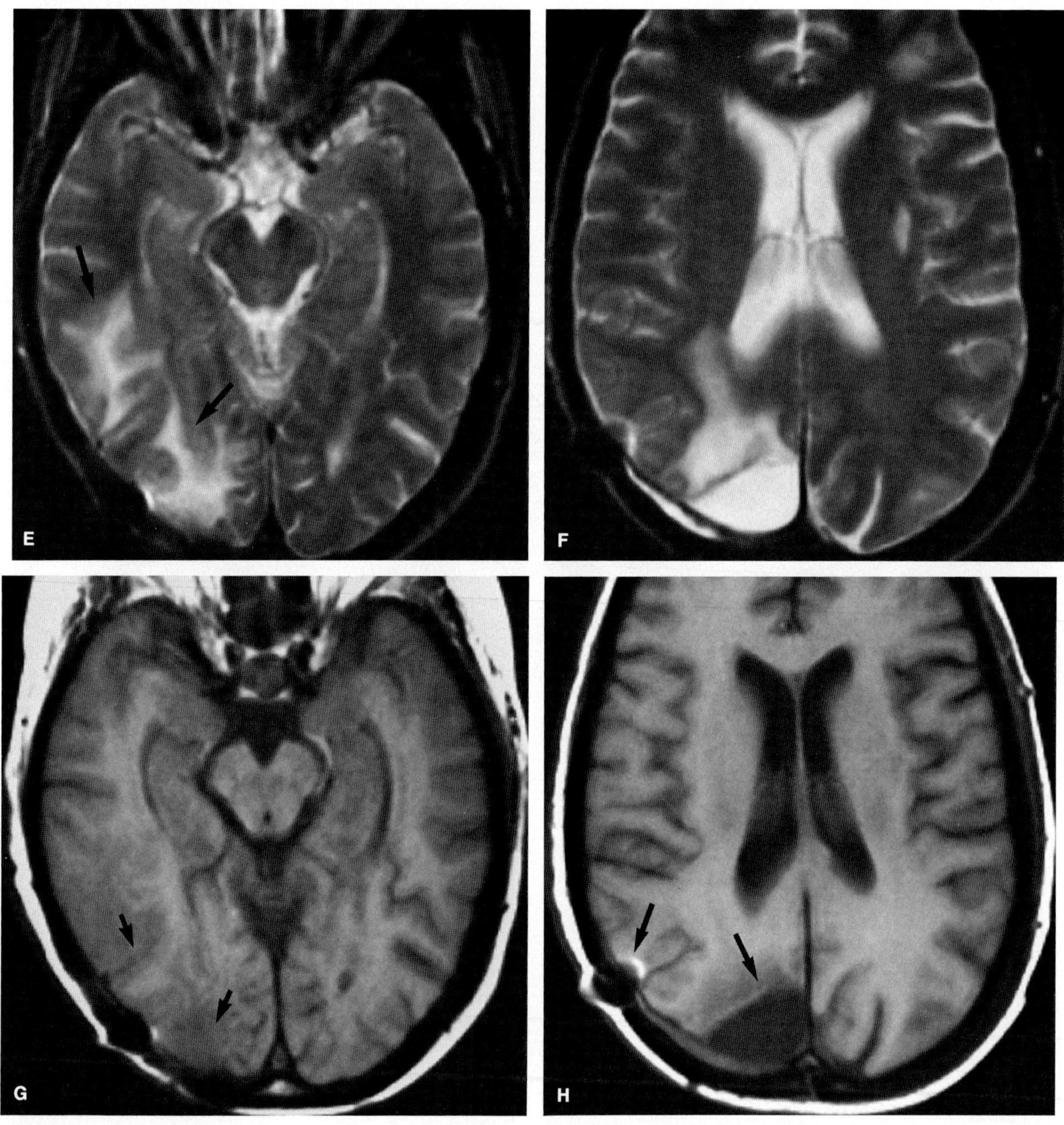

administration was interpreted as normal, with the exception of postoperative changes. (*B*) A single postcontrast CT image, at the level of the frontal horns and atria, is depicted. Intermediate (*C and D*) and heavily (*E and F*) T2-weighted MR images at two anatomic levels demonstrate multiple areas of abnormal hyperintensity both adjacent to the dura posteriorly on the right (*arrows in C and E*) and in white matter on the left (*open arrows in D*). The peripheral changes are primarily adjacent to the site of previous craniotomy. (*G and H*) Precontrast T1-weighted images reveal both postoperative changes (*arrows in H*) and effacement of sulci (*short arrows in G*) in the right occipital lobe. (*I and J*) Postcontrast T1-weighted images demonstrate tumor seeding and recurrence (*arrows in I*) along the dura on the right and three new intraparenchymal metastases (*open arrows in J*) on the left. Edema, seen as abnormal high signal intensity on the T2-weighted examination, serves to mark only two of the three metastatic lesions visualized on the left postcontrast. The abnormalities noted on T2-weighted scans adjacent to the dura, as well as the sulcal effacement noted on the T1-weighted scan (*G*), prove to represent primarily edema associated with neoplastic disease rather than postoperative changes.

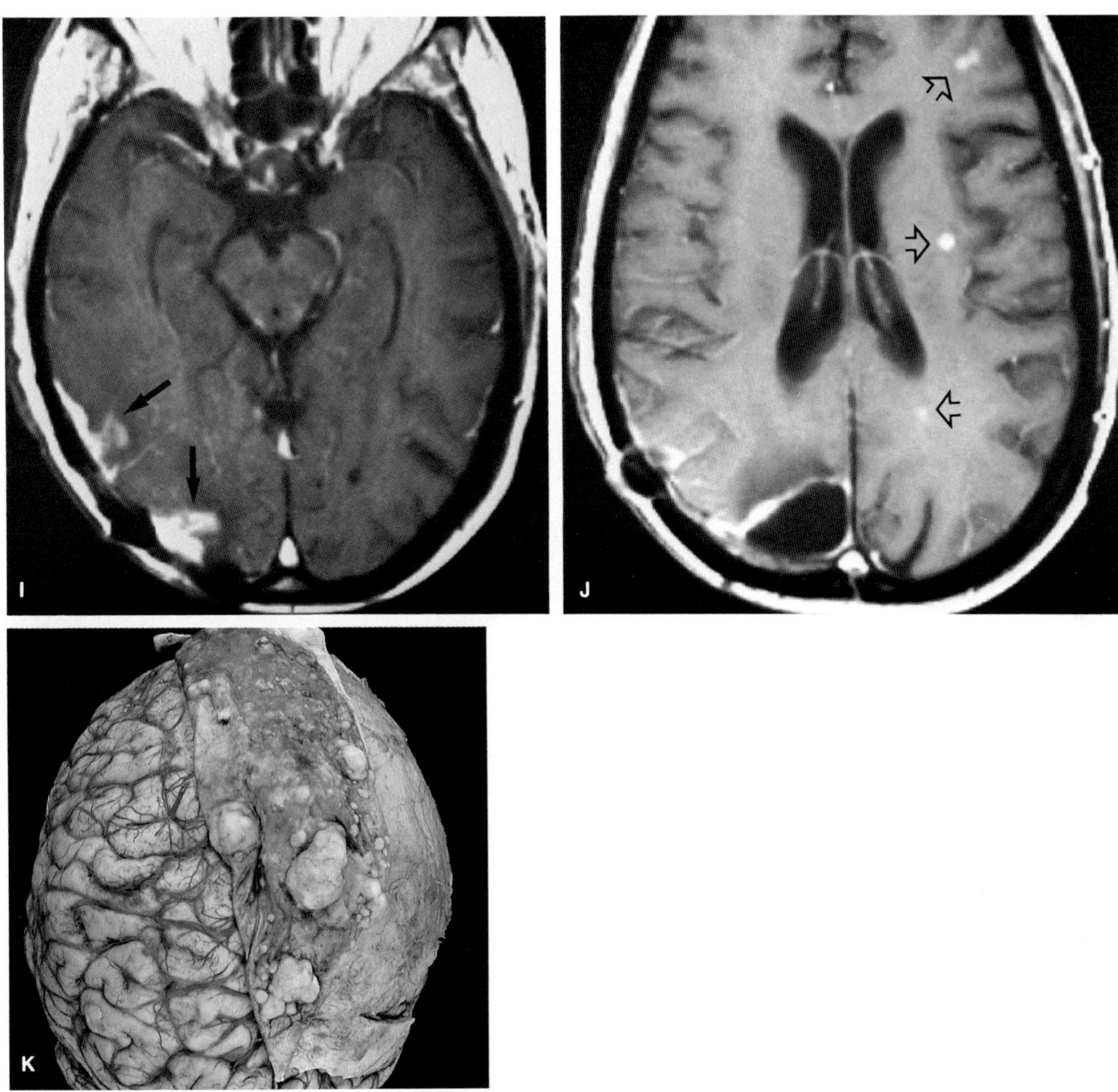

DIAGNOSIS

Meningeal carcinomatosis (focal) and intraparenchymal brain metastases from breast carcinoma

DISCUSSION

CT and MR were compared for efficacy in diagnosis of leptomeningeal brain metastases in a study of 14 patients with positive CSF studies.[1] Contrast-enhanced MR proved superior to contrast-enhanced CT, with detection of abnormal meningeal or parenchymal foci in 10 as compared with 5 patients respectively. The demonstration of abnormal dural, tentorial, sulcal, ependymal, and cisternal enhancement was also superior by MR. Neither study demonstrated abnormalities in the 4 remaining patients.

Although contrast administration markedly improves the ability of MR to detect leptomeningeal metastases, imaging studies (encompassing both the head and the spine) may give negative results in patients with proven cytologic evidence of disease.[2] Conversely, negative cytologic results also represent a clinical problem, with repeated lumbar or even cisternal puncture required for detection of neoplastic cells.[3] Negative cytologic findings with positive MR has also been reported.[3] Although lumbar puncture should be performed first, delineation of the anatomic extent of neoplastic seeding in both the head and spine is possible only by contrast-enhanced MR. Such demarcation of disease is of clinical importance in radiation therapy planning.

MR Technique

Contrast-enhanced T1-weighted imaging is the technique of choice for detection of leptomeningeal metastases.

Pitfalls in Image Interpretation

Abnormal contrast enhancement, by itself, is not diagnostic of leptomeningeal metastatic disease on MR, particularly in the postoperative state. Contrast-enhanced MR is sensitive to meningeal disease but, unfortunately, nonspecific with regard to etiology. Findings on enhanced MR, used in context with clinical information, can lead to rapid diagnosis and thus treatment of leptomeningeal neoplastic disease.

Pathologic Correlate

K demonstrates the gross appearance of dural metastases in a patient with breast carcinoma. In this case, metastatic disease was limited to the dura, without direct infiltration of underlying cortex.

Clinical References

1. Chamberlain MC, Sandy AD, Press GA. Leptomeningeal metastasis: a comparison of gadolinium-enhanced MR and contrast-enhanced CT of the brain. Neurology 1990; 40(3):435–438.
2. Yousem DM, Patrone PM, Grossman RI. Leptomeningeal metastases: MR evaluation. J Comput Assist Tomogr 1990; 14:255–261.
3. Rodesch G, VanBogaert P, Mavroudakis N, et al. Neuroradiologic findings in leptomeningeal carcinomatosis: the value interest of gadolinium-enhanced MRI. Neuroradiology 1990;32:26–32.

(K from Okazaki H, Scheithauer B. Slide atlas of neuropathology. New York, Gower Medical Publishing, 1988. By permission of Mayo Foundation.)

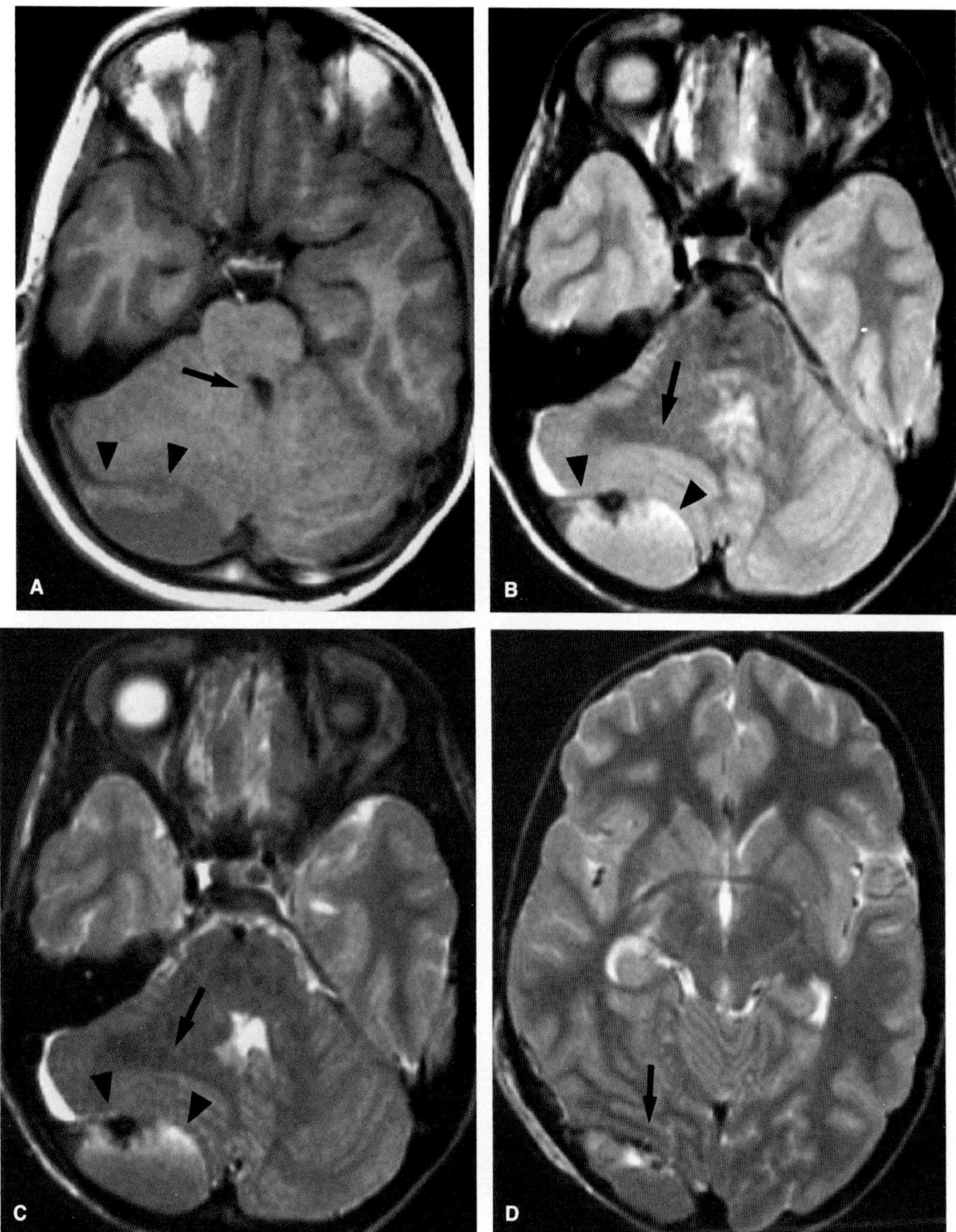

HISTORY

A 9-year-old with headache, nausea, and vomiting 2 days after a 10-ft fall off a bridge. A right occipital bone fracture was noted on CT.

FINDINGS

T1-weighted (*A*), intermediate (*B*) and heavily (*C*) T2-weighted axial images demonstrate a heterogeneous, biconvex, elliptic fluid collection (*black arrowheads*) posterior to, and compressing, the right cerebellar hemisphere. The fluid collection is causing a mass effect, which is reflected by distortion of the fourth ventricle (*black arrow in A*) and the right cerebellar hemisphere (*black arrows in B and C*). T2-weighted axial image at a higher level (*D*), and the T1-weighted sagittal image (*E*) show extension of the lesion above the level of the tentorium (*arrows in D and E*) indicating that it is located in the extradural space.

This heterogeneous fluid collection does not have the classic signal intensity characteristics of any hemoglobin degradation product and is likely to be diluted by CSF.

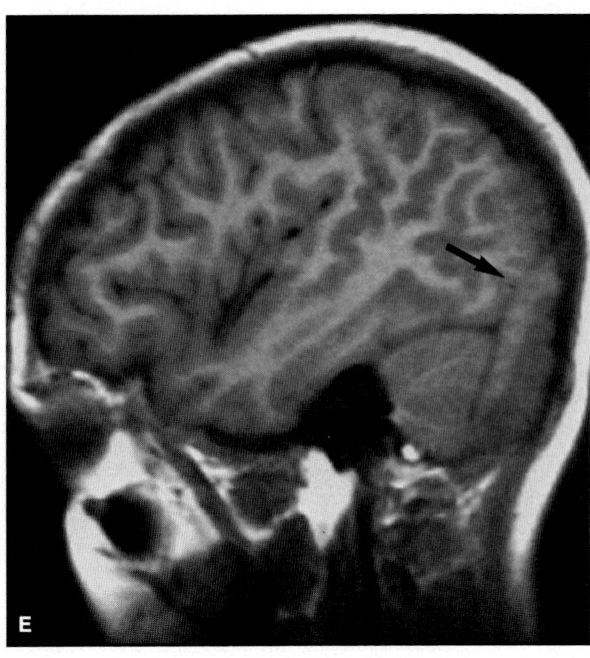

DIAGNOSIS

Epidural hematoma

DISCUSSION

The dura is strongly adherent to the skull and represents the periosteum of the inner table. An epidural hematoma accumulates within the potential space between the inner table of the skull and the dura, usually as the result of a skull fracture and accompanying laceration of a blood vessel. Fracture of the temporal or parietal bone with laceration of branches of the middle meningeal artery is the most common cause. Epidural hematomas in the posterior fossa are less common, and coexist with a supratentorial epidural hematoma in 20% of cases.[1] An occipital bone fracture is usually present, and the disrupted transverse sinus is the usual source of the bleeding.

Epidural hematomas may not become symptomatic until several hours ("lucid interval") after the trauma and often have an acute, rapidly progressing clinical course.[2] Because the source of the bleeding in posterior fossa epidural hematomas is usually venous, clinical manifestations may develop more slowly than expected.[1] Headache, nausea, and vomiting are signs of increased intracranial pressure caused by the enlarging intracranial hematoma.

Somnolence after the lucid interval is an ominous sign of deteriorating neurologic status. The Glasgow Coma Scale score at the time of injury is not a reliable indicator for development of subsequent deterioration.[2]

CT remains the first diagnostic step in evaluating an acutely injured, or rapidly deteriorating trauma patient, because of its relative insensitivity to motion and compatibility with life-support systems.[3] However, MR is much more sensitive than CT for detection of subacute hemorrhages and coexistent nonhemorrhagic parenchymal changes, such as shearing injuries, which have prognostic significance.[3] An epidural hematoma most commonly appears as a biconvex, elliptic fluid collection adjacent to a fracture site. The venous sinuses are displaced away from the inner table of the skull. The MR appearance of an epidural hematoma changes with time and often is the manifestation of a mixture of hemoglobin degradation products.

Clinical References

1. Pozzati E, Tognetti F, Cavallo M, et al. Extradural hematomas of the posterior cranial fossa. Surg Neurol 1989; 32:300–303.
2. Knuckey N, Gelbard S, Epstein M. The management of "asymptomatic" epidural hematomas. J Neurosurg 1989; 70:392–396.
3. Zimmerman R, Bilaniuk L, Hackney D, et al. Head injury: early results of comparing CT and high-field MR. AJNR 1986;7:757–764.

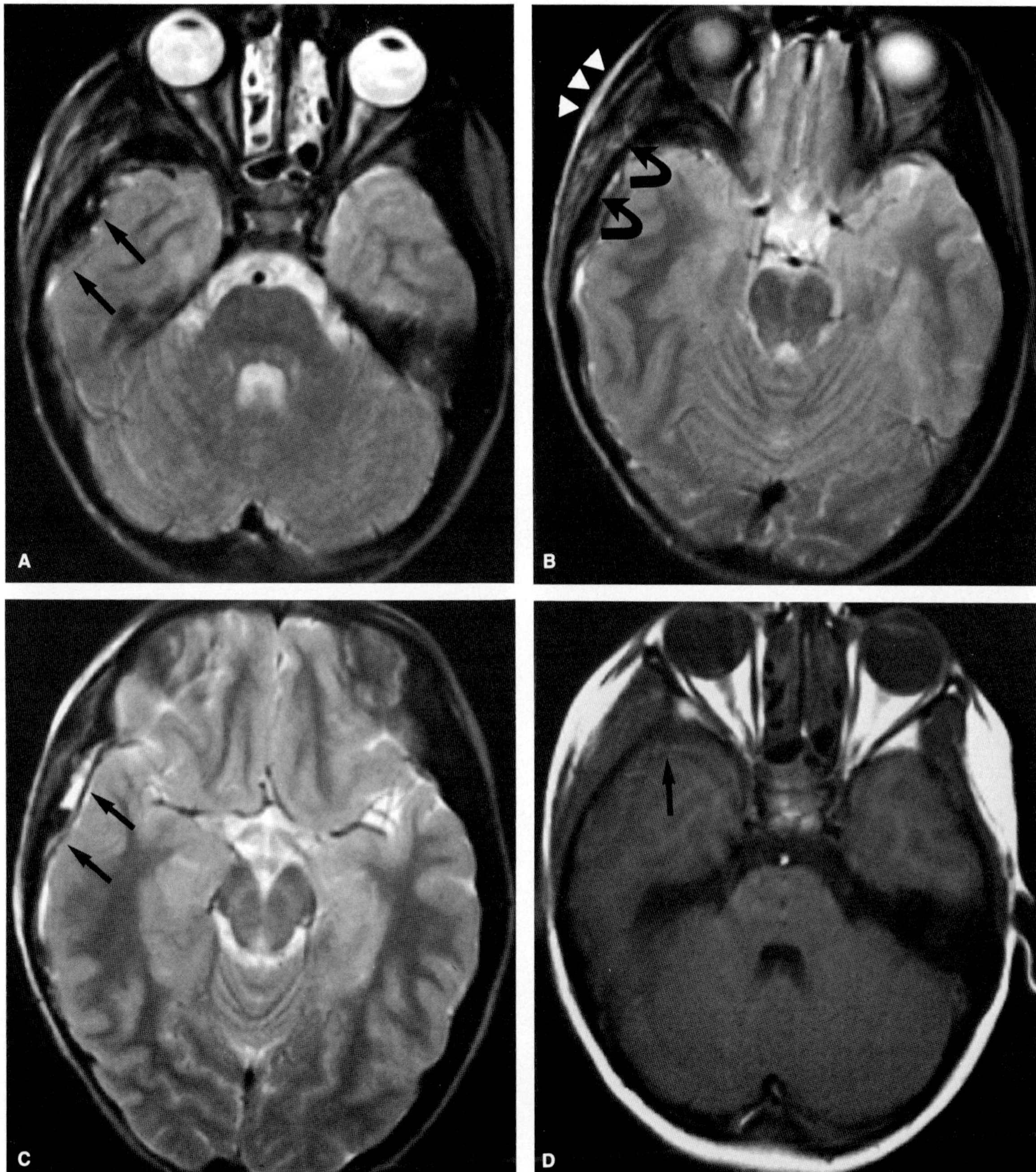

HISTORY

A 7-year-old with chronic uncontrolled seizures, who 3 days before the current examination rode her bike over an embankment of 30 ft and landed on a pavement with loss of consciousness

FINDINGS

(*A to C*) T2-weighted images reveal abnormal high signal intensity, due to edema, within both the subcutaneous tissue (*arrowheads*) and the temporalis muscle (*curved arrows*) on the right. There is incidental inflammatory ethmoid sinus disease. An extraaxial fluid collection is noted adjacent to the right temporal lobe. This fluid has predominantly low signal intensity on the lowest image (*arrows in A*) and a mixture of hypointensity and hyperintensity on the highest image (*arrows in C*). (*D to F*) On the corresponding T1-weighted images, the fluid collection (*arrow*) is isointense with brain and somewhat difficult to identify, particularly on the lowest section.

DIAGNOSIS

Acute subdural hematoma

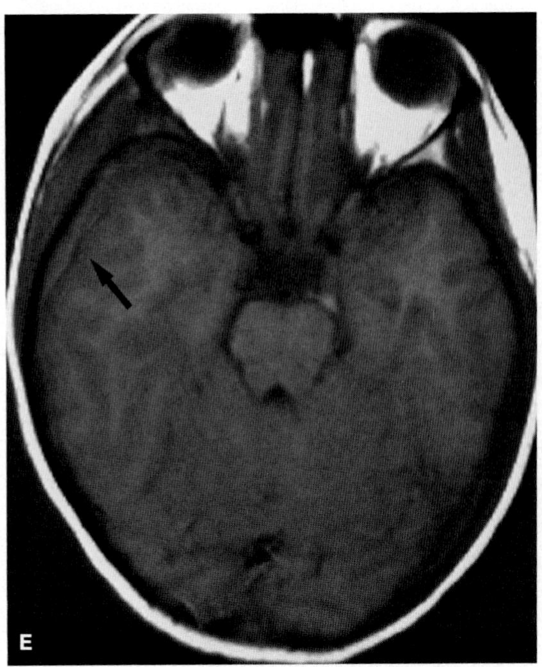

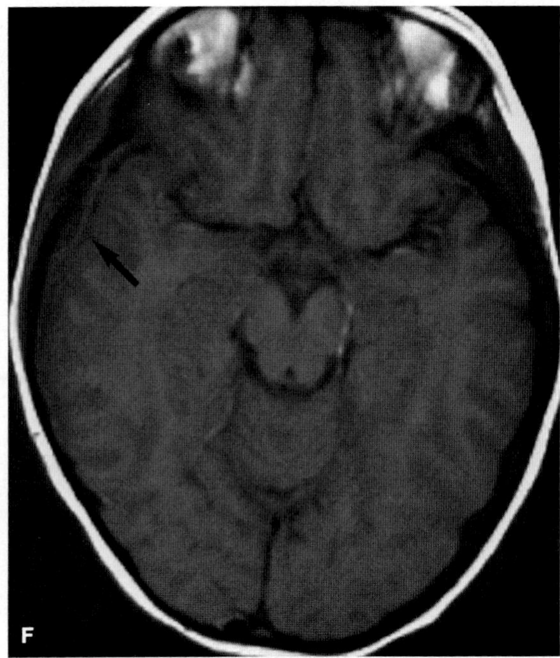

DISCUSSION

Acute, early subacute, late subacute, and chronic subdural hematomas can be differentiated on MR by their characteristic signal intensities on T1- and T2-weighted images.[1] As with intraparenchymal hematomas, hypointensity on T2-weighted scans is noted in the acute time frame (due to deoxyhemoglobin), which progresses to hyperintensity on T1-weighted and hypointensity on T2-weighted images (early subacute phase, due to the presence of intracellular methemoglobin), followed by hyperintensity on both images (late subacute phase, due to the presence of extracellular methemoglobin). In the chronic phase, however, subdural hematomas differ markedly from intraparenchymal hematomas, being hypointense to isointense with gray matter on T1-weighted images and typically without hemosiderin deposition.

In the case presented, the mixture of signal intensities seen within the fluid collection on T2-weighted images could be due to the presence of oxyhemoglobin (which should be hyperintense) in addition to deoxyhemoglobin (which should be hypointense). Alternatively, the nondependent portion could represent proteinaceous serum, with intact red blood cells in the more dependent portion. The convex inward border, as well as extension of the collection over the right frontal lobe (*images not shown*), favors a subdural location. However, a low-signal-intensity border is present (although incomplete) medially on both T1- and T2-weighted images, a finding more characteristic of epidural hematomas, and in that instance corresponding to the fibrous dura mater.

Pitfalls in Image Interpretation

In the setting of acute trauma, close inspection of T2-weighted images and their comparison with T1-weighted images are necessary to detect small extraaxial hematomas. The hypointensity of these fluid collections on T2-weighted images, and their proximity to the inner table of the skull (which is also hypointense), can make recognition difficult.

Clinical References

1. Fobben ES, Grossman RI, Atlas SW, et al. MR characteristics of subdural hematomas and hygromas at 1.5T. AJR 1989; 153:589–595.

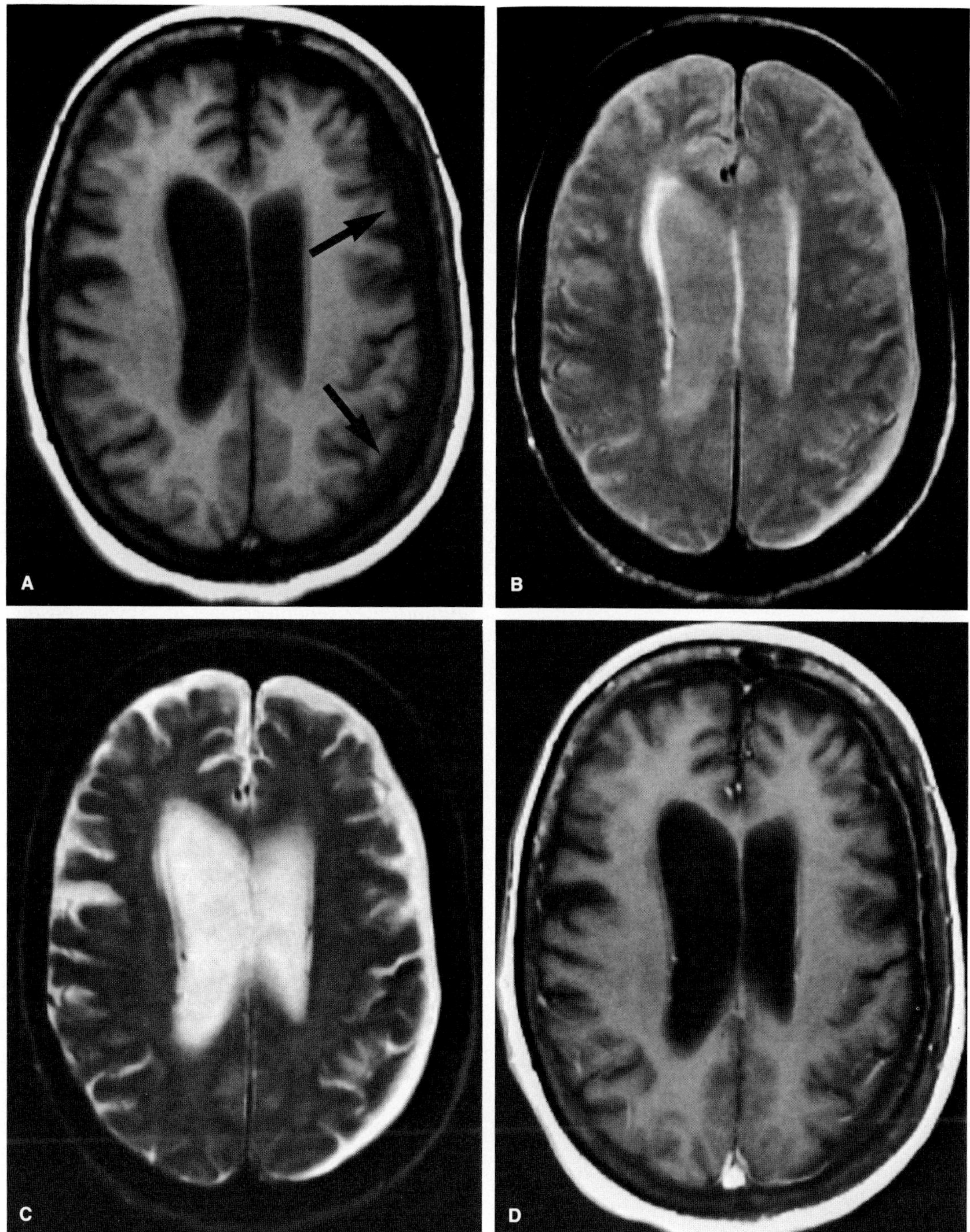

HISTORY

A 72-year-old with dementia

FINDINGS

(*A*) The T1-weighted axial image demonstrates an extraaxial fluid collection (*arrows*) surrounding the entire left cerebral hemisphere. The signal intensity of the fluid is slightly greater on the T1-weighted image than CSF in the lateral ventricles. On the intermediate (*B*) and heavily (*C*) T2-weighted axial images the anterior portion of the fluid collection has the same signal intensity as CSF. However, the posterior aspect of the fluid collection, along the parietal lobe, is hyperintense on both echoes (*B and C*) when compared with CSF. (*D*) Postcontrast T1-weighted axial image shows diffuse enhancement of the

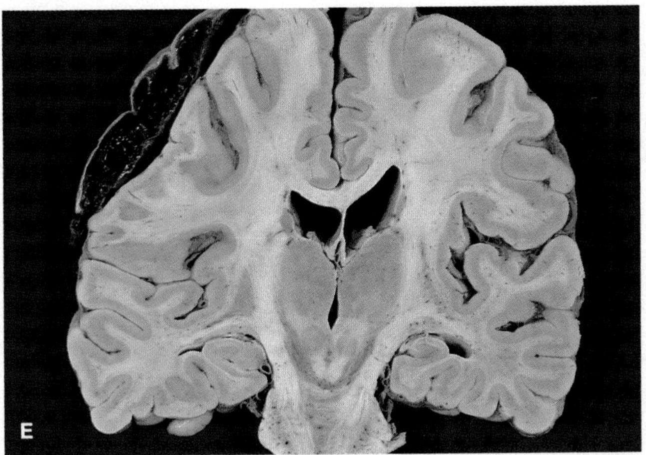

dura adjacent to the fluid collection. The lateral ventricles are slightly enlarged, right greater than left, and there is high signal intensity surrounding the ventricles on *B*. Both of these findings are manifestations of chronic deep white matter ischemia.

DIAGNOSIS

Chronic subdural hematoma

DISCUSSION

The subdural space is a potential space that differs from the brain parenchyma both physiologically and anatomically.[1] Because the dura lacks a blood–brain barrier, macrophages may freely enter any fluid, including blood, which lies within the subdural space. Therefore, the appearance of a chronic subdural hematoma differs significantly from a chronic intraparenchymal hematoma. Chronic intraparenchymal hematomas typically have a hyperintense center with a hypointense hemosiderin rim on both T1- and T2-weighted images. The signal intensity of chronic subdural hematomas, on the other hand, is very low but usually slightly higher than CSF on T1-weighted images due to persistence of proteins and a low concentration of hemoglobin degradation products. The signal intensity of chronic subdural hematomas is isointense to slightly hyperintense compared with CSF on T2-weighted images. Hemosiderin is rare in chronic subdural hematomas because blood products are resorbed into the bloodstream. The presence of hemosiderin usually indicates rehemorrhage and thickened membranes in the subdural space.[1]

Patients with chronic subdural hematomas may present with mental status changes, dementia, neurologic deficit, or seizures.

Pathologic Correlate

(*E*) A fixed and stained coronal gross section demonstrates a large chronic subdural hematoma compressing the adjacent brain. Subdural hematomas are often located near the cerebral convexity because of tearing of bridging veins that drain toward the superior sagittal sinus.

Clinical References

1. Fobben E, Grossman R, Atlas S, et al. MR characteristics of subdural hematomas and hygromas at 1.5T. AJR 1989; 153:589–595.

(E from Okazaki H, Scheithauer B. Slide atlas of neuropathology. New York, Gower Medical Publishing, 1988. By permission of Mayo Foundation.)

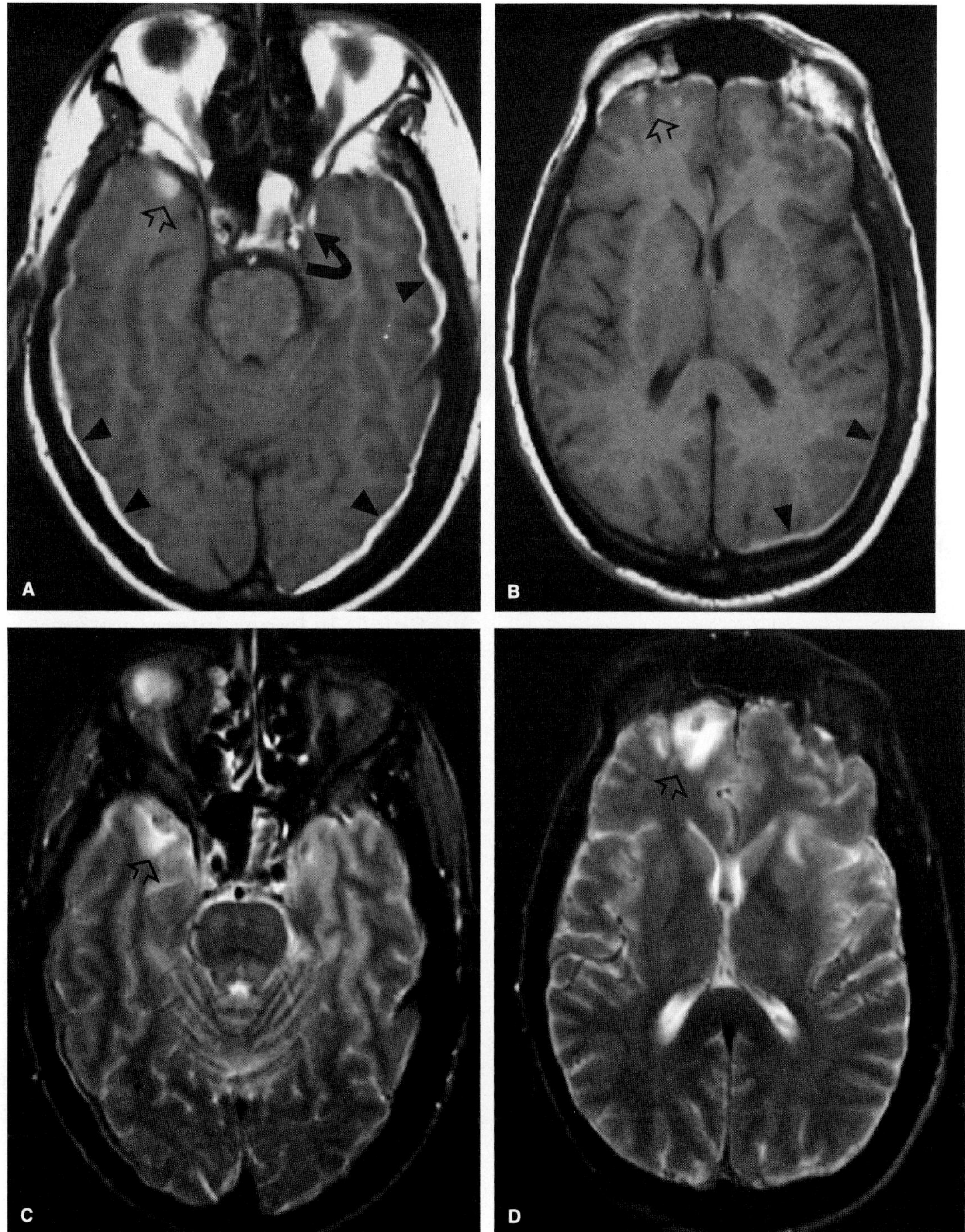

HISTORY

A 56-year-old man 9 days following a hard fall to the pavement, which time the patient suffered a 15-minute loss of consciousness with subsequent nausea and vomiting

FINDINGS

(*A and B*) Abnormal hyperintensity, consistent with methemoglobin, is noted on T1-weighted images in the subdural space (*arrowheads in A and B*), sphenoid sinus

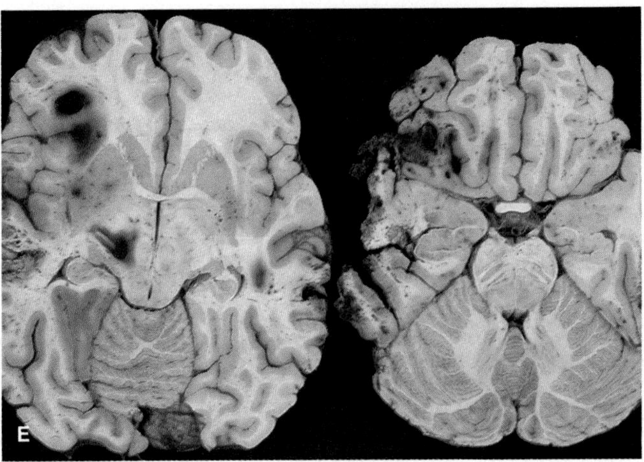

(*curved arrow in A*), right temporal tip (*open arrow in A*), and right low frontal lobe (*open arrow in B*). (*C and D*) On the corresponding T2-weighted images (TE = 90 msec), these areas are principally of low signal intensity, compatible with methemoglobin, which is intracellular in location. Edema with high signal intensity (*open arrows in C and D*) is also noted adjacent to the two sites of intraparenchymal hemorrhage. CT (*not shown*) results were negative.

DIAGNOSIS

Frontal and temporal lobe contusions, with subacute intraparenchymal and subdural hemorrhage

DISCUSSION

A cortical contusion is, by definition, a bruise of the brain's surface. Coup contusions are those in which the injury lies immediately beneath the area of impact, as in the present case. Contrecoup contusions, which are due to acceleration effects, occur in brain remote from and along a direct line opposite to the site of impact. In accidents due to impaction of the head against an unyielding surface, the inferior frontal and temporal poles are particularly vulnerable.

In a large prospective study of MR and CT for the evaluation of closed head trauma,[1] both modalities proved comparable for detection of hemorrhagic intraaxial lesions. However, MR proved markedly superior for detection of nonhemorrhagic lesions. The only advantage of CT is its ability to provide rapid assessment of unstable patients. A second head trauma study[2] also demonstrated MR to be markedly superior to CT for the diagnosis of extracerebral fluid collections, providing improved estimation of size and detection of small collections. A further advantage of MR is its ability to differentiate chronic subdural hematomas from hygromas.

Pitfalls in Image Interpretation

A CT scan with negative results does not rule out the possibility of significant brain trauma. Beam-hardening artifacts on CT also tend to result in underestimation of the size of extracerebral fluid collections and relative insensitivity to cortical contusions, particularly in the low frontal and temporal regions. Care must be exercised in comparing an initial CT examination to follow-up MR. Better visualization of subdural or epidural blood on MR may lead incorrectly to the conclusion that an interval increase in size of the extracerebral collection has occurred.

Pathologic Correlate

(*E*) Gross pathologic sections are from a 35-year-old patient who sustained a head injury in a 30-ft fall onto concrete. The patient died 27 hours after the fall. Extensive brain contusion is present in the frontal and temporal lobes.

Clinical References

1. Gentry LR, Godersky JC, Thompson B, Dunn VD. Prospective comparative study of intermediate-field MR and CT in the evaluation of closed head trauma. AJR 1988;150:673–682.
2. Snow RB, Zimmerman RD, Gandy SE, Deck MD. Comparison of magnetic resonance imaging and computed tomography in the evaluation of head injury. Neurosurgery 1986;18:45–52.

(E *from Okazaki H, Scheithauer B. Slide atlas of neuropathology. New York, Gower Medical Publishing, 1988. By permission of Mayo Foundation.)*

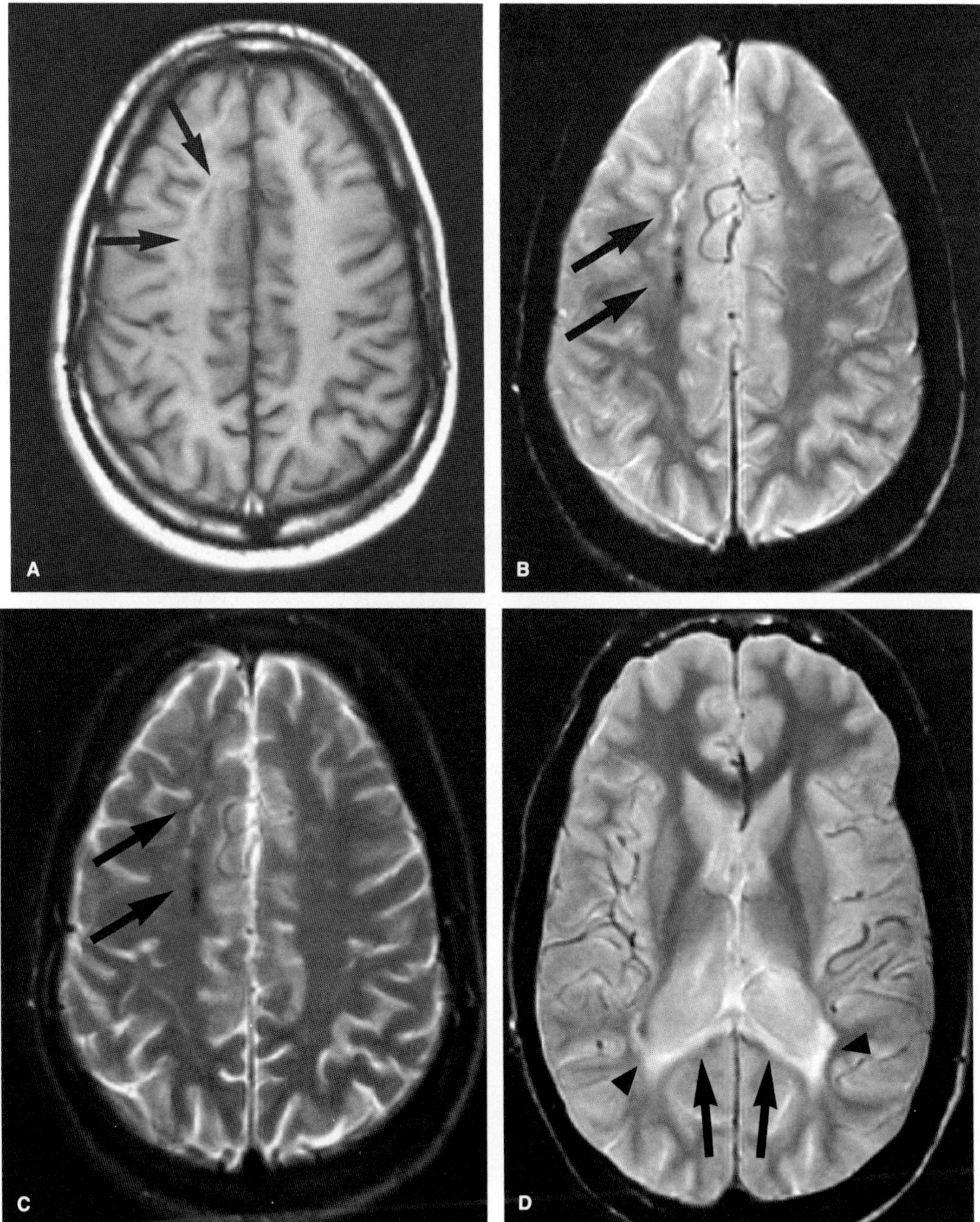

HISTORY

A 24-year-old with neurobehavioral changes and a history of a severe automobile accident 2 years previously

FINDINGS

(*A*) The T1-weighted axial image shows several irregular foci of low signal intensity (*arrows*) within the subcortical white matter of the right frontal lobe. On the intermediate (*B*) and heavily (*C*) T2-weighted axial images the lesions (*arrows*) have a mixture of both low and high signal intensity. Intermediate (*D*) and heavily (*E*) T2-weighted images at a lower level demonstrate abnormal high signal intensity in the splenium of the corpus callosum (*arrows*) and in the periatrial white matter (*arrowheads*).

DIAGNOSIS

Diffuse axonal injury

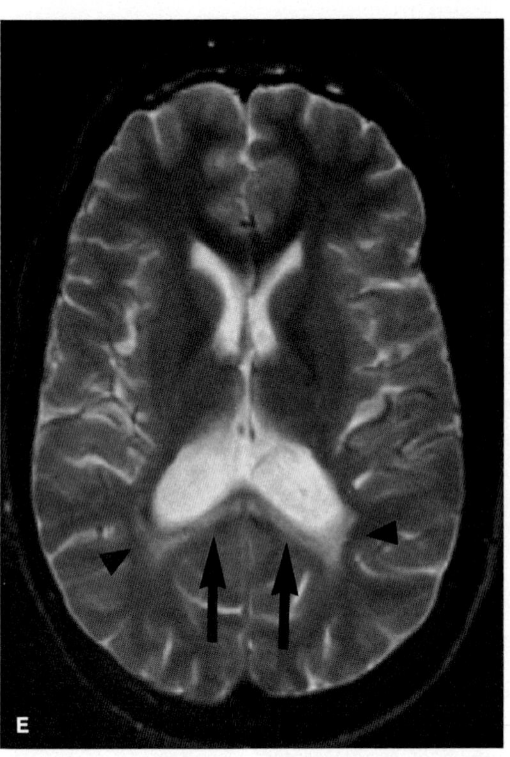

DISCUSSION

Primary intraaxial traumatic lesions of the brain have been classified into four types based on their location: diffuse axonal injury (DAI), cortical contusion, subcortical gray matter injury, and primary brain stem injury.[1] Of these, diffuse axonal injury is the most common. DAI is characterized by multiple, small, abnormal, ovoid to elliptic foci limited to the white matter tracts. Typically, the lesions are located at the gray–white matter junction (corticomedullary interface), and spare the overlying cortex.

DAI occurs as a result of rotationally induced shear-strain forces, and is commonly caused by motor vehicle accidents. Shear-strain is greatest at the junction of tissues with different rigidity and density.[1] Thus, the most common location for DAI is within the parasagittal white matter of the frontal lobes and white matter of the temporal lobes, usually at the gray–white matter interface. Lesions in the corona radiata are less common. The corpus callosum is the second most common area involved in DAI but rarely occurs without lobar white matter involvement. Most callosal lesions occur in the splenium,[2] because it is more fixed in position than the body and genu, and thus is subject to greater shear forces. Intraventricular hemorrhage is commonly seen in patients with corpus callosum DAI, probably as a result of shearing injury to nearby subependymal veins.

Nonhemorrhagic DAI lesions have low signal intensity on T1-weighted images, and high signal intensity on T2-weighted images. In old lesions, the high signal intensity on T2-weighted images represents gliosis and demyelination. Approximately 20% of DAI lesions have a hemorrhagic component. Old lesions typically contain hemosiderin, which has low signal intensity on T1-weighted images, and very low signal intensity on T2-weighted images.

Clinical References

1. Gentry L, Godersky J, Thompson B. MR imaging of head trauma: review of the distribution and radiopathologic features of traumatic lesions. AJNR 1988;9:101–110.
2. Gentry L, Thompson B, Godersky J. Trauma to the corpus callosum: MR features. AJNR 1988;9:1129–1138.

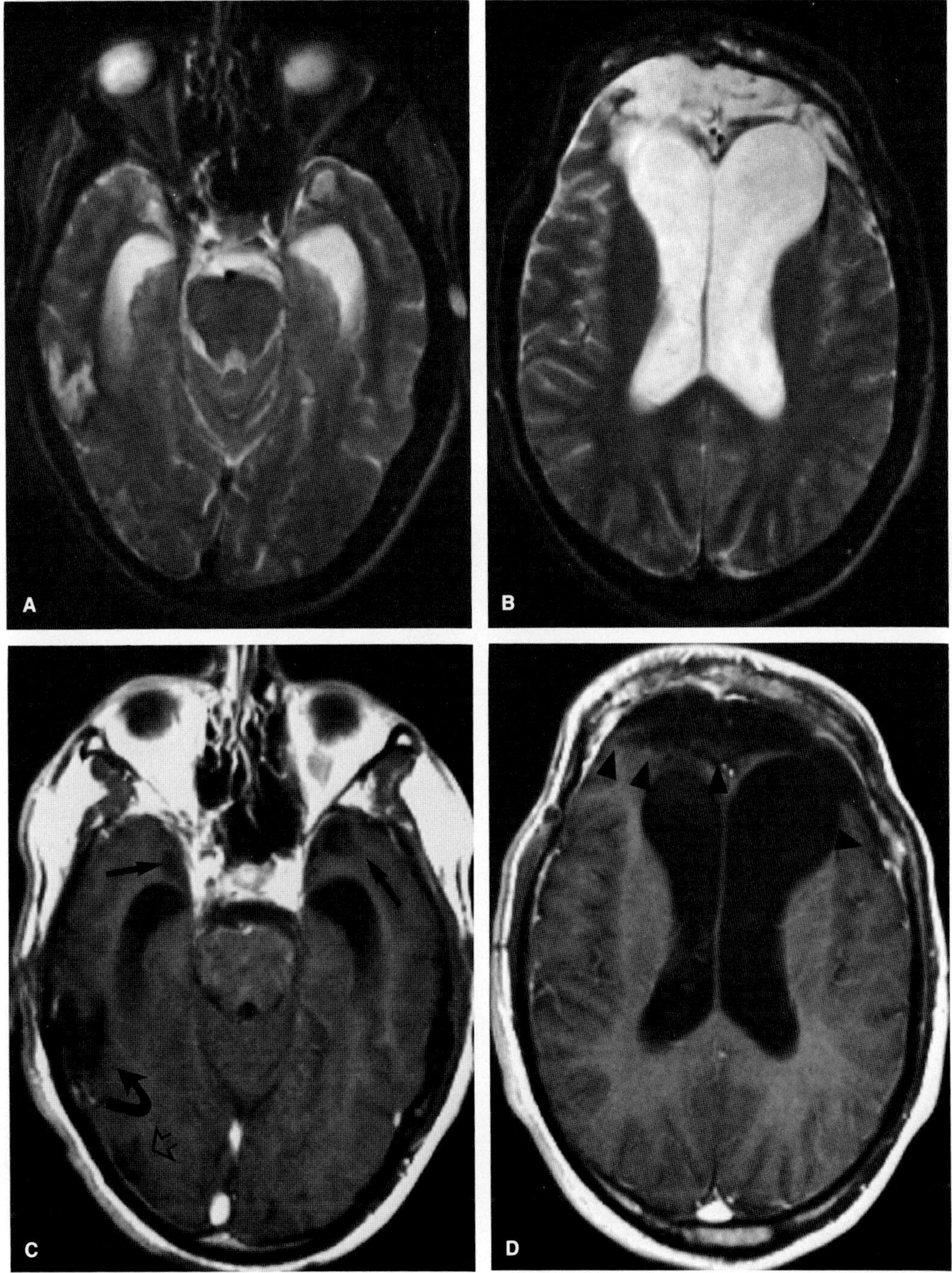

HISTORY

A 29-year-old with a severe head injury 8 months prior to this examination

FINDINGS

Precontrast T2-weighted (TE = 90 msec) (*A and B*) and postcontrast T1-weighted (*C and D*) images reveal cystic changes in the temporal tips (*arrows*), in brain immediately above the right petrous bone (*curved arrow*), in the right occipital lobe (*open arrow*), and in the frontal lobes bilaterally (*arrowheads*). On the T2-weighted images, abnormal low signal intensity, consistent with hemosiderin or ferritin deposition, is seen at the periphery of all but one lesion. There is generalized ventriculomegaly, with striking enlargement of the frontal horns due to adjacent loss of brain substance. (*E*) The intermediate T2-weighted scan (TE = 45 msec) permits differentiation of gliosis, with high signal intensity (*open arrow*), from adjacent cystic changes, which are isointense to CSF in the

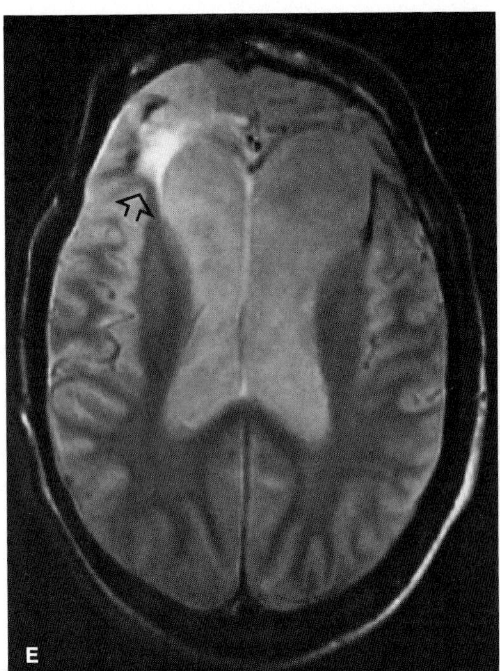

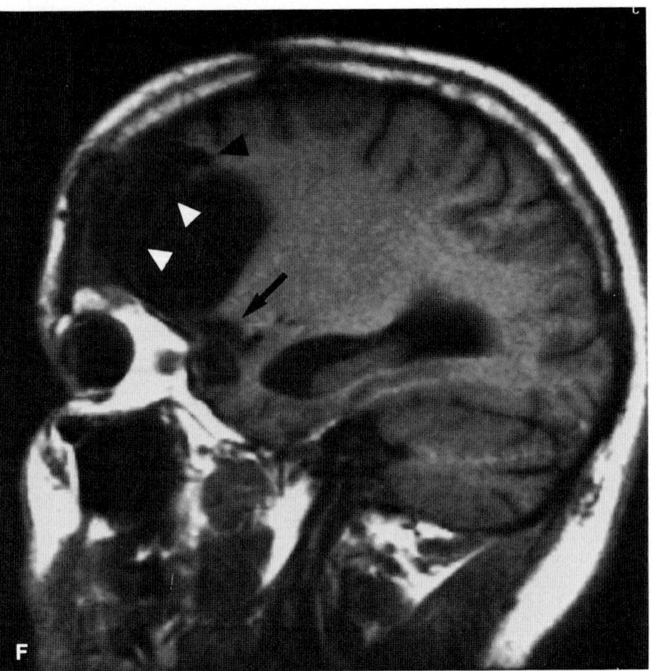

ventricular system. The presence of blood degradation products (with marked hypointensity) is confirmed. (*F*) A single slice from the precontrast sagittal T1-weighted scout image provides correlation in a perpendicular plane of the chronic injury to the left frontal lobe (*white and black arrowheads*) and temporal tip (*arrow*).

DIAGNOSIS

Chronic head injury

DISCUSSION

Findings which can be seen in chronic head injury include shear injuries, focal contusional ecephalomalacia, generalized atrophy, diffuse gray–white matter damage, and evidence of old hemorrhage.[1] The cystic changes noted in the current case are the end result of cortical contusions. Such lesions most commonly involve the inferior, lateral, and anterior portions of the frontal and temporal lobes.[2]

In acute head trauma, both CT and MR well depict recent hemorrhage. However, only MR is sufficiently sensitive to demonstrate accompanying chronic hematomas or infarction. In subacute head trauma, MR is markedly superior to CT for the detection and characterization of brain injury, including specifically shear injuries, contusions, and subdural hematomas. In chronic head trauma, MR and CT equally demonstrate atrophic changes. However, evidence of previous hemorrhage and parenchymal abnormalities are best identified by MR. CT remains the modality of choice only for evaluation of acute cases, primarily due to its greater speed. The sensitivity of MR, however, is key to the assessment of prognosis in subacute and chronic injury.

MR Technique

Multiplanar imaging is particularly important in brain trauma, as this greatly facilitates lesion localization.

Pitfalls in Image Interpretation

Without two different imaging planes, differentiation of cortical contusions from diffuse axonal injury involving the gray–white matter junction can be difficult.

Clinical References

1. Zimmerman RA, Bilaniuk LT, Hackney DB, et al. Head injury: early results of comparing CT and high-field MR. AJR 1986;14:1215–1222.
2. Gentry LR, Godersky JC, Thompson B. MR imaging of head trauma: review of the distribution and radiopathologic features of traumatic lesions. AJR 1988;150:663–672.

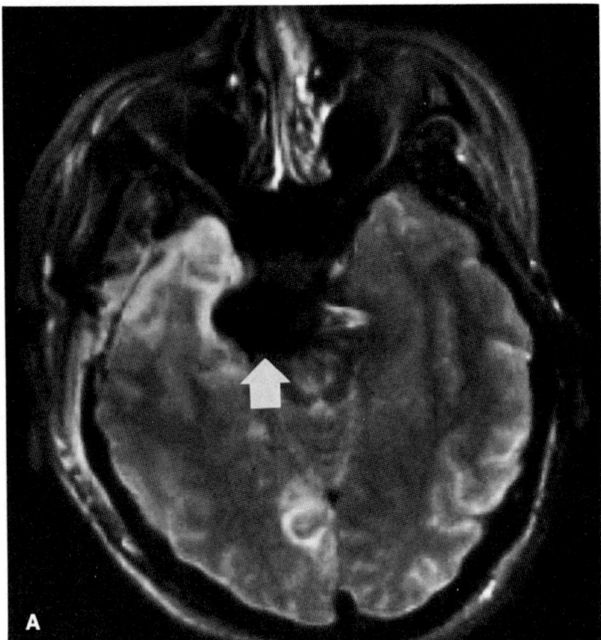

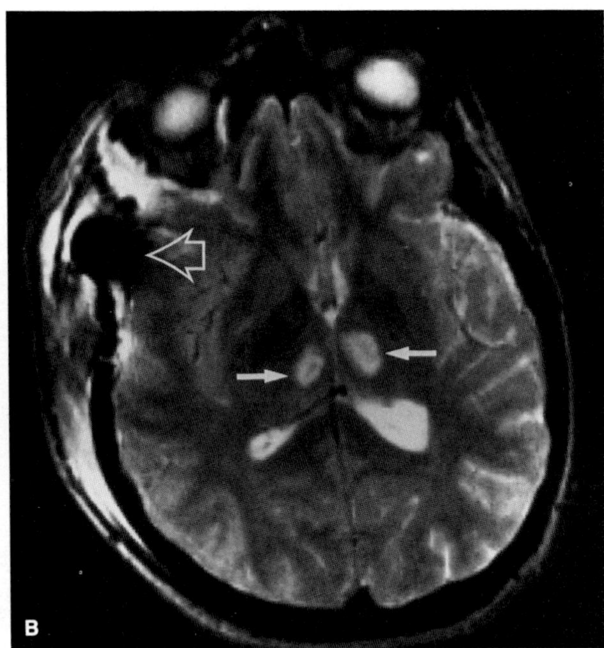

HISTORY

A comatose 35-year-old after brain surgery

FINDINGS

(*A and B*) Two T2-weighted axial sections are presented. The lower level (*A*) depicts a large signal dropout (*arrow*) in the region of the basilar artery, for which reason the case is included. Abnormal high signal intensity is also seen in the vascular territory of the right posterior cerebral artery, consistent with a subacute infarct. (*B*) At the higher level, an additional metallic artifact (*open arrow*) is present, probably because of a dural clip. Additional infarcts (*arrows in B*), which occurred as a complication of surgery, are noted in the thalami bilaterally, in the distribution of the deep penetrating arteries.

DIAGNOSIS

Intracranial aneurysm clip (nonmagnetic, placed for a basilar artery aneurysm)

DISCUSSION OF SAFETY ISSUES IN MR

The presence of an intracranial aneurysm clip represents a potential, but not absolute, contraindication to MR.[1] Nonferromagnetic or weakly ferromagnetic aneurysm clips (Sugita, Heifetz Elgiloy, Yasargil, and Vari-angle McFadden) do not experience strong deflection in a magnetic field and thus should be safe for study. Ferromagnetic clips (Sundt-Kees, McFadden, Drake, Mayfield, Kapp, Heifetz (pre-1984), Vari-angle Micro, Vari-angle Spring, Pivot, Sundt-Kees Multi-angle, and Scoville-Lewis) experience significant deflection and torque in a magnetic field and have the potential to dislodge. The presence of a ferromagnetic aneurysm clip thus does represent an absolute contraindication to MR. As illustrated, the image distortion produced by a nonferromagnetic aneurysm clip is relatively small in dimension (diameter of several centimeters), allowing good visualization of adjacent brain tissue. The artifact produced by a ferromagnetic clip is much larger, often obscuring almost an entire axial section.

The reader is referred to a current compilation of biomedical implants, materials, and devices in regard to contraindications for MR.[2] Risks with metal implants include movement or dislodgement, electrical current induction, heating, and artifacts that may render the scan nondiagnostic. Particular concern arises with metal adjacent to or within vital neural, vascular, or soft tissue structures. MR is contraindicated in patients who have electrically, mechanically, or magnetically activated implants, as the operation of these may be affected. Included in this list are cardiac pacemakers (internal or external), implantable cardioverter defibrillators, neurostimulators, bone-growth stimulators, cochlear implants, and implantable drug infusion pumps. Of particular concern are intracardiac wires of any type, in which a current could potentially be induced, leading to fibrillation or thermal injury. Potential risks exist with temporary pacing wires, residual external pacing wires, thermodilution Swan-Ganz catheters, and similar devices. That the patient has previously undergone MR safely does not preclude the possibility of injury, emphasizing the need for active and thorough screening.

The presence of any one of the additional following implants, materials, or devices represents a contraindication to MR: ferromagnetic aneurysm clips (as previously noted); Poppen-Blaylock carotid artery vascular clamp; Starr-Edwards pre-6000 heart valve prosthesis; ferromagnetic intravascular coils, filters, and stents (within several weeks of implantation or if possibly loose); certain ocular implants (specifically the Fatio eyelid spring and the martensitic retinal tack); cochlear implants; the McGee stapedectomy piston prosthesis; ferromagnetic pellets, bullets, and shrapnel; the Dacomed Omniphase penile implant; and the triple-lumen thermodilution Swan-Ganz catheter (also previously noted). The presence of a ferromagnetic object (foreign body) within the globe represents an absolute contraindication to MR because of the potential for hemorrhage. Plain radiography is considered an acceptable screen for excluding potentially hazardous intraocular metallic foreign bodies.[3] Bullets, shrapnel, or other types of metal fragments can pose a risk for MR, depending on the ferromagnetic properties of the substance, location near vital structures, magnetic field strength, and fixation by adjacent tissue or scar. Certain medical devices are magnetically activated, including cochlear implants, ocular prostheses, tissue expanders, and dental implants. MR in these patients is also potentially hazardous. Movement, alteration of operation, and damage to these devices are all possible. Gating leads, halo vests, and physiologic monitoring equipment, depending on the specific type of equipment used and setup, can also present a risk to the patient during MR study. Care should be taken so that unused gating leads or other external wires be removed, even if disconnected. Loops in external wiring should be avoided and an insulator (such as a cloth towel) should be placed between the patient and any external wires or cables, such as that used with a surface coil. MR-compatible halo vests are now commercially available and routinely used in many centers.

Current FDA guidelines require labeling for MR units that states that the safety for the fetus "has not been established."[3] Few studies have been performed in this area, and a number of mechanisms exist that could potentially result in adverse biologic effects. MR imaging is typically performed only in a pregnant woman, given informed consent, when there is no appropriate alternative diagnostic examination and the results of MR could substantially affect patient care before delivery.

Last but not least, any review of MR safety issues and patient concerns would not be complete without mention of the "tapping" made by the magnet. Acoustic noise is produced by activation of the gradient coils and is greater with higher static magnetic field strengths. Newer pulse sequences with faster repetition rates and greater applied gradient strengths also tend to raise the level of acoustic noise. Routine use of earplugs or of recently available antinoise systems is encouraged for patient comfort.

Clinical References

1. Becker RL, Norfray JF, Teitelbaum GP, et al. MR imaging in patients with intracranial aneurysm clips. AJNR 1988;9:885–889.
2. Shellock FG, Curtis JS. MR imaging and biomedical implants, materials, and devices: an updated review. Radiology 1991;180:541–550.
3. Shellock FG, Kanal E. Policies, guidelines, and recommendations for MR imaging safety and patient management. J Magn Reson Imaging 1991;1:97–101.

(A and B from Runge VM. Clinical magnetic resonance imaging. Philadelphia, JB Lippincott, 1990.)

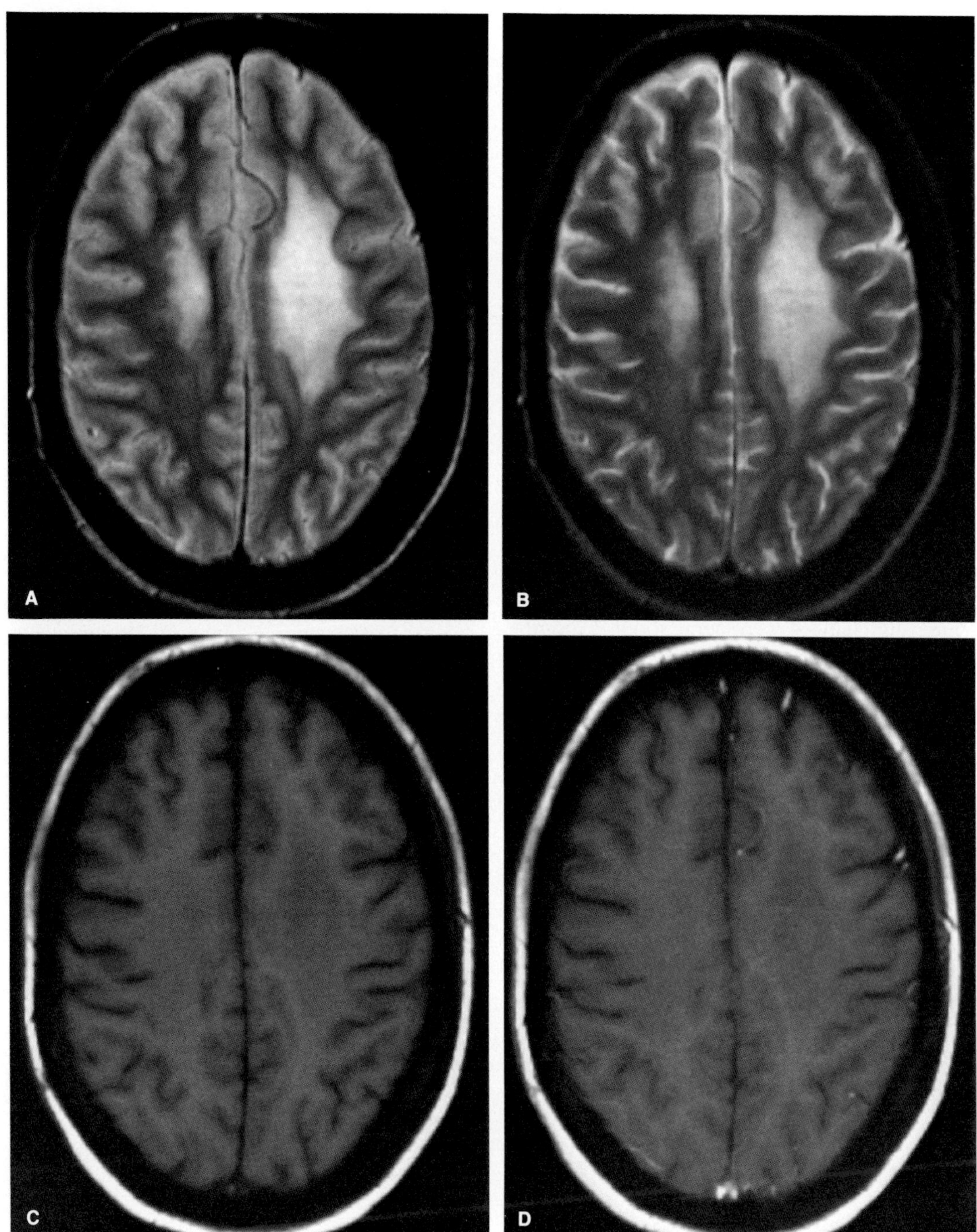

HISTORY

A 44-year-old patient who received a total of 6510 cGy for a grade 2/3 astrocytoma about 11 months earlier

FINDINGS

Increased signal intensity in the white matter of the centrum semiovale is identified on the first (*A*) and second (*B*) echoes of the axial T2-weighted sequence. (*C*) The corresponding axial T1-weighted image demonstrates subtle low signal intensity in these areas. (*D*) On the axial postcontrast T1-weighted image no abnormal enhancement is seen in the centrum semiovale.

DIAGNOSIS

Radiation white matter changes

DISCUSSION

The white matter changes secondary to radiation therapy can be either permanent or transient. The early changes consist primarily of white matter vasogenic edema resulting from damage to the capillary endothelium and are of limited clinical consequence.[1] The endothelium is the most radiosensitive tissue in the brain.

The diffuse white matter hyperintensity on T2-weighted images postradiation that does not demonstrate enhancement is due to demyelination of axons. Demyelination leads to increased water content of the affected brain tissues and explains the prolonged T2 relaxation time.[2] These radiation changes typically are symmetric and affect most of the periventricular white matter.

Radiation necrosis appears as regions of hyperintensity on T2-weighted sequences that demonstrate enhancement. Increased radiation dose correlates with increased incidence of radiation necrosis.

The time of onset of radiation lesions varies greatly from case to case. In single-dose radiation experiments, MR signal intensity changes were seen about 7 months after treatment.[3] In patients, radiation changes are variable and can be noted over a wide dose range but appear with increased frequency with higher total doses.

Pitfalls in Image Interpretation

Although MR can depict radiation changes to the brain with a high sensitivity, the T1 and T2 relaxation times of radiation demyelination, radiation necrosis, and recurrent brain tumor are all increased and are not significantly different from one another. Follow-up studies are necessary to exclude residual tumor.

Clinical References

1. Hecht-Leavitt CM, Grossman RI, Curran WJ, et al. MR of brain radiation injury: experimental studies in cats. AJNR 1987;8:427–430.
2. Dooms GC, Hecht SH, Brant-Zawadzki M, et al. Brain radiation lesions: MR imaging. Radiology 1986;158:149–155.
3. Grossman RI, Hecht-Leavitt CM, Evans SM, et al. Experimental radiation injury: combined MR imaging and spectroscopy. Radiology 1988;169:305–309.

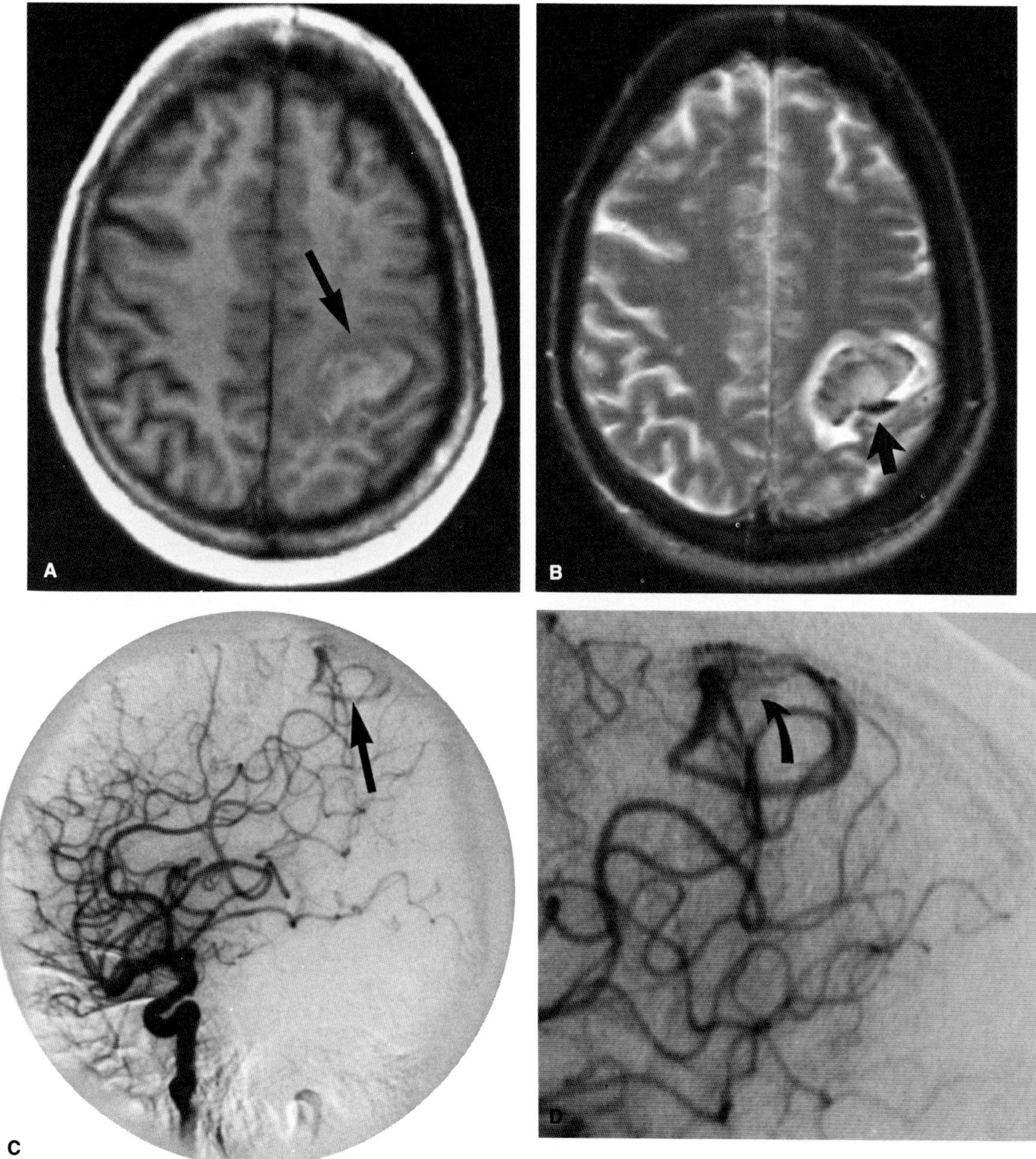

HISTORY

A 63-year-old with right-sided weakness

FINDINGS

(*A*) T1-weighted axial image demonstrates an irregular mass (*arrow*) in the left parietal lobe that has a slightly greater signal intensity than the surrounding brain. There is a subtle low-signal-intensity rim surrounding the lesion. (*B*) On the T2-weighted axial image the lesion is more heterogeneous, although predominantly high signal intensity compared with brain. Along the posterolateral border of the mass is a very low signal intensity tubular structure (*arrow*) that represents signal void in a vessel. The high-signal-intensity rim surrounding the lesion is due to vasogenic edema. (*C*) The arterial phase from a conventional angiogram (performed by a left common carotid artery injection) reveals abnormal early filling of a large cortical vein (*arrow*) in the left parietal region, which drains into the superior sagittal sinus. (The superior sagittal sinus was depicted on venous phase images [not shown]). (*D*) A magnified view from the angiogram reveals small abnormal feeding arteries (*curved arrow*).

DIAGNOSIS

Dural arteriovenous fistula, with parenchymal hematoma

DISCUSSION

Dural arteriovenous fistulas are acquired vascular malformations that most commonly occur in the posterior fossa and usually involve venous sinuses. It is believed that the development of a dural arteriovenous fistula begins with thrombosis or occlusion of the involved venous sinus.[1] The extensive arterial network in the walls of the venous sinus subsequently attempts to recanalize the occluded sinus by forming numerous new direct artery-to-sinus feeding vessels.[1] These direct feeding vessels are very small and often visible using conventional angiography but are not seen with MR.

The diagnosis of a dural arteriovenous fistula may be difficult to make with MR. In fact, findings may be normal using routine MR in a patient with a dural arteriovenous fistula. However, the diagnosis should be suspected when large, superficial, dural-based draining veins are present without a parenchymal vascular nidus.

Concomitant thrombus within an adjacent venous sinus also points to the diagnosis. Complications associated with dural arteriovenous fistulas are common and include venous infarction, parenchymal hemorrhage, and subdural hematoma, all of which are best seen with MR. Patients present with nonspecific signs and symptoms such as headache or neurologic deficit caused by one of the aforementioned complications.

Carotid artery–cavernous sinus fistulas are unique dural arteriovenous fistulas which form as a result of traumatic laceration of the internal carotid artery, or rupture of an aneurysm, within the cavernous sinus. The clinical findings of pulsatile exophthalmos, audible bruit over the eye, diplopia, and headache are highly suggestive of the diagnosis. On MR, there is enlargement of the ipsilateral cavernous sinus and superior ophthalmic vein, due to either increased flow or thrombosis.[2]

Clinical References

1. DeMarco J, Dillon W, Halbach V, et al. Dural arteriovenous fistulas: evaluation with MR imaging. Radiology 1990; 175:193–199.
2. Castillo M, Silverstein M, Hoffman J, et al. Spontaneous thrombosis of a direct carotid cavernous sinus fistula: confirmation by Gd-DTPA–enhanced MR. AJNR 1989;10:S75–S76.

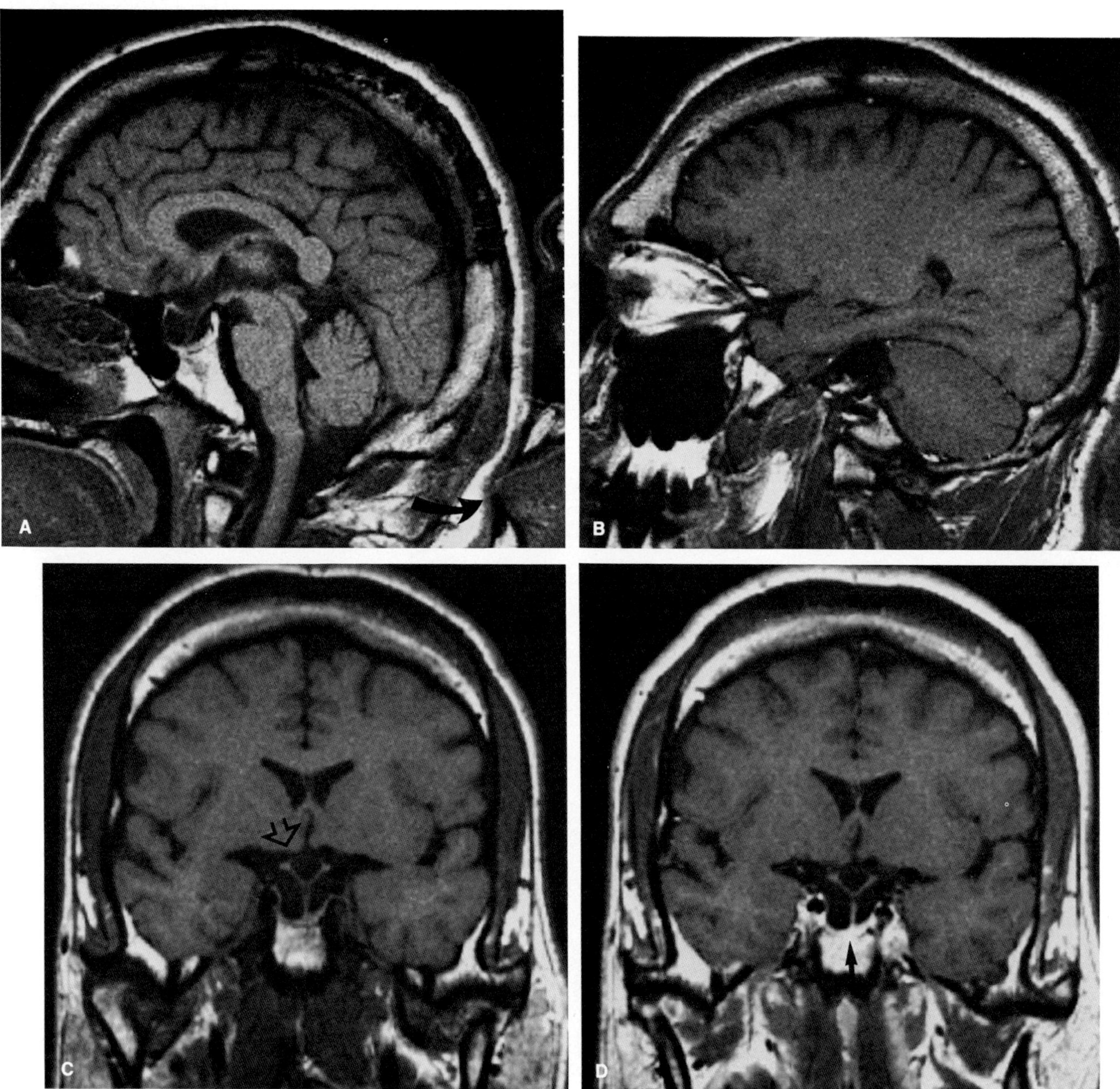

HISTORY

An older gentleman with coarse facial features who previously had transsphenoidal surgery

FINDINGS

(*A*) The midline T1-weighted sagittal image reveals an enlarged sella turcica, which contains principally CSF. The frontal sinus appears slightly enlarged. The skull is markedly thickened, with an enlarged diploic space. Posterior to the head, a soft tissue structure can be seen, which overlaps the brain slightly. On second glance, the patient's nose and very large jaw (*curved arrow*) can be recognized, which appear posteriorly because of aliasing. (*B*) On a sagittal T1-weighted section off midline, enlargement of the maxillary sinus can be noted. Precontrast (*C*) and postcontrast (*D*) thin-section coronal T1-weighted images demonstrate draping of the optic chiasm (*open arrow in C*) into the sella and minimal residual enhancing pituitary tissue (*arrow in D*).

DIAGNOSIS

Acromegaly

DISCUSSION

Growth hormone excess produces acromegaly in adults, a chronic debilitating disease with bony and soft tissue overgrowth.[1] In most cases, a pituitary adenoma (the source of excess growth hormone) can be identified by imaging means, either CT or MR. Common secondary features seen in head imaging include prognathism (abnormal forward projection of the jaw), paranasal sinus enlargement, and skull thickening.

The therapy of choice in acromegaly is surgical excision of the adenoma using a transsphenoidal approach, with cure possible if complete resection is achieved. Predictors of positive surgical outcome include preoperative growth hormone levels less than 40 μg/L and an adenoma under 10 mm in diameter. Tumor regrowth and recurrent symptoms are common.

MR Technique

Head imaging is typically performed with a field-of-view (FOV) of 25 cm or less, in order to achieve high (approximately 1 × 1 mm) in-plane spatial resolution. In patients with exceptionally large heads, this choice of FOV can lead to wraparound, particularly in the sagittal plane, with the nose (or jaw, as in this instance) overlapping the posterior part of the head. Wraparound or aliasing is caused by undersampling. To eliminate wraparound, oversampling can be employed in the frequency encoding dimension at no cost in scan time or S/N. Oversampling in the phase encoding direction, although possible, would lead to increased scan time and is not commonly employed.

In the past few years, the coils used for head imaging on most MR equipment have been redesigned to maximize S/N. In addition to employing quadrature technology (which should theoretically lead to a 40% increase in S/N), the length and diameter of these coils have been reduced, with smaller coils (being closer to the object of interest) generally producing higher S/N. Note that the images in this case appear somewhat "grainy," the result of poor S/N. The patient's head did not fit in the standard coil, and thus an older linear polarized design of larger internal dimensions, with poorer S/N had to be employed.

Clinical References

1. Ezzat S, Melmed S. Acromegaly: etiology, diagnosis and management. Compr Ther 1991;17(7):31–35.

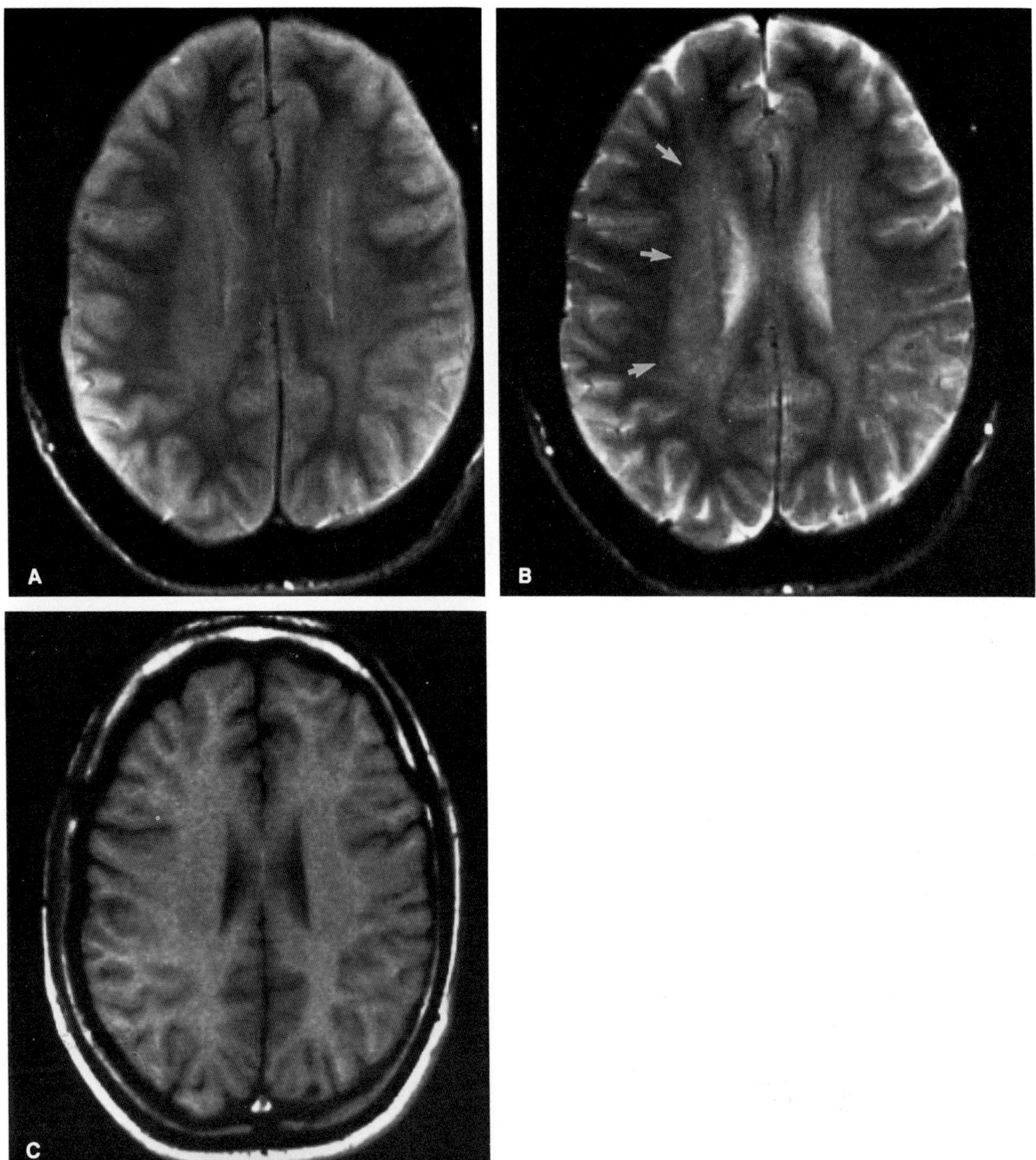

HISTORY

A 22-year-old chronic abuser of toluene-based spray paint. Neurologic symptoms included cognitive impairment, cerebellar ataxia, and corticospinal tract dysfunction.

FINDINGS

The first (TE = 45 msec) (*A*) and second (TE = 90 msec) (*B*) echoes from a T2-weighted examination reveal diffuse central white matter abnormal hyperintensity (*arrows in B*). (*C*) No white matter abnormality is evident on the corresponding T1-weighted scan. There is mild cortical atrophy, a significant finding given the patient's age.

DIAGNOSIS

Diffuse white matter injury due to chronic toluene abuse

DISCUSSION

Toluene (methyl benzene), a major component of many spray paints and glues, is a widely used and abused organic solvent. Chronic abuse is by vapor inhalation of a commercially available product. Neurologic abnormalities include cognitive, behavioral, pyramidal, brain stem and cerebellar findings. MR studies of toluene abusers have revealed the following abnormalities attributed to chronic high-dose exposure: diffuse atrophy (cerebral, cerebellar, and brain stem), loss of gray-white matter differentiation, and abnormal periventricular white matter hyperintensity on T2-weighted images.[1] Study of patients following abstinence suggests that the white matter changes demonstrated on MR are irreversible. The degree of white matter abnormality on T2-weighted scans strongly correlates with neuropsychologic impairment.[2] Dementia appears to relate to the degree of cerebral white matter damage, which by MR is most severe in long-term abusers. T2-weighted scans can be normal in patients with a relatively short duration of abuse (less than 3 years). The long-term effect on painters or other workers exposed to organic solvents at low levels is unclear. Brain stem auditory evoked response testing may detect early injury to the central nervous system due to toluene inhalation when MR is normal.[3]

Toluene is an organic solvent with high lipophilicity, which becomes concentrated in lipid-rich tissues following inhalation. The distribution of toluene within the CNS correlates with regional lipid content. High concentrations have been shown in both central white matter and spinal nerves. The encephalopathy seen clinically with toluene abuse, including dementia, is likely due to the high uptake of this chemical in central white matter. Peripheral nerves appear spared.[4] The effect of other potentially neurotoxic solvents, such as glue, has not been well defined, with many solvent abusers inhaling commercial products with multiple potentially neurotoxic components.

Pitfalls in Image Interpretation

In addition to toluene abuse, the differential diagnosis for diffuse white matter hyperintensity on T2-weighted scans includes the leukodystrophies (in which an enzyme deficiency results in progressive destruction of myelin) and radiation therapy (where radiation-induced arteritis can lead to widespread leukomalacia). Characteristics possibly specific for radiation-induced injury include diffuse involvement of white matter up to the cortical gray matter junction, with sparing of the corpus collosum.[5]

Clinical References

1. Rosenberg NL, Kleinschmidt-DeMasters BK, Davis KA, et al. Toluene abuse causes diffuse central nervous system white matter changes. Ann Neurol 1988;23:611–614.
2. Filley CM, Heaton RK, Rosenberg NL. White matter dementia in chronic toluene abuse. Neurology 1990;40:532–534.
3. Rosenberg NL, Spitz MC, Filley CM, et al. Central nervous system effects of chronic toluene abuse—clinical, brainstem evoked response and magnetic resonance imaging studies. Neurotoxicol Teratol 1988;10:489–495.
4. Gospe SM Jr. Toluene dementia. Neurology 1990;40:1320–1321.
5. Edwards MK, Smith RR. White matter diseases. Top Magn Reson Imaging 1989;2:41–48.

(A to C from Runge VM. Clinical magnetic resonance imaging. Philadelphia, JB Lippincott, 1990.)

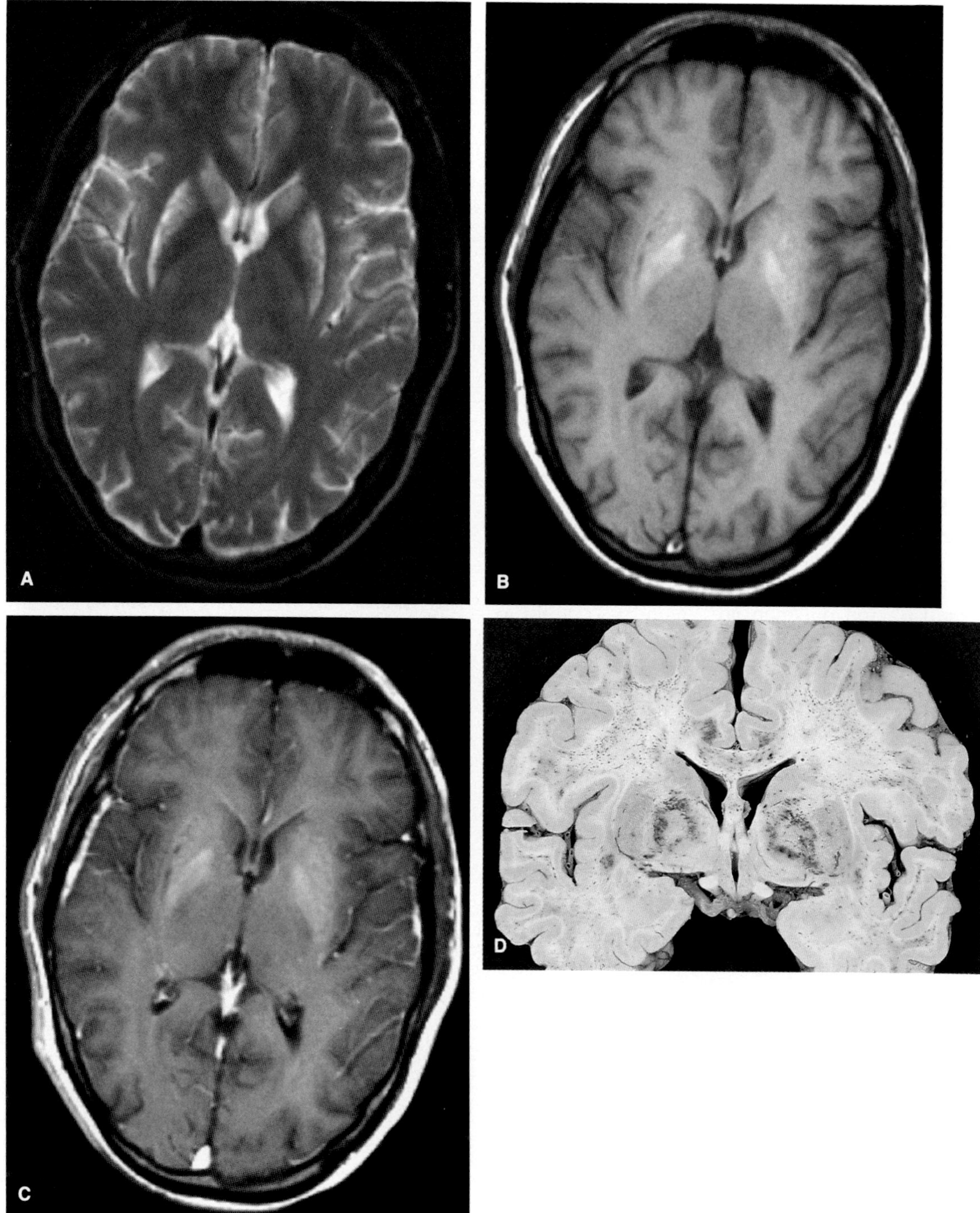

HISTORY

A 26-year-old man with a 2-day history of upper gastrointestinal bleeding that required 12 units of packed red blood cells and 6 units of frozen plasma. The patient had an episode of asystole during his initial hospital course. Oral intubation was not successful and a tracheostomy tube was placed. The patient received total parenteral nutrition for a short time during his hospital stay. All of this occurred about 1 month before this study.

FINDINGS

(*A*) Axial T2-weighted image demonstrates abnormal hyperintensity in the putamen and caudate nuclei bilaterally. (*B*) On the axial T1-weighted image, tram-track foci of abnormal hypointensity are present in the lateral aspect of the putamen bilaterally. Abnormal hyperintensity of the globus pallidus is also seen bilaterally on *B*. This may be secondary to the patient receiving total parenteral nutrition (TPN). (*C*) Subtle contrast enhancement is present in the putamen bilaterally on the axial T1-weighted postcontrast image.

DIAGNOSIS

Anoxic brain injury

DISCUSSION

Cerebral anoxia is the result of inadequate oxygen delivered to the brain. It can occur secondary to hypoxia (decreased oxygen content in the blood) or ischemia (hypoperfusion).[1] The entire brain is not uniformly affected by an anoxic–ischemic insult. Gray matter is more vulnerable than white matter. The watershed zones between arterial circulations are particularly vulnerable, as these regions are the last to be perfused. Neurons are the cells most sensitive to anoxia–ischemia, and in general small neurons are more sensitive than larger ones. The hippocampus, cerebral cortex, cerebellum (notably Purkinje cells), caudate, and putamen are highly susceptible to anoxic–ischemic injury. The globus pallidus, thalamus, hemispheric white matter, brain stem, and spinal cord are less sensitive to anoxia.[2] In children following severe anoxic insults, iron deposition can occur in the basal ganglia and thalamus, resulting in abnormal hypointensity on T2-weighted images.[3]

Abnormal hyperintensity has been observed in the globus pallidus bilaterally on T1-weighted images in patients receiving long-term TPN therapy. This may be secondary to deposition of intravenously administered paramagnetic trace elements (in particular manganese), which increases the rate of T1 relaxation.[4]

Pathologic Correlate

(*D*) A coronal section of a partially fixed brain demonstrates early infarction of the globus pallidus bilaterally in addition to white matter petechiae in an elderly man with carbon monoxide poisoning. Patients who die from carbon monoxide poisoning show pink-red discoloration of their skin and organs.

Clinical References

1. Stark DD, Bradley WG. Magnetic resonance imaging, 2nd ed. St Louis, Mosby–Year Book, 1992:662–664.
2. Davis RL, Robertson DM. Textbook of neuropathology. Baltimore, Williams & Wilkins:1991:461–474.
3. Dietrich RB, Bradley WG. Iron accumulation in the basal ganglia following severe ischemic-anoxic insults in children. Radiology 1988;168:203–206.
4. Mirowitz SA, Westrich TJ, Hirsh JD. Hyperintense basal ganglia on T1 weighted MR images in patients receiving parenteral nutrition. Radiology 1991;181:117–120.

(D *from Okazaki H, Scheithauer B. Slide atlas of neuropathology. New York, Gower Medical Publishing, 1988. By permission of Mayo Foundation.*)

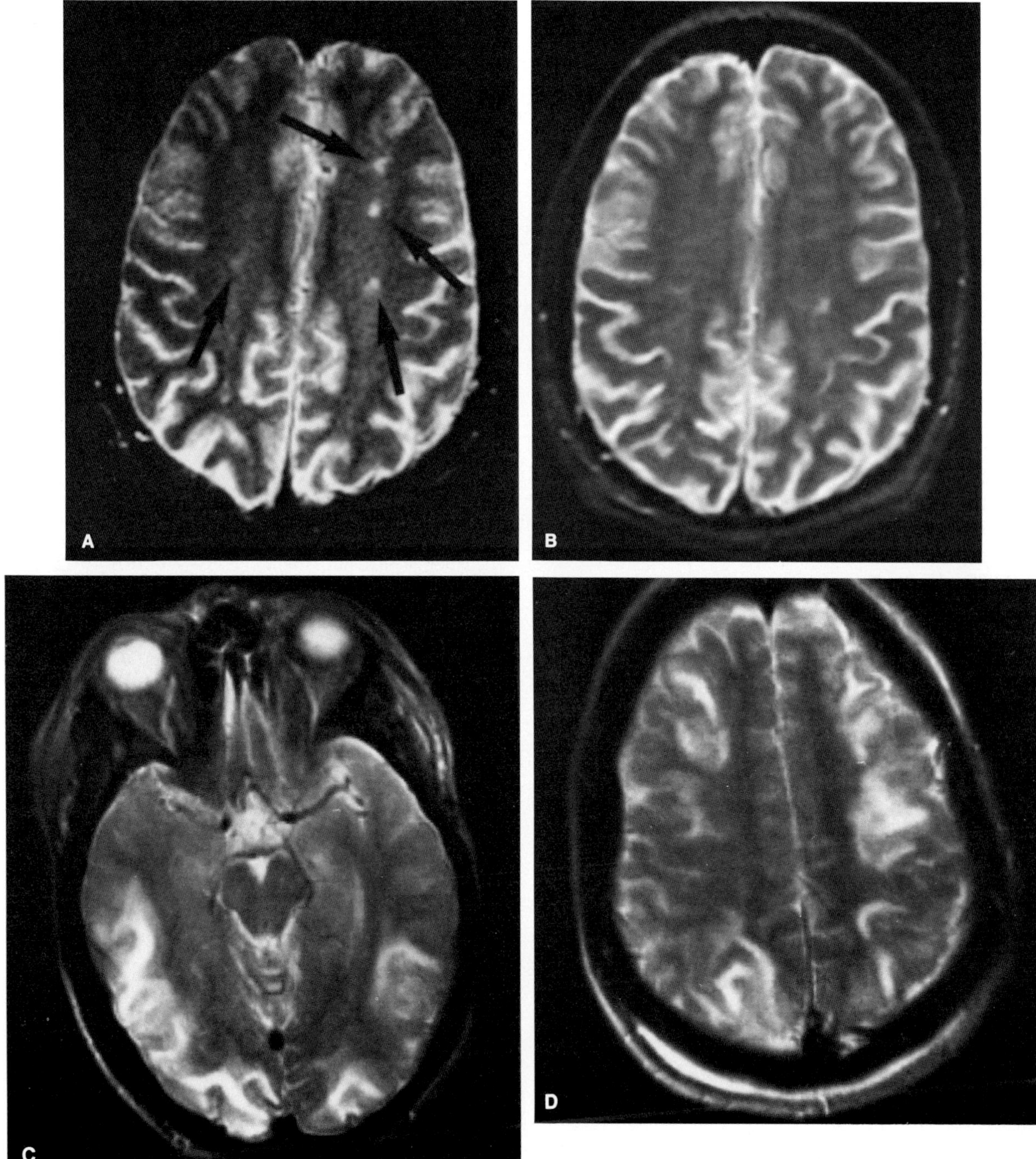

HISTORY

Patient 1: A 34-year-old man presenting acutely with seizures

Patient 2: A 19-year-old woman with nephritis

FINDINGS

Patient 1: (*A*) On the axial T2-weighted scan just above the ventricular system, four punctate white matter lesions (*arrows*) can be identified. (*B*) Four months later, after treatment with steroids, only one lesion is clearly identified.

Patient 2: *C* and *D* are two sections from the axial T2-weighted scan that demonstrate multiple bilateral parenchymal abnormalities in the anterior, middle, and posterior cerebral artery territories involving both gray and white matter.

DIAGNOSIS

Systemic lupus erythematosus (SLE)

DISCUSSION

Approximately 40% of all SLE patients demonstrate CNS involvement clinically.[1] CNS symptoms can be diffuse (generalized seizures) or focal (stroke).

On MR, lesions in SLE can be noted that involve (1) gray matter (exclusively), (2) subcortical white matter, (3) deep white matter, and (4) both gray and white matter (similar to a territorial infarct).[2,3] Resolution of parenchymal abnormalities in the first three locations has been observed on follow-up MR (after aggressive corticosteroid treatment), suggesting that the hyperintensity observed on T2-weighted images is due to either edema or inflammatory infiltrates. Changes that are chronic in nature presumably correspond to macroinfarction or microinfarction. Blood–brain barrier disruption can also be demonstrated in certain cases on postcontrast MR. CT is less sensitive than MR for both lesion detection and demarcation.[4]

MR Technique

T2-weighted scans are favored for detection of parenchymal lesions in SLE, which are seen as regions of abnormal hyperintensity relative to normal brain.

Pitfalls in Image Interpretation

In the differential diagnosis of a young patient with deep white matter and periventricular lesions on MR, multiple sclerosis, neurosarcoidosis, Behçet's syndrome, polyarteritis nodosa, and other vasculitides should be considered in addition to CNS lupus erythematosus.

Clinical References

1. Van Dam AP. Diagnosis and pathogenesis of CNS lupus. Rheumatol Int 1991;11:1–11.
2. Jacobs L, Kinkel PR, Costello PB, et al. Central nervous system lupus erythematosus: the value of magnetic resonance imaging. J Rheumatol 1988;15:601–606.
3. Aisen AM, Gabrielsen TO, McCune WJ. MR imaging of systemic lupus erythematosus involving the brain. AJR 1985;144:1027–1031.
4. Sibbitt WL Jr, Sibbitt RR, Griffey RH, et al. Magnetic resonance and computed tomographic imaging in the evaluation of acute neuropsychiatric disease in systemic lupus erythematosus. Ann Rheum Dis 1989;48:1014–1022.

(A and B courtesy of Clifford Wolf, MD; C and D from Runge VM. Clinical magnetic resonance imaging. Philadelphia, JB Lippincott, 1990.)

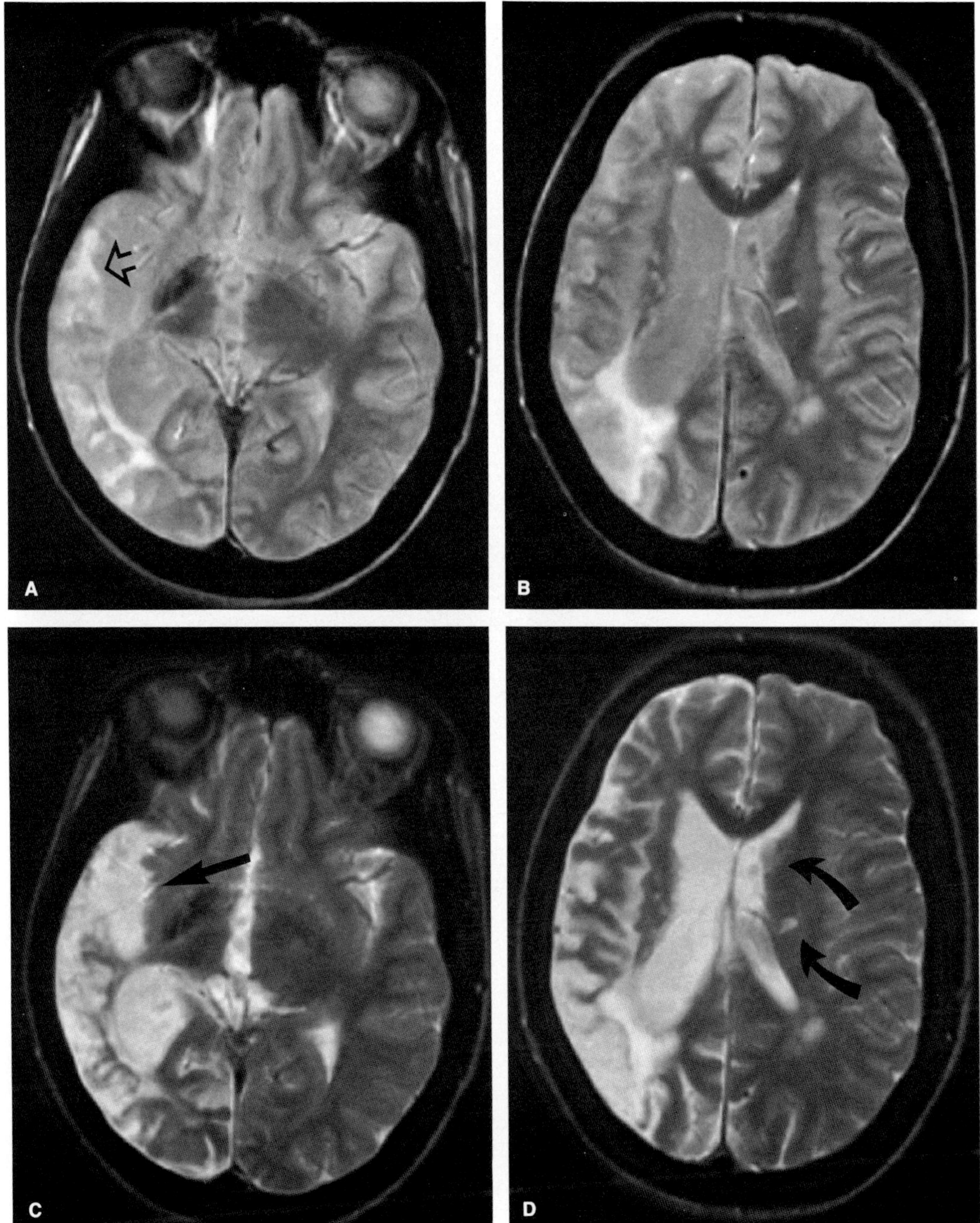

HISTORY

A 27-year-old patient with seizures and dysarthria, who has suffered multiple strokes in the past, the most severe of which resulted in left hemiparesis

FINDINGS

Intermediate (TE = 45 msec) (*A and B*) and heavily (TE = 90 msec) (*C and D*) T2-weighted images reveal a large, old, right middle-cerebral-artery infarct, which includes the watershed region with the posterior cerebral artery. There is both cystic encephalomalacia (*arrow in C*) and gliosis (*open arrow in A*), the latter best recognized on the intermediate T2-weighted images. There is compensatory dilatation of the right ventricle. Lacunar infarcts are noted in the left caudate nucleus and internal capsule (*curved arrows in D*). (*E and F*) The postcontrast T1-weighted scans also depict these abnormalities. (*G*) 3D TOF MRA demonstrates occlusion of the internal ca-

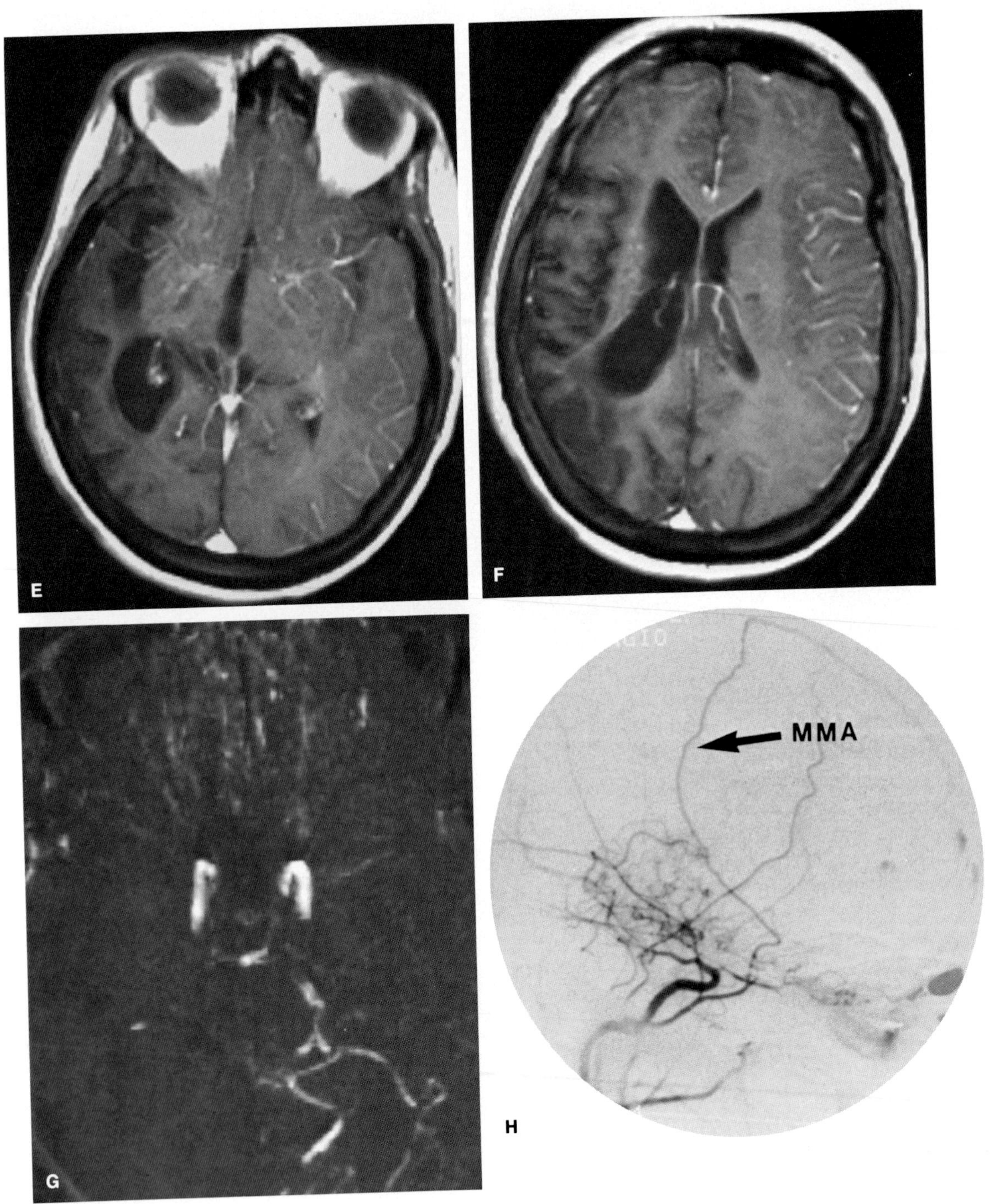

rotid arteries at the origin of the anterior and middle cerebral arteries.

(*H*) Digital contrast angiography reveals bilateral distal internal artery occlusions (the right carotid injection is shown). The right posterior cerebral artery has a fetal origin and fills from the right internal carotid artery. Collateral circulation includes a hypertrophied right middle meningeal artery (MMA). There are dilated thalamoperforate and thalamolenticular arteries which reconstitute flow to the basal ganglia and thalamus.

DIAGNOSIS

Moyamoya disease

DISCUSSION

In moyamoya disease, hemispheric infarctions and subcortical infarctions, the latter in the centrum semiovale, occur in hemodynamically compromised brain.[1] The distribution of cerebral infarction is bilateral, multiple, and affects predominantly the carotid circulation in watershed areas. Infarcts in the caudate nucleus, putamen, globus pallidus, and internal capsule have also been described. Infarction occurs as a result of occlusion or stenosis of the terminal internal carotid artery and proximal anterior and middle cerebral artery branches.[2] A network of small anastomotic vessels ("cloud of smoke") may be present at the base of the brain. Brain atrophy and venticulomegaly may occur secondary to the primary disease. These features are all well depicted by MR, which has proved superior to CT.[3] The disease is most common in childhood, with an increased incidence in the Japanese population, and rarely progresses after the initial illness.

Clinical References

1. Bruno A, Yuh WT, Biller J, et al. Magnetic resonance imaging in young adults with cerebral infarction due to moyamoya. Arch Neurol 1988;45:303–306.
2. Fujisawa I, Asato R, Nishimura K, et al. Moyamoya disease: MR imaging. Radiology 1987;164:103–105.
3. Suto Y, Caner BE, Nakatsugawa S, et al. Evaluation of MRI in moyamoya disease. Radiat Med 1990;8(3):92–95.

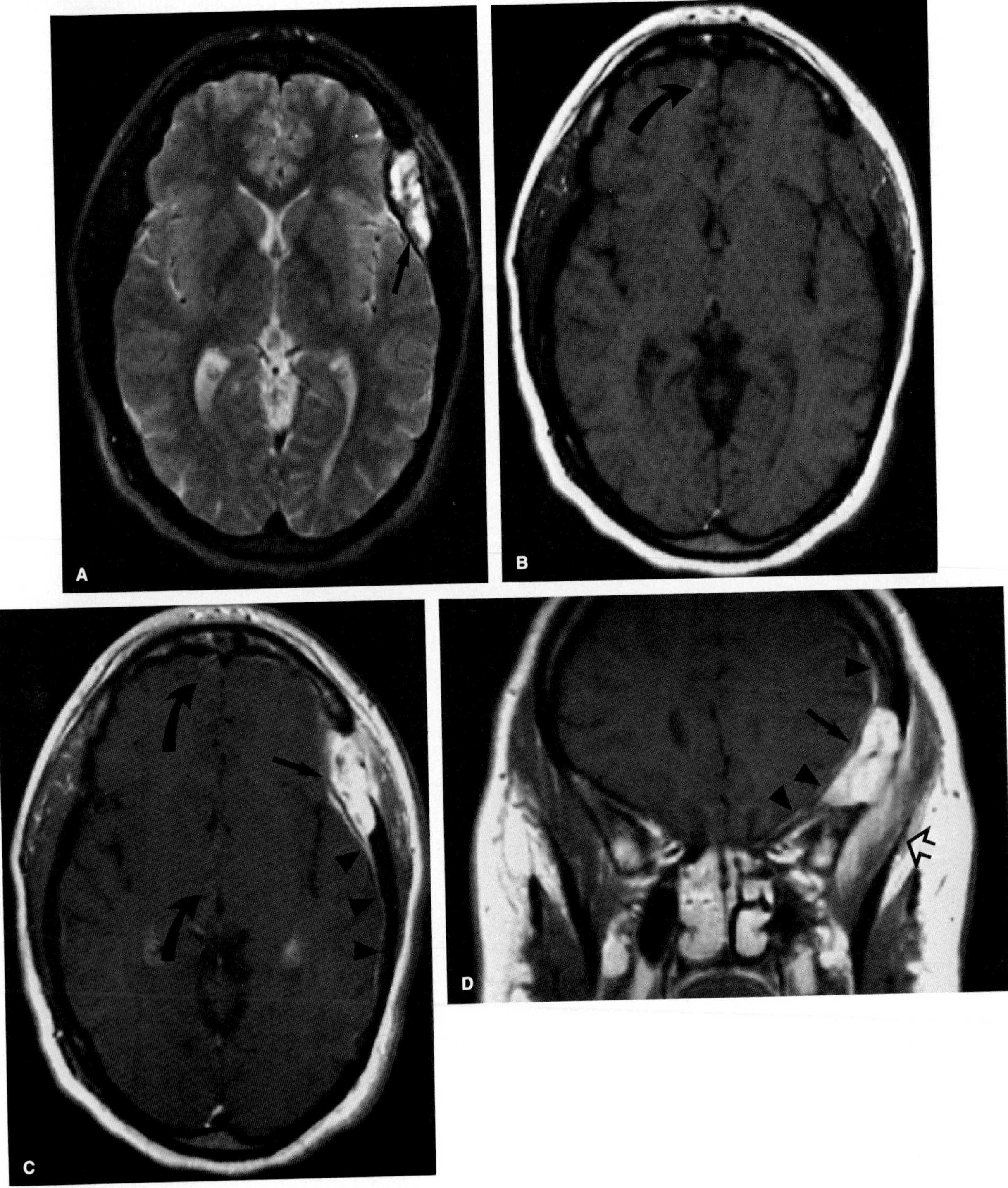

HISTORY

A 20-year-patient with diabetes insipidus and biopsy-proven disease of the scapula and ribs, who now presents with swelling and tenderness in the left frontal region. A lytic bone lesion was noted on the skull radiograph (not shown).

FINDINGS

(*A*) T2-weighted (TE = 90 msec) axial image discloses a high-signal-intensity lesion (*arrow*) located principally within the diploic space. Comparison of precontrast (*B*) and postcontrast (0.2 mmol/kg gadoteridol) (*C*) axial T1-weighted images reveals intense enhancement of both the lesion (*arrow*) and adjacent dura (*arrowheads*). (*D*) Abnormal enhancement of adjacent temporalis muscle (*open arrow*) is best seen on the postcontrast coronal image. This plane of section also confirms the intradiploic nature of the lesion (*arrow*) and adjacent dural reaction (*arrowheads*).

DIAGNOSIS

Multifocal Langerhans cell (eosinophilic) granulomatosis

DISCUSSION

Langerhans cell (eosinophilic) granulomatosis is the term currently preferred for reference to the eosinophilic granuloma syndromes. This replaces older nomenclature including the term *histiocytosis X,* which referred to a spectrum of diseases now known to include both this benign entity and malignant lymphoma.

Unifocal Langerhans cell granulomatosis is a disease of children and young adults, predominantly males, who present with a solitary osteolytic lesion (most often in the femur, skull, vertebrae, ribs, or pelvis). Diagnosis requires biopsy, with treatment being simple excision. Multifocal Langerhans cell granulomatosis also presents in childhood, with multiple bony lesions in virtually any site. Diabetes insipidus occurs in one third as a result of hypothalamic involvement. *Hand-Schuller-Christian syndrome* was previously used in reference to patients who manifested the disease triad of destructive bone lesions, diabetes insipidus, and exophthalmos. Only 25% of patients with multifocal Langerhans cell (eosinophilic) granulomatosis have this triad, which can also be caused by malignant lymphoma and carcinoma. Although benign, treatment of multifocal disease is with methotrexate, vinblastine, or prednisone. In the case presented, the patient had previously received radiation therapy to the hypothalamic region.

MR is the imaging technique of choice for staging disease involvement, both skull and brain, in multifocal Langerhans cell (eosinophilic) granulomatosis.[1] Intradiploic lesions are well delineated. Complete resolution of hypothalamic lesions can be observed after effective therapy.

MR Technique

Gradient moment refocusing (or nulling; GMR, sometimes also referred to as motion compensation) is a software technique commonly employed to decrease artifacts on MR caused by pulsatile blood flow. In the case presented, GMR was not used on the T1-weighted scans, accounting for the prominent pulsation artifact (*curved arrow in B*) from the superior sagittal sinus. Flow artifacts are typically accentuated on postcontrast scans (*curved arrows in C*), also exemplified by this case. The use of GMR and other similar techniques is strongly recommended, particularly postcontrast.

Clinical References

1. Moore JB, Kulkarni R, Crutcher DC, Bhimani S. MRI in multifocal eosinophilic granuloma: staging disease and monitoring response to therapy. Am J Pediatr Hematol Oncol 1989;11:174–177.

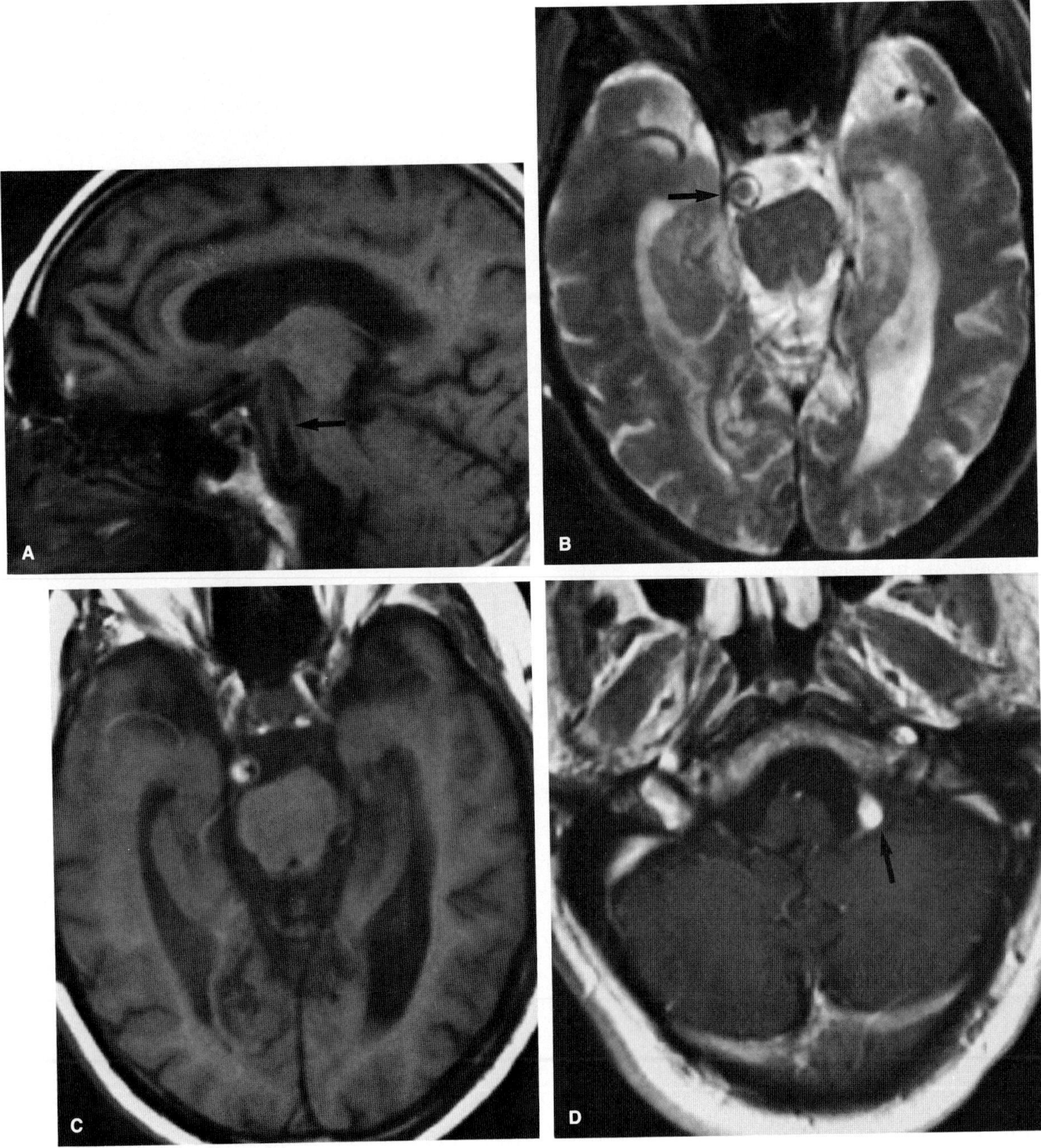

HISTORY

A 69-year-old hypertensive man

FINDINGS

(*A*) The sagittal T1-weighted image to the right of midline reveals a tubular structure (*arrow*), just anterior to the middle cerebellar peduncle, which extends superiorly to impinge on the optic tracts. This same structure can be identified in cross section (*arrow*) on axial precontrast (TE = 90 msec) T2-weighted (*B*) and T1-weighted (*C*) images at the level of the pons. The mass appears to be compressing the right pons with resultant deformity. Incidentally noted is mild cortical atrophy and hydrocephalus. (*D to F*) Postcontrast axial T1-weighted images at three levels again identify this structure (*arrows*), which demonstrates intense uniform enhancement and has a maximum diameter of 10 mm. (*G*) A coronal reformatted image from a 3D MRA reveals dilated and tortuous left vertebral and basilar arteries (*arrowheads*).

DIAGNOSIS

Vertebrobasilar dolichoectasia

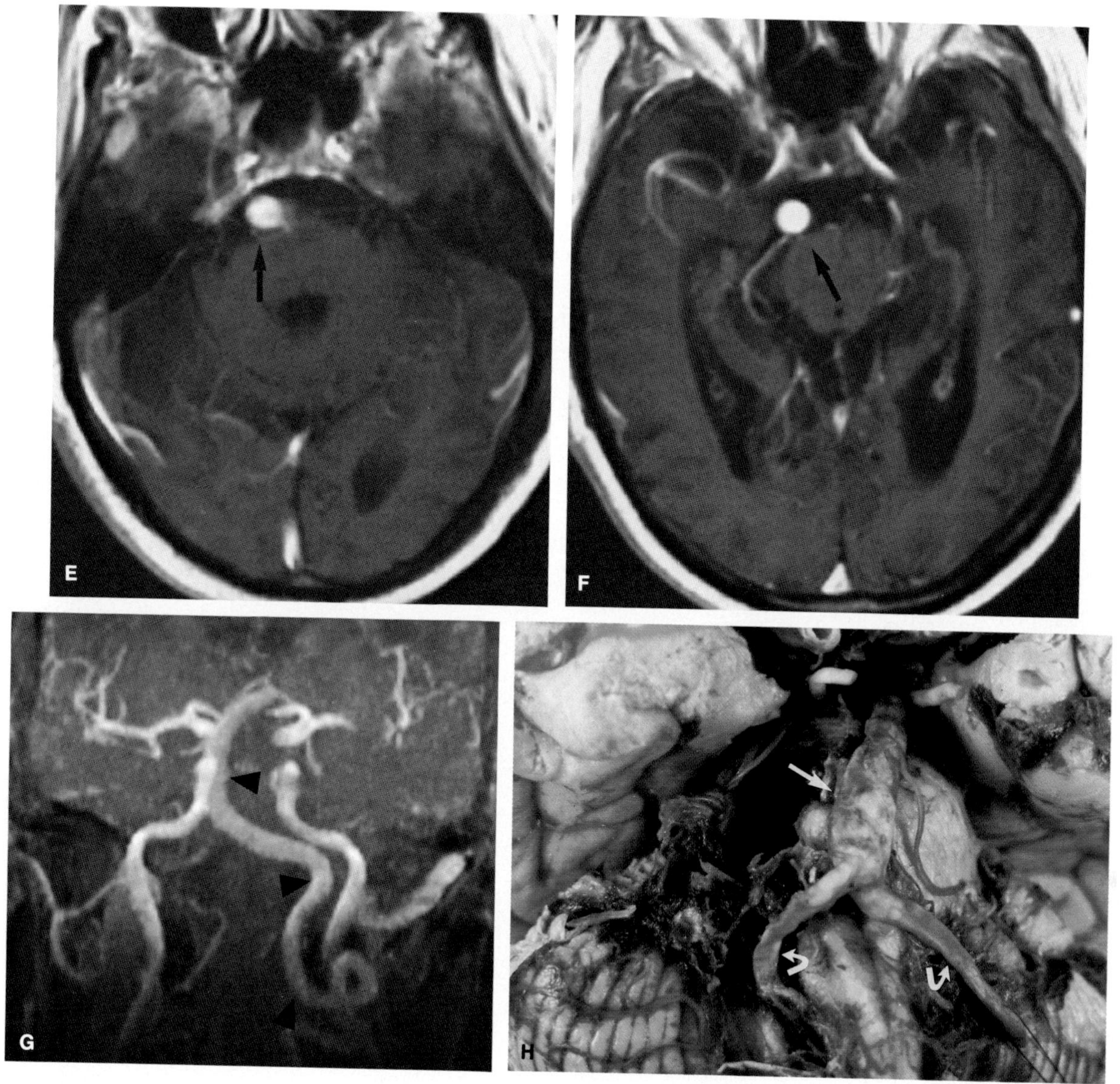

DISCUSSION

Dolichoectasia, as literally translated from its Greek roots, refers to elongation and distention. Basilar artery elongation is strictly defined radiologically by the presence of the basilar artery lateral to either the clivus or dorsum sellae or by bifurcation above the suprasellar cistern.[1] A basilar artery greater than 4.5 mm in diameter is defined as ectatic.

In a retrospective study of 20 patients with symptomatic vertebrobasilar dolichoectasia,[1] two different patient populations were identified: those with isolated cranial nerve involvement (third, sixth, or seventh) and those with multiple neurologic deficits. The latter population included patients with combinations of cranial nerve deficits (due to compression), CNS deficits (due to compression or ischemia), and hydrocephalus. A tortuous but normal-caliber basilar artery was more likely to produce isolated cranial nerve involvement, while ectasia was more likely to cause multiple deficits of either compressive or ischemic etiology. If x-ray angiography is required in patients with vertebrobasilar dolichoectasia, digital subtraction techniques are advised because of the increased risk of brain stem ischemia.

Other abnormalities that have been reported with basilar artery ectasia include subarachnoid hemorrhage (due to aneurysmal rupture), trigeminal neuralgia (due to compression of the fifth cranial nerve), and visual field defects (due to compression of the visual pathway by the distal end of an elongated basilar artery).

In the case presented, the vertebral and basilar arteries are of uniform hyperintensity throughout their course on the postcontrast T1-weighted images. This occurred in part because of the use of gradient moment nulling, a software technique employed to compensate for motion that occurs during TE. As a result of differences in flow rate and other factors, however, the signal intensity of arterial flow on routine SE imaging is highly variable, adding to the complexity in scan interpretation.

Pitfalls in Image Interpretation

A contour deformity of the pons, due to basilar artery ectasia, is a common incidental finding on MR in the elderly population. This finding is often unrelated to both the patient's symptoms and the reason for clinical referral, as in the present case.

Pathologic Correlate

(*H*) Gross pathologic specimen, viewed from the base, reveals a fusiform aneurysm of the basilar artery. The term *fusiform aneurysm* has unfortunately been used interchangeably in the scientific literature with dolichoectatic change and ectasia, all referring to diffuse tortuous enlargement and elongation of an artery. Dolichoectasia occurs with greatest frequency in the vertebrobasilar system but may also involve the intracranial internal carotid and middle cerebral arteries. Ectasia of the basilar artery can lead to traction or displacement of the cranial nerves, most commonly cranial nerves VII and VIII, with resultant symptoms. The lower cranial nerves can be affected by ectasia of the vertebral artery. In *H,* there is enlargement of both vertebral arteries (*curved arrows*), in addition to the basilar artery (*arrow*).

Clinical References

1. Smoker WR, Corbett JJ, Gentry LR, et al. High resolution computed tomography of the basilar artery. Pt. 2. Vertebrobasilar dolichoectasia: clinical-pathologic correlation and review. AJNR 1986;7:61–72.

(H *courtesy of Daron G. Davis, MD.*)

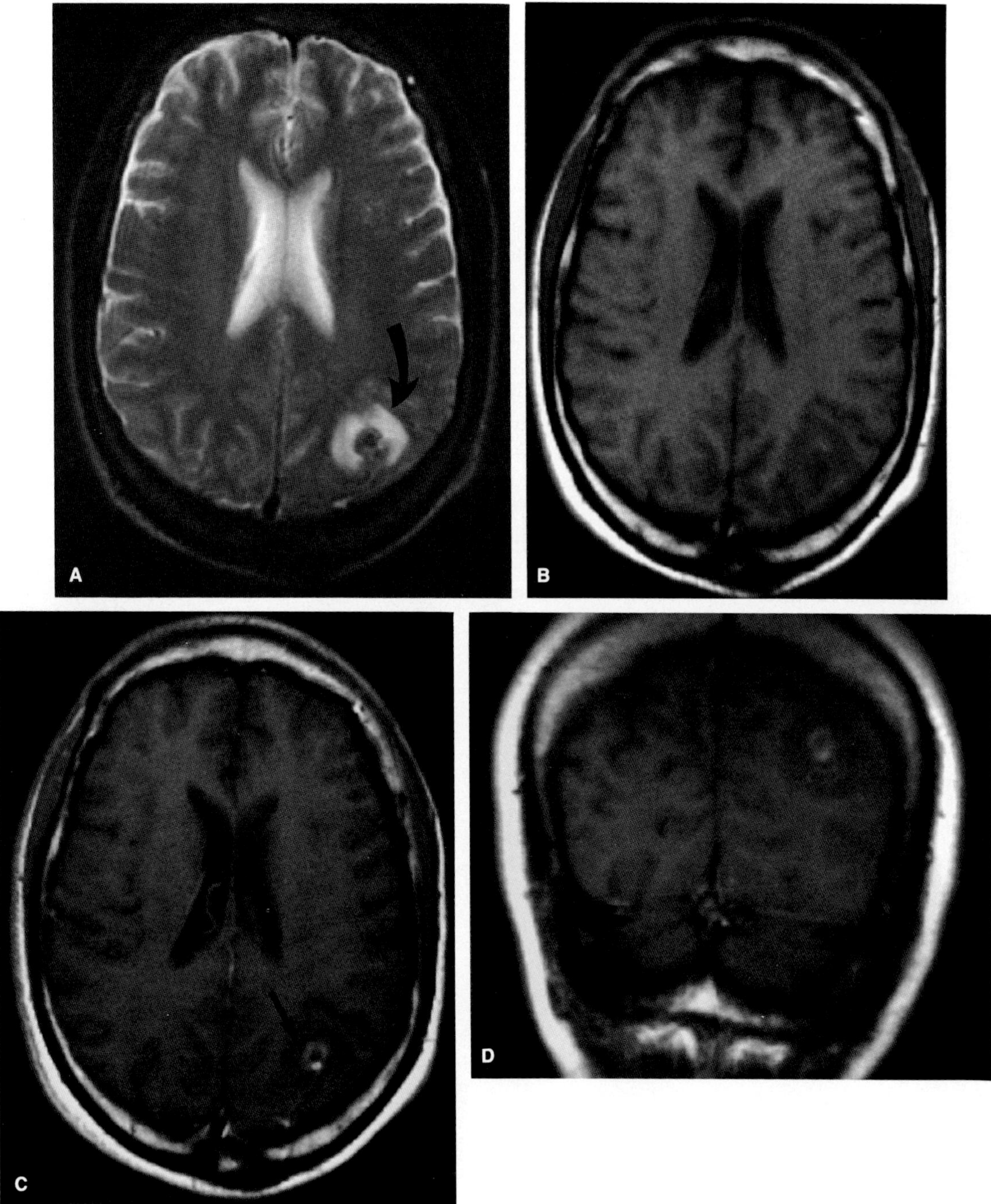

HISTORY

A 42-year-old IV drug abuser being treated for endocarditis

FINDINGS

(*A*) The T2 weighted scan (TE = 90 msec) demonstrates an abnormal low-signal-intensity focus in the left parietal lobe with surrounding edema, the latter with high signal intensity (*curved arrow*). Comparison of axial precontrast (*B*) and postcontrast (*C*) T1-weighted images reveals central enhancement (*arrow in C*). (*D*) Lesion enhancement, with surrounding cerebral edema, is also well depicted on the postcontrast coronal T1-weighted image. A second abnormality (*images not shown*), virtually identical in appearance to the first, was identified in the left temporal lobe. MRA (*images not shown*) revealed blood flow within the central portion of each lesion.

DIAGNOSIS

Mycotic aneurysm

DISCUSSION

Mycotic aneurysms arise as a result of septic emboli and are typically located more peripherally (in intermediate to small cerebral arteries) than congenital aneurysms.[1] A history of blood-borne infection or evidence of hemorrhage, either intraparenchymal or subarachnoid in location, gives clues to this diagnosis.

The term *mycotic aneurysm* has traditionally been used to refer to both bacterial and fungal (or true mycotic) aneurysms, although clinically the great majority are bacterial in origin.[2] Treatment (surgical versus medical) remains controversial, with antibiotic therapy favored. Serial angiography is recommended, specifically looking for lesion enlargement, because of the high mortality associated with rupture. Regression of aneurysms has been demonstrated during antibiotic therapy.

MR Technique

MRA is a useful adjunct in the evaluation of space occupying lesions in the brain. The time required for a 3D TOF examination with current instrumentation is less than 5 minutes, making routine application possible. The information gained may, as in this case, lead to improved diagnosis.

Pitfalls in Image Interpretation

The differential diagnosis on MR for multiple enhancing parenchymal masses, with accompanying cerebral edema, is extensive. Specific diagnosis is often not possible. Neoplastic disease, infection, inflammation (demyelinating disease), subacute multifocal infarction, and vascular lesions must all be considered.

Clinical References

1. Bowen BC, Post MJD. Intracranial infection. In: Atlas S, ed. Magnetic resonance imaging of the brain and spine. New York, Raven Press, 1991;501–538.
2. Frazee JG. Inflammatory intracranial aneurysms. In: Wilkins RH, Rengachary SS, eds. Neurosurgery. New York, McGraw-Hill, 1985;1440–1443.

(A to D courtesy of Mark Traill, MD.)

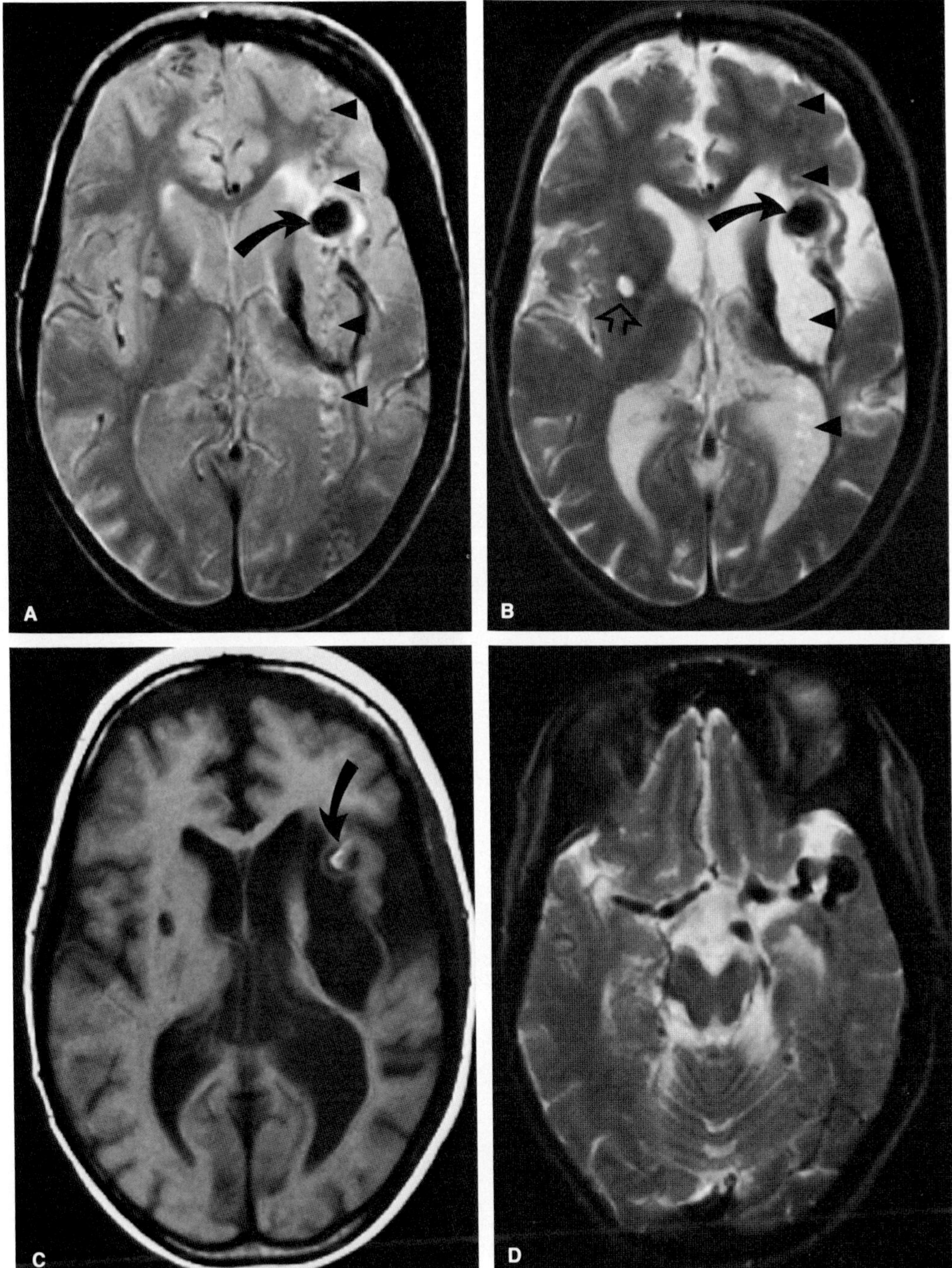

HISTORY

A 26-year-old woman with right hemiparesis, 10 years after cranial radiation for acute leukemia and 6 years after bilateral cerebral infarction

FINDINGS

(*A and B*) On both echoes (TE = 45,90) of the T2-weighted examination, an abnormal flow void (*curved arrow*) is noted just lateral to the left frontal horn, with a prominent associated pulsation artifact (*arrowheads*). (*C*) The T1-weighted image shows the lesion (*curved arrow*) to be a mixture of high and low signal intensity. (*D*) A lower section from the T2-weighted examination suggests continuity of the lesion with the left middle cerebral artery. Also noted are chronic cavitated infarcts bilaterally—a small lacune on the right (*open arrow in B*) and a larger, hemosiderin- or ferritin-lined, left-sided infarct involving the putamen and middle cerebral artery territory. (*E and F*) 3D TOF MRA reveals ectatic intracranial vessels, a 1-cm aneurysm (*curved white arrow*), a suggestion of multiple focal vessel stenoses, and dolichoec-

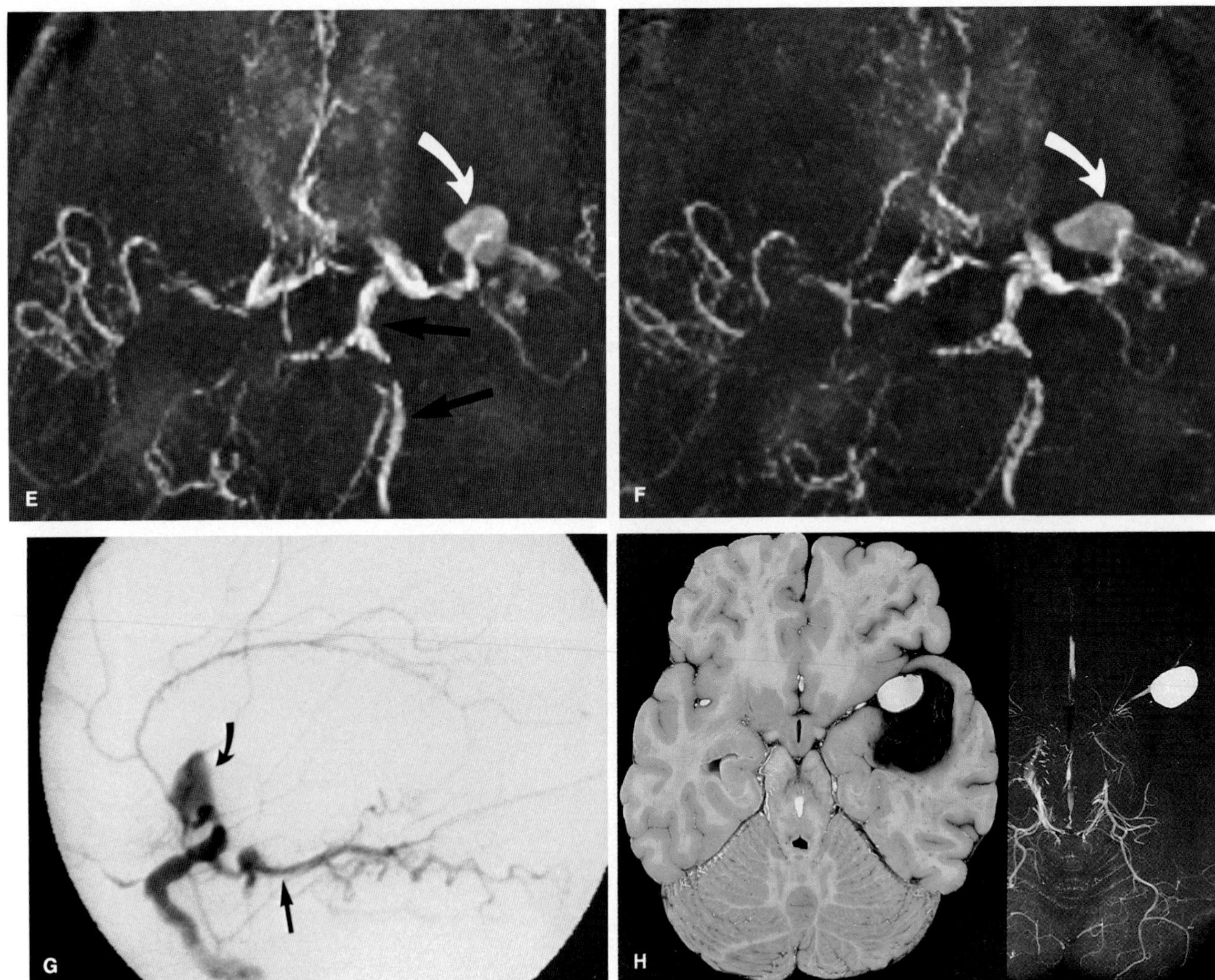

tasia (*arrows in E*) of the left posterior communicating artery and the proximal left posterior cerebral artery. These findings were confirmed on cerebral arteriography. (*G*) A single lateral projection from the cerebral arteriogram depicts the aneurysm (*curved arrow*) and dolichoectatic posterior cerebral artery (*arrow*).

DIAGNOSIS

Middle cerebral artery bifurcation aneurysm

DISCUSSION

Arterial flow on conventional SE MR images can be visualized as either high or low signal intensity, although the latter (a flow "void") is more common. Pulsation artifacts, which propagate along the phase encoding axis, serve to confirm the vascular nature of lesions such as aneurysms and arteriovenous malformations. These and other characteristic flow effects allow for definitive diagnosis of aneurysms on MR, unlike CT.

SE MR imaging clearly delineates the size, residual lumen, and location of large aneurysms.[1] MRA permits detection of intracranial aneurysms in the vicinity of the circle of Willis as small as 3 to 4 mm.[2]

Vasculitis due to radiation injury was thought to be a likely causal factor in the development of cerebral infarction in this patient.

Pathologic Correlate

H shows a middle cerebral artery aneurysm on gross section, together with the corresponding postmortem angiogram. When such a lesion ruptures, bleeding can be either limited to the subarachnoid space or extend into the parenchyma (specifically the frontal or temporal lobes). Fatal cases more often demonstrate parenchymal hemorrhage. Fibrin thrombus, as in this case, can seal the point of rupture.

Clinical References

1. Biondi A, Scialfa G, Scotti G. Intracranial aneurysms: MR imaging. Neuroradiology 1988;30:214–218.
2. Ross JS, Masaryk TJ, Modic MT, et al. Intracranial aneurysms: evaluation by MR angiography. AJR 1990;155:159–165.

(H from Okazaki H, Scheithauer B. Slide atlas of neuropathology. New York, Gower Medical Publishing, 1988. By permission of Mayo Foundation.)

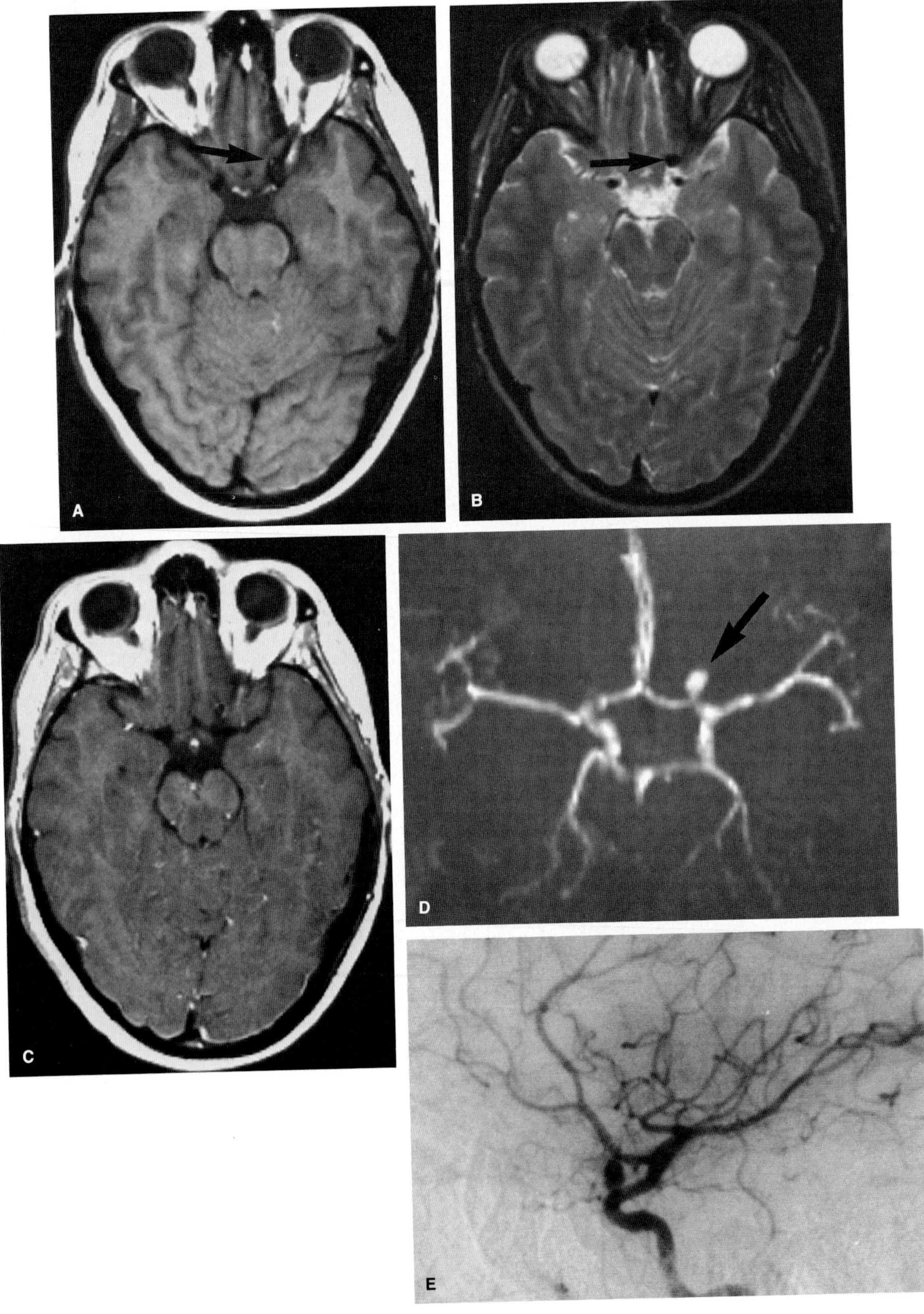
A
B
C
D
E

HISTORY

A 73-year-old woman

FINDINGS

Axial T1-weighted (*A*) and T2-weighted (*B*) images identify a small round signal void (*black arrow*) anterior to the supraclinoid segment of the left internal carotid artery. (*C*) There is enhancement of the rim of this lesion on the axial T1-weighted image postcontrast. (*D*) MRA shows a small aneurysm (*black arrow*) just medial and anterior to the extracavernous, intracranial segment of the left internal carotid artery. (*E*) A left ophthalmic artery aneurysm is identified on digital subtraction angiography.

DIAGNOSIS

Ophthalmic artery aneurysm

DISCUSSION

Intracranial berry aneurysms are present in 1% to 8% of the population. In the United States about 20,000 aneurysms rupture per year; approximately 8% of these patients die before they reach the hospital, and 50% die within the first month of rupture.[1] Berry aneurysms are associated with adult polycystic kidney disease, Marfan's syndrome, and aortic coarctation.

Intracranial aneurysms are multiple in 15% to 20% of cases. The reported frequency of occurrence varies. General percentages are as follows: 20% to 30% occur at the origin of the posterior communicating artery, 30% arise from the anterior communicating artery, 20% from the middle cerebral artery bifurcation, and 15% are in the posterior fossa circulation.[2]

Both TOF and phase-contrast (PC) techniques are commonly used in clinical MRA. In TOF methods, vessel enhancement depends on inflow effects of moving spins.[3] PC MRA relies on phase changes in the transverse magnetization of spins moving along a magnetic field gradient. Signals arising from stationary material have no flow-induced phase shift and can be differentiated from signals arising from moving material.[2] Disadvantages to MRA include inferior spatial resolution when compared with conventional arteriography.

Pitfalls in Image Interpretation

Slow-flow vascular pathology such as giant intracranial aneurysms are poorly visualized on 3D TOF MRA secondary to saturation of moving spins (which reside for too long within the excited volume).

Clinical References

1. Ross JS, Masaryk TJ, Modic MT, et al. Intracranial aneurysms: evaluation by MR angiography. AJNR 1990;11:449–456.
2. Osborn AG. Introduction to cerebral angiography. Philadelphia, Harper & Row, 1980.
3. Dumoulin CL, Cline HE, Souza SP, et al. Three-dimensional time-of-flight magnetic resonance angiography using spin saturation. Magn Reson Med 1989;11:35–46.

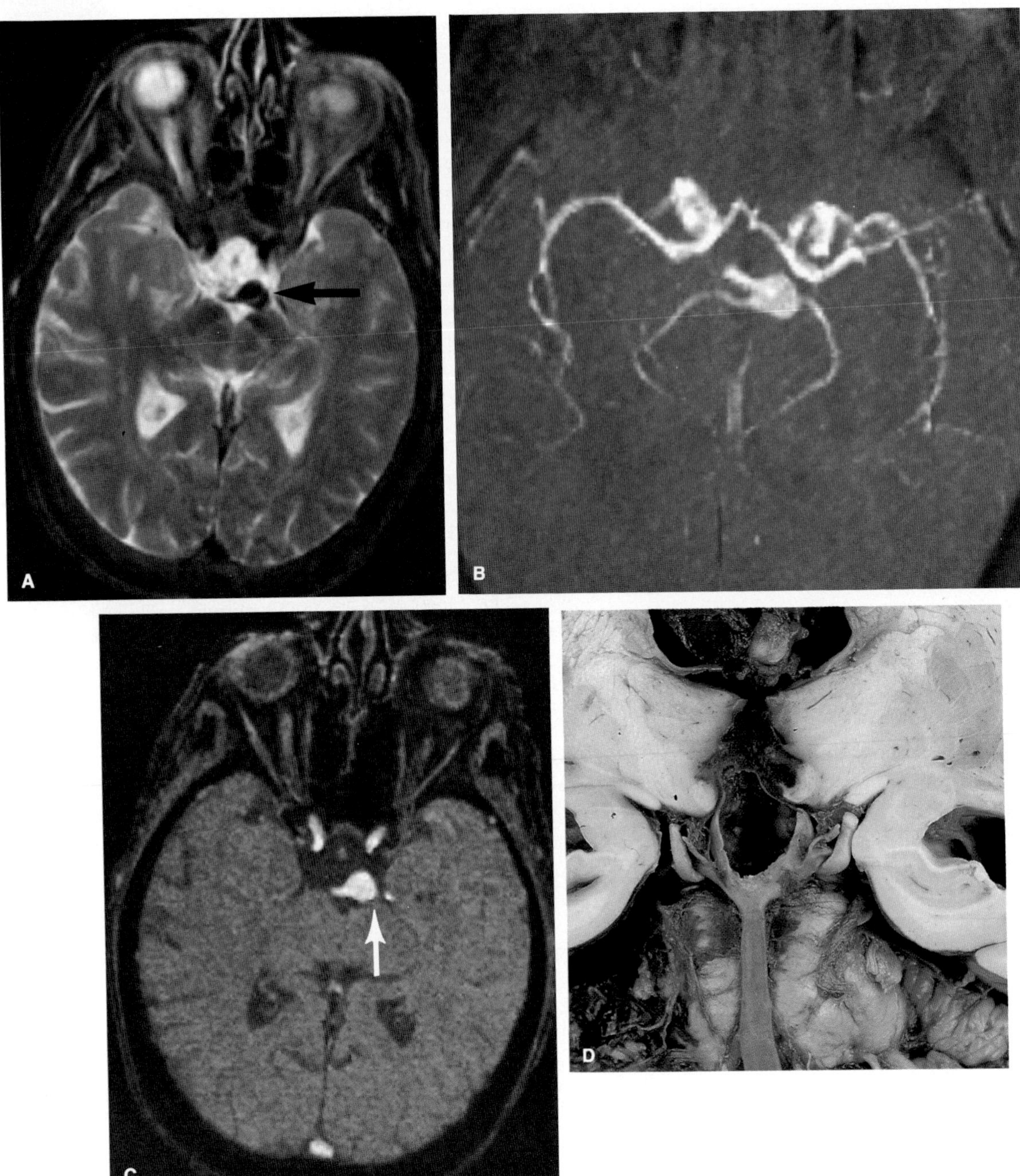

HISTORY

A 59-year-old with sixth nerve palsy

FINDINGS

(*A*) On the axial T2-weighted scan there is an oval signal void (*black arrow*) in the prepontine cistern just superior to the basilar artery. (*B*) MRA demonstrates a large aneurysm arising from the tip of the basilar artery. (*C*) The raw data image from MRA identifies the aneurysm (*white arrow*) as a high-signal-intensity structure in the prepontine cistern.

DIAGNOSIS

Basilar artery aneurysm

DISCUSSION

Aneurysms of the posterior fossa represent 5% to 15% of all intracranial aneurysms. In the vertebral-basilar system, saccular aneurysms are most common at the apex or dome of the basilar artery, with the second most common site at the origin of the posterior inferior cerebellar artery. Anterior inferior cerebellar artery aneurysms are rare. Regardless of location, intracranial aneurysms are more common at arterial branching points.

Although basilar artery aneurysms can result in compression of the 5th through 10th cranial nerves, the most common clinical presentation is subarachnoid hemorrhage.[1]

Increasing age correlates with increased number of aneurysms. Intracranial saccular aneurysms are not found in childhood. The incidence of intracranial aneurysms is higher among relatives of patients with ruptured aneurysms. Aneurysms predominate in females at a ratio of 3:2. The maximum diameter of ruptured saccular aneurysms tends to be larger than that of unruptured ones.[2]

Pitfalls in Image Interpretation

CSF motion transmitted from vascular structures can result in focal signal loss on MR imaging, which must be distinguished from an aneurysm.

Pathologic Correlate

D is the gross specimen of a large nonthrombosed saccular basilar artery aneurysm. Hemorrhage secondary to rupture of a basilar artery aneurysm commonly extends into the third ventricle by way of its thin floor.

Clinical References

1. Bryce W. Aneurysm affecting the nervous system. Baltimore, Williams & Wilkins, 1987:21.
2. Davis RL, Robertson DM. Textbook of neuropathology. Baltimore, Williams & Wilkins: 1991:631–633.

(D *from Okazaki H, Scheithauer B. Slide atlas of neuropathology. New York, Gower Medical Publishing, 1988. By permission of Mayo Foundation.*)

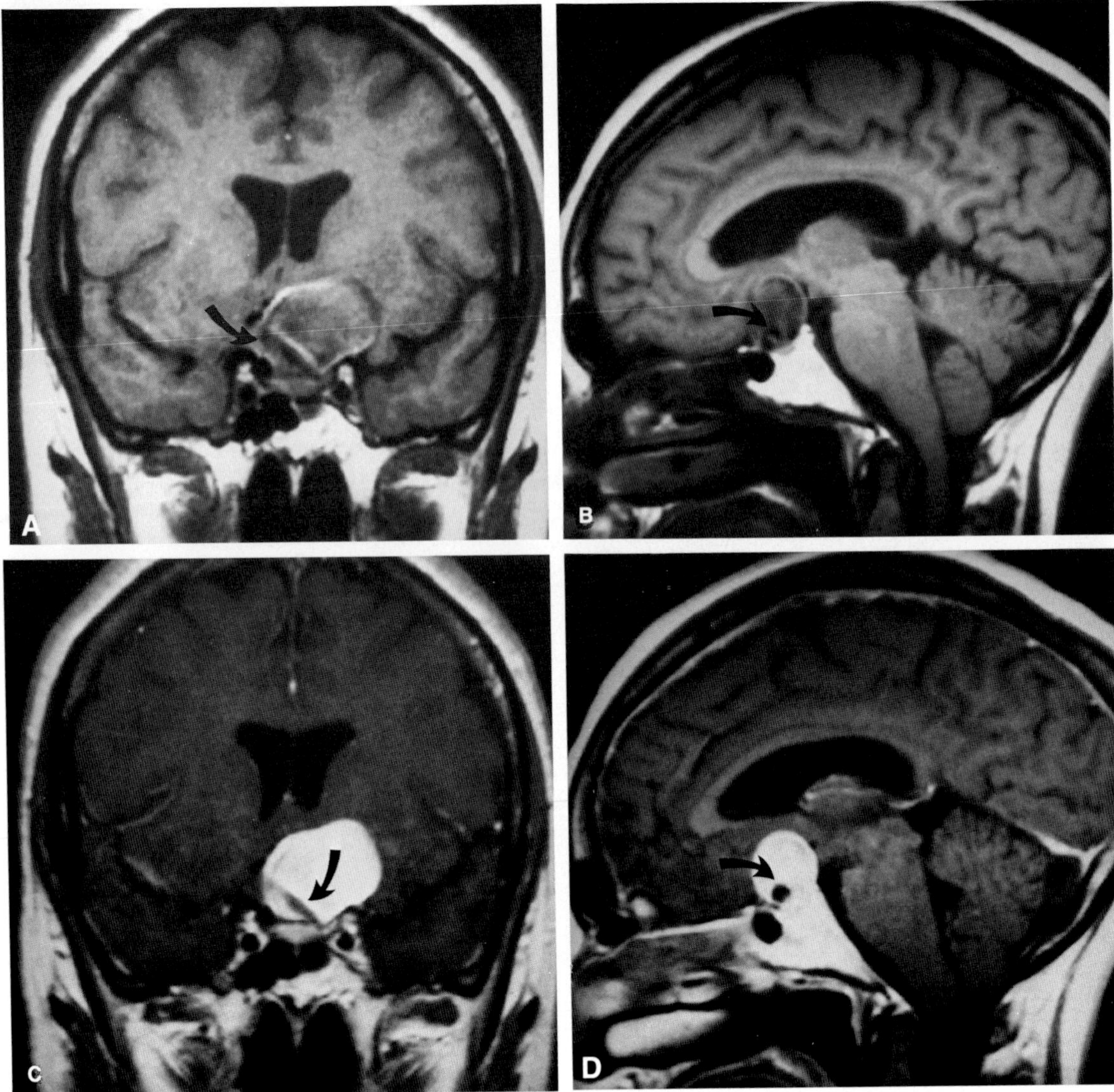

HISTORY

A 60-year-old woman with a visual field defect

FINDINGS

T1-weighted coronal (*A*) and sagittal (*B*) images demonstrate a large heterogeneous suprasellar mass. On the postcontrast coronal (*C*) and sagittal (*D*) images, there is intense enhancement of the majority of the mass, with a persistent low-signal-intensity focus (*curved arrows in A to D*) in the inferior aspect. (*E*) On the coronal T2-weighted image this region is also of low signal intensity (*curved arrow*). In *E* can be seen multiple "ghosts" (*small arrows*) due to pulsation artifact, along the phase encoding direction on both sides of the mass. (*F*) MRA shows only faintly increased signal intensity in the region of the mass, which lies directly adjacent to the supraclinoid portion of the left internal carotid artery. (*G*) The conventional digital angiogram reveals a large contrast-filled aneurysm extending off the internal carotid artery just distal to the origin of the ophthalmic artery (*arrow*).

DIAGNOSIS

Giant intracranial aneurysm

DISCUSSION

A saccular, or berry, aneurysm whose diameter is greater than 25 mm is termed a *giant aneurysm.*[1] Giant aneurysms account for approximately 2.5% to 5% of all intracranial aneurysms and occur most commonly in middle-aged women. These lesions typically present with signs and symptoms of a space occupying mass lesion such as

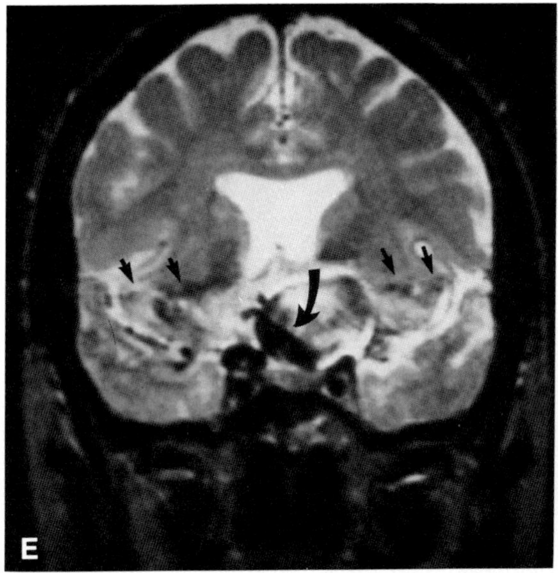

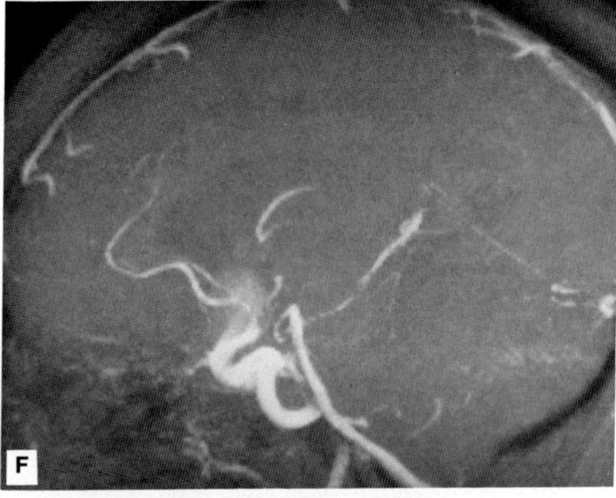

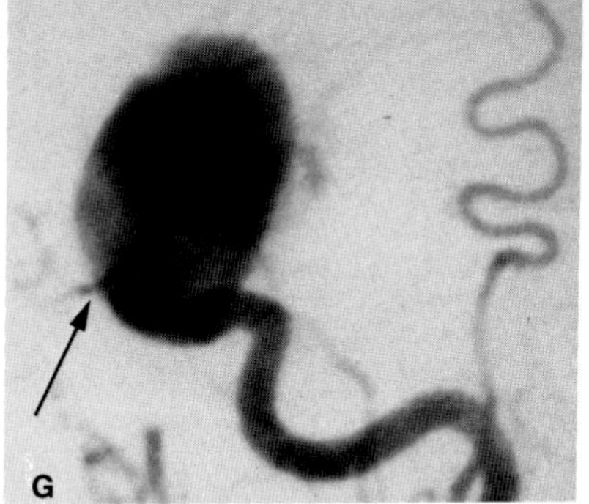

visual changes, cranial nerve palsies, and seizures rather than subarachnoid hemorrhage, although rupture can occur. Giant aneurysms most commonly arise from the cavernous and supraclinoid portions of the internal carotid artery and at the bifurcation or trifurcation of the middle cerebral artery.

Most giant aneurysms have a complex, but characteristic, appearance on MR because of the presence of both flowing blood and thrombus. A flow void is usually present near the center of the aneurysm on both T1- and T2-weighted images representing the residual patent lumen with flowing blood. Low signal intensity on all pulse sequences is characteristic for fast or turbulent blood flow and allows for differentiation of an aneurysm from solid tumors. Mixed signal intensity along the periphery of the aneurysm lumen represents thrombus in various stages of hemoglobin degradation.[2] In the case illustrated, the entire lumen of the aneurysm is patent and shows enhancement after contrast infusion as a result of slow flow within the lesion. One portion of the aneurysm, however, is low signal intensity on all sequences, including post-contrast, because of rapid flow as the "jet" of blood enters the aneurysm.

Another differential diagnostic clue to the vascular nature of a giant aneurysm on routine SE images is the presence of pulsation artifacts emanating from it along the phase encoding direction. MRA is useful for detecting flow in an aneurysm and for determining the site of origin. 3D TOF technique, which is best for depicting rapid arterial flow, was used for the MRA illustrated, and the full extent of the aneurysm is not well seen. 2D TOF or phase-contrast (PC) techniques are better for depiction of slow flow in the lumen of a large aneurysm or in venous structures.

Pitfalls in Image Interpretation

The differential diagnosis for a parasellar mass includes meningioma, craniopharyngioma, and pituitary adenoma, all of which may look like a giant aneurysm on enhanced CT. MR allows differentiation of a giant aneurysm from these entities based on the signal intensity characteristics of blood flow and clot.

Clinical References

1. Olsen W, Brant-Zawadzki M, Hodes J, et al. Giant intracranial aneurysms: MR imaging. Radiology 1987;163:431–435.
2. Atlas S. Intracranial vascular malformations and aneurysms: current imaging applications. Radiol Clin North Am 1988; 26:821–837.

(A to G *from Runge VM. Magnetic resonance imaging: clinical principles. Philadelphia, JB Lippincott, 1992.)*

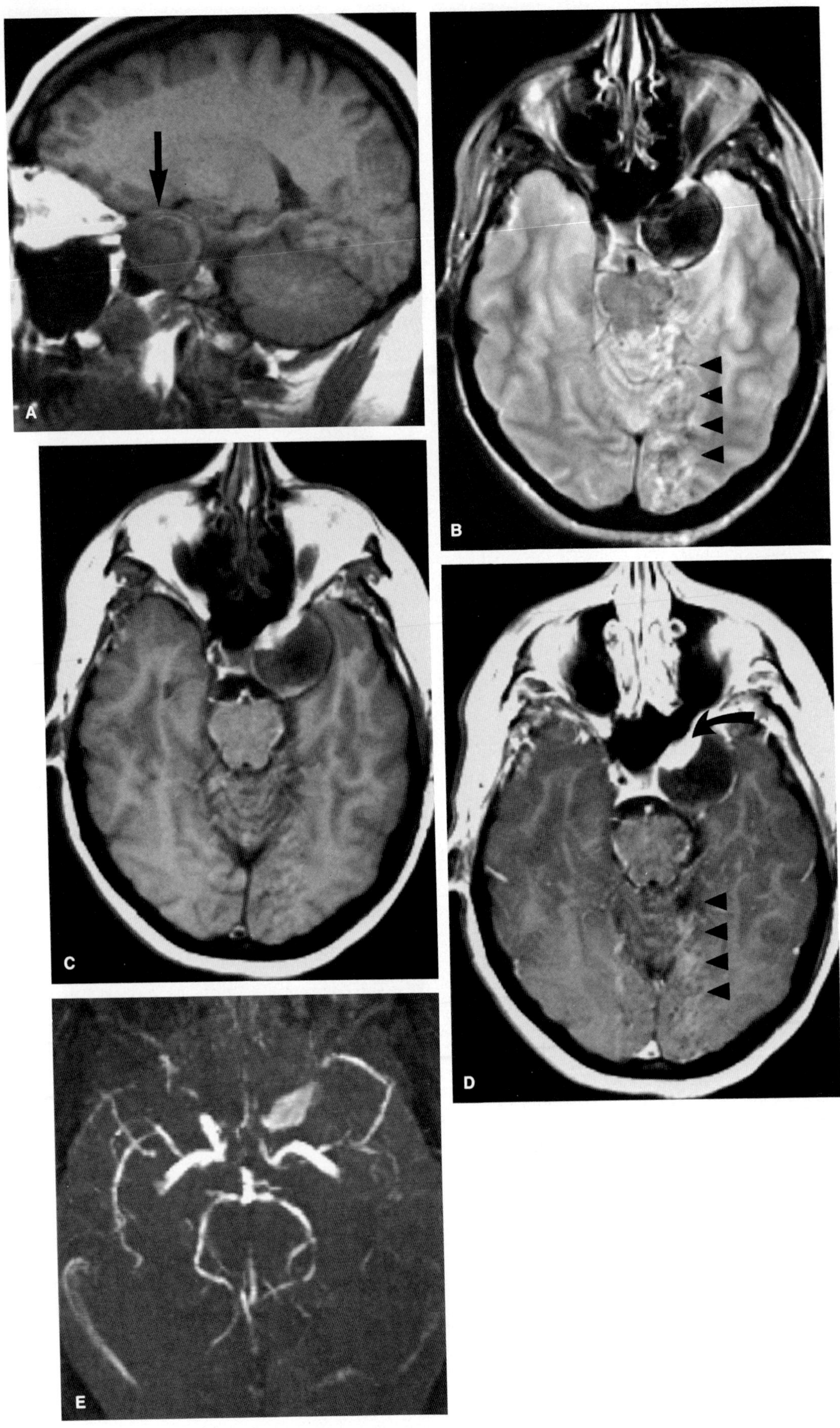
A
B
C
D
E

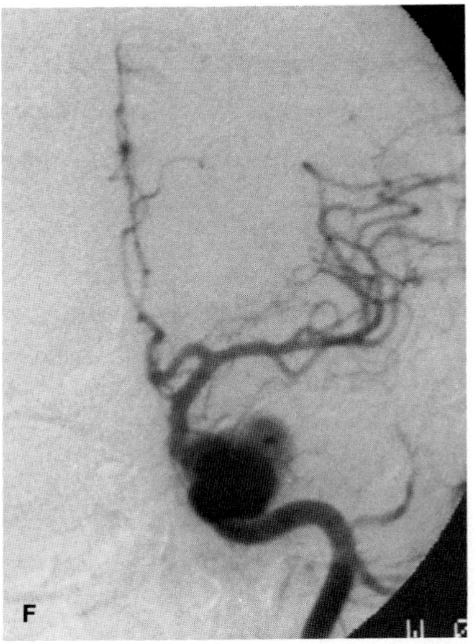

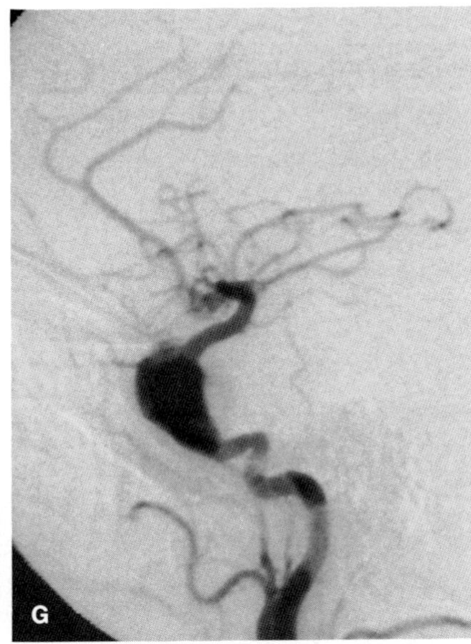

HISTORY

A 49-year-old patient with left retroorbital and facial pain

FINDINGS

(*A*) On the sagittal precontrast T1-weighted examination a soft tissue mass (*arrow*), with suggestion of laminated signal intensity, is noted in the region of the cavernous sinus. (*B*) On the first echo of the T2-weighted examination (TE = 45 msec), the mass is principally of low signal intensity. A pulsation artifact (*arrowheads*) is noted in the phase encoding direction, emanating from only the more medial portion of the mass. Comparison of precontrast (*C*) and postcontrast (*D*) T1-weighted images reveals enhancement (*curved arrow in D*) in only the most anterior and medial portion of the lesion. The abnormal pulsation artifact, which is more prominent on the postcontrast study (*arrowheads in D*), remains limited in right to left dimension. 3D TOF MRA in the craniocaudad projection (*E*) reveals a patent lumen within the mass, corresponding in position to that suggested by the pulsation artifact and contrast enhancement. Anteroposterior (*F*) and lateral (*G*) views from a conventional contrast arteriogram reveal a giant aneurysm of the cavernous and distal petrous carotid artery, with the crescent of residual lumen corresponding to that depicted by MRA.

DIAGNOSIS

Partially thrombosed giant aneurysm of the cavernous carotid artery

DISCUSSION

MR plays a significant role in diagnosis and characterization of giant aneurysms.[1] Findings in partially thrombosed lesions include a flow void in the residual patent lumen. A high-signal-intensity rim (*not seen in the current case*), representing methemoglobin, may be present adjacent to the signal void. Mixed laminated signal intensity in the clotted portion of the lesion corresponds to different stages of organized clot. Perianeurysmal hemorrhage and cerebral edema may be present. Old thrombus is reported to be isointense on T1-weighted images and hyperintense on T2-weighted images, unlike the present case.

Treatment of giant aneurysms is surgical. Approaches include ligation at the neck, use of intravascular balloons, and ipsilateral internal carotid artery ligation, with the last option performed in this patient.

MR Technique

IV contrast enhancement can improve the depiction of flowing blood on conventional SE images, providing supplemental diagnostic information in patients with intracranial aneurysms and vascular malformations.

Pitfalls in Image Interpretation

The use of 3D TOF MRA, although adequate in the present study, may underestimate the patent lumen of giant aneurysms because of poor sensitivity to slow flow.

Clinical References

1. Maiuri F, Corriero G, Damico L, Simonetti L. Giant aneurysm of the pericallosal artery. Neurosurgery 1990;26:703–706.

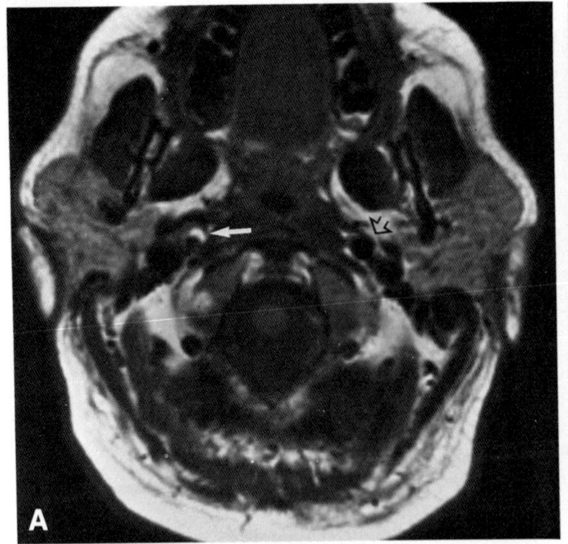

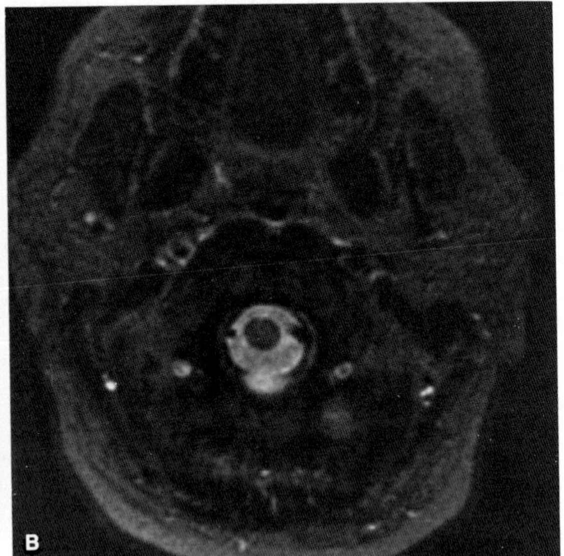

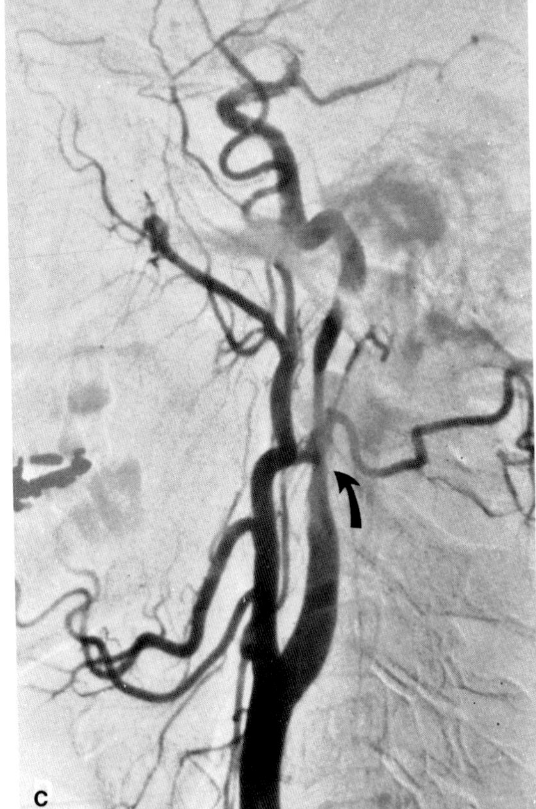

HISTORY

A young man with acute neck pain and visual loss in the right eye

FINDINGS

(*A*) The T1-weighted examination demonstrates a flow void which corresponds to the right internal carotid artery and is markedly smaller than that of the left internal carotid (*open arrow*). Also present just anterior on the right is an abnormal crescent of hyperintensity (*arrow*). (*B*) The asymmetry in size of the carotids is confirmed on the T2-weighted (TE = 90 msec) examination. (*C*) The lateral view from a right common carotid arteriogram reveals moderate narrowing (*curved arrow*) of the mid and distal cervical segments of the internal carotid artery.

DIAGNOSIS

Subacute internal carotid artery dissection

DISCUSSION

MR is sensitive in the detection of subacute dissection involving the cervical internal carotid artery.[1] In a subacute hematoma, the presence of methemoglobin leads to abnormal hyperintensity on T1-weighted images, and hypointensity (if intracellular) or hyperintensity (if extracellular) on T2-weighted images. Hemorrhage within a dissection is thus easily visualized and can be noted to expand the wall of the vessel and compromise the lumen. Follow-up MR may demonstrate spontaneous resolution, which is typically observed several months later if complete occlusion has not occurred.

Before the advent of MR, carotid dissection was diagnosed on the basis of clinical findings and indirect (and presumptive) signs on angiography. Clinical signs are frequently nonspecific, and include pain in the neck, face, or anterior head, with Horner's syndrome (ptosis, miosis, and anhidrosis) common. Surgery is generally not indicated unless a pseudoaneurysm is present or there are progressive neurologic deficits. Early diagnosis is important, with institution of anticoagulation advised to prevent possible stroke from an embolus arising at the site of dissection.

MR Technique

Of all possible planes, axial imaging best demonstrates the anatomic and signal intensity abnormalities in a dissection involving the cervical internal carotid artery.

Pitfalls in Image Interpretation

Occlusion of the carotid artery can be more difficult to diagnose on MR than dissection, particularly if MRA or specific flow sequences are not employed. With regard to the carotid artery siphon, isointensity with adjacent brain on MR can indicate either occlusion or very slow flow.[2] Hyperintense intraluminal signal (on proton density and T2-weighted scans) can be due to either occlusion or high-grade stenosis.[3] Furthermore, the presence of a normal flow void does not exclude the possibility of significant carotid disease.

Clinical References

1. Goldberg HI, Grossman RI, Gomoro JM, et al. Cervical internal carotid artery dissecting hemorrhage: diagnosis using MR. Radiology 1986;158:157–161.
2. Brant-Zawadzki M. Routine MR imaging of the internal carotid artery siphon: angiographic correlation with cervical carotid lesions. AJR 1990;155:359–363.
3. Lane JI, Flanders AE, Doan HT, Bell RD. Assessment of carotid artery patency on routine spin-echo MR imaging of the brain. AJNR 1991;12:819–826.

(A to C from Runge VM. Magnetic resonance imaging: clinical principles. Philadelphia, JB Lippincott, 1992.)

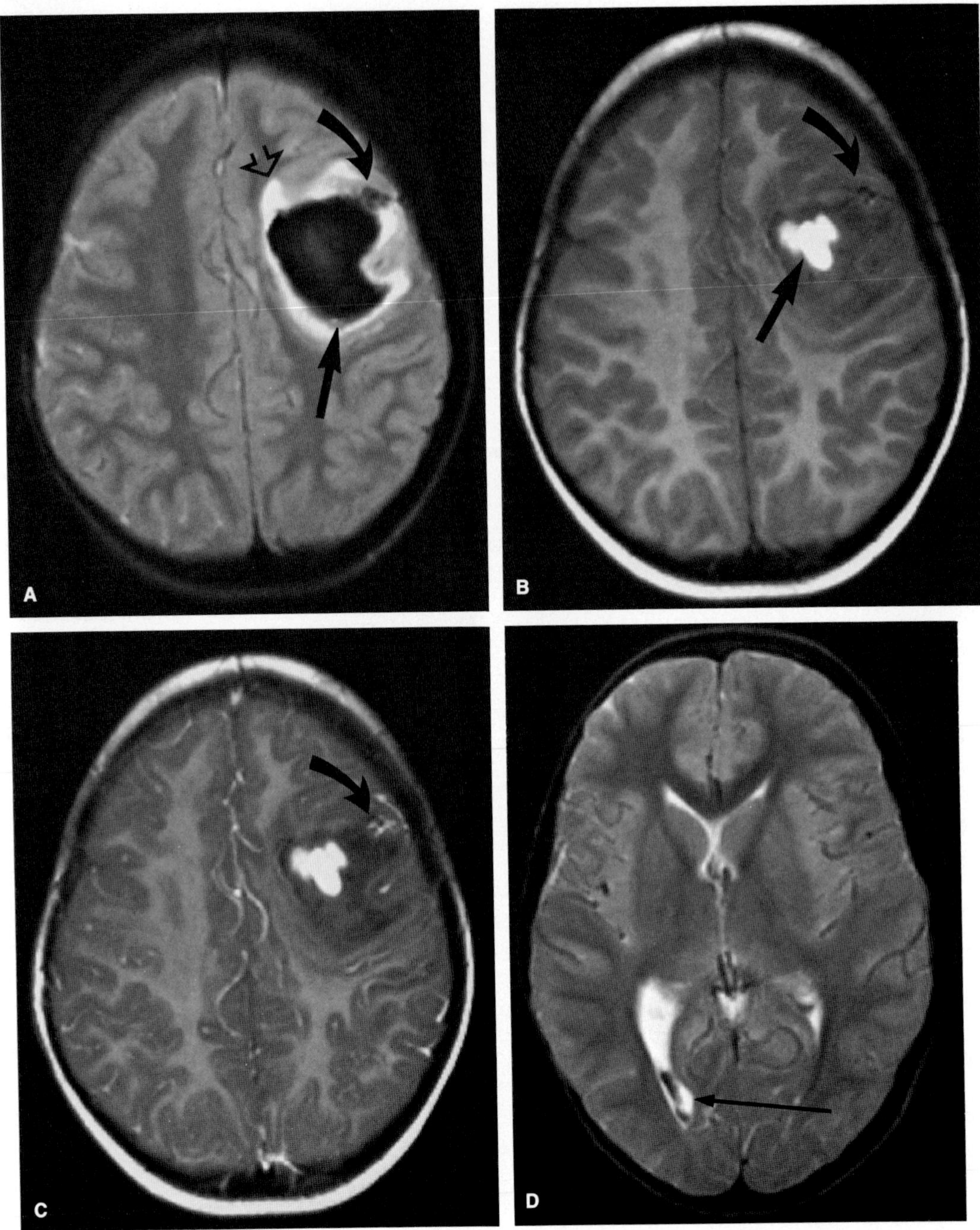

HISTORY

A 7-year-old girl with sudden onset of severe headache, nausea, vomiting, decreased level of consciousness, and right-sided hemiparesis

FINDINGS

Axial T2-weighted (TE = 90 msec) (*A*) and T1-weighted (*B*) precontrast MR images reveal a large left frontal mass with marked hypointensity, relative to gray matter, on the T2-weighted image (*arrow in A*) and central hyperintensity on the T1-weighted image (*arrow in B*). Surrounding cerebral edema (*open arrow in A*) with high signal intensity is well delineated on the T2-weighted image. Just lateral and anterior to the primary lesion, a second smaller serpiginous abnormality is noted. This displays low signal intensity on all precontrast scans (*curved arrows in A and B*). (*C*) On the postcontrast T1-weighted image, the secondary lesion shows enhancement (*curved arrow*). (*D*) At the ventricular level on the T2-weighted image, a low-signal-intensity abnormality is noted within the right occipital horn (*long arrow in D*). The T1-weighted image at this level (*not shown*) was normal. (*E*) Unenhanced x-ray CT, performed emergently, demon-

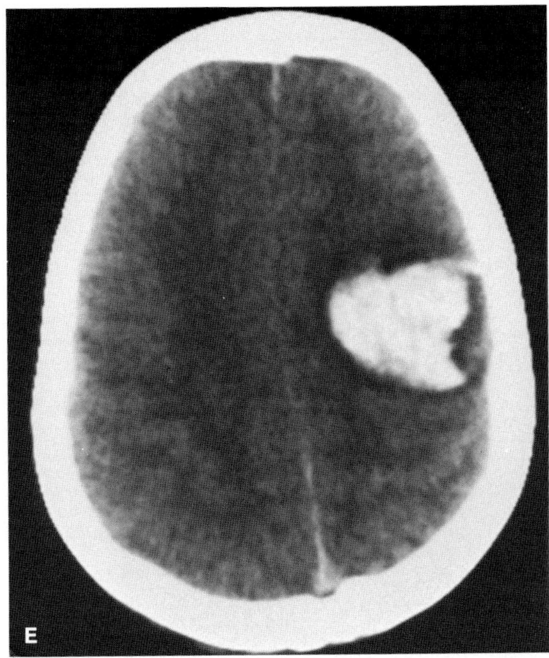

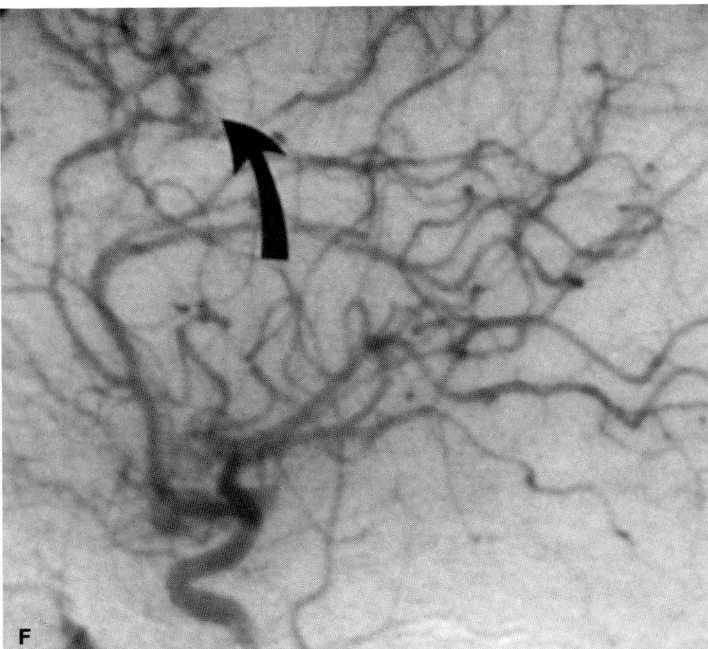

strates a large hyperdense mass. (*F*) X-ray contrast digital angiography in the lateral projection reveals a 1-cm nidus of abnormal vessels (*curved arrow*) in the posterior frontal lobe, corresponding to the serpiginous abnormality noted on MR. The blood supply is from both the anterior and middle cerebral arteries.

DIAGNOSIS

AVM with subacute intraparenchymal and intraventricular hemorrhage

DISCUSSION

Six days after presentation, surgery was performed with resection of the AVM and evacuation of the adjacent clot. Postoperatively, there was residual paresis of the right hand.

On MR, the nidus of the AVM (*curved arrows in A and B*) is seen as a flow void precontrast, with enhancement postcontrast. The intraparenchymal hemorrhage consists of both deoxyhemoglobin (low signal intensity on T2-weighted and isointense on T1-weighted MR) and intracellular methemoglobin (high signal intensity on T1-weighted MR). The intraventricular hemorrhage (*long arrow in D*) represents deoxyhemoglobin.

Intraparenchymal hemorrhage evolves on MR in a defined sequence of signal intensity patterns, with its appearance predominantly determined by the chemical degradation of hemoglobin.[1] A high magnetic field strength (1.5 T) improves detection of both acute and chronic hemorrhage by visualization of deoxyhemoglobin and hemosiderin, respectively.

Angiography remains the standard for depiction of AVMs, with patent vascular malformations, however, well depicted on conventional MR because of flow-related phenomena.[2] TOF MRA can be used in conjunction with SE methods to demonstrate the nidus of an AVM and its feeding vessels.[3] Incomplete rephasing and slow flow may lead to incomplete visualization of feeding vessels and venous drainage, respectively, with 3D TOF techniques.[4]

MR Technique

Recognition and depiction of AVMs are improved on MR by both the utilization of IV contrast enhancement with conventional planar imaging and implementation of MRA techniques.

Pitfalls in Image Interpretation

In the presence of intracranial hemorrhage, the MR examination should be checked specifically for delineation of an underlying cause, such as an aneurysm, AVM, or neoplasm.

Clinical References

1. Grossman RI, Gamori JM, Goldberg HI, et al. MR imaging of hemorrhagic conditions of the head and neck. Radiographics 1988;8:441–454.
2. Hyman RA, Black KS. Aneurysms and vascular malformations. Top Magn Reson Imaging 1989;2:49–62.
3. Edelman RR, Wentz KU, Mattle HP, et al. Intracerebral arteriovenous malformations: evaluation with selective MR angiography and venography. Radiology 1989;173:831–837.
4. Marchal G, Bosmans H, Van Fraeyenhoven L, et al. Intracranial vascular lesions: optimization and clinical evaluation of three-dimensional time-of-flight MR angiography. Radiology 1990;175:443–448.

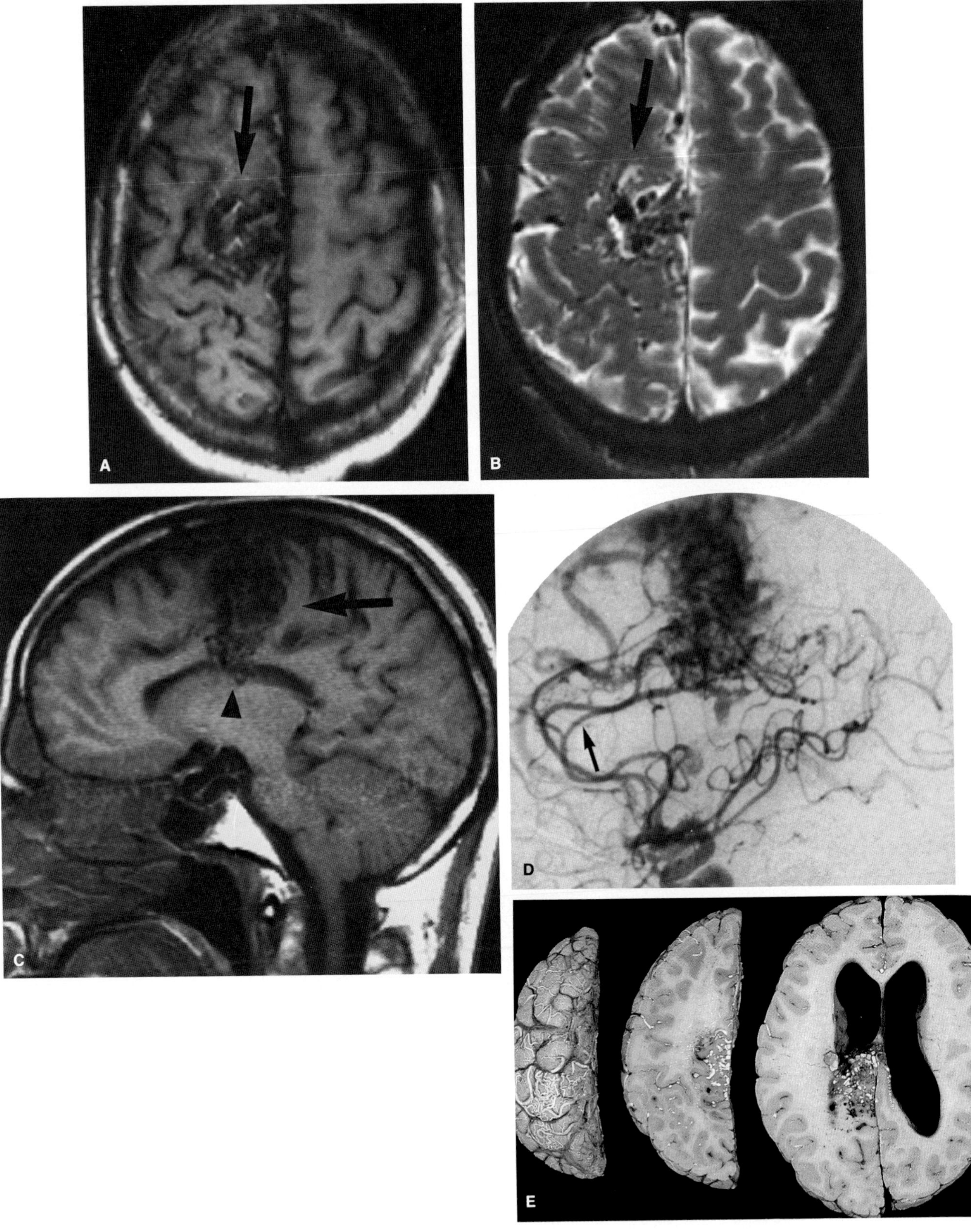
A
B
C
D
E

HISTORY

New onset seizures; remote history of intracranial bleeding

FINDINGS

T1-weighted (*A*) and T2-weighted (*B*) axial images demonstrate a large mass lesion composed of multiple serpiginous structures, most of which have low signal intensity because of blood flow. The lesion (*arrows in A and B*) is noted within the posterior right frontal lobe, with no surrounding edema and little mass effect on adjacent structures. (*C*) The T1-weighted sagittal image, approximately 1.5 cm to the right of midline, demonstrates the transcortical course of the lesion (*arrow*) and its extension to the body of the right lateral ventricle (*arrowhead*). (*D*) Injection of the left common carotid artery on cerebral arteriography reveals a large abnormal tangle of dilated arteries and draining veins, with enlarged feeding vessels including the pericallosal artery (*arrow*).

DIAGNOSIS

Arteriovenous malformation

DISCUSSION

The vascular malformations of the brain are divided into AVM, venous angioma, cavernous angioma, and capillary telangiectasia. Of these, AVM is the most common symptomatic lesion. AVMs are congenital, and usually detected between the ages of 20 and 40 years. Eighty percent are symptomatic by age 50. Patients present with subarachnoid hemorrhage, headache, seizure, or neurologic deficit. AVMs may occur in any location, although 90% are supratentorial. The most common sites are the parietal and frontal lobes, involving the peripheral branches of the anterior or middle cerebral arteries.

The nidus of an AVM is a tangle of tightly packed dilated, tortuous arteries and veins without an intervening capillary network, resulting in arteriovenous shunting. Aneurysms involving the feeding arteries are present in 7% to 9% of cases. AVMs are usually solitary. Calcification is common on CT (25% to 50%). A variable amount of gliosis, edema, or ischemia may accompany the lesion.

Risk of hemorrhage from an AVM is approximately 2% to 3% per year, and each hemorrhagic episode carries a 30% risk of death. Elimination of risk of intracranial hemorrhage is the primary indication for treatment.[1] The size of the AVM *nidus,* and the precise anatomic location of the lesion, especially with respect to vital areas of the brain, are important for treatment planning, and are best evaluated by MR.[1,2] However, MR and MRA have not yet supplanted conventional cerebral angiography for evaluation of the arterial feeders and venous drainage.[3]

Pitfalls in Image Interpretation

The use of gradient moment nulling on conventional planar imaging may mask a small AVM.

Pathologic Correlate

E shows multiple views of an AVM that extends from the surface of the cerebral hemisphere down into the brain parenchyma adjacent to the body of the lateral ventricle. Large AVMs often produce seizures or other neurologic signs long before resulting in intracranial bleeding.

Clinical References

1. Smith H, Strother C, Kikuchi Y, et al. MR imaging in the management of supratentorial intracranial AVMs. AJR 1988;150:1143–1153.
2. Noorbehesht B, Fabrikant J, Enzmann D. Size determination of supratentorial arteriovenous malformation by MR, CT, and angio. Neuroradiology 1987;29:512–518.
3. Edelman R, Wentz K, et al. Intracerebral arteriovenous malformations: evaluation with selective MR angiography and venography. Radiology 1989;173:831–837.

(E *from Okazaki H, Scheithauer B. Slide atlas of neuropathology. New York, Gower Medical Publishing, 1988. By permission of Mayo Foundation.)*

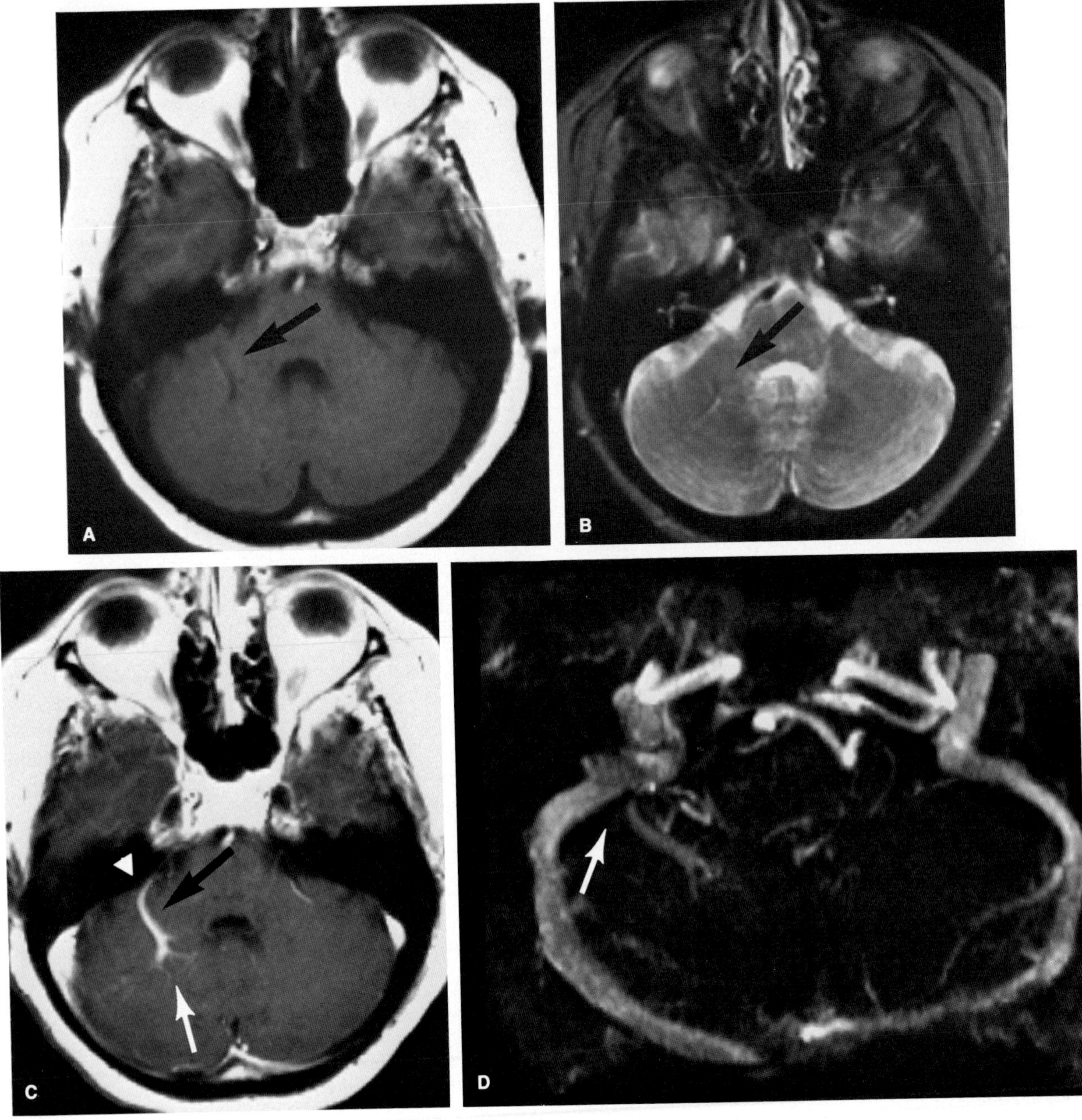

HISTORY

A 52-year-old woman

FINDINGS

(*A*) The T1-weighted axial image demonstrates a linear, tubular flow void (*black arrow*) within the right cerebellar hemisphere, with a suggestion of feeding branches. (*B*) No surrounding edema, or associated parenchymal abnormality, is evident on the heavily T2-weighted image at the same level, and the lesion (*arrow*) is not well seen. (*C*) The T1-weighted axial image obtained after IV gadolinium chelate infusion shows intense enhancement of the lesion (*black arrow*), with improved visualization of the medial feeding branches (*white arrow*) and lateral course of the lesion to the cerebellar border (*white arrowhead*). (*D*) MR venography (2D fast low-angle shot [FLASH]) from a different patient demonstrates direct communication of a similar lesion with the sigmoid sinus (*arrow*).

DIAGNOSIS

Venous angioma

DISCUSSION

An intracranial venous angioma is a collection of abnormal veins representing a developmental anomaly of the venous drainage of the periependymal zones not involving the arterial system. The stellate or umbrella configuration, "caput medusae," represents peripheral dilated medullary veins, usually extending to a ventricular wall, and the longer, larger linear structure represents a central dilated draining vein with a transcortical course. Contrast-enhanced MR and MRA have replaced CT and conventional angiography as the procedure of choice for diagnosis.[1] The main purpose of MR should be to demonstrate the medullary veins, and the central draining vein.[2,3]

Venous angioma is the most common asymptomatic vascular malformation of the brain. Headache, seizure, and vertigo are the most commonly reported symptoms. Acute hemorrhage and hemorrhagic infarction are rare complications, occurring most often with posterior fossa lesions. The frontal lobe is the most common site for a venous angioma, accounting for about 40% of cases, followed by the cerebellum (25%). Lesions are usually solitary. Surgery is performed only if the venous angioma is hemorrhagic or the cause of an intractable seizure disorder.

Intracranial venous angiomas can be missed on routine nonenhanced MR, with approximately 30% of lesions nonvisualized,[1] or recognized only in retrospect, before IV contrast infusion.

MR Technique

Contrast enhancement or MR venography is suggested for visualization.

Clinical References

1. Wilms G, Demaerel P, Marchal G, et al. Gadolinium-enhanced MR imaging of cerebral venous angiomas with emphasis on their drainage. J Comput Assist Tomogr 1991;15:199–206.
2. Toro V, Geyer C, Sherman J, et al. Cerebral venous angiomas: MR findings. J Comput Assist Tomogr 1988;12:935–940.
3. Uchino A, Imada H, Ohno M. Magnetic resonance imaging of intracranial venous angiomas. Clin Imaging 1990;14:309–314.

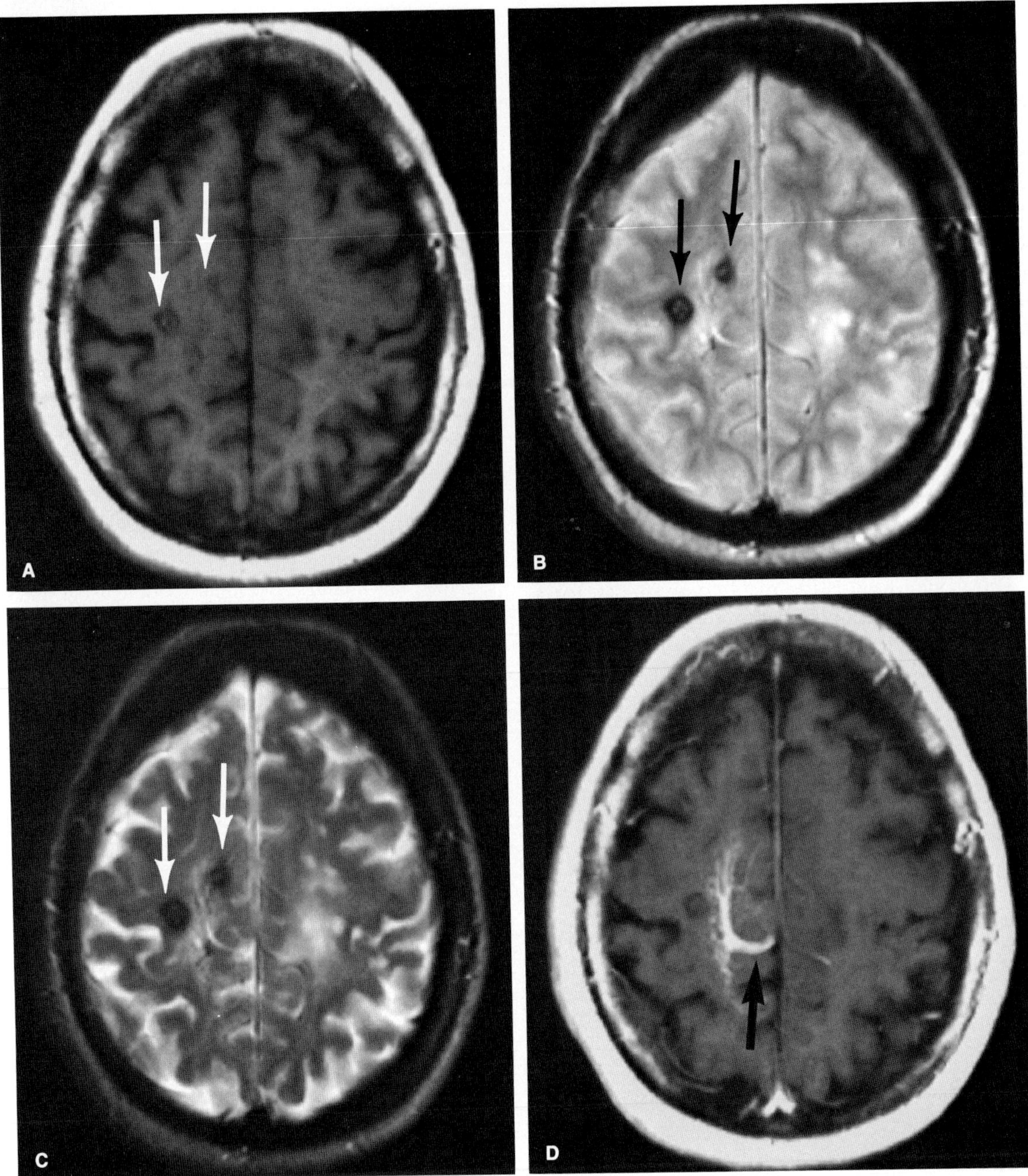

HISTORY

A 63-year-old woman with numbness in the left lower extremity

FINDINGS

(*A*) Two lesions of decreased signal intensity (*white arrows*) are identified in the right frontal lobe on the axial T1-weighted image. As seen on the first (*B*) and second (*C*) echoes of the T2-weighted sequence these two lesions (*arrows*) show a further decrease in signal intensity with increasing T2 weighting. These hypointense abnormalities presumably correspond to sites of hemosiderin or ferritin deposition. (*D*) On the axial postcontrast T1-weighted image there is abnormal enhancement of numerous tiny vessels and a solitary large draining vein (*black arrow*) is identified in the right frontal lobe. The solitary draining vein extends to the midline and was seen to drain into the superior sagittal sinus (*images not shown*).

DIAGNOSIS

Venous angioma with evidence of previous hemorrhage

DISCUSSION

The clinical significance of venous angiomas is controversial. Most are clinically asymptomatic. Reported symptoms in supratentorial lesions include seizures and headache and in the posterior fossa include vestibular complaints (tinnitus, dizziness, vertigo), headache, diplopia, ataxia, and nystagmus. In most cases, the correlation between symptoms and the lesion is weak; in a minority of cases, the clinical presentation can be acute secondary to venous infarction or acute hemorrhage.[1]

Cerebral venous angiomas are composed of dilated medullary veins that are located in the white matter and converge toward a central draining vein, with a transhemispheric course. Most supratentorial venous angiomas have a draining vein that extends to the ventricular wall. The lesion is the result of abnormal venous development during embryogenesis.[2]

As in this case, many venous angiomas are demonstrated only on conventional MR imaging after IV contrast infusion.

Clinical References

1. Wilms G, Demaerel P, Marchal G, et al. Gadolinium-enhanced MR imaging of cerebral venous angiomas with emphasis on their drainage. J Comput Assist Tomogr 1991; 15:199–206.
2. Wilms G, Marchal G, Van Hecke P, et al. Cerebral venous angiomas. Neuroradiology 1990;32:81–85.

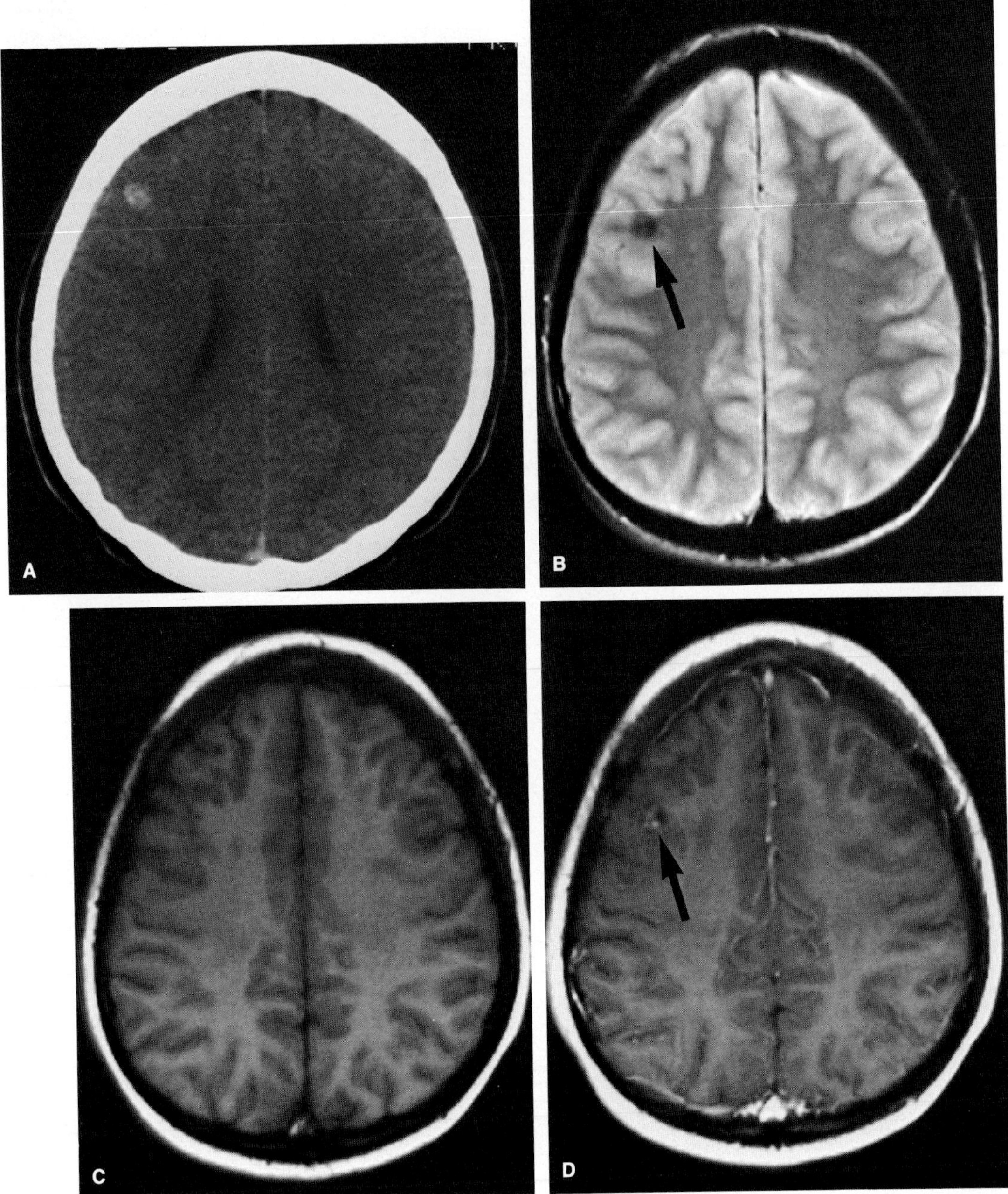

HISTORY

A 21-year-old man with a generalized seizure 1 day before the initial MR examination. *A* to *D* are preoperative; *E* to *G* are postoperative.

FINDINGS

(*A*) Unenhanced CT reveals a right frontal 1-cm calcified lesion (this did not enhance postcontrast). (*B*) On the T2-weighted image the lesion (*arrow*) is predominantly low signal intensity, with contrast enhancement demonstrated by comparison of precontrast (*C*) and postcontrast (*D*) T1-weighted images. The lesion is identified by the arrow in *D*. (*E to G*) On follow-up MR, a surgical defect is noted (*open arrow in E*), filled with bloody fluid, with the primary lesion still noted just posteriorly (*curved arrows in E and G*).

DIAGNOSIS

Cavernous angioma

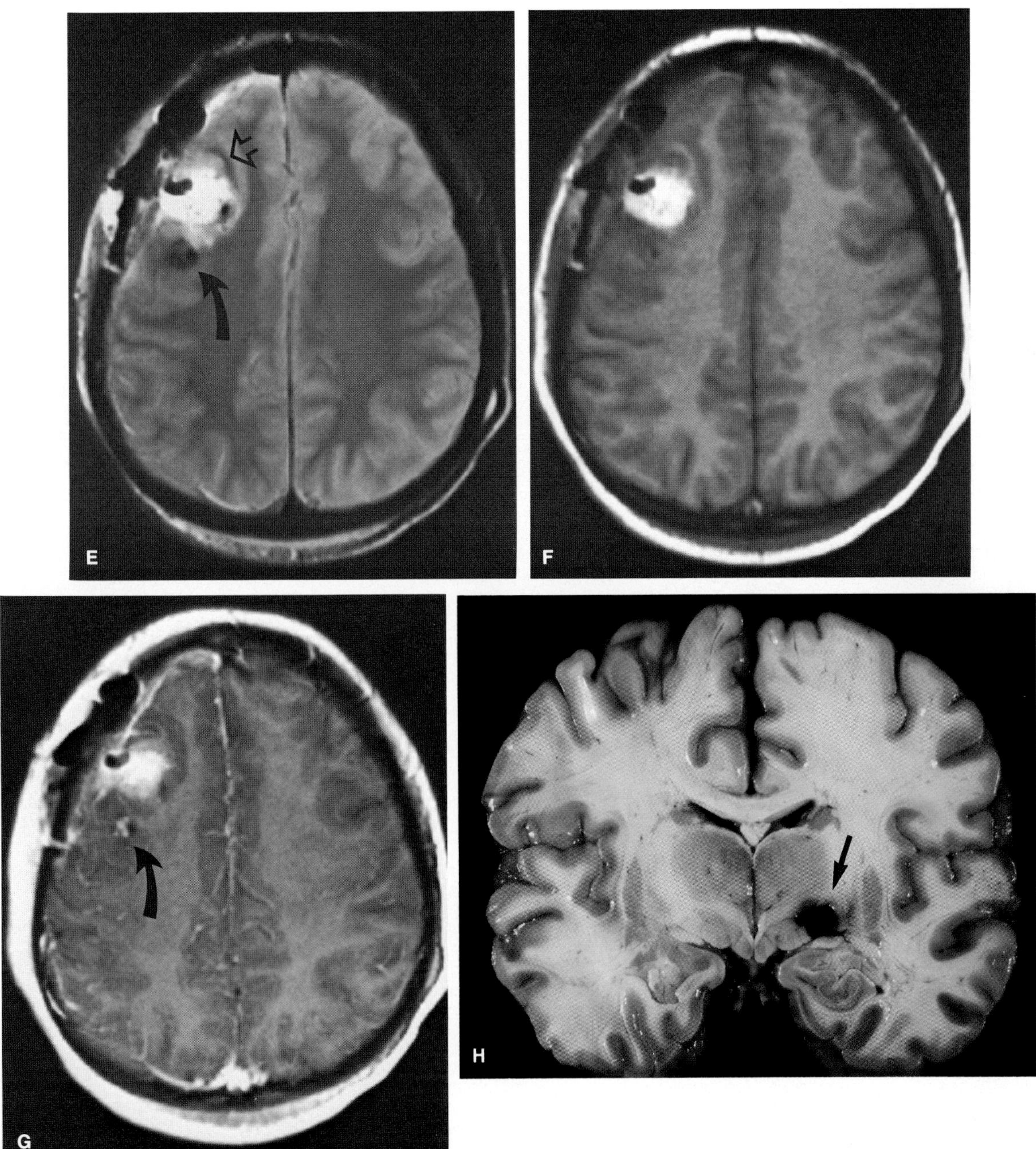

DISCUSSION

Cavernous angiomas (hemangiomas) of the brain are vascular malformations that can present with seizures, hemorrhage, or as a space-occupying mass. These lesions are classically high density on unenhanced CT (if detected), occult or "cryptic" on angiography, and mixed high and low signal intensity[1] with a hypointense (hemosiderin) rim on both T1- and T2-weighted images on MR. Contrast enhancement on MR is a common finding. These lesions are liable to spontaneous hemorrhage, which can be recurrent and life threatening. Surgical resection is often successful. Most lesions are seen in the third to fifth decades, with 75% of cases supratentorial in location. In the cerebrum, many are subcortical in location. Multiplicity of lesions is common (25%). Size is variable, with lesions characteristically well defined and consisting of a honeycomb of vascular spaces separated by fibrous strands (without intervening normal brain parenchyma).

In the case presented, no pathologic alterations were identified in tissue specimens obtained at initial surgery. The patient underwent reoperation, with resection of the mass (confirmed by a third MR examination) and tissue specimens consistent with a cavernous angioma.

MR Technique

GRE techniques[2] with long echo times (≥ 30 msec) and low flip angles (15° or less) emphasize susceptibility-based contrast and thus demonstrate improved sensitivity to blood-breakdown products. Such scans should be employed, as a supplement to conventional SE techniques, for detection of occult vascular malformations, metastases prone to hemorrhage, injury due to prior head trauma, and hemorrhage.

Pitfalls in Image Interpretation

Postoperative films must be interpreted in comparison with preoperative films, particularly following surgical resection. Residual abnormal tissue may be difficult to identify with certainty on the postoperative examination alone, due to superimposed postsurgical changes.

Pathologic Correlate

(*H*) Coronal gross section from an autopsy case demonstrates a cavernous angioma (*arrow*). The finding was incidental in this 35-year-old man, who died in a bicycle–automobile accident. On gross pathology, cavernous angiomas are usually red or black and well circumscribed, and may demonstrate calcification or ossification. Histologically, in the case of prior hemorrhage, there may be hemosiderin containing macrophages and gliosis at the periphery of the lesion.

Clinical References

1. Rapacki TFX, Brantley MJ, Furtlow TW, et al. Heterogeneity of cerebral cavernous hemangiomas diagnosed by MR imaging. J Comput Assist Tomogr 1990;14:18–25.
2. Atlas SW, Mark AS, Grossman RI, Gomori JM. Intracranial hemorrhage: gradient-echo MR imaging at 1.5T. Radiology 1988;168:803–807.

(H *courtesy of Daron G. Davis, MD.*)

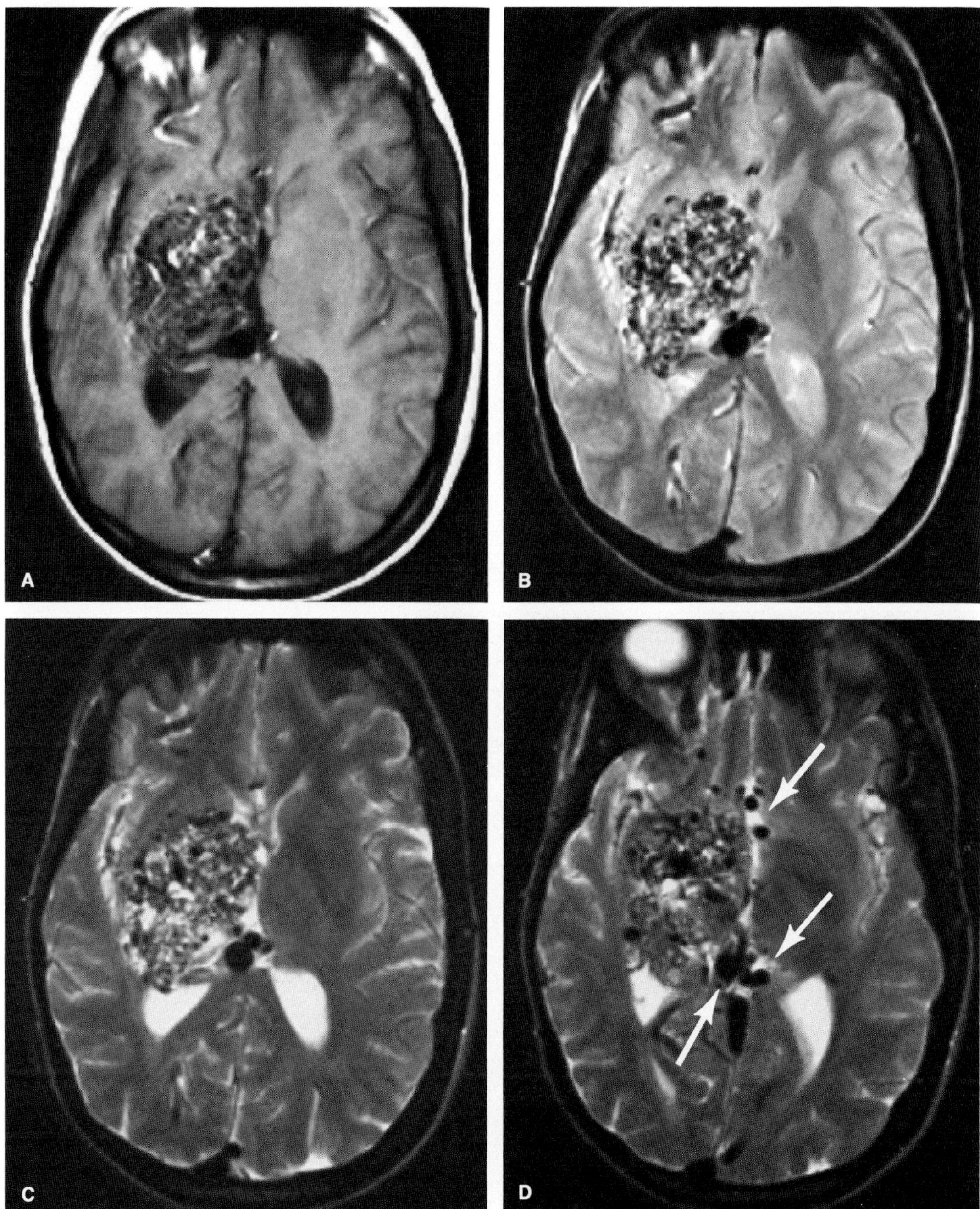

HISTORY

A 27-year-old with history of a seizure at age 13. No recent symptoms were noted.

FINDINGS

T1-weighted axial image (*A*), intermediate (*B*), and heavily (*C*) T2-weighted axial images at the level of the basal ganglia demonstrate a large heterogeneous mass in the expected region of the right basal ganglia and thalamus. The mass consists of innumerable serpiginous structures, most of which have low signal intensity on both T1- and T2-weighted images, representing signal void due to fast flowing blood. (*D and E*) T2-weighted axial images obtained at lower levels show enlarged central draining veins (*white arrows in D*) and a large vein of Galen (*white arrow in E*). The proximal middle and anterior cerebral arteries (*arrowheads in E*) are enlarged.

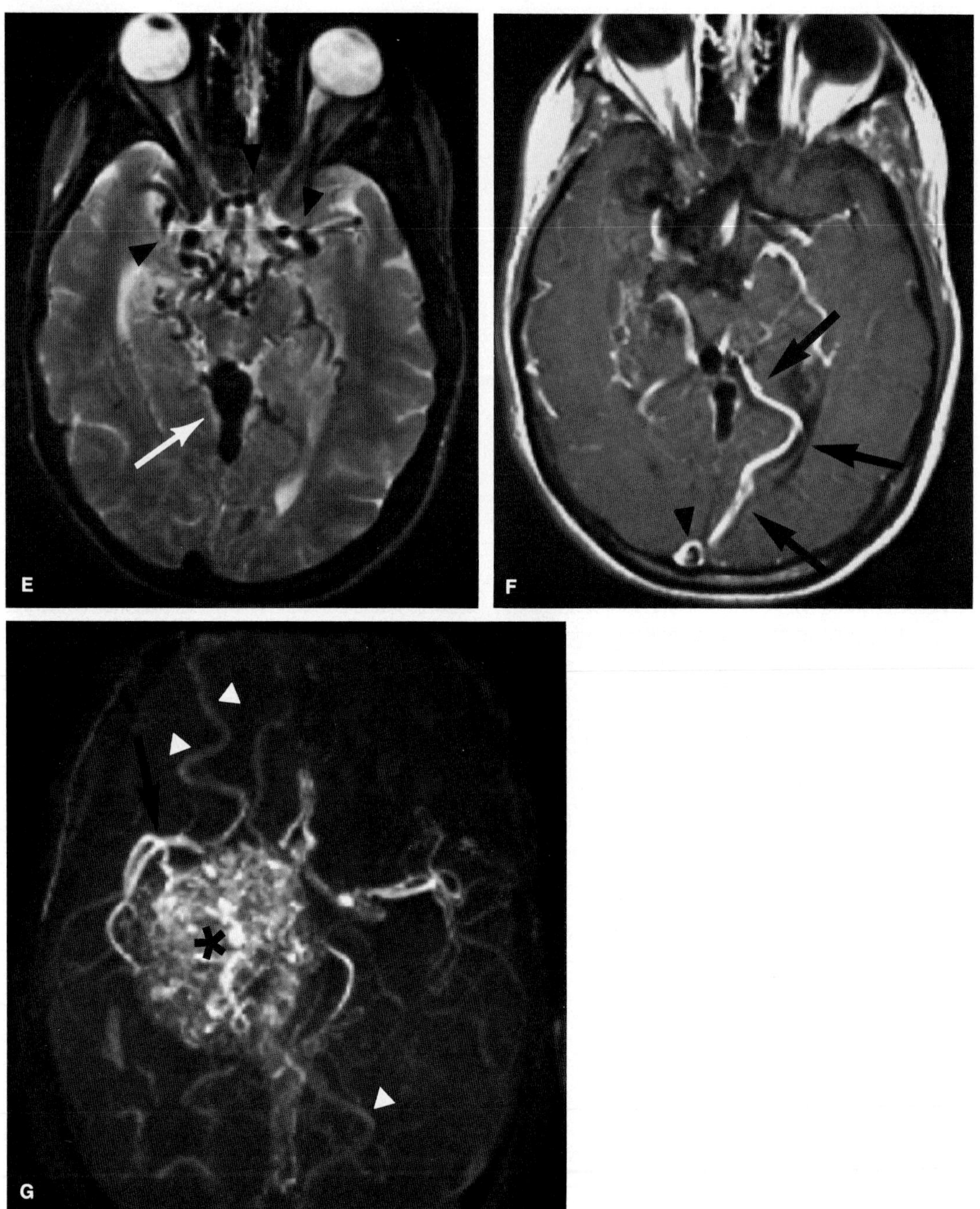

(*F*) On a postcontrast T1-weighted axial image a large contralateral vein (*arrows*) draining into the superior sagittal sinus (*arrowhead*) is well visualized. (*G*) MRA reveals the branches of the right middle cerebral artery (*arrow*) to be enlarged and draped around the vascular malformation (*asterisk*). Several enlarged veins draining peripherally are also depicted (*white arrowheads*).

DIAGNOSIS

Arteriovenous malformation (AVM)

DISCUSSION

AVMs consist of a tortuous nidus of abnormally dilated arteries and veins. Brain tissue is not found intervening within the vascular nidus. Mass effect is usually absent or minimal, unless hemorrhage has occurred. Approximately 18% of AVMs are situated deep within the brain, involving the basal ganglia and internal capsule. These lesions can be fed by any of the arteries which normally supply the basal ganglia, including the anterior choroidal artery off the internal carotid artery, lenticulostriate arteries off the middle cerebral artery, and the thalamoperforating arteries arising from the posterior cerebral artery. Feeding arteries are enlarged on SE images and have a prominent flow void on T2-weighted images.

Draining veins of deep AVMs typically include the thalamostriate veins, which, together with the septal vein, form the internal cerebral veins that feed the vein of Galen. Other enlarged veins may drain into the superior sagittal sinus. Markedly dilated draining veins may cause mass effect, particularly on the brain stem, even in the absence of hemorrhage.[1]

MR Technique

Three-dimensional MRA is useful for noninvasive visualization of the arterial component of an AVM. Large abnormal veins with high flow may also be depicted by 3D volumetric methods. In general, however, venous structures are best seen with 2D sequential multislice MR "venography."[2]

Clinical References

1. Brown R, Wiebers D, Forbes G, et al. The natural history of unruptured intracranial arteriovenous malformations. J Neurosurg 1988;68:352–357.
2. Edelman R, Wentz K, Mattle H, et al. Intracerebral arteriovenous malformations: evaluation with selective MR angiography and venography. Radiology 1989;173:831–837.

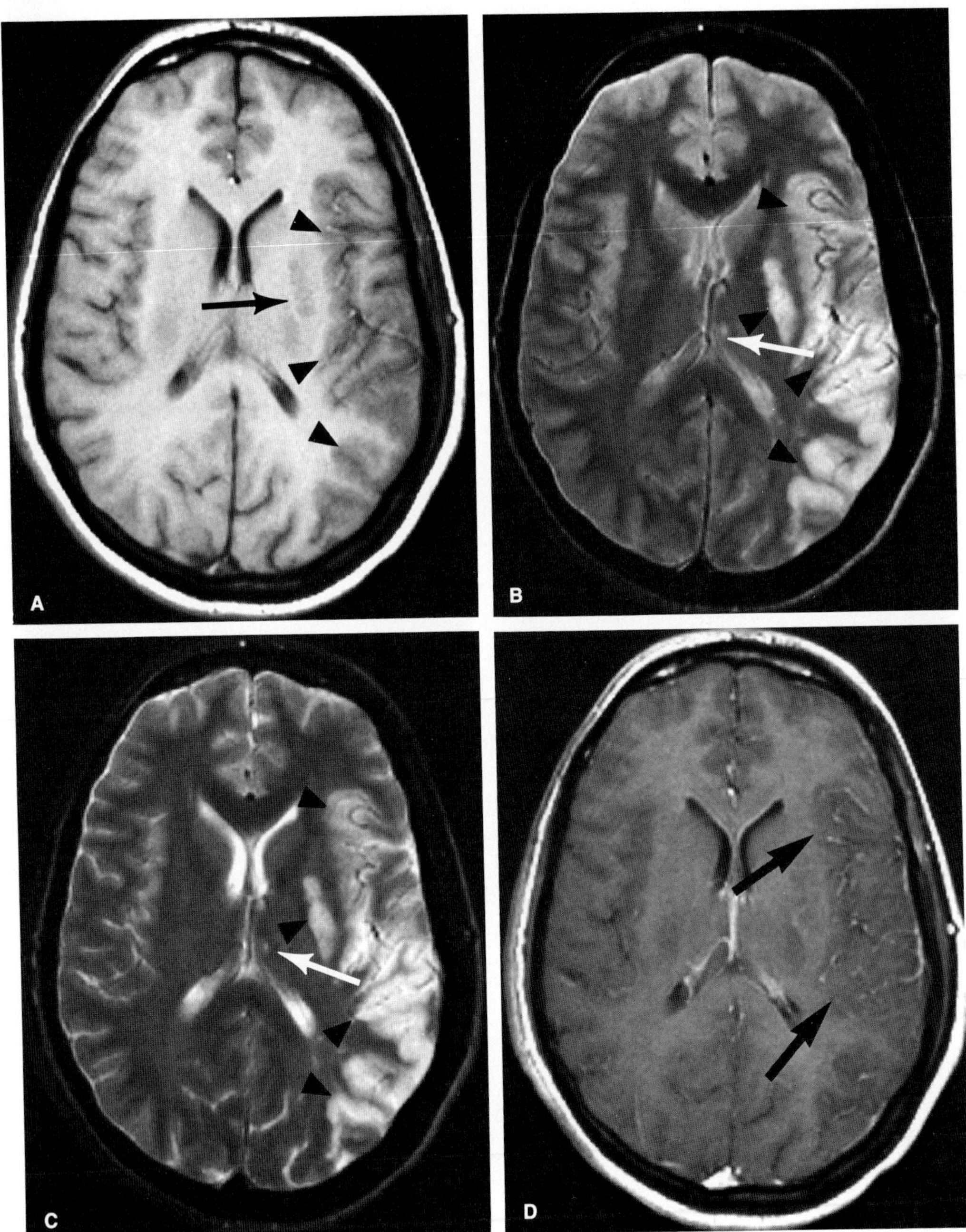

HISTORY

A 27-year-old with acute right hemiparesis, with receptive and expressive aphasia. Vegetations were noted on the aortic valve by transesophageal echocardiography.

FINDINGS

(*A*) On the T1-weighted axial image, the gyri (*arrowheads*) of the left temporal and parietal lobes are thickened and have abnormal decreased signal intensity. The signal intensity of the left putamen (*small white arrow*) is also abnormally low. On the intermediate (*B*) and heavily (*C*) T2-weighted axial images, there is high signal intensity (*arrowheads*) in the same regions, all corresponding to the distribution of the left middle cerebral artery. (*D*) The T1-weighted axial image obtained after IV gadolinium chelate infusion demonstrates increased signal intensity (enhancement) within the blood vessels (*arrows*) in the affected areas. The brain parenchyma does not enhance.

A punctate abnormality (*white arrows in B and C*) with high signal intensity is also present in the left thalamus on the T2-weighted images.

DIAGNOSIS

Acute cerebral infarction (2 days postictus) in the left middle cerebral artery territory and thalamus

DISCUSSION

Cerebral infarction progresses in steps from ischemia with its potential risk to actual infarction with brain cell death.[1] MR is much more sensitive than CT in detecting acute (less than 48 hours) ischemia, routinely demonstrating changes by 4 to 6 hours postictus. Enhancement after IV gadolinium chelate infusion varies with time after ictus. Intravascular enhancement, demonstrated in this case, reflects slow arterial flow and is the earliest recognized pattern of enhancement. This pattern may occur up to 7 days postictus and temporally precedes both meningeal and parenchymal enhancement.[1,2]

Stroke in young people is often embolic in etiology. Cardiac lesions, such as valve vegetations with endocarditis or left atrial thrombus due to atrial fibrillation, are the most common cause of showers of emboli, producing acute infarction in more than one vascular territory.

Infarction of the left precentral gyrus, or primary motor strip, causes right hemiparesis. Expressive aphasia is the result of infarction of Broca's area, located immediately anterior to the primary motor cortex and immediately above the sylvian fissure.

Clinical References

1. Elster A, Moody D. Early cerebral infarction: gadopentetate dimeglumine enhancement. Radiology 1990;177:627–632.
2. Yuh W, Crain M, Loes D, et al. MR imaging of cerebral ischemia: findings in the first 24 hours. AJR 1991;157:565–574.

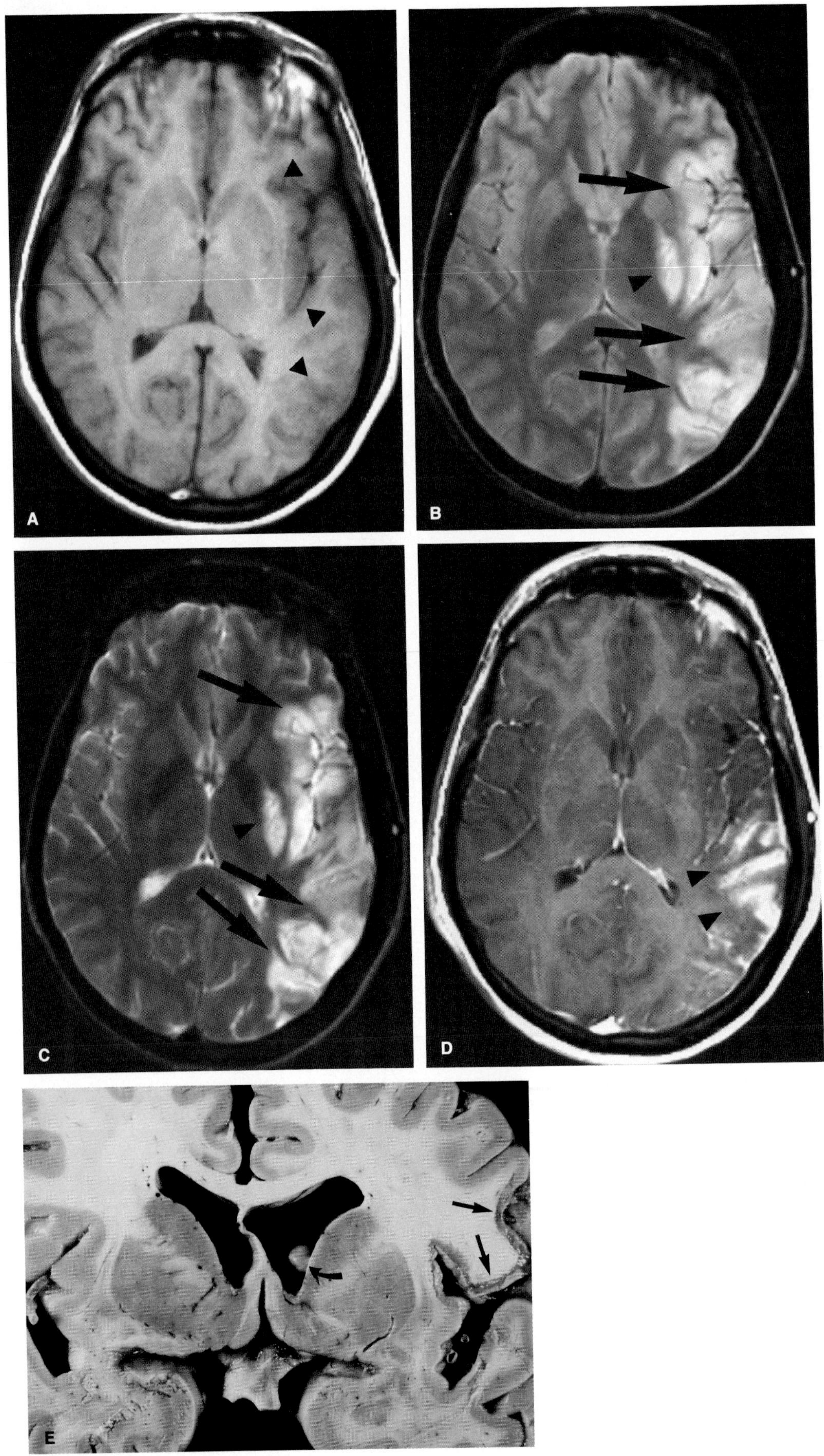
A
B
C
D
E

HISTORY

Same patient as case 1.781-1, now with persistent receptive aphasia 6 days postictus

FINDINGS

(*A*) T1-weighted axial image demonstrates subtle narrowing of the sulci (*arrowheads*) of the left temporal lobe. On the intermediate (*B*) and heavily (*C*) T2-weighted axial images there is abnormal high signal intensity in the cortex and subcortical white matter of the left temporal lobe (*arrows*) and in the left putamen (*arrowhead*). (*D*) The T1-weighted axial image obtained after contrast infusion shows parenchymal enhancement (*arrowheads*) in a gyriform pattern in the posterosuperior left temporal lobe.

DIAGNOSIS

Subacute cerebral infarction in the left middle cerebral artery territory

DISCUSSION

Cerebral infarction (stroke) is a leading cause of morbidity and mortality in the United States. Stroke is usually associated with atherosclerosis, which commonly involves the carotid bifurcation, the internal carotid artery, and the middle cerebral artery. Acute neurologic deficit is the presenting symptom.

Stroke may involve both gray and white matter with the lesion usually sharply demarcated and confined to a specific vascular territory. MR findings in subacute cerebral infarction reflect increased water content, with low signal intensity on T1-weighted images and high signal intensity on T2-weighted images. The increased water content of the infarcted brain reflects vasogenic (extracellular) edema caused by breakdown of the blood–brain barrier and is manifested best by signal intensity changes on T2-weighted images.[1] Vasogenic edema is first seen approximately 8 hours after the ischemic event. Cytotoxic edema is abnormal accumulation of intracellular water and may be detected by MR as early as 2 hours after the ischemic event. Cytotoxic edema is manifested by parenchymal swelling with no signal intensity abnormality, best seen on T1-weighted images.[1]

The posterior superior temporal lobe comprises the general interpretative area, or Wernicke's area. Infarction of this area in the dominant hemisphere causes loss of intellectual functions associated with language or symbolism (ie, receptive aphasia). Parenchymal enhancement of Wernicke's area is demonstrated in this case. Parenchymal enhancement in completed cortical infarction is usually not seen before 6 days postictus, is the predominant pattern of enhancement in the subacute phase (7 to 30 days), slowly fades in the chronic phase (more than 30 days), and may persist for 6 to 8 weeks.[2]

Pathologic Correlate

(*E*) A subacute middle cerebral artery infarct (*black arrows*) is shown on a coronal gross section from an autopsy specimen. At this stage in its evolution, the infarcted tissues begin to look smaller in size than contralateral normal tissues, and the gray matter takes on a granular, glassy appearance. Incidental note is made of a subependymoma (*curved arrow*) within the ventricular system. Subependymomas are asymptomatic tumors, frequently found in older men, with multiplicity, sharp demarcation, and lobulation characteristic. These benign tumors are noted for their slow growth, with location in the fourth ventricle most common, followed by the lateral ventricles.

Clinical References

1. Yuh W, Crain M, Loes D, et al. MR imaging of cerebral ischemia: findings in the first 24 hours. AJR 1991;157:565–574.
2. Crain M, Yuh W, Greene G, et al. Cerebral ischemia: evaluation with contrast-enhanced MR imaging. AJR 1991; 157:575–538.

(*E courtesy of Daron G. Davis, MD.*)

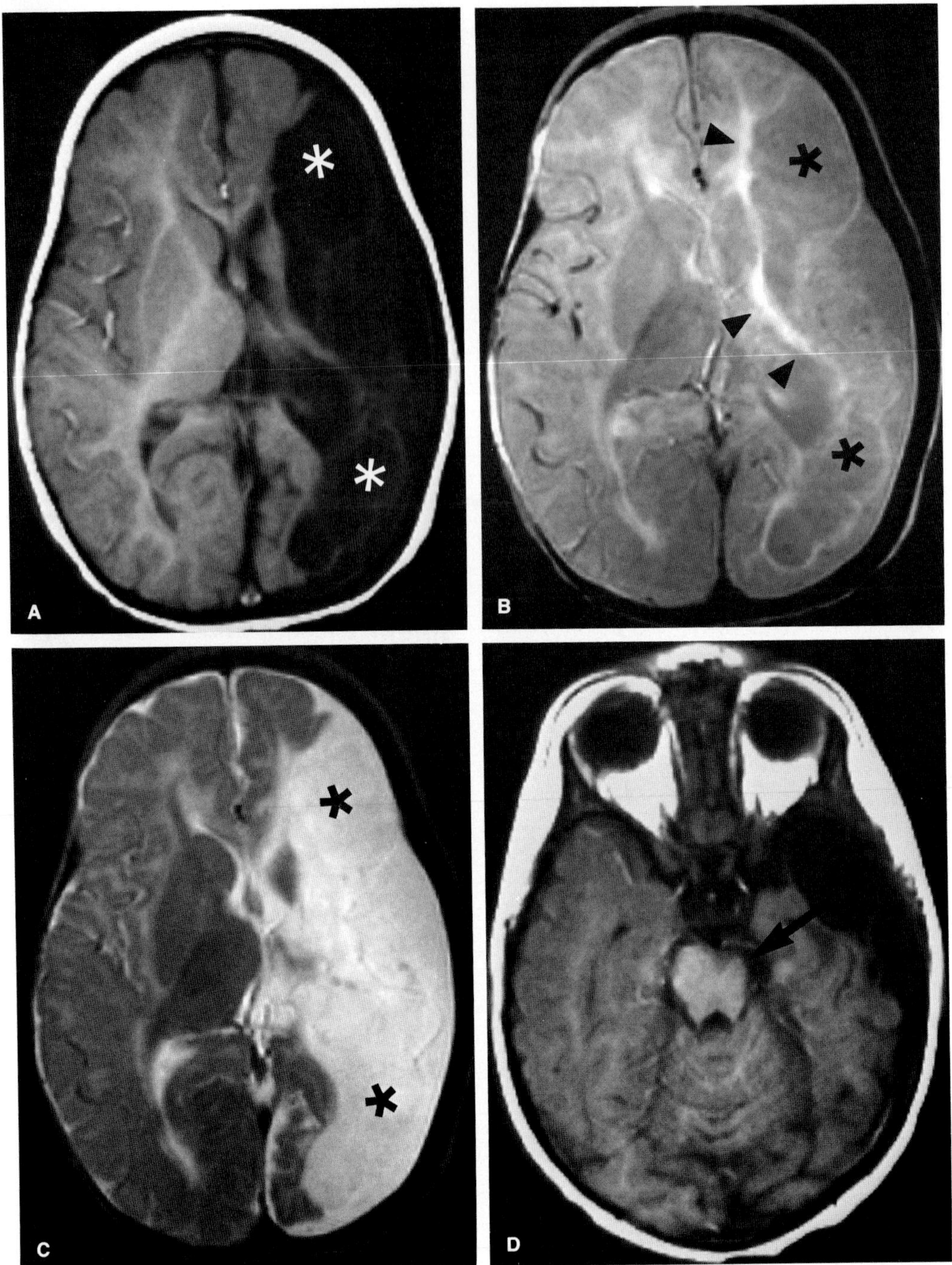

HISTORY

A 10-month-old with history of a neonatal cerebrovascular accident

FINDINGS

T1-weighted axial (*A*), intermediate (*B*), and heavily (*C*) T2-weighted axial images demonstrate replacement of most of the left cerebral hemisphere by large cystic spaces (*asterisks*). The cystic spaces have the signal intensity of CSF on all images, and replace the brain normally perfused by the left middle cerebral artery (MCA). On the intermediate T2-weighted image (*B*), a high-signal-intensity rim (*black arrowheads*), within the remaining brain, surrounds the cystic spaces. (*D*) The T1-weighted axial image at a lower level shows atrophy of the left side of the pons (*arrow*). (*E*) The corresponding T2-weighted axial image demonstrates abnormal high signal intensity in the left pons (*arrow*). (*F*) On MRA the left middle cerebral artery (*arrow*) is small, and there are minimal peripheral branches.

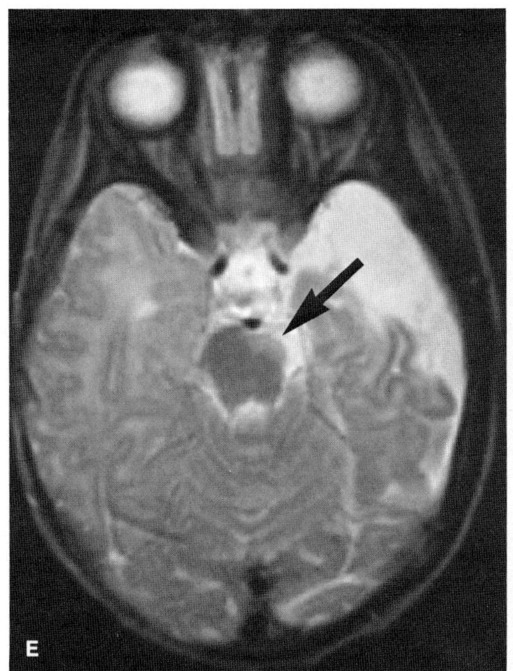

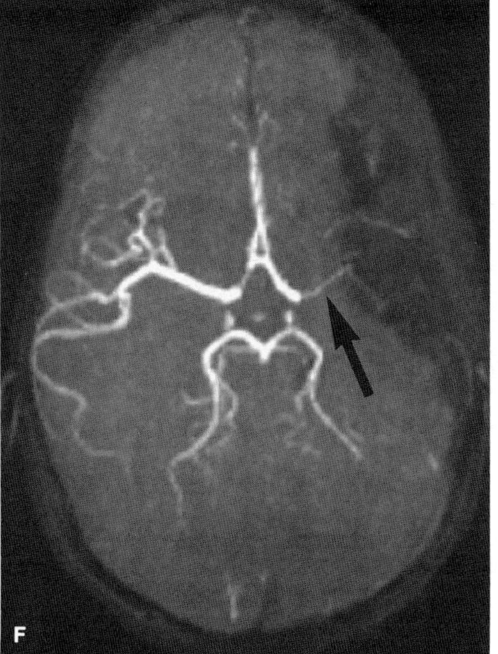

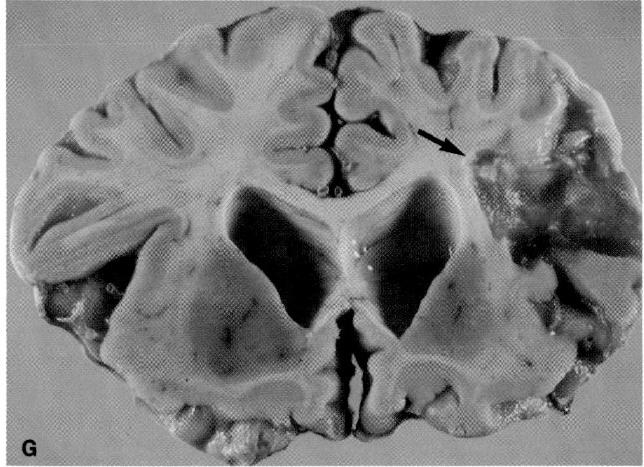

DIAGNOSIS

Chronic left MCA infarct

DISCUSSION

Chronic stroke is defined loosely as a cerebral infarction at least 30 days old. The hallmarks of chronic stroke are cerebral atrophy, encephalomalacia, and gliosis confined to a discrete vascular territory.[1] Gliosis has high signal intensity on both intermediate and heavily T2-weighted images and often surrounds the encephalomalacic region, which has the signal intensity of CSF on all pulses sequences. Atrophy is manifested as widened sulci and ex vacuo dilatation of the ventricles.

White matter atrophy may include wallerian degeneration, a term used for anterograde degeneration of axons and their myelin sheaths secondary to injury or death of the proximal neuron or axon.[2] Wallerian degeneration causes abnormally low signal intensity on T1-weighted images, abnormally high signal intensity on T2-weighted images, and shrinkage along the course of the white matter fibers. It does not enhance after contrast infusion.

Wallerian degeneration is often seen in the corticospinal tract in old, large infarcts involving the motor cortex. The corticospinal tract descends from the motor cortex progressively into the corona radiata, posterior limb of the internal capsule, cerebral peduncle, anterior pons, and anterior medulla, where approximately 90% of the fibers decussate to the contralateral spinal cord.

MR Technique

Gliosis surrounding an old cavitated stroke is best seen on intermediate T2-weighted images. CSF and gliosis cannot be differentiated on heavily T2-weighted images because both have the same high signal intensity.

Pathologic Correlate

(*G*) Coronal gross section demonstrates cavitation of the brain parenchyma (*arrow*) just superior to the sylvian fissure, in the posterior frontal lobe. The gray and white matter are both affected. These changes correspond to a chronic infarct in the left MCA distribution.

Clinical References

1. DeWitt L, Kistler J, Miller D, et al. NMR—neuropathologic correlation in stroke. Stroke 1987;18:342–351.
2. Kuhn M, Johnson K, Davis K. Wallerian degeneration: evaluation with MR imaging. Radiology 1988;168:199–202.

(G courtesy of Daron G. Davis, MD.)

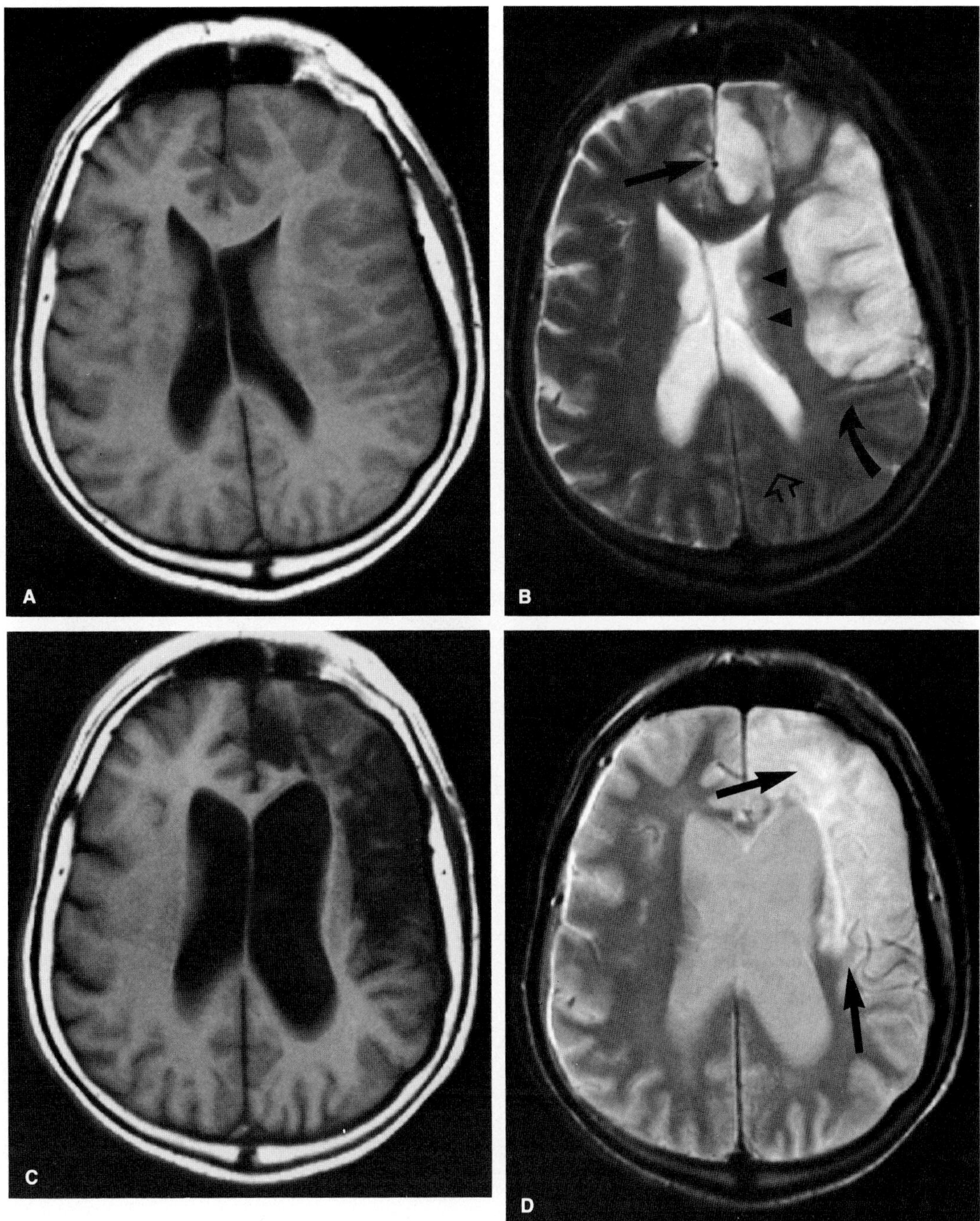

HISTORY

Abrupt onset of paralysis involving the right face, arm, leg, and foot. The patient demonstrated partial recovery of function on clinical follow-up. The MR examination was repeated 18 months later because of new paralysis of the right hand.

FINDINGS

(*A and B*) Initial MR examination. A lesion is identified with abnormal low signal intensity on the T1-weighted image (*A*), and high signal intensity on the T2-weighted image (*B*) (TE = 90 msec) involving principally gray matter in both the left anterior cerebral artery (ACA) (*arrow*) and middle cerebral artery (MCA) (*curved arrow*) territories. The gray matter thickness in these regions is increased over that of normal, reflecting in part cytotoxic edema, with mass effect noted on the lateral ventricle. The more posterior distribution (*open arrow in B*) of the ACA is uninvolved. The head and body of the left caudate nucleus are abnormal (*arrowheads in B*), an area also supplied by the ACA. (*C through I*) Subsequent MR examination. T1-weighted image (*C*) and T2-weighted images (*D*) (TE = 45 msec) and (*E*) (TE = 90 msec) at the

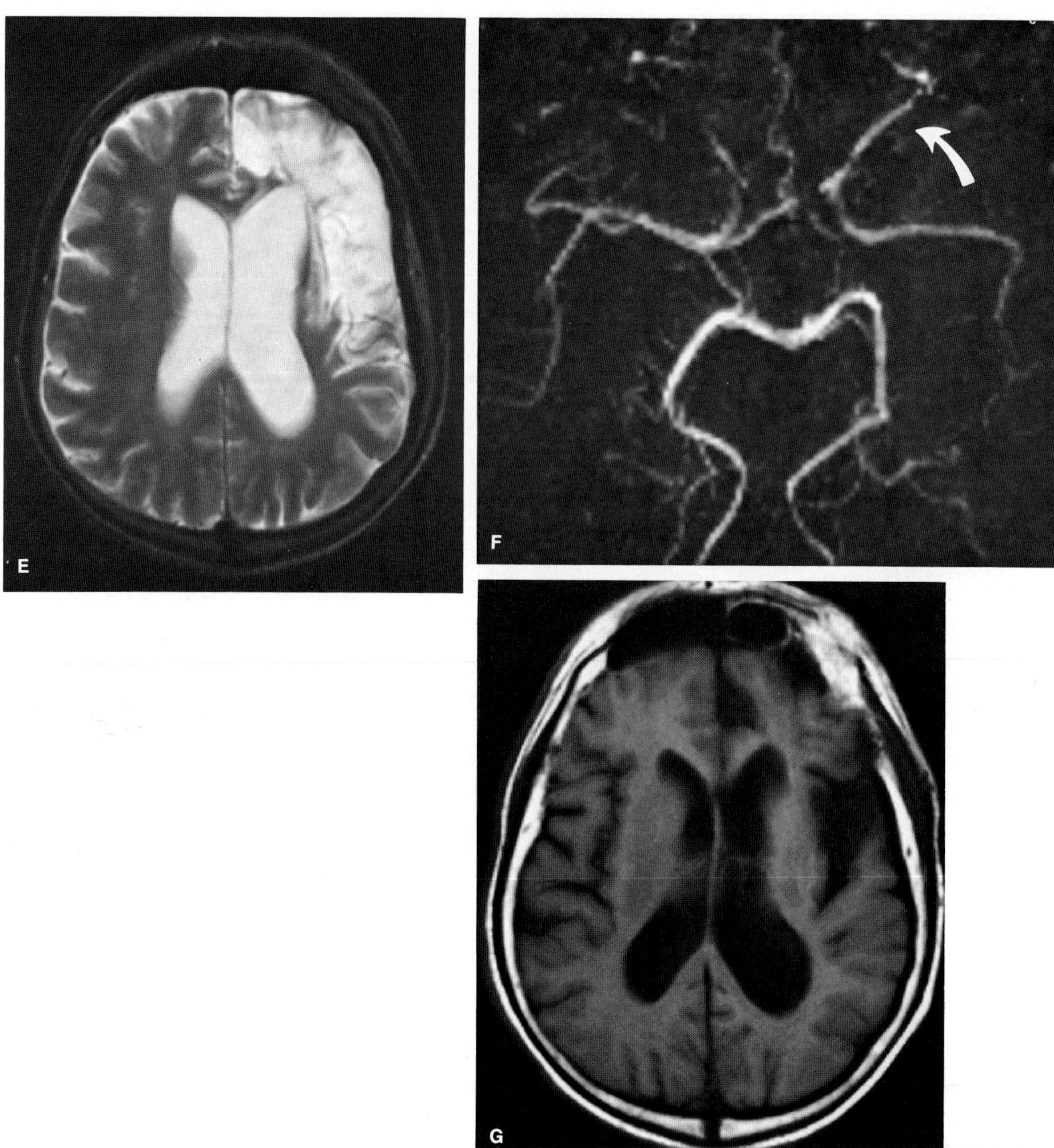

same anatomic level reveal atrophic changes predominantly. There is minimal gliosis, seen best on the intermediate T2-weighted image (*D*) with abnormal high signal intensity (*arrows*), at the periphery of the involved region. (*F*) 3D TOF MRA (craniocaudal projection) reveals a dilated ophthalmic artery on the left (*white curved arrow*), which serves to provide collateral flow from the external carotid artery to the supraclinoid internal carotid artery. T1-weighted image (*G*) and T2-weighted images (*H*) (TE = 45 msec) and (*I*) (TE = 90 msec) at a level just inferior to images *C to E* reveal an additional abnormality (*arrow in H*) in the posterior limb of the left internal capsule. The hyperintensity of the lesion relative to CSF on the first echo of the T2-weighted image (*H*) suggests that the lesion is either recent, or that gliosis is present. This abnormality was not seen on comparable sections of the initial MR examination (*not illustrated*).

DIAGNOSIS

1. Anterior cerebral artery infarction (partial)
2. Middle cerebral artery infarction
3. Lacunar infarction, left posterior internal capsule (subacute)

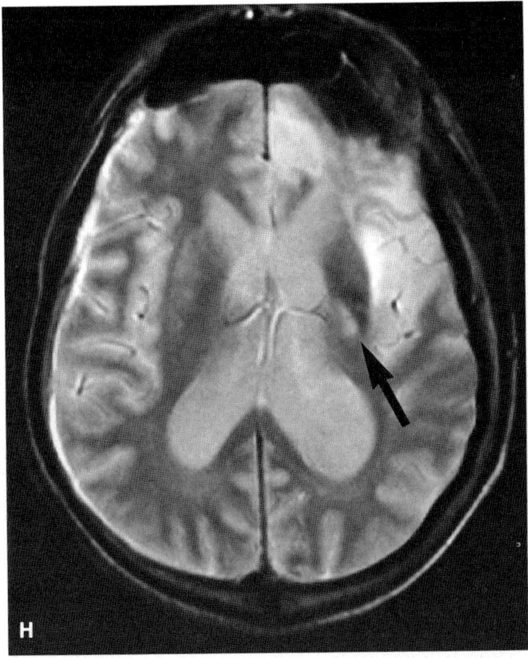

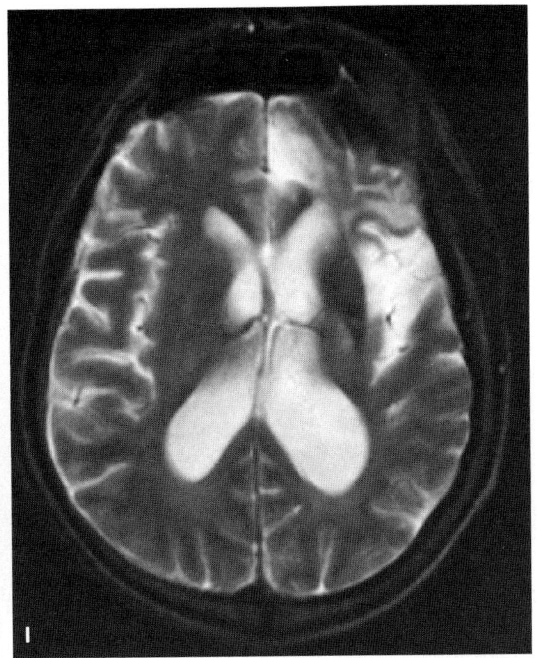

DISCUSSION

The patient in this case presented at the initial MR with a subacute left ACA and MCA infarct. Follow-up MR 18 months later reveals atrophic changes (chronic infarction) and a new left internal capsule lacunar infarct. MRA at this time illustrates the collateral arterial pathway that serves the remaining brain in the ACA and MCA territories.

Occlusion of the ACA is rare, representing only 3% of all cerebral infarctions in a large CT study.[1] Mechanisms for occlusion include emboli in patients with increased flow in the anterior communicating artery, propagation of thrombus from the internal carotid artery, hemodynamic disturbances (spasm, emboli, or thrombosis) associated with an aneurysm of the anterior communicating artery, and stenosis or a small-caliber vessel (ACA) accompanying bilateral internal carotid artery disease.[1,2] Infarction of both the ACA and MCA territories is seen as a result of thrombosis of the distal internal carotid artery with ineffective cervical or circle of Willis anastomoses.

Three major groups of vessels arise from the ACA.[3,4] The first group is that of the medial lenticulostriate arteries, which includes the artery of Heubner (supplying the anterior part of the putamen, caudate nucleus, and inferior internal capsule) and the basal branches of the ACA (supplying the hypothalamus and dorsal chiasm). The second group is composed of the pericallosal branches which supply the corpus callosum. Infarction of these vessels results in isolation of the left (language dominant) and right (left motor) hemispheres. The third group is that of the hemispheric branches, which supply the medial surface of the hemisphere. Collateral supply is common from the contralateral hemispheric branches. From anterior to posterior, these branches supply brain which mediates (1) judgment, insight, and mood, (2) motor synchronization, (3) motor function, (4) sensory function, and (5) memory and emotion.

MR Technique

T2-weighted images with intermediate TE values (40 to 50 msec, with TR = 2500 to 3000 msec) permit ready identification and differentiation of gliosis from adjacent cystic encephalomalacic change in chronic infarction.

Pitfalls in Image Interpretation

In the setting of chronic brain infarction, the MR examination must be carefully reviewed and compared with previous examinations to detect recent ischemic events and to differentiate these from chronic disease. In the patient with a history of cerebral infarction, a common reason for repeated MR examination is recent clinical symptoms suggestive of new ischemic disease.

Clinical References

1. Gacs G, Fox AJ, Barnett HJM, Vinuela F. Occurrence and mechanisms of occlusion of the anterior cerebral artery. Stroke 1983;14:952–959.
2. Rodda RA. The arterial patterns associated with internal carotid disease and cerebral infarcts. Stroke 1986;17:69–75.
3. Berman SA, Hayman LA, Hinck VC. Correlation of CT cerebral vascular territories with function. I. Anterior cerebral artery. AJR 1980;135:253–257.
4. Naheedy MH, Azar KB, Fine M. Radiology of anterior cerebral artery infarction. Comput Radiol 1984;8:183–192.

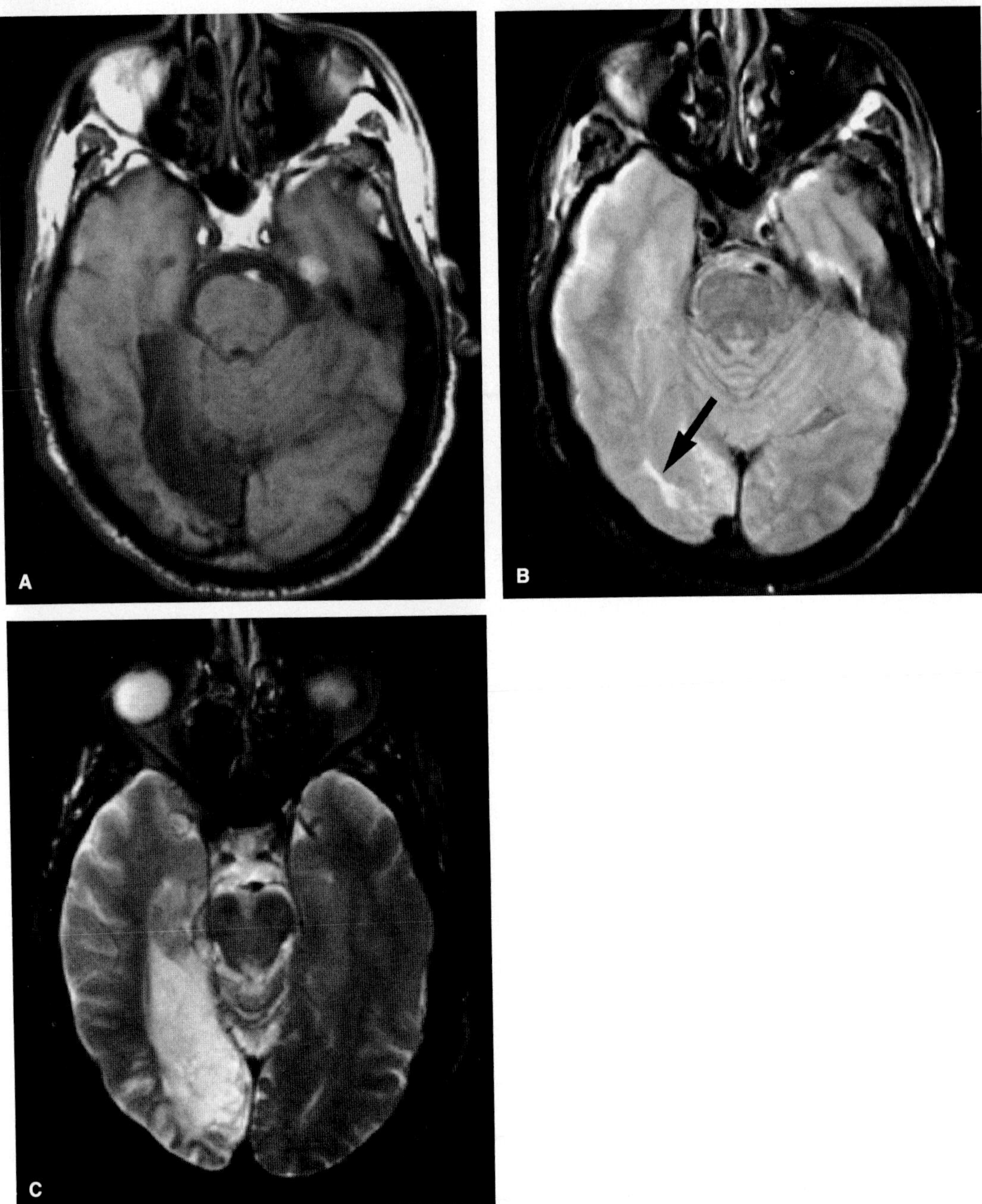

HISTORY

A 51-year-old man with chronic atrial fibrillation. Two years earlier, the patient presented with acute confusion, unsteady gait, and difficulty reading.

FINDINGS

(*A*) Axial T1-weighted image identifies changes of focal atrophy and abnormal decreased signal intensity in the distribution of the right posterior cerebral artery. The lesion is of CSF signal intensity on the first (*B*) and second (*C*) echoes of the T2-weighted sequence. A rim of increased signal intensity (*arrow in B*), corresponding to gliosis, is present surrounding the region of brain substance loss on the scan with intermediate T2 weighting.

DIAGNOSIS

Chronic posterior cerebral artery infarction

DISCUSSION

The posterior cerebral artery can originate from either the basilar tip or the internal carotid artery (fetal origin of the posterior cerebral artery). Branches arising from this vessel perfuse the posteroinferior temporal lobe, hippocampal formation, most of the occipital lobe, medial portion of the parietal lobe, calcarine cortex, and portions of the brain stem, thalamus, and internal capsule.[1,2] The tip of the temporal lobe is supplied by the middle cerebral artery.

In chronic infarction there is glial proliferation with loss of brain tissue. Gliosis results in increased water content and therefore prolongation of T1 and T2 relaxation times. Brain atrophy leads to enlarged sulci and adjacent subarachnoid and ventricular spaces. Chronic cystic changes, referred to as encephalomalacia, are of CSF signal intensity on all pulse sequences. Enhancement by gadolinium chelate injection is uncommon more than 6 weeks after the ischemic event.[3]

MR Technique

The intermediate T2-weighted sequence best differentiates gliosis from encephalomalacic changes, both of which can be observed in chronic infarction.

Clinical References

1. Osborne AG. Introduction to cerebral angiography. Philadelphia, Harper & Row, 1980:295–325.
2. Berman SA, Hayman LA, Hink. Correlation of CT cerebral vascular territories with function. II. Posterior cerebral artery. AJR 1981;137:13–19.
3. Brant-Zawadzki M, Weinstein P, Bartkowski, et al. MR imaging and spectroscopy in clinical and experimental cerebral ischemia: a review. AJR 1987;148:579–588.

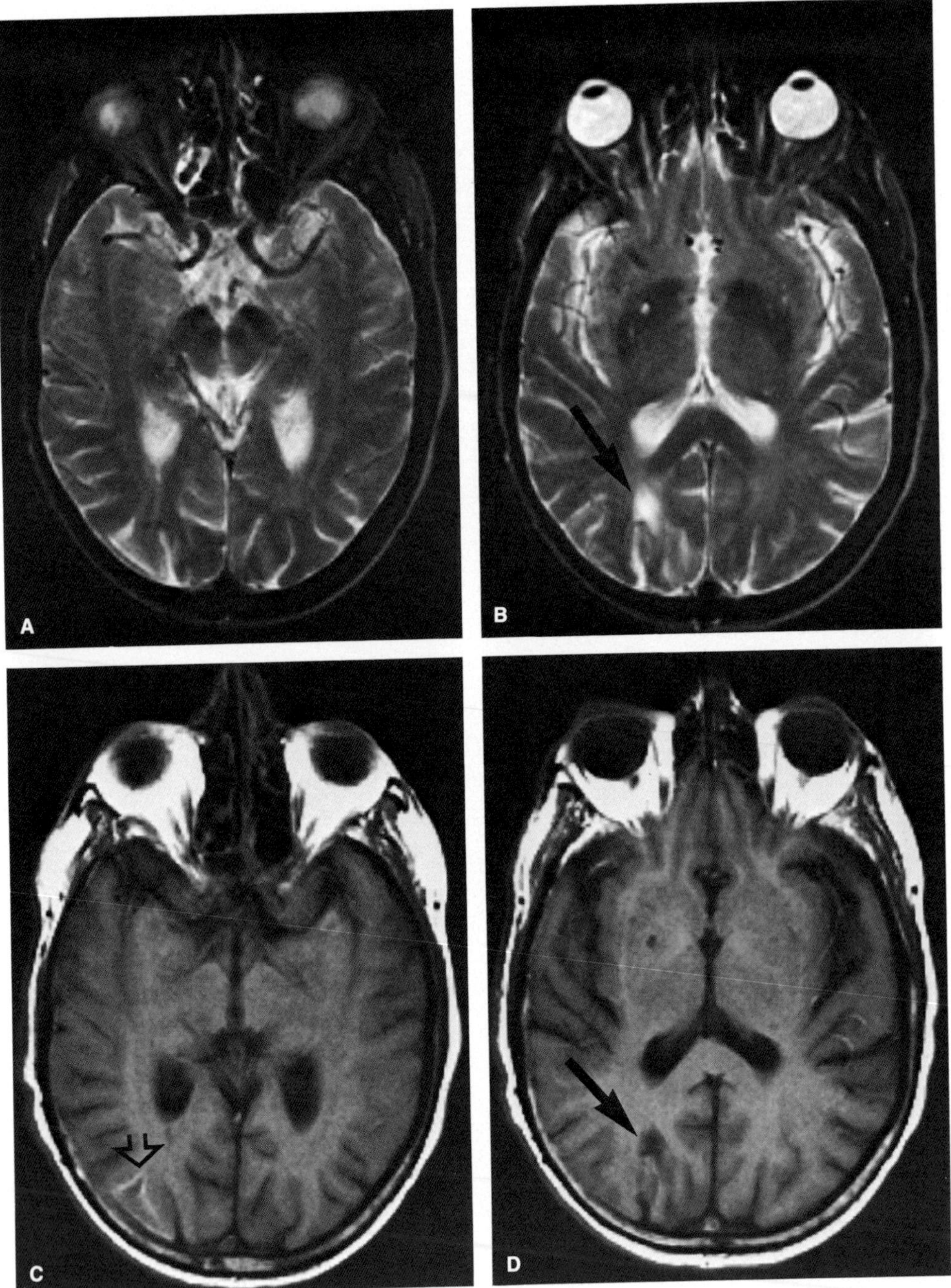

HISTORY

A 62-year-old hypertensive man with diabetes with a 1-week history of left-sided weakness

FINDINGS

Axial T2-weighted (*A and B*) and T1-weighted (*C and D*) images depict focal atrophy and gliosis (*arrows in B and D*) in the right posterior watershed territory, between the vascular distributions of the middle and posterior cerebral arteries. Subtle abnormal hyperintensity (*open arrow in C*), corresponding to methemoglobin, is noted within gray matter on the more inferior T1-weighted section. Abnormal contrast enhancement (*curved arrows in C and D*) is identified in the watershed territory on axial T1-weighted images (*E and F*) after administration of a gadolinium chelate.

DIAGNOSIS

Right posterior watershed subacute infarction superimposed on chronic infarction

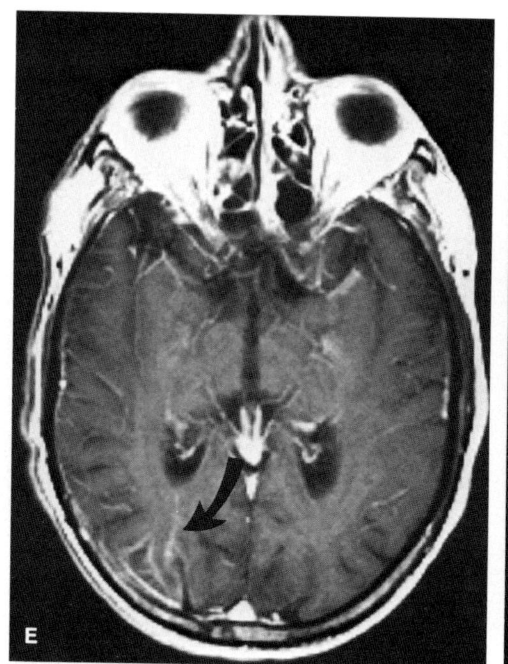

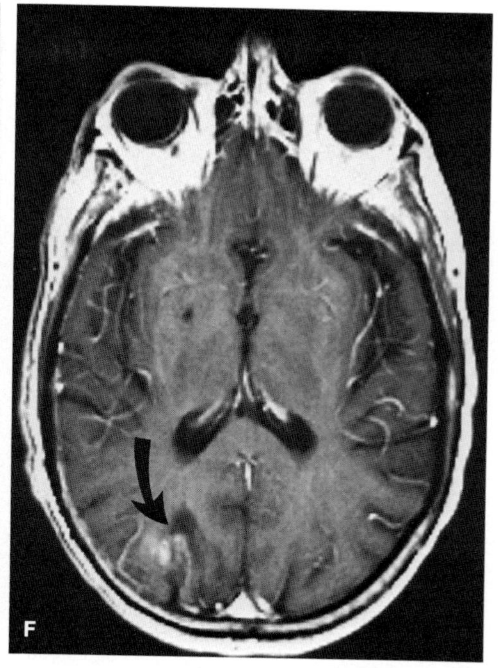

DISCUSSION

Three types of abnormal contrast enhancement have been described in cerebral infarction:

Vascular enhancement of vessels supplying the zone of infarction. This is the earliest type of abnormal enhancement identified and has been reported as early as 2 hours after the vascular insult.[1] It is frequently seen in 1- to 3-day-old infarcts and is uncommon after the first postinfarct week.[2]

Meningeal enhancement adjacent to the damaged tissue is observed in the first week, with a peak occurrence at 1 to 3 days postictus.

Two types of *parenchymal enhancement* of ischemic brain tissue have been described: slowly progressive enhancement and early or intense enhancement. Abnormal parenchymal contrast enhancement can be seen as early as 2 to 3 days postictus and depends on blood–brain barrier breakdown.[3] It is consistently identified by day 6 and is almost universally seen in 1- to 2-week-old infarcts. This enhancement may persist for up to 6 to 8 weeks.

Clinical References

1. Yuh WT, Crain MR, Loes DJ, et al. MR imaging of cerebral ischemia: findings in the first 24 hours. AJR 1991;157:565–573.
2. Elster AD, Moody DM. Early cerebral infarction: gadopentetate dimeglumine enhancement. Radiology 1990;177:627–632.
3. Brant-Zawadzki M, Weinstein P, Bartkowski H, et al. MR imaging and spectroscopy in clinical and experimental cerebral ischemia: a review. AJR 1987;148:579–588.

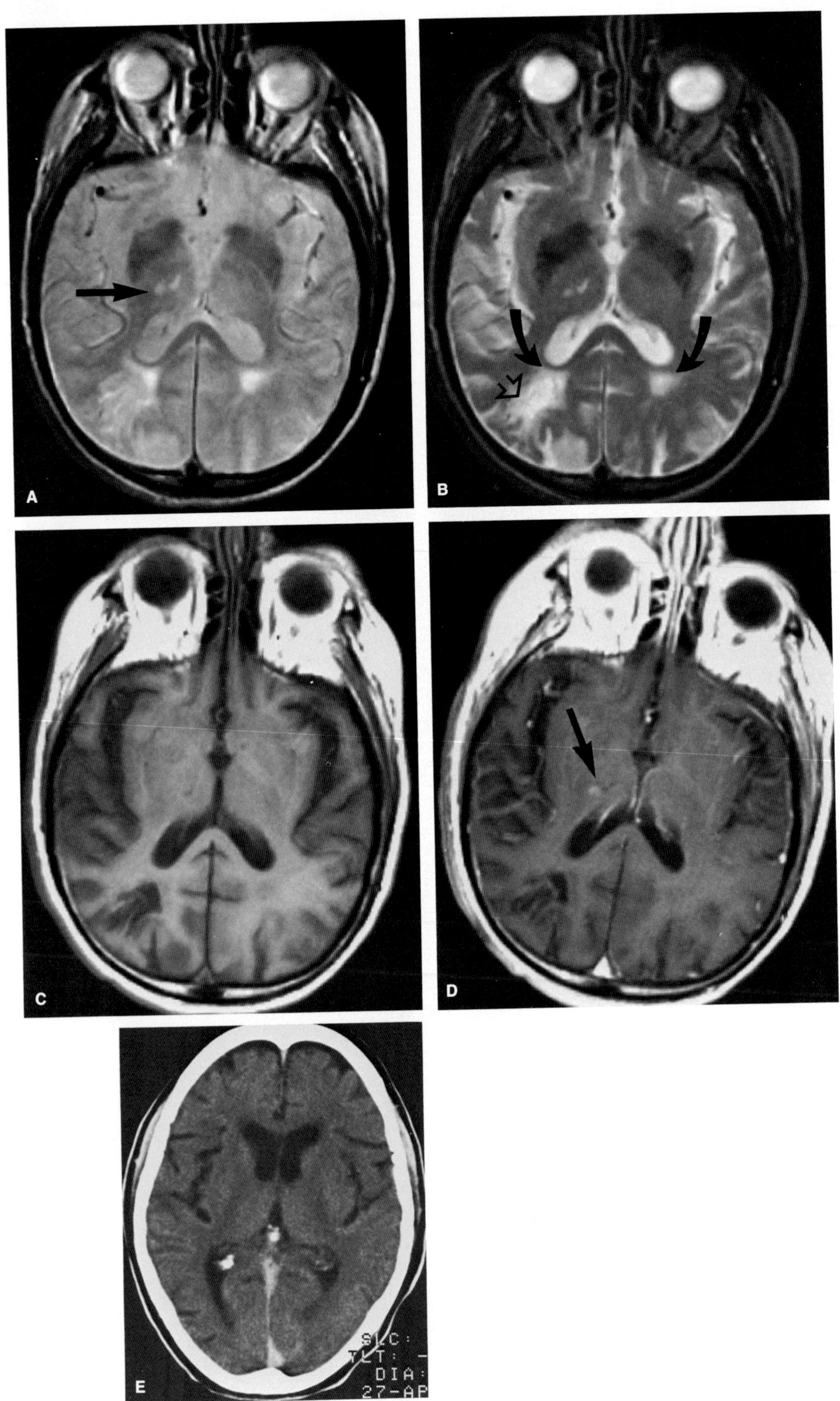
A
B
C
D
E

HISTORY

A 76-year-old man with transient ischemic attacks, hypertension, and non–insulin dependent diabetes mellitus. He was admitted to a local hospital 10 days before MR with hemiparesis, which has resolved.

FINDINGS

(*A*) On the first echo (TE = 45 msec) of the T2-weighted examination, an abnormal focus of hyperintensity (*arrow*) is noted on the right in the region of the posterior limb of the internal capsule and lateral thalamus. (*B*) The second echo (TE = 90 msec) of the T2-weighted examination depicts well the ischemic changes (*curved arrows*) adjacent to the atria of the lateral ventricles and an old right watershed infarction (*open arrow*) at the junction of the vascular distribution of the middle cerebral and posterior cerebral arteries. (*C*) The precontrast T1-weighted image reveals prominent atrophic changes bilaterally in the region of the sylvian fissure. (*D*) On the enhanced T1-weighted image contrast enhancement of the capsular lesion (*arrow*), caused by blood–brain barrier disruption, is noted. (*E*) CT was performed without IV contrast to rule out the presence of intraparenchymal blood. Neither the lesion in the internal capsule nor the chronic watershed infarct was visualized (only the section at the level of the capsular lesion is displayed).

DIAGNOSIS

Subacute right internal capsule lacunar infarction

DISCUSSION

Two clinical studies[1,2] have documented the marked superiority of MR compared with CT for the detection of lacunar infarcts. In the larger study,[1] published in the neurology literature, MR was positive in 78% of cases, compared with 30% by CT. The authors concluded by recommending MR for all patients presenting with symptoms suggestive of lacunar infarction.

Acute lacunar infarcts (within 1 week of symptom onset) are best seen on T2-weighted images, whereas chronic lesions can be well seen on both T1- and T2-weighted images. In a recent study of 100 prospective patients hospitalized with lacunar infarction (79 with classic lacunar syndrome, 21 with less typical lacunar syndromes), designed to evaluate the detection capability of MR, at least one lacunar infarct compatible with symptoms was detected in 89 patients.[3]

Lesion enhancement is consistently demonstrated on MR following gadolinium chelate administration in recent lacunar infarcts. In 9 patients studied on the same day by both enhanced CT and enhanced MR,[4] lesion enhancement was seen in only 4 patients on CT as compared with 8 patients on MR. Lesion enhancement was consistently poor on CT and excellent on MR. In only 1 patient, examined 4 weeks after ictus, was enhancement of the lacunar infarct not noted.

MR Technique

IV administration of a gadolinium chelate is mandatory when recent lacunar infarction is questioned clinically. In a study of 9 patients with recent lacunar stroke,[4] lesion identification was possible only on enhanced MR in 4 patients. Contrast administration also makes possible, as illustrated in this case, differentiation of recent infarcts from chronic ischemia or gliosis.

Pitfalls in Image Interpretation

Small deep-seated arteries or veins, such as the lenticulostriate arteries, can be visualized postcontrast on MR. When cut in cross section, enhancement of such normal vessels can mimic, and should not be confused with, a very small lacunar infarct.

Clinical References

1. Arboix A, Marti-Vilalta JL, Pujol J, Sanz M. Lacunar cerebral infarct and nuclear magnetic resonance. Eur Neurol 1990;30:47–51.
2. Brown JJ, Hesselink JR, Rothrock JF. MR and CT of lacunar infarcts. AJR 1988;151:367–372.
3. Hommel M, Besson G, Le-Bas JF, et al. Prospective study of lacunar infarction using magnetic resonance imaging. Stroke 1991;21:546–554.
4. Miyashita K, Naritomi H, Sawada T, et al. Identification of recent lacunar lesions in cases of multiple small infarctions by magnetic resonance imaging. Stroke 1988;19:834–839.

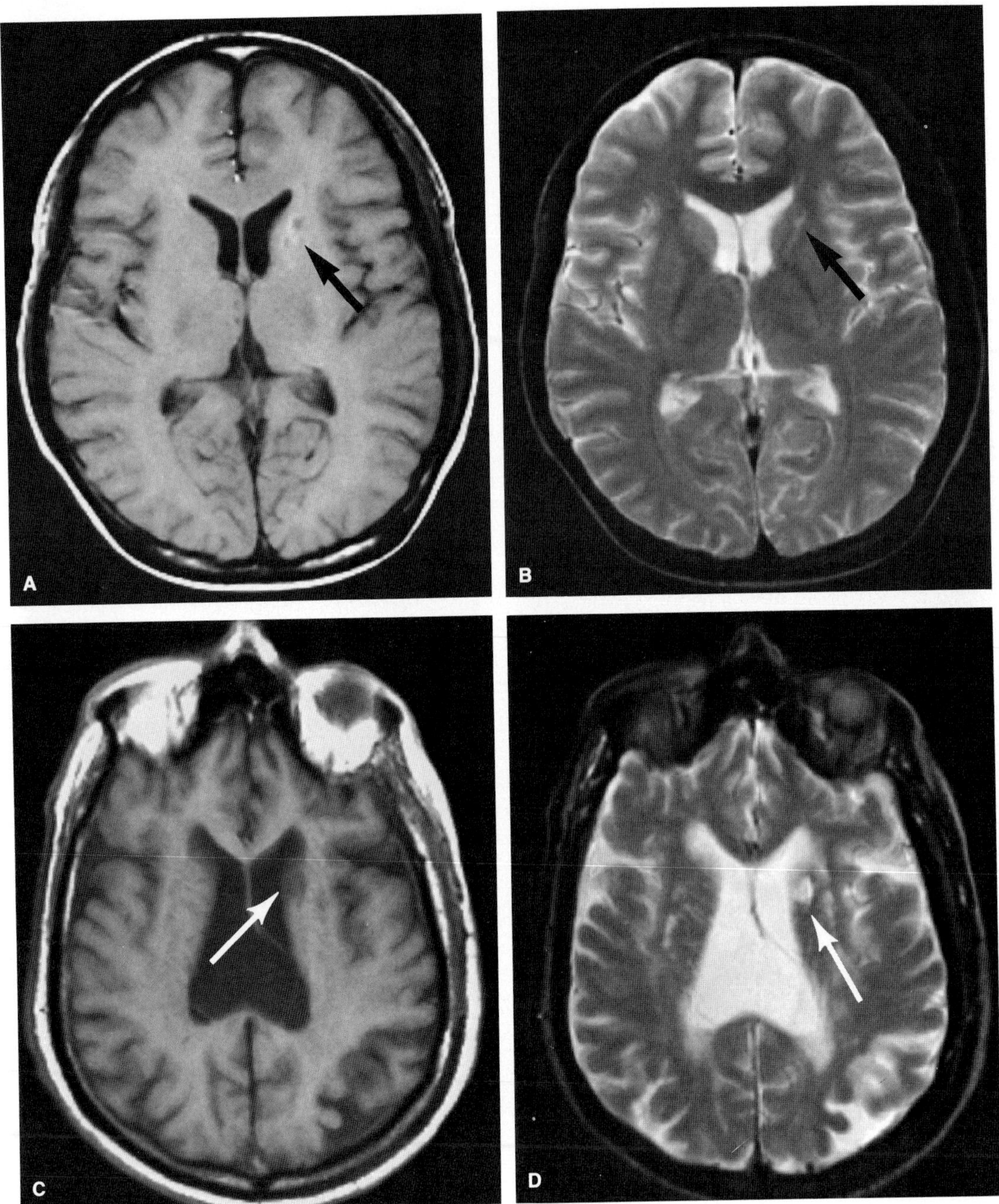

HISTORY

All three patients have a history of hypertension.

FINDINGS

Patient 1: A slitlike lesion (*black arrows in A and B*) of decreased signal intensity on the axial T1-weighted image (*A*) and increased signal intensity on the axial T2-weighted image (*B*) is identified in the anterior limb of the left internal capsule. No enhancement was noted (*images not shown*).

Patient 2: (*C*) Axial T1-weighted image demonstrates a small round hypointense lesion (*white arrow*) in the head of the left caudate nucleus. (*D*) On the axial T2-weighted image this lesion (*white arrow*) is hyperintense. No contrast enhancement was seen (*images not shown*).

Patient 3: (*E*) On the axial T1-weighted image a small round lesion (*curved arrow*) of decreased signal intensity is present in the left globus pallidus. (*F*) On the axial T2-weighted image, the lesion (*curved arrow*) is hyperin-

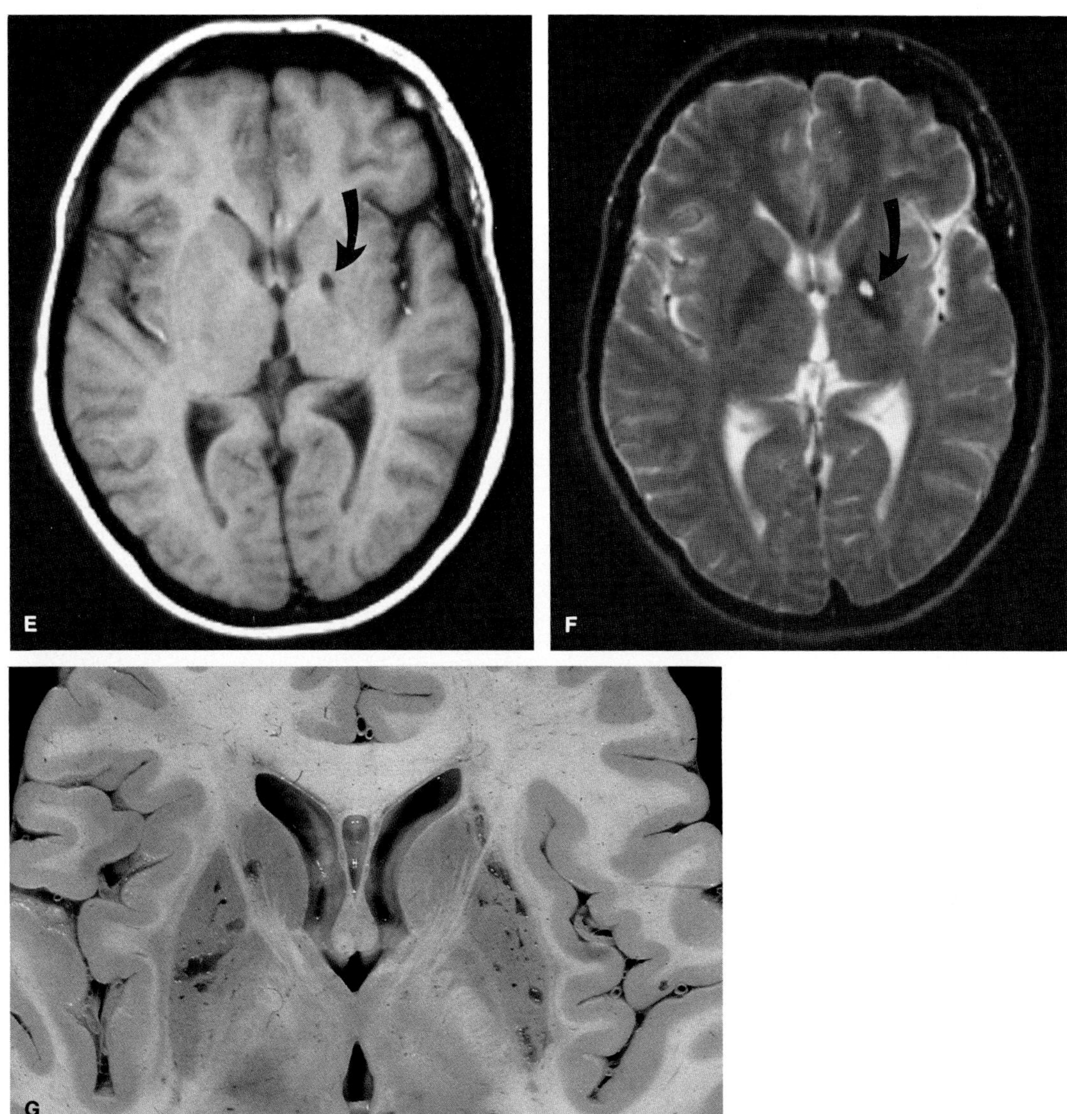

tense. No contrast enhancement was noted (*images not shown*).

DIAGNOSIS

Patient 1: Lacunar infarct, anterior limb of left internal capsule

Patient 2: Lacunar infarct, left caudate nucleus

Patient 3: Lacunar infarct, left globus pallidus

DISCUSSION

Lacunar infarcts are small, deep cerebral infarcts, most frequently seen in patients with hypertension. They result from occlusion of small penetrating branches that arise from the major cerebral arteries, including the middle and posterior cerebral arteries, the basilar artery, and the anterior cerebral and vertebral arteries. Lacunae most commonly involve the basal ganglia, internal capsule, thalamus, and brain stem.[1]

The following description details the vascular supply to the basal ganglia, internal capsule, and thalamus.[2–5]

CAUDATE NUCLEUS

- Recurrent artery of Heubner (arises from the A1 segment of the anterior cerebral artery) supplies the anterior and medial portions of the caudate nucleus.
- Lenticulostriate arteries (arise from the middle cerebral artery) supply the bulk (body and head) of the caudate nucleus.
- Lateral posterior choroidal artery (arises from the P2 segment or from various cortical posterior cerebral artery branches) perfuses a small portion of the caudate nucleus.

INTERNAL CAPSULE

- Recurrent artery of Heubner supplies the anteroinferior portion.
- Lenticulostriate arteries supply the anterior two thirds.
- Anterior choroidal artery (arises from the internal carotid artery just above the posterior communicating artery) supplies a large portion of the posterior limb.
- Thalamoperforating arteries (arise from the posterior cerebral artery) supply a portion of the posterior limb.

THALAMUS

Typically, four perforating branches (the premamillary, thalamoperforators, thalamogeniculate, and posterior choroidal arteries and cingulate branches) of the posterior cerebral artery supply the thalamus. However, the arterial supply to the thalamus is variable, as follows:

- Premamillary branches supply the anterior thalamus.
- Thalamoperforating arteries supply the medial ventral thalamus.
- Thalamogeniculate arteries supply the lateral ventral thalamus.
- Medial and lateral posterior choroidal arteries and cingulate branches supply the posterior and superior thalamus.
- Anterior choroidal artery supplies the lateral thalamus.

GLOBUS PALLIDUS

- Lenticulostriate arteries supply the lateral segment.
- Recurrent artery of Heubner supplies the anteroinferior portion.

PUTAMEN

- Lenticulostriate arteries supply the lateral segment.
- Recurrent artery of Heubner supplies the anteroinferior portion.

Pathologic Correlate

(*G*) Axial gross specimen shows multiple small, old, bilateral lacunar infarcts in the basal ganglia (primarily in the putamen and caudate nuclei).

Clinical References

1. Brown JJ, Hesselink JR, Rothrock JF. MR and CT of Lacunar infarcts. AJR 1988;151:367–372.
2. Osborn AG. Introduction to cerebral angiography. Philadelphia, Harper & Row, 1980:167–326.
3. Berman SA, Hayman LA, Hinck VC. Correlation of CT cerebral vascular territories with function. 1. Anterior cerebral artery. AJNR 1980;1:259–263.
4. Berman SA, Hayman LA, Hinck VC. Correlation of CT cerebral vascular territories with function. 3. Middle cerebral artery. AJR 1984;142:1035–1040.
5. Berman SA, Hayman LA, Hinck VC. Correlation of CT cerebral vascular territories with function. 2. Posterior cerebral artery. AJR 1981;137:13–19.

(G from Okazaki H, Scheithauer B. Slide atlas of neuropathology. New York, Gower Medical Publishing, 1988. By permission of Mayo Foundation.)

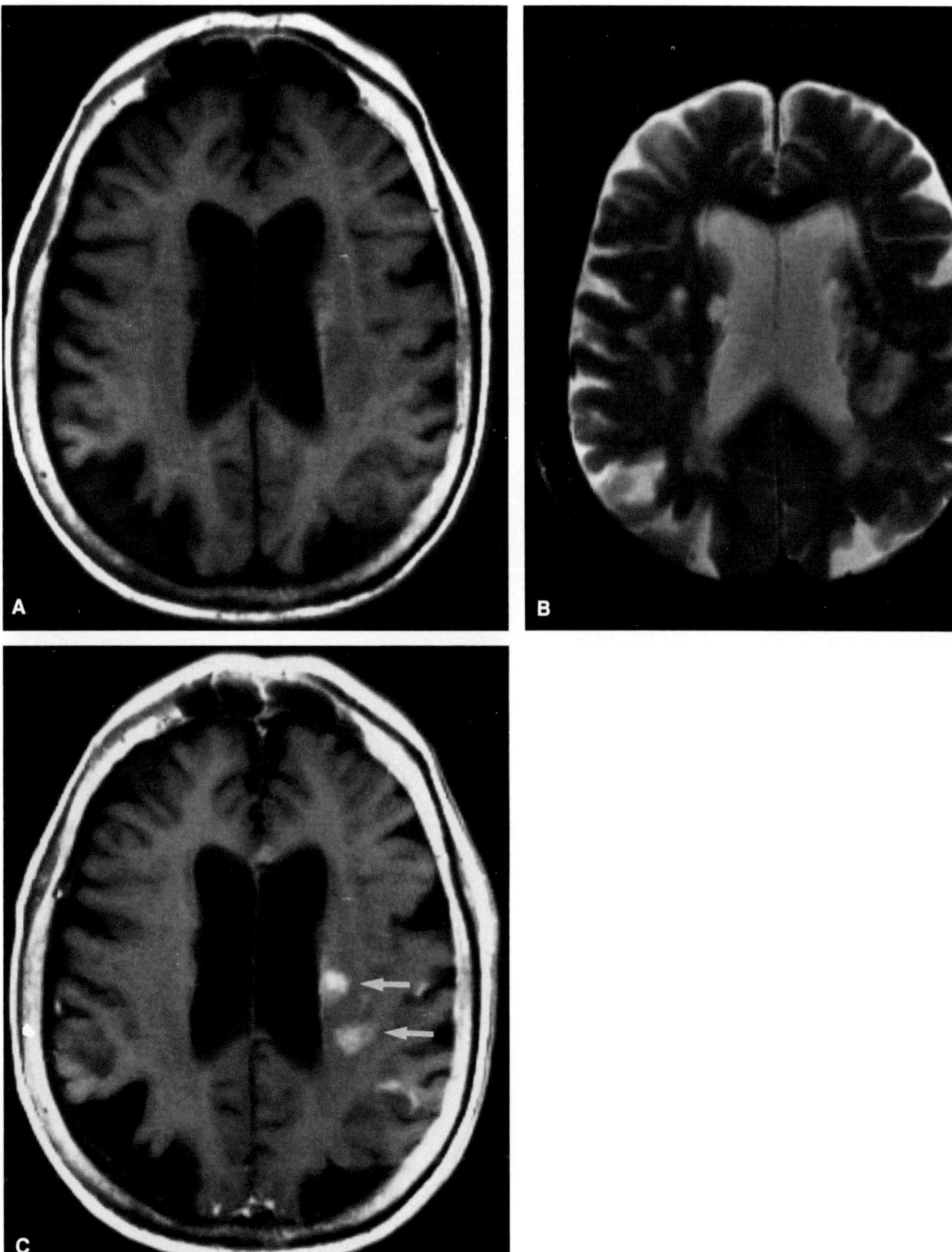

HISTORY

A 78-year-old with a 20-year history of hypertension and recent onset of right hemiparesis

FINDINGS

(*A*) The T1-weighted axial image demonstrates an old cavitated lacunar infarct in the right periventricular white matter, just posterior to the superior portion of the head of the caudate. There is also subtle low signal intensity in the white matter adjacent to the posterior body of the left lateral ventricle. (*B*) The heavily T2-weighted axial image shows multiple periventricular high-signal-intensity foci. (*C*) On the postcontrast T1-weighted axial image, two of the lesions enhance (*white arrows*), with more peripheral gyriformlike enhancement also noted.

DIAGNOSIS

Subacute infarction superimposed on chronic ischemic changes

DISCUSSION

High-signal-intensity foci, both punctate and confluent, are common on T2-weighted images in the periventricular and subcortical white matter of elderly patients. Most of these "lesions" are caused by chronic, low-grade vascular insufficiency and are usually asymptomatic. These "ischemic/gliotic" changes may occur in patients with no cardiovascular risks, but the incidence and severity are increased in patients with hypertension, diabetes mellitus, heart disease, or history of a completed stroke, all of which are associated with atherosclerotic vascular disease.[1]

Symptomatic lacunar infarcts of the brain stem, and deep cerebral gray and white matter may be superimposed on chronic ischemic/gliotic changes. The use of IV contrast material allows for distinction of subacute infarction from chronic ischemic/gliotic foci. Parenchymal enhancement of infarcts typically occurs from 3 days to 3 months postictus and is a reliable indicator of subacute age.[2] Intravascular and meningeal enhancement may be seen in the more acute stage.[2] Chronic lacunar infarcts may cavitate and have very low signal intensity on T1-weighted images.

Pitfalls in Image Interpretation

Multiple sclerosis (MS) with enhancing plaques may mimic subacute lacunar infarcts superimposed on chronic ischemic white matter changes. However, MS lesions have a predilection for specific areas of white matter, which aids in diagnosis. Furthermore, the patient populations are generally different, with MS seen most commonly in young women.

Clinical References

1. Braffman B, Zimmerman R, Trojanowski J, et al. Brain MR: pathologic correlation with gross and histopathology. 2. Hyperintense white-matter foci in the elderly. AJR 1988; 151:559–566.
2. Elster A. MR contrast enhancement in brainstem and deep cerebral infarction. AJR 1992;158:173–178.

(A to C from Runge VM. Clinical magnetic resonance imaging. Philadelphia, JB Lippincott, 1990.)

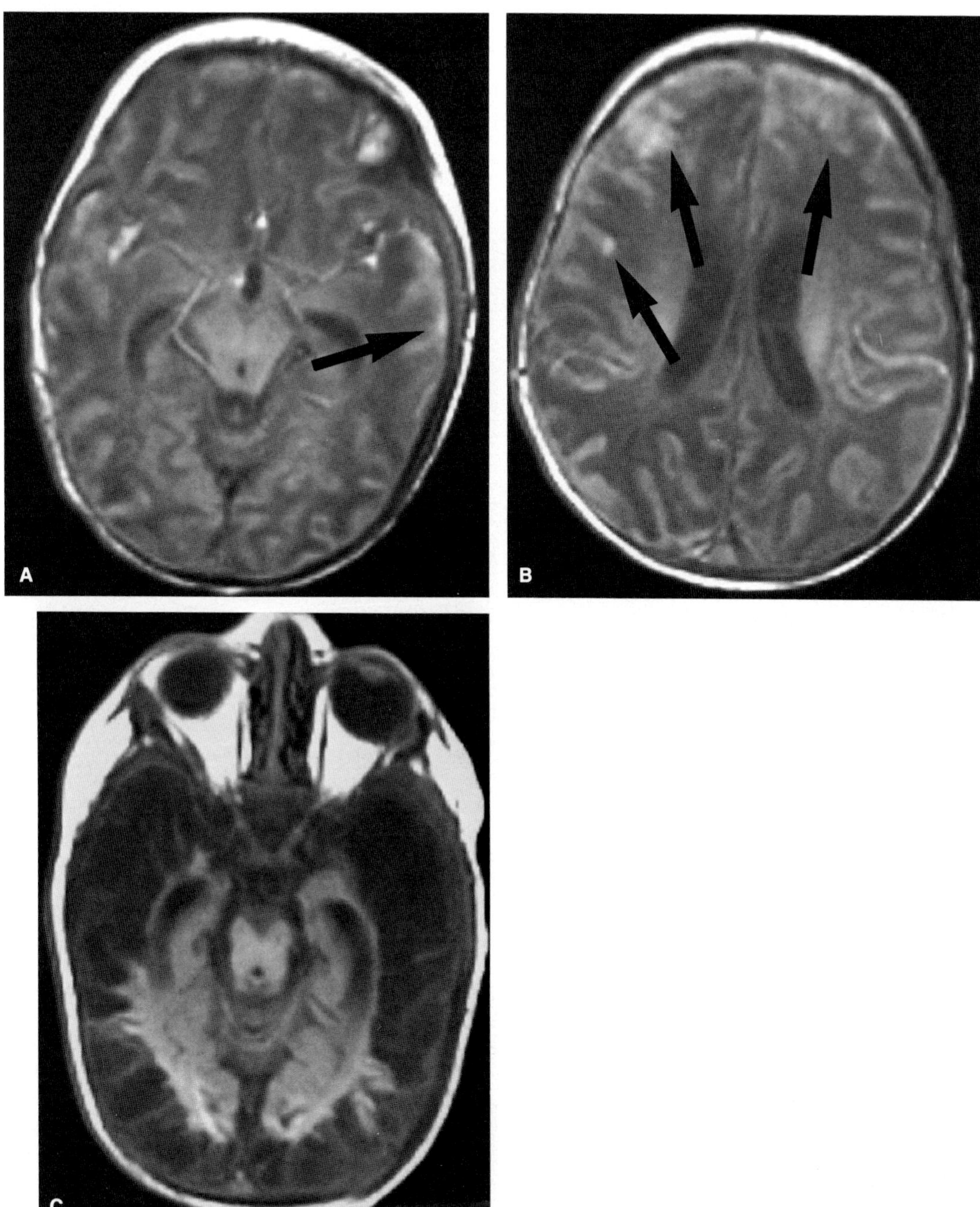

HISTORY

A neonate with possible hypoxic brain injury

FINDINGS

The first MR examination was obtained at 1 month of age, with T1-weighted images (*A and B*) at two anatomic levels presented for interpretation. The white matter is hypointense relative to gray matter, the normal pattern for young infants. However, the hypointensity of white matter is more marked than usual. Furthermore, the overlying mantel of cortical gray matter appears too thin. Multiple abnormal high-signal-intensity foci (*arrows*), consistent with methemoglobin, are also noted. T2-weighted scans (*not shown*) were grossly normal.

MR was repeated at 2 months of age, with T1-weighted (*C to E*) and T2-weighted (*F to H*) images presented from this examination. There is now global loss of cortical gray matter and underlying white matter, with residual cystic changes. Central gray matter and white matter are for the most part spared. Marked hypointensity (*curved arrow in H*) on the more superior T2-weighted

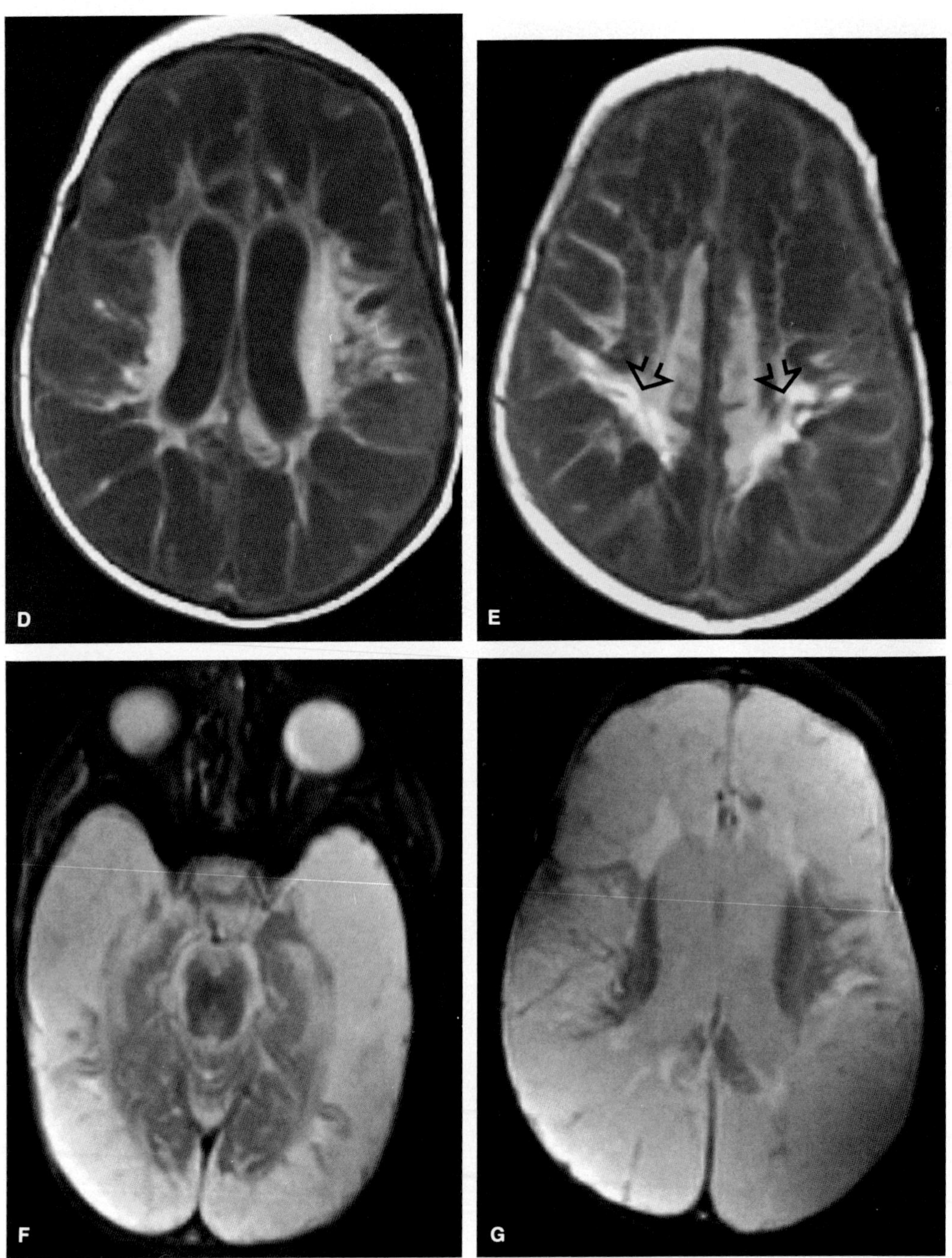

image is consistent with hemosiderin, the residual of previous hemorrhage. Abnormal hyperintensity (*open arrows in E*) on the T1-weighted examination is consistent with dystrophic calcification.

DIAGNOSIS

Global cerebral infarction in the neonate

DISCUSSION

In premature neonates, because of the high water content of white matter, ultrasonography can be more sensitive than CT or MR for detection of ischemic changes.[1] However, after about 37 weeks' gestational age, MR is superior. MR is more sensitive than CT or ultrasonography in the detection of hemorrhage. MR may also play an important role in the neonate with regard to predicting neurologic outcome, by its ability to depict myelination.

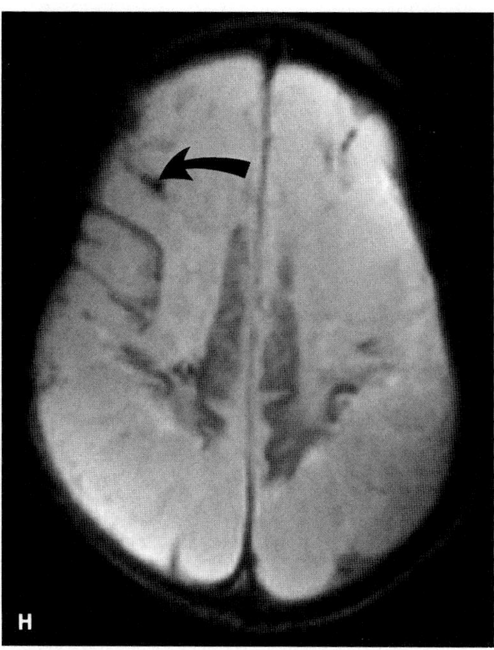

In the case presented, the first MR depicts global gray and white matter edema (due to ischemia), with accompanying petechial hemorrhage. By the time of the second examination, there has been severe loss of brain tissue with global cystic change.

MR Technique

Special attention to imaging technique is required in the neonate and infant because of increased brain water content. TE≥90 msec and TR≥3500 msec are recommended for T2-weighted SE scans, with TE≤10 msec and TR≤500 msec for T1-weighted SE scans. Inversion recovery scans can be used to provide greater T1 contrast.[2] T2-weighted fast spin echo (FSE) scans can be employed to provide increased lesion contrast and reduced motion artifact, as a result of the long TRs (5000 msec or longer) typically used and the short scan time (compared with conventional T2-weighted SE imaging).

Pitfalls in Image Interpretation

Infarction can be masked by the normal increased water content of the neonate's brain,[3] with edema and gliosis difficult to detect. If ischemia is global, as in the case presented, detection may be even more difficult, because of the symmetry of disease involvement. T1-weighted images can be particularly valuable, with changes less evident on T2-weighted images.

Clinical References

1. McArdle CB, Richardson CJ, Hayden CK, et al. Abnormalities of the neonatal brain: MR imaging. Part II. Hypoxic-ischemic brain injury. Radiology 1987;163:395–403.
2. Johnson MA, Pennock JM, Bydder GM, et al. Serial MR imaging in neonatal cerebral injury. AJNR 1987;8:83–92.
3. Moore JB, Parker CP, Smith RJ, Goethe BD. Concealment of neonatal cerebral infarction on MRI by normal brain water. Pediatr Radiol 1987;17:314–315.

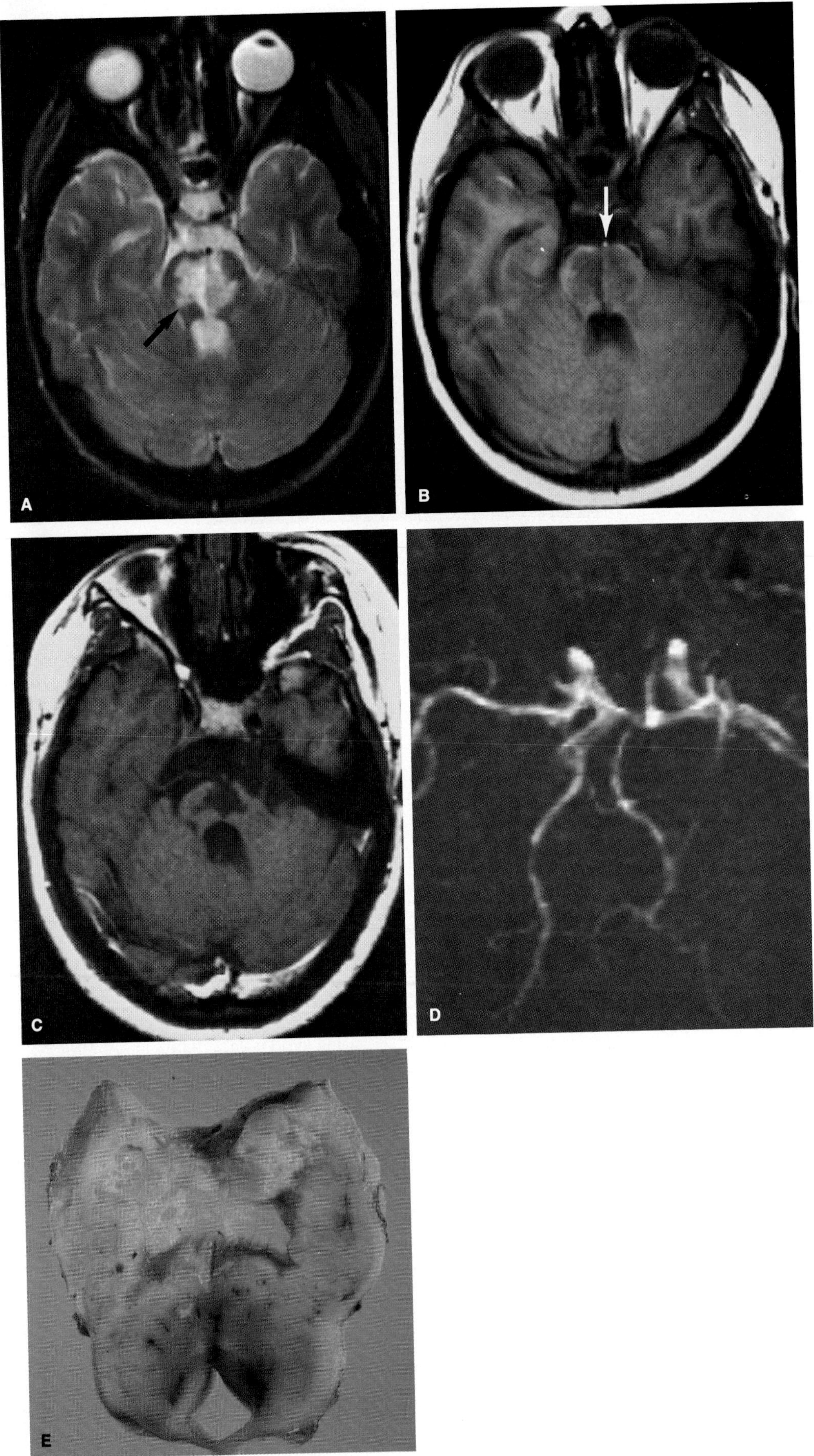
A
B
C
D
E

HISTORY

An 11-year-old with headache, vomiting, and dizziness

FINDINGS

(*A*) Axial T2-weighted image reveals a high-signal-intensity lesion (*arrow*) centrally in the pons. (*B*) The lesion is of low signal intensity on the axial T1-weighted image. No abnormal contrast enhancement was noted (*images not shown*). Increased signal intensity is identified in the basilar artery (*white arrow in B*), indicating either slow flow or occlusion. (*C*) The follow-up study performed 6 months later demonstrates a smaller, now cavitated, lesion on T1-weighted imaging. (*D*) No flow is identified in the basilar artery on MRA, confirming occlusion.

DIAGNOSIS

Bilateral pontine infarction

DISCUSSION

Infarcts of the brain stem that involve tissue both to the right and left of midline are relatively uncommon. When they do occur, they most frequently involve the mesencephalon (midbrain). Such infarcts result from occlusion of the thalamoperforate arteries, which originate from the tip of the basilar artery, and from adjacent interpeduncular precommunicating segments of the posterior cerebral arteries.[1]

The MR criteria used to diagnose thrombosis of the basilar artery include the presence of an isointense structure (corresponding to the course of the basilar artery) in the prepontine cistern on T1-weighted images, and the lack of a normal flow void on T2-weighted images.[2] However, MRA and other specific flow techniques are more accurate for documentation of vessel occlusion.

Pitfalls in Image Interpretation

The differential diagnosis for a large central pontine lesion with high signal intensity on T2-weighted images includes central pontine myelinolysis, which tends to be more symmetric in appearance than pontine infarction.

Pathologic Correlate

(*E*) Cut gross section in a different patient demonstrates a chronic cavitated bilateral infarct of the pons.

Clinical References

1. Savoiardo M, Bracchi M, Passerini A, et al. The vascular territories in the cerebellum and brainstem: CT and MR study. AJNR 1987;8:199–209.
2. Knepper L, Biller J, Adams HP, et al. MR imaging of basilar artery occlusion. J Comput Assist Tomogr 1990;14:32–35.

(E *courtesy of Daron G. Davis.*)

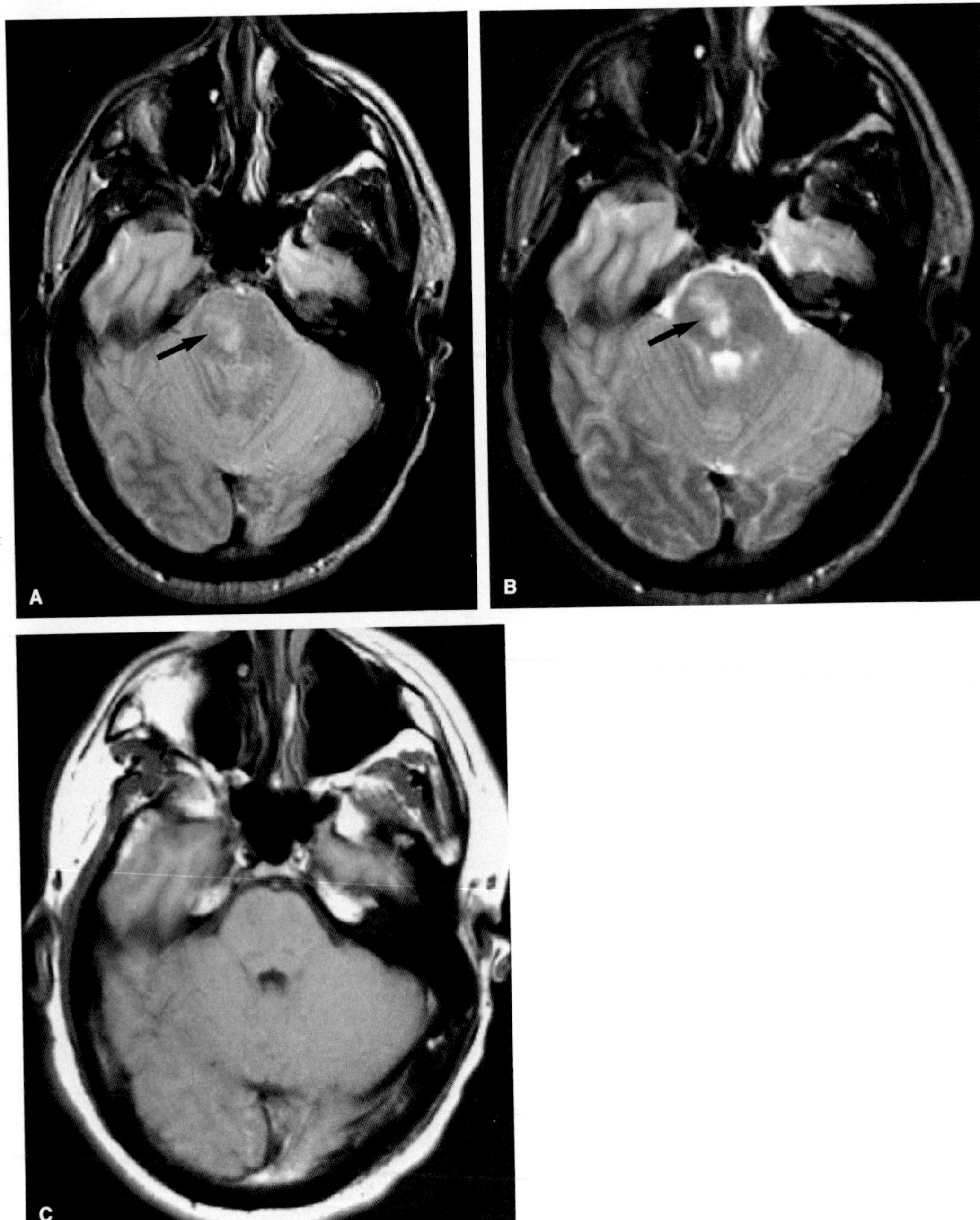
A
B
C

HISTORY

A 20-year-old man with left-sided lower and upper extremity weakness and decreased coordination

FINDINGS

First (*A*) and second (*B*) echoes of the axial T2-weighted scan reveal an irregular lesion (*arrows*) of increased signal intensity in the right pons that is sharply marginated at the midline. (*C*) The lesion is difficult to visualize on the corresponding axial T1-weighted image. No abnormal contrast enhancement was noted (*images not shown*).

DIAGNOSIS

Unilateral pontine infarction

DISCUSSION

The brain stem is supplied by penetrating vessels that arise from the basilar artery.[1] These vessels are divided into paramedian, lateral, and dorsal branches, based on their place of entry and the territory supplied. Infarcts involving the pons are most frequently small, unilateral, and sharply marginated at the midline. This location reflects the distribution of the paramedian penetrating arteries, which are paired branches of the basilar and distal vertebral arteries. Lateral pontine infarcts (in contrast to paramedian infarcts) are uncommon and occur in the distribution of the short circumferential arteries that penetrate the brain stem laterally.[2] A true dorsal vascular territory does not exist in the pons, as it does in the medulla.

MR Technique

Thin-section axial and sagittal imaging is suggested for improved detection and depiction of small infarcts in the brain stem.

Clinical References

1. Savoiardo M, Bracchi M, Passerini A, et al. The vascular territories in the cerebellum and brainstem: CT and MR study. AJNR 1987;8:199–209.
2. Knepper L, Biller J, Adams HP, et al. MR imaging of the basilar artery occlusion. J Comput Assist Tomogr 1990; 14:32–35.

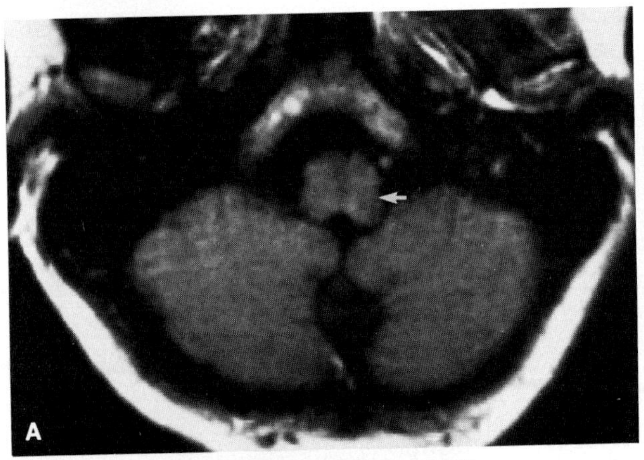
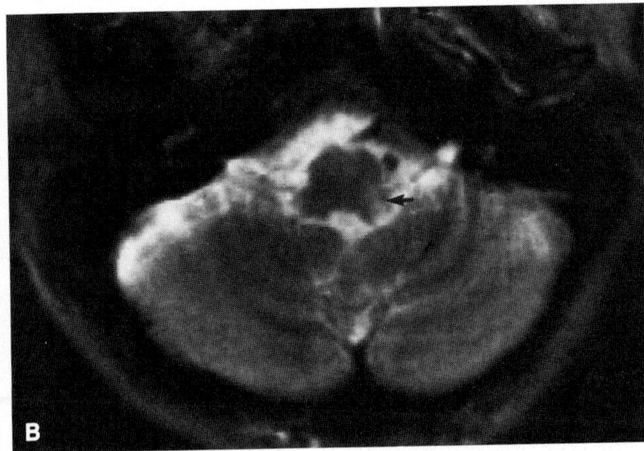
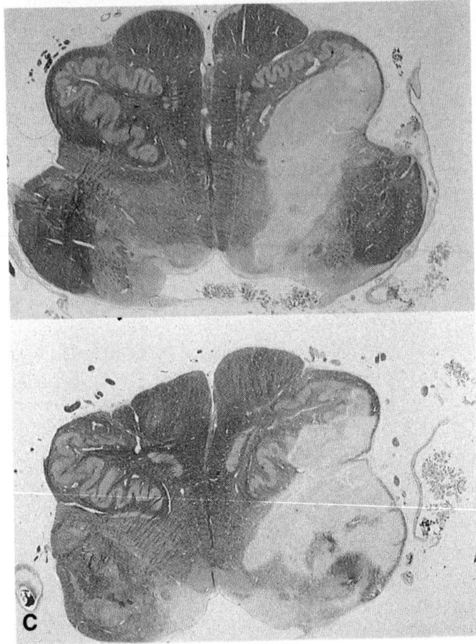

HISTORY

A 55-year-old with acute loss of pain and thermal sense over the right side of the body and Horner's syndrome on the left side

FINDINGS

(*A*) On the axial T1-weighted scan, there is abnormal hypointensity in the left lateral medulla (*white arrow*). (*B*) The T2-weighted (TR/TE = 3000/90) scan reveals abnormal hyperintensity (*black arrow*) in the same region. On cerebral angiography (*not shown*), there was occlusion of the left posteroinferior cerebellar artery.

DIAGNOSIS

Lateral medullary infarction

DISCUSSION

In lateral medullary infarction (Wallenberg's syndrome), clinical features include dysarthria, dysphagia, vertigo, nystagmus, ipsilateral Horner's syndrome (ptosis, miosis, and anhidrosis), and contralateral loss of pain and temperature sense (over the body). In the acute phase following lateral medullary infarction, respiratory and cardiovascular complications, presumably related to autonomic dysfunction, are major hazards.[1] Recurrent strokes are uncommon. Vessel occlusion is usually due to atherosclerosis (thrombus), with embolic occlusion uncommon. Vertebrobasilar artery distribution infarction, and specifically lateral medullary infarction, has been reported in otherwise healthy young individuals following chiropractic neck manipulation. Such manipulation can cause dissection of the vertebral artery near the atlantoaxial joint.[2]

In medial medullary infarction, there is characteristically contralateral hemiparesis (sparing the face), accompanied in some patients by contralateral disturbance of deep sensation and ipsilateral hypoglossal nerve palsy. In patients with an atypical presentation, MR is critical for diagnosis and also provides prognostic information.[3] Infarction involving the upper one third of the medulla is typically due to occlusion of the vertebral artery or its branches and carries a good prognosis. Infarction involving the lower two thirds is caused by occlusion of the anterior spinal artery or its branches, and carries a poor prognosis.

Not surprisingly, MR is markedly more sensitive than CT for the detection of medullary infarction. Coexisting cerebellar infarction may also be visualized by MR, and go undetected by CT.[4]

MR Technique

Acquisition of thin-section (3 mm or less), motion artifact–free, axial T2-weighted images is critical for detection of infarction involving the medulla.

Pitfalls in Image Interpretation

Plaques in multiple sclerosis not uncommonly involve the medulla and may mimic the appearance of ischemic disease on MR sections at this level, although the presence of characteristic abnormalities elsewhere typically permits differentiation.

Pathologic Correlate

(*C*) Gross pathologic section of a lateral medullary infarction. The extent of this lesion, which typically results from occlusion of the vertebral artery proximal to the origin of the posteroinferior cerebellar artery, can vary substantially from case to case.

Clinical References

1. Norrving B, Cronqvist S. Lateral medullary infarction: prognosis in an unselected series. Neurology 1991;41:244–248.
2. Frumkin LR, Baloh RW. Wallenberg's syndrome following neck manipulation. Neurology 1990;40:611–615.
3. Sawada H, Seriu N, Udaka F, Kameyama M. Magnetic resonance imaging of medial medullary infarction. Stroke 1990;21:963–966.
4. Ross MA, Biller J, Adams HP, Dunn V. Magnetic resonance imaging in Wallenberg's lateral medullary syndrome. Stroke 1986;17:542–545.

*(*A *and* B *from Runge VM. Clinical magnetic resonance imaging. Philadelphia, JB Lippincott, 1990;* C *from Okazaki H, Scheithauer B. Slide atlas of neuropathology. New York, Gower Medical Publishing, 1988. By permission of Mayo Foundation.)*

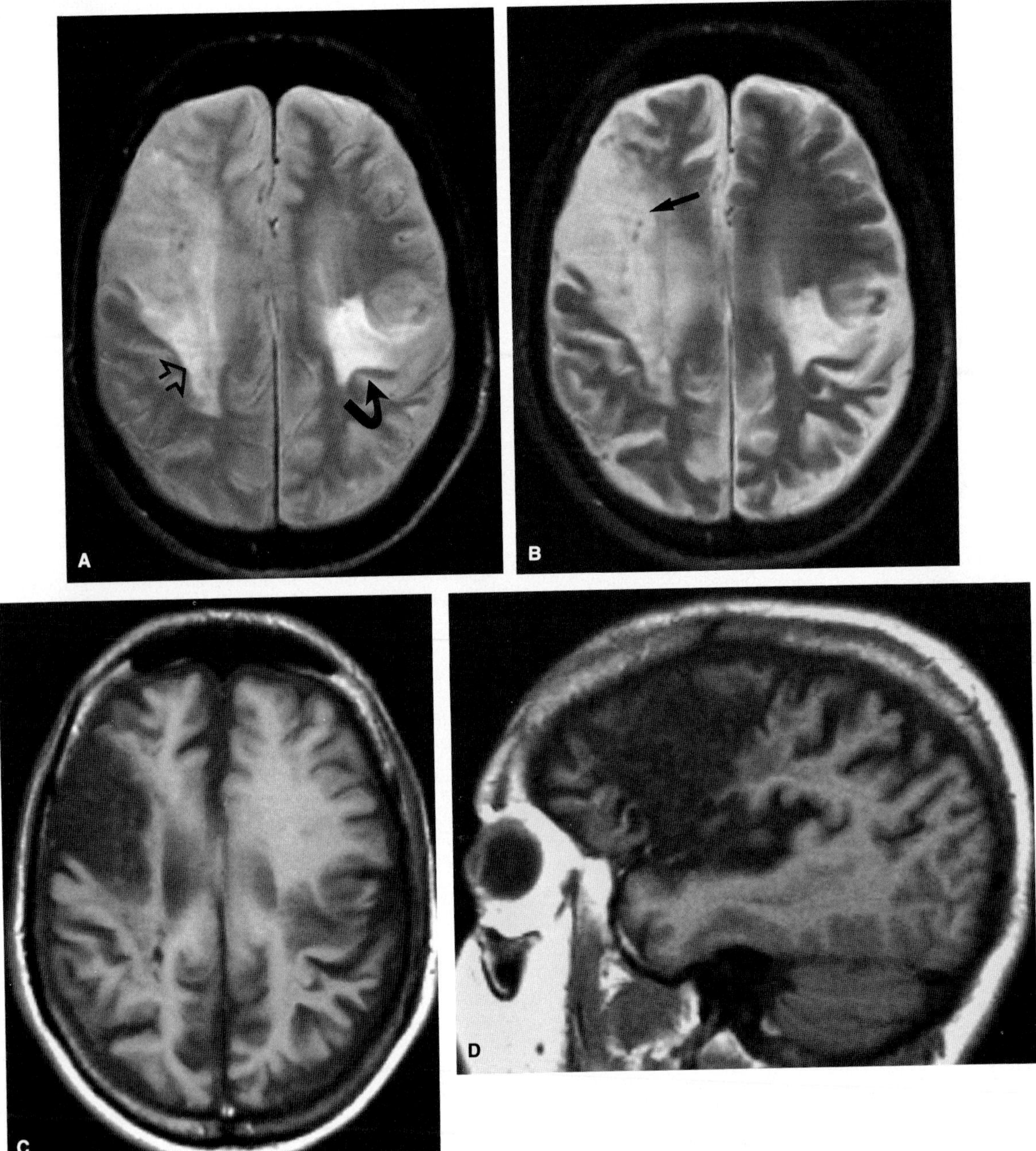
A
B
C
D

HISTORY

A 41-year-old IV drug abuser

FINDINGS

First (TE = 45 msec) (*A*) and second (TE = 90 msec) (*B*) echoes of the T2-weighted study reveal cystic encephalomalacia (*arrow in B*), with surrounding gliosis (*open arrow in A*), in the vascular territory of the anterior division of the right middle cerebral artery and gliosis (*curved arrow in A*) in the vascular territory of the posterior division of the left middle cerebral artery. (*C*) The corresponding precontrast T1-weighted image demonstrates mild generalized cerebral atrophy with an increase in size of the cortical sulci bilaterally. (*D*) An off-midline precontrast sagittal T1-weighted image shows cerebral atrophy, enlargement of the sylvian fissure, and cystic changes in the right hemisphere. No abnormal contrast enhancement was noted (*images not shown*).

DIAGNOSIS

Bilateral middle cerebral artery infraction (chronic), complication of drug abuse

DISCUSSION

Cerebral infarction is a known complication of the ingestion or abuse of certain drugs. Anticoagulants, oral contraceptives, ergot alkaloids, cocaine, amphetamines, phenylpropanolamine, and xanthines have all been implicated.[1] Hemorrhagic and ischemic infarcts occur.[2] Both cocaine and amphetamines can cause sympathetically mediated vasoconstriction or vasculitis. Amphetamines are a frequent contaminant of illegally obtained cocaine, with the two agents demonstrated to have a synergistic vasoconstrictive effect.[3] Both can also cause transient arterial hypertension.

MR Technique

In cerebrovascular disease, T1-weighted images provide an assessment of cerebral and cerebellar atrophy. T2-weighted images provide sensitivity to edema and gliosis. Both techniques demonstrate cystic change well. Mildly T2-weighted images best differentiate cystic changes from either gliosis or edema.

Clinical References

1. Uldry PA, Regli F. Cerebrovascular accidents in relation to drug consumption or drug abuse. Schweiz Rundsch Med Prax 1989;78:663–666.
2. Diez-Tejedor E, Tejada J, Frank A. Neurologic complications caused by use of cocaine, amphetamines and sympathomimetics. Arch Neurobiol (suppl) 1989;1:162–182.
3. Wang AM, Suojanen JN, Colucci VM, et al. Cocaine- and methamphetamine-induced acute cerebral vasospasm: an angiographic study in rabbits. AJNR 1990;11:1141–1146.

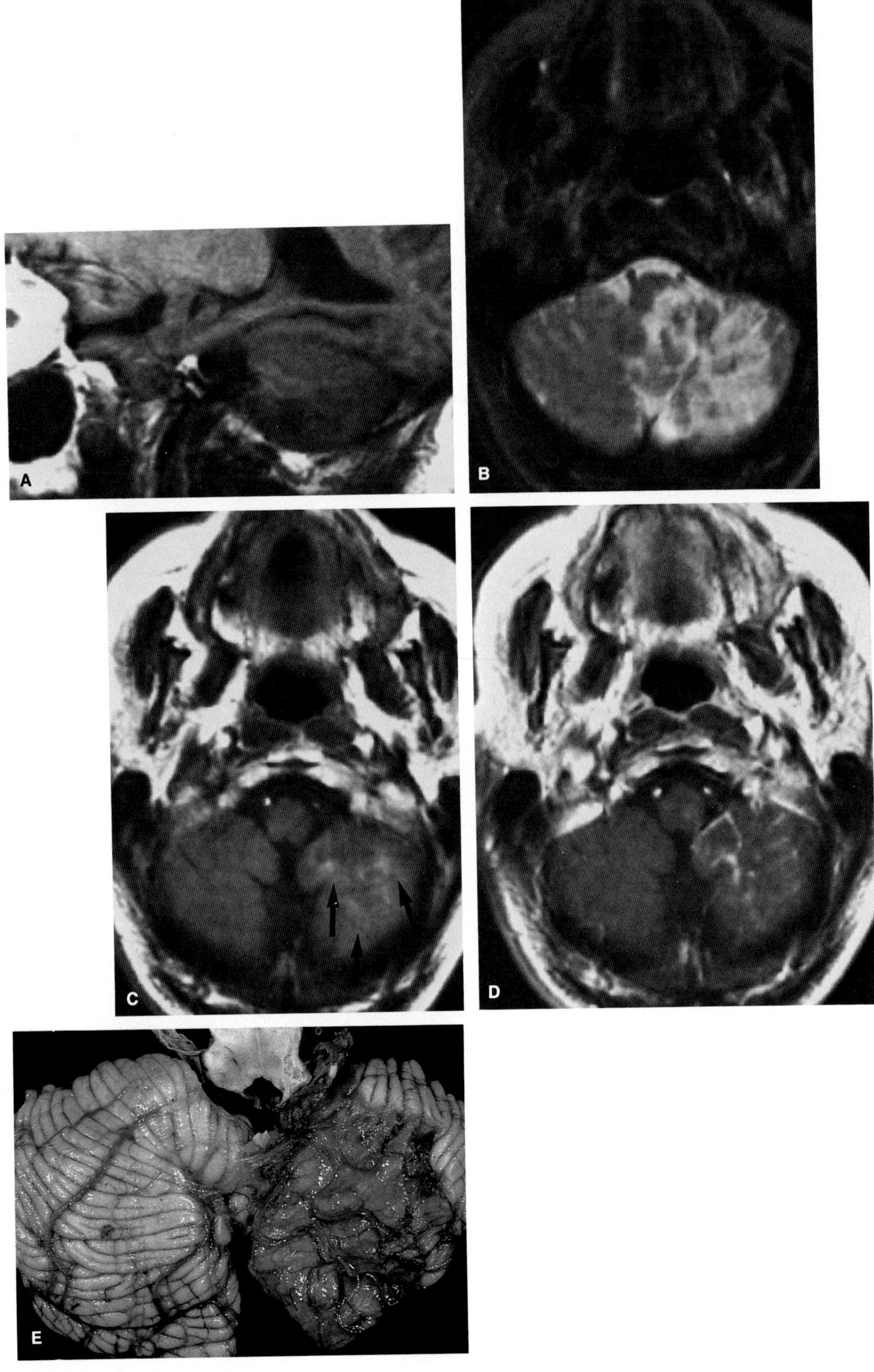
A
B
C
D
E

HISTORY

A 74-year-old man with sudden onset of nausea, vomiting, and dizziness, 6 days before the MR examination

FINDINGS

(*A*) Sagittal T1-weighted image depicts a lesion of decreased signal intensity in the left inferior cerebellum. (*B*) This lesion is of increased signal intensity on the axial T2-weighted image. (*C*) Numerous foci of slightly increased signal intensity (*arrows*) are identified within the lesion on the axial T1-weighted image (presumably corresponding to methemoglobin). (*D*) Axial postcontrast T1-weighted image shows areas of predominantly curvilinear enhancement.

DIAGNOSIS

Subacute hemorrhagic posteroinferior cerebellar artery (PICA) infarction

DISCUSSION

The PICA arises from the distal vertebral artery and supplies the retroolivary portion of the medulla, the ipsilateral inferior vermis, cerebellar tonsil, and the inferior lateral posterior surface of the cerebellar hemisphere. There is some overlap of vascular territories with the anterior inferior cerebellar artery (AICA).[1]

The PICA is variable in its route and site of origin. The PICA and AICA are in equilibrium with one another; the larger the PICA territory, the smaller the AICA territory, and the smaller the PICA territory, the larger the AICA territory.

The lateral medullary syndrome is sometimes seen in patients with PICA infarctions. The short circumferential medullary arteries supplying the lateral medulla usually arise from the distal vertebral artery, but can originate from the PICA or the AICA. The most frequent cause of a PICA infarct is thrombosis of the vertebral artery.

MR Technique

Sagittal images best delineate the vascular territory of the PICA in the inferior cerebellum.

Pathologic Correlate

(*E*) Gross specimen viewed from below shows an extensive chronic infarct in the vascular distribution of the PICA. In many cases, such lesions are not recognized clinically, with demonstration only in the chronic state at autopsy. Infarction of the ventral aspect of the cerebellar hemisphere (PICA territory) is accompanied in this case by infarction of the lateral medullary region. Thus, the involved vessel would have been either the vertebral artery proximal to the PICA or the proximal portion of the PICA.

Clinical References

1. Savoiardo M, Bracchi M, Passerini A, et al. The vascular territories in the cerebellum and brainstem: CT and MR study. AJNR 1987;8:199–209.

(E *from Okazaki H, Scheithauer B. Slide atlas of neuropathology. New York, Gower Medical Publishing, 1988. By permission of Mayo Foundation.)*

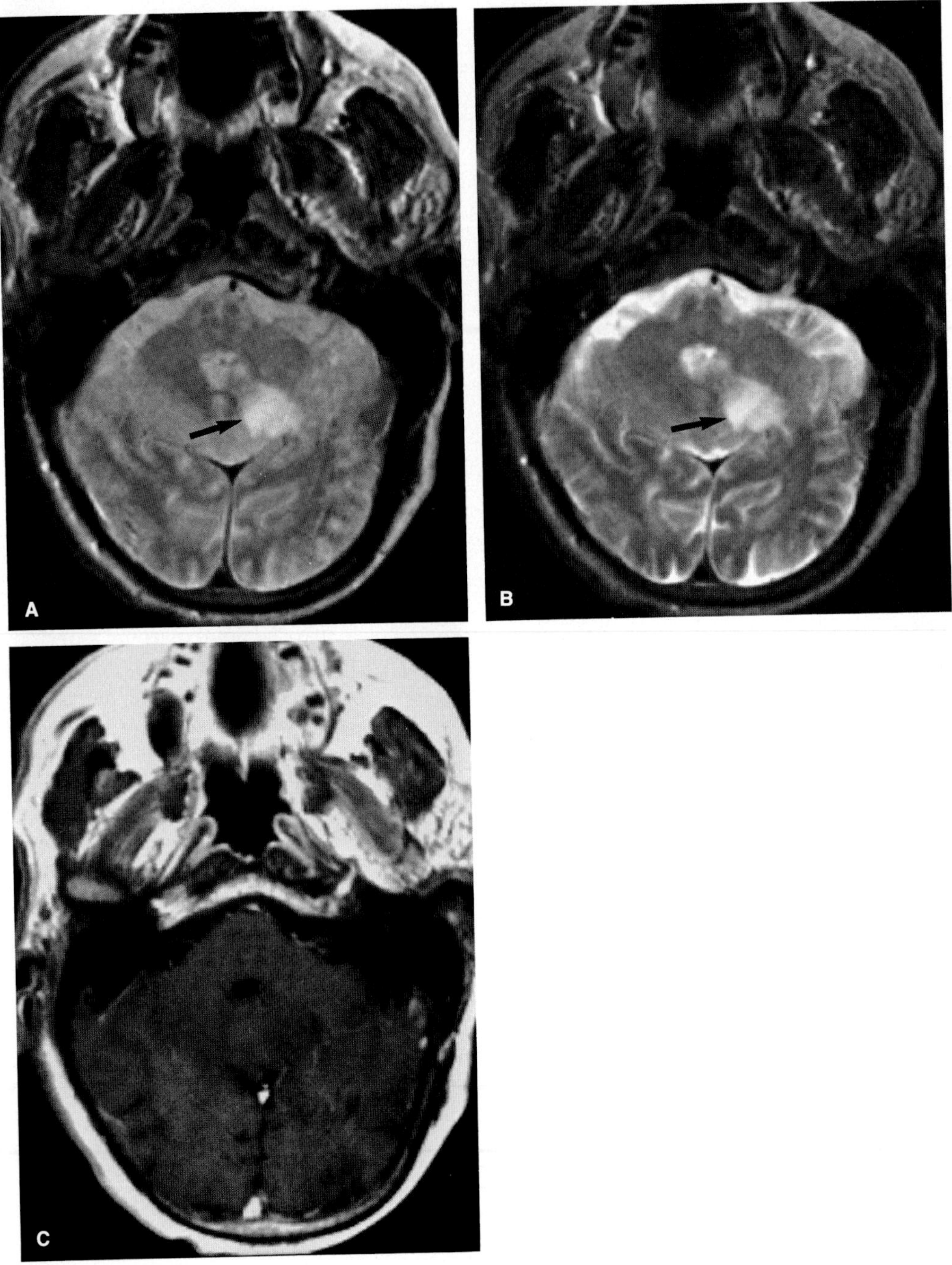

HISTORY

A 70-year-old man presents 1 day before MR examination with sudden onset of severe headache, followed by vertigo, nausea, and vomiting, all of which occurred in conjunction with a 15-minute loss of upper and lower extremity limb control

FINDINGS

Intermediate (*A*) and heavily (*B*) T2-weighted images demonstrate a wedge-shaped region of abnormal high signal intensity (*arrow*) in the left superior cerebellum. There is slight mass effect on the fourth ventricle. (*C*) On the postcontrast T1-weighted image, there is no abnormal enhancement and the lesion is poorly demonstrated, being just slightly lower in signal intensity than adjacent normal cerebellar tissue.

DIAGNOSIS

Acute left superior cerebellar artery infarction

DISCUSSION

MR is the modality of choice for visualization of brain infarction, with T2-weighted images demonstrating high signal intensity in ischemic tissue within several hours of ictus.[1] Within the first 48 hours, x-ray CT may be normal. The superiority of MR becomes even more pronounced in the examination of posterior fossa disease, as seen in this case.

Transient ischemic attacks in the proximal basilar distribution can produce dizziness (lightheadedness). Occlusion of the superior cerebellar artery with subsequent infarction can cause ipsilateral cerebellar ataxia (loss of muscular coordination), nausea and vomiting, dysarthria (difficulty in articulation), and contralateral loss of pain and temperature sensation. The superior cerebellar artery supplies the superior aspect of the cerebellum, the pons, and the pineal body.

Pitfalls in Image Interpretation

At high field strengths, vascular pulsation artifacts can be quite prominent in the posterior fossa and should not be confused with pathology. This is not a problem in the present case because of lesion size.

Clinical References

1. Bryan RN. Imaging of acute stroke. Radiology 1990; 177:615–616.

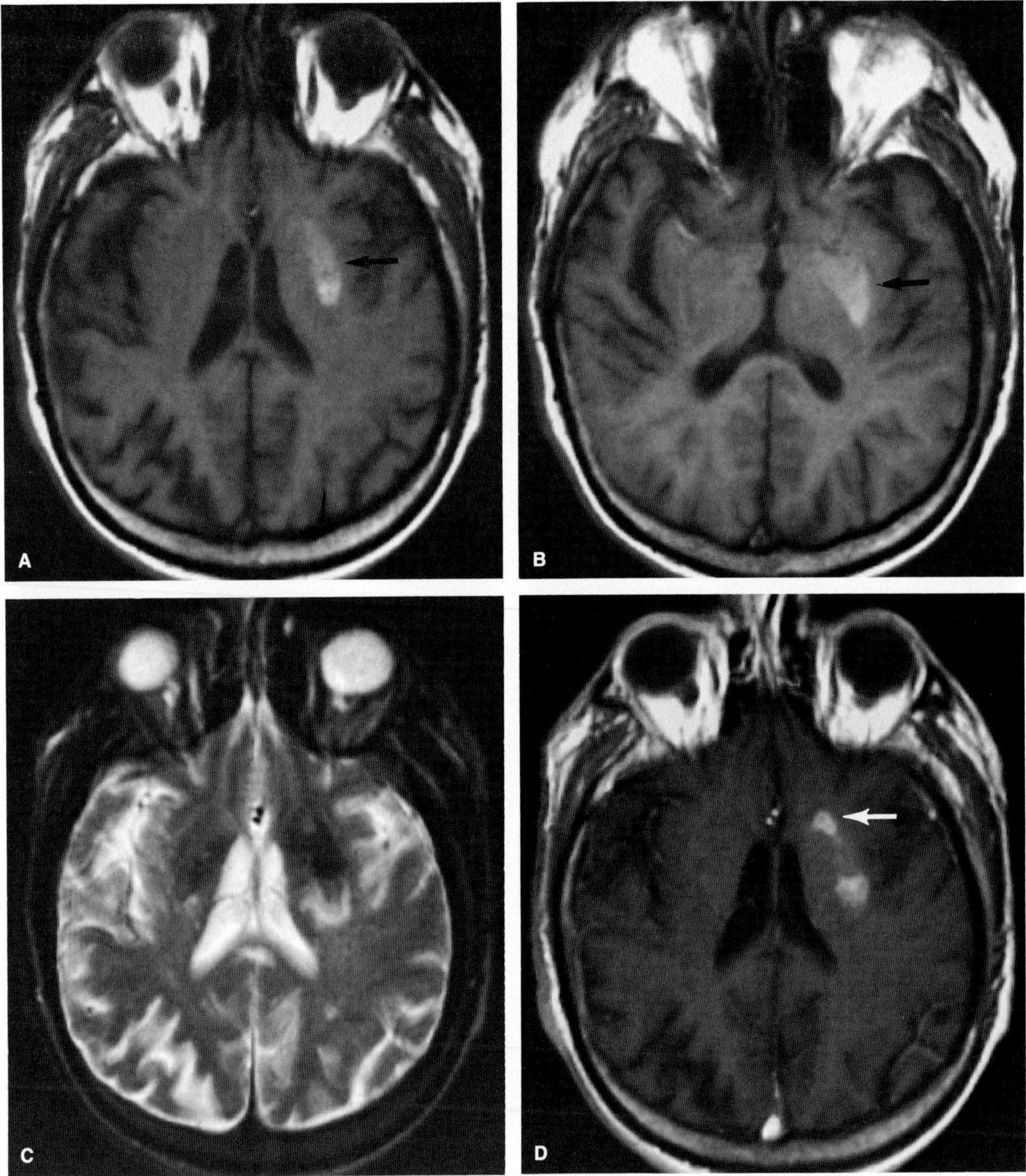

HISTORY

A 65-year-old man with a history of hypertension, diabetes mellitus, atrial fibrillation, and coronary artery disease who presented acutely 1 week earlier with confusion and right-sided extremity weakness

FINDINGS

(*A and B*) Axial precontrast T1-weighted images identify increased signal intensity (*black arrows*) in the left putamen and lateral globus pallidus. (*C*) This lesion is principally of decreased signal intensity on the axial T2-weighted image (corresponding to intracellular methemoglobin). On axial (*D*) and coronal (*E*) T1-weighted postcontrast images, abnormal enhancement (*white arrows*) is present in the left caudate nucleus.

DIAGNOSIS

Subacute left caudate infarction
Subacute left lentiform nucleus infarction with petechial hemorrhage

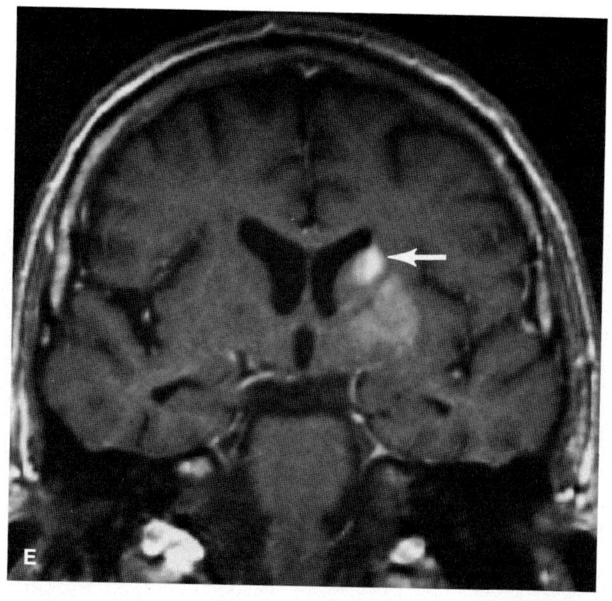

DISCUSSION

The recurrent artery of Heubner and the lenticulostriate arteries perfuse the caudate, globus pallidus, and putamen. This vascular distribution explains the infrequent occurrence of ischemic events in only one of these basal ganglia without involvement of the others.[1,2]

One cause of increased signal intensity on precontrast T1-weighted images in the basal ganglia is the presence of methemoglobin. Intracellular methemoglobin is of increased signal intensity on T1-weighted images and decreased signal intensity on T2-weighted images. The decreased signal intensity on the T2-weighted sequences is secondary to the inhomogeneous distribution of paramagnetic methemoglobin within red blood cells. This inhomogeneous distribution leads to a large magnetic susceptibility effect resulting in shortening of the T2 relaxation time.[3]

The presence of methemoglobin 1 week after the ischemic event is consistent with the usual 3- to 4-day time course of oxidation of deoxyhemoglobin to methemoglobin. These lesions probably represent petechial hemorrhagic infarcts rather than true hematomas. Methemoglobin can at times be seen earlier than 3 to 4 days after an ischemic insult. This rapid formation of methemoglobin in ischemic sites can be explained by the exposure of oxyhemoglobin and deoxyhemoglobin to free radicals in the ischemic site. Free radicals accelerate the oxidation of hemoglobin to methemoglobin. Ischemic areas with reperfusion have been experimentally shown to have increased free radical concentration.[4,5]

Clinical References

1. Berman SA, Hayman LA, Hinck VC. Correlation of CT cerebral vascular territories with function. 1. Anterior cerebral artery. AJNR 1980;1:259–263.
2. Berman SA, Hayman LA, Hinck VC. Correlation of CT cerebral vascular territories with function. 3. Middle cerebral artery. AJR 1984;142:1035–1040.
3. Brooks RA, Di Chiro G, Patromas N. MR imaging of cerebral hematomas at different field strengths: theory and applications. J Comput Assist Tomogr 1989;13:194–206.
4. Atlas SW. Magnetic resonance imaging of the brain and spine. New York, Raven Press, 1991:420.
5. Moon KL Jr, Brant-Zawadzki M, Pitts LH, et al. Nuclear magnetic resonance imaging of CT-isodense subdural hematomas. AJNR 1984;5:319–322.

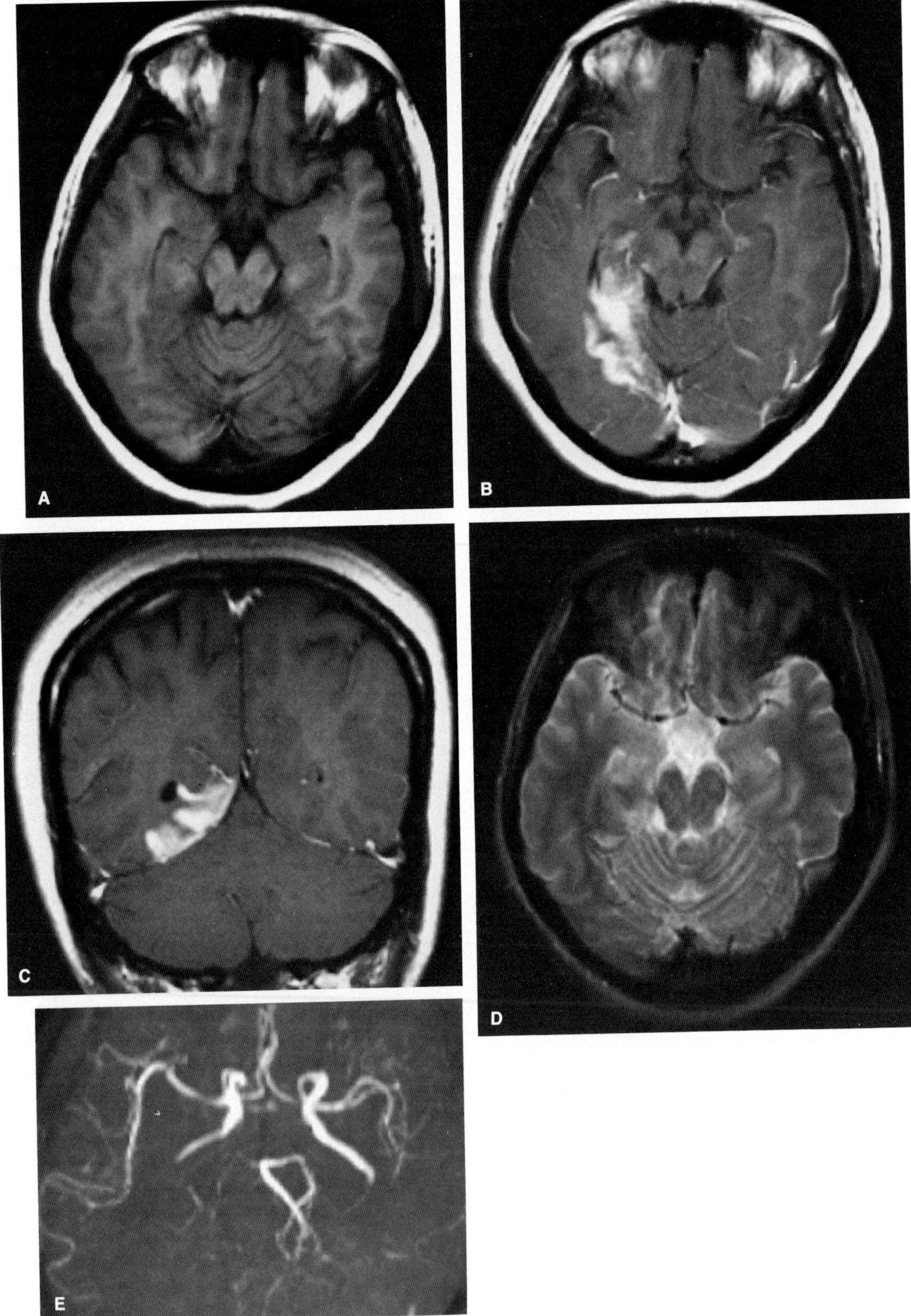
A
B
C
D
E

HISTORY

A 44-year-old woman with a severe headache 19 days before the current examination

FINDINGS

(*A*) The axial precontrast T1-weighted image is essentially normal. Axial (*B*) and coronal (*C*) postcontrast T1-weighted images demonstrate gyriform enhancement in the right temporal and occipital lobes, in the distribution of the posterior cerebral artery. (*D*) On the axial precontrast T2-weighted image only a subtle signal abnormality is identified in this vessel distribution. (*E*) MRA reveals a normal left posterior cerebral artery. The right posterior cerebral artery is not seen and is presumably occluded.

DIAGNOSIS

Subacute right posterior cerebral artery infarction

DISCUSSION

The ability of MR to detect parenchymal abnormalities in ischemic stroke depends on anatomic distortion (best seen on T1-weighted images) or signal abnormalities (best seen on T2-weighted images). The first type of edema seen in cerebral infarction is cytotoxic edema. In this state, there is a shift of water from an extracellular to intracellular location. The overall water content is unchanged and thus no gross signal abnormalities are noted on T2-weighted scans. The abnormal high signal intensity seen in acute to subacute cerebral infarction on T2-weighted images is secondary to the onset of vasogenic edema, which develops subsequently. Before the development of vasogenic edema, there may be insufficient change in water content to produce signal intensity changes,[1] as just noted. There have also been a few reported cases of isointense subacute infarction. Gyriform enhancement of subacute infarcts is well documented and can be used for lesion identification in this instance.

Three-dimensional TOF MRA is a common clinically used MRA technique. When projection images are desired, a maximum intensity projection (MIP) algorithm can be used. Several artifacts can occur with the use of MIP. The most common observed distortion is an apparent reduction in vessel width. The edges of a vessel are less intense than its center, and these regions can be obscured by background fluctuations resulting in a vessel appearing narrower on MIP images than it actually is. The pixel intensities are less at the edge of a vessel secondary to both slower laminar flow along vessel walls and partial volume averaging of the marginal pixels with the lower intensity background. Local differences in blood-flow streamline patterns such as stagnant blood flow along one edge of a vessel also allow blood to become saturated and thus appear dark.

When a vessel is smaller than the size of a pixel, the vessel may disappear altogether. This is the primary reason for the frequent nonvisualization of the posterior communicating artery on MIP projections. Overestimation of the degree of vascular stenosis can also occur. Flow turbulence leads to decreased signal intensity and can also result in overestimation of vascular stenosis.[2]

Clinical References

1. Crain MR, Yuh WTC, Greene GM, et al. Cerebral ischemia: evaluation with contrast-enhanced MR imaging. AJR 1991; 157:575–583.
2. Anderson CM, Saloner D, Tsuruda JS, et al. Artifacts in maximum-intensity-projection display of MR angiograms. AJR 1990;154:623–629.

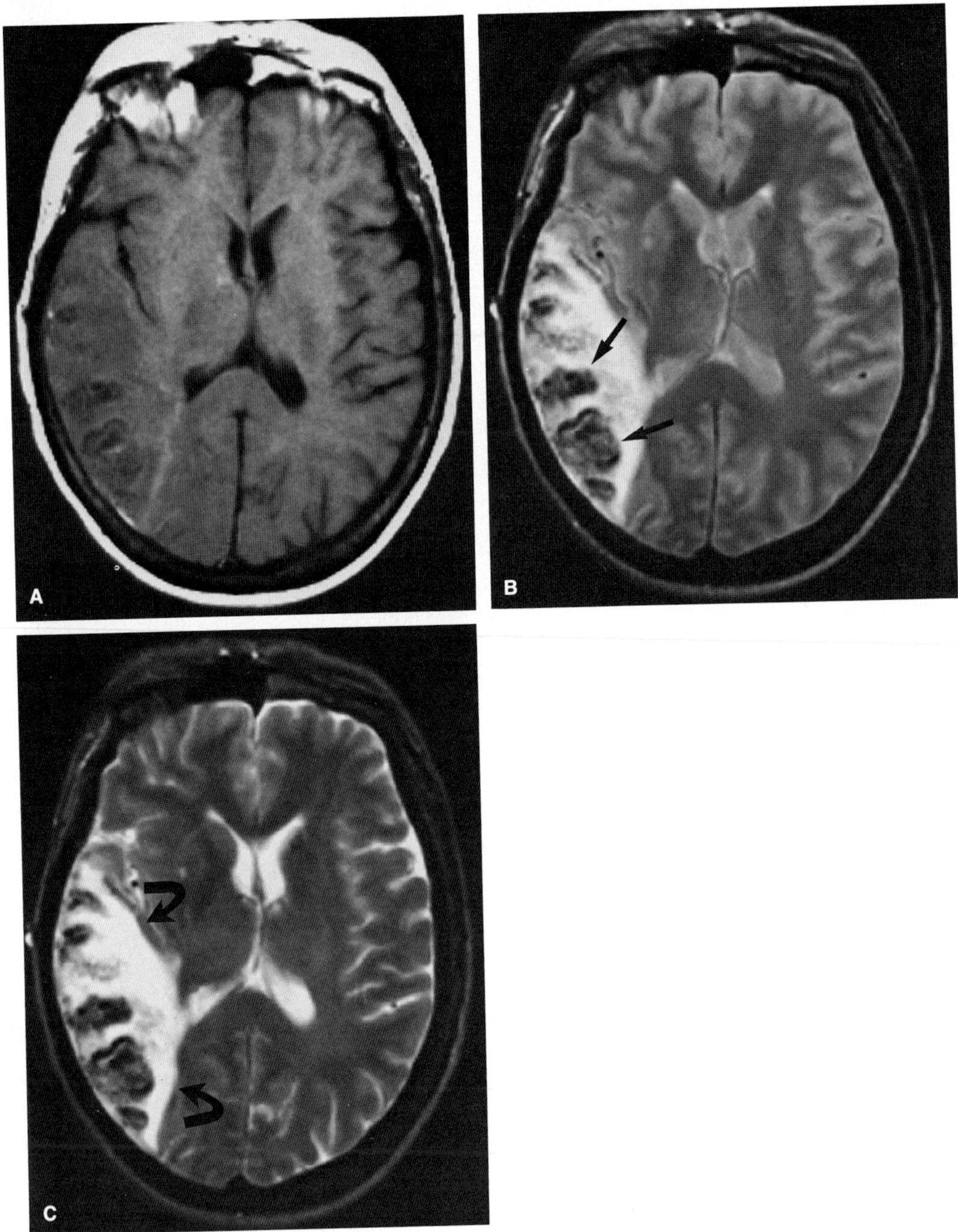

HISTORY

A 61-year-old hypertensive diabetic who, 6 days before examination, presented with the worst headache of her life, accompanied by severe nausea and vomiting

FINDINGS

(*A*) On the T1-weighted scan, there is sulcal effacement in the vascular territory of the posterior division of the right middle cerebral artery (MCA), with slight midline shift and compression of the frontal horn and atrium of the right lateral ventricle. First (TE = 45 msec) (*B*) and second (TE = 90 msec) (*C*) echoes of the T2-weighted examination reveal gyriform areas of low signal intensity (*arrows*) consistent with deoxyhemoglobin staining of cortical gray matter, and surrounding high signal intensity (*curved arrows*) consistent with edema. MR was performed at high field (1.5 T).

DIAGNOSIS

Hemorrhagic (deoxyhemoglobin) MCA (posterior division) infarction

DISCUSSION

High field MR is capable of distinguishing acute, subacute, and chronic hemorrhagic cortical infarcts on the basis of signal intensity patterns.[1] Acute hemorrhagic infarction appears isointense (to slightly hypointense) on T1-weighted scans, with mild cortical hypointensity outlined by subcortical hyperintensity (edema) on T2-weighted scans. Subacute hemorrhagic infarction demonstrates cortical hyperintensity first on T1-weighted scans, and subsequently on T2-weighted scans, highlighted by subcortical hyperintensity (edema). Chronic hemorrhagic infarction demonstrates persistent cortical hypointensity on T2-weighted scans, predominantly in deep infolded gyri. The hypointensity on T2-weighted scans in hemorrhagic infarction may be due to the presence of blood products, with deoxyhemoglobin present in the acute state and hemosiderin chronically. The high signal intensity noted in the subacute stage initially on T1-weighted images and subsequently on T2-weighted images is thought to result from the autooxidation of hemoglobin to methemoglobin, which is seen first intracellularly and then in its free state after red blood cell lysis.

Pitfalls in Image Interpretation

Low field MR scanners (1 T or less) are relatively insensitive to the presence of deoxyhemoglobin and hemosiderin. The visualization of both blood products also depends on the sensitivity to magnetic susceptibility of the imaging technique used. GRE scans can be used to improve the sensitivity at low field to these blood products. However, such scans are rarely used in routine head imaging. SE scans appear normal. Conversely, at high field (1.5 T), routine T2-weighted SE sequences readily depict deoxyhemoglobin and hemosiderin.
On GRE techniques at high field, the loss in signal intensity due to susceptibility (T2•) effects is further accentuated.

Clinical References

1. Hecht-Leavitt C, Gomori JM, Grossman RI, et al. High-field MRI of hemorrhagic cortical infarction. AJNR 1986;7:581–585.

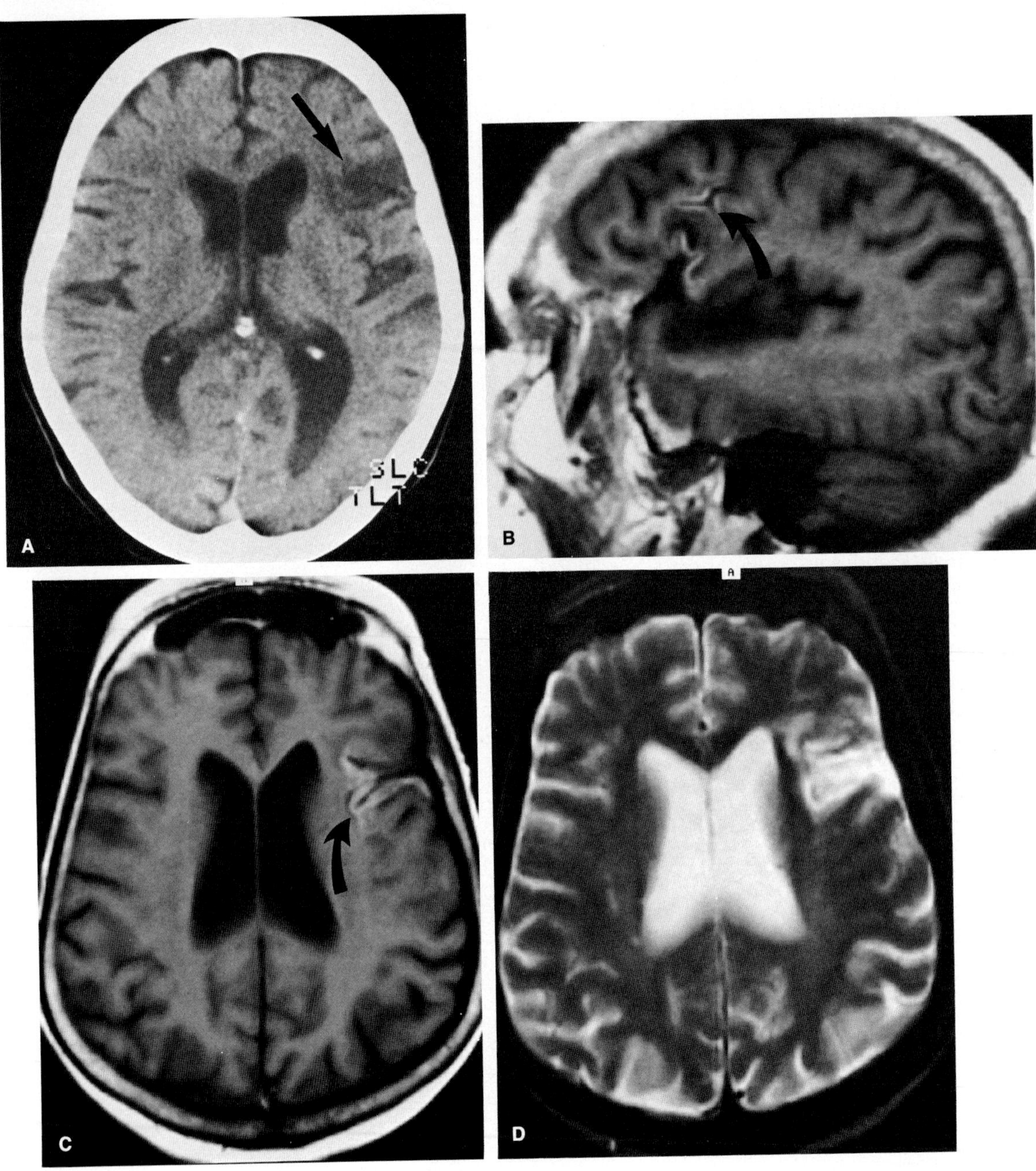

HISTORY

A 60-year-old with two recent transient ischemic attacks

FINDINGS

(*A*) CT without contrast enhancement reveals an area of low attenuation in the left middle cerebral artery (MCA) distribution (*arrow*). There was no discernible enhancement postcontrast (*image not shown*). Because of the apparent compensatory dilatation of the frontal horn, the scan was interpreted as consistent with an old infarct. Sagittal (*B*) and axial (*C*) T1-weighted images reveal petechial hemorrhage (methemoglobin) within cortical gray matter (*curved arrows*). (*D*) There is also localized increased signal intensity on the T2-weighted image (TE = 90 msec) because of a combination of extracellular methemoglobin and edema. Abnormal gyriform enhancement was noted following IV gadolinium chelate administration (*image not shown*). The left internal cerebral artery appeared isointense with brain on all pulse sequences (*images not illustrated*). Both MR and CT were performed on the same day. Angiography (*not il-*

lustrated) revealed occlusion of the left common carotid artery at its origin from the aortic arch, with an aplastic left A1 segment of the anterior cerebral artery and filling of the branches of the left internal carotid artery from the posterior circulation by way of the posterior communicating artery.

DIAGNOSIS

Hemorrhagic (methemoglobin) subacute MCA (anterior division) infarction

DISCUSSION

About one fifth of all infarcts are hemorrhagic, as defined by findings on pathologic testing, which shows red softening.[1] Hemorrhage is typically confined to the cortex; however, the adjacent pia mater may also be stained by hemoglobin pigments. Hemorrhage occurs in ischemic brain that is reperfused. This can be the result of (1) lysis of an embolus, (2) opening of collaterals, (3) restoration of normal blood pressure following a hypotensive episode, or (4) intermittent compression of the posterior cerebral artery due to transtentorial herniation of the temporal lobe. Other conditions predisposing to hemorrhage include hypertension and anticoagulation.

Pitfalls in Image Interpretation

Although methemoglobin appears hyperintense on T1-weighted images, whether intracellular or extracellular in distribution, the appearance on T2-weighted scans can be confusing. Intracellular methemoglobin is markedly hypointense, and extracellular methemoglobin is hyperintense, on T2-weighted SE scans at high field (1.5 T).

Particularly in the setting of infarction, the carotid arteries should be inspected closely for evidence of slow flow or occlusion. Isointensity with adjacent brain on all pulse sequences is compatible with occlusion.[2]

Clinical References

1. Hecht-Leavitt C, Gomori JM, Grossman RI, et al. High-field MRI of hemorrhagic cortical infarction. AJNR 1986;7:581–585.
2. Lane JI, Flanders AE, Doan HT, Bell RD. Assessment of carotid artery patency on routine spin echo MR imaging of the brain. AJNR 1991;12:819–826.

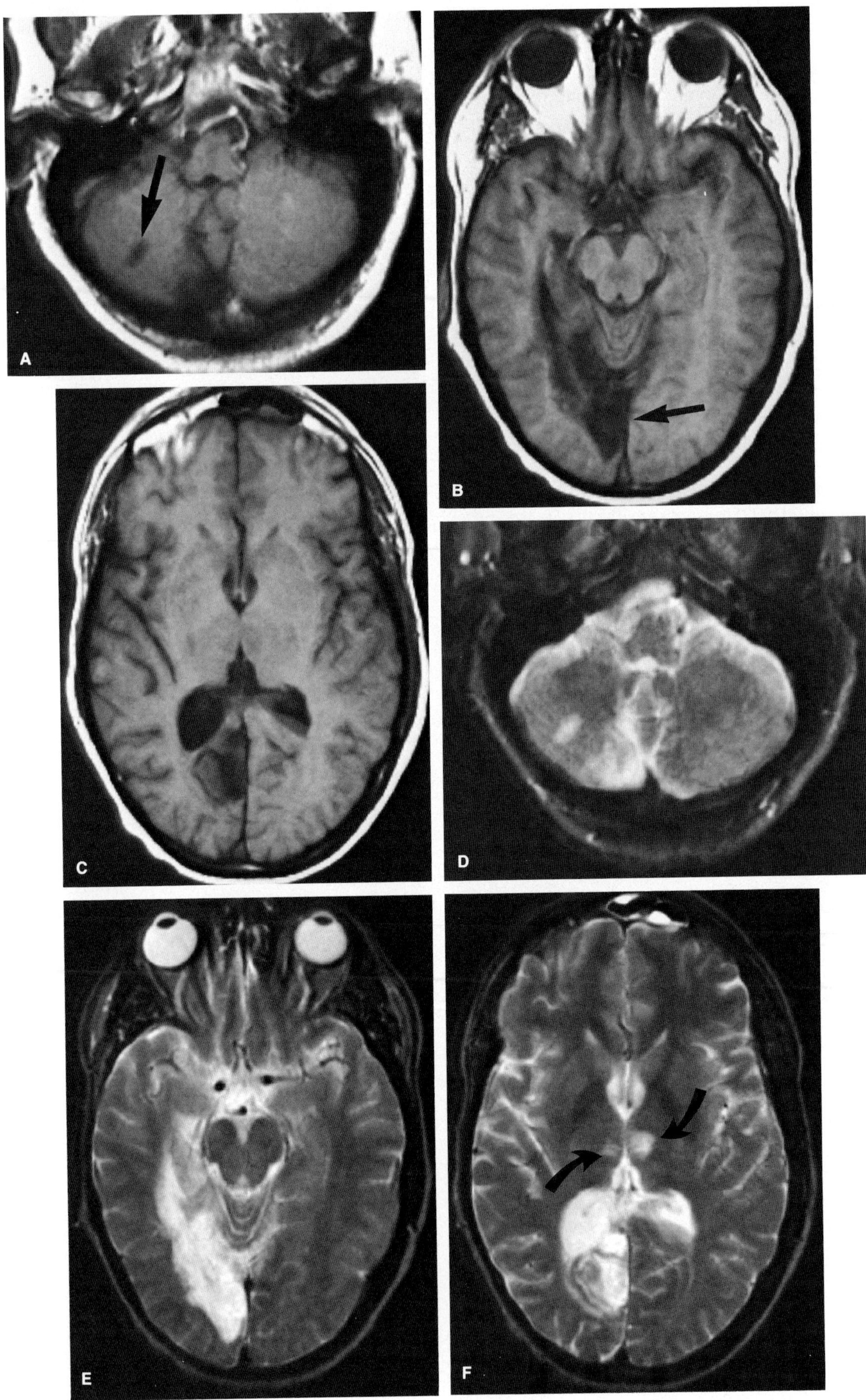
A
B
C
D
E
F

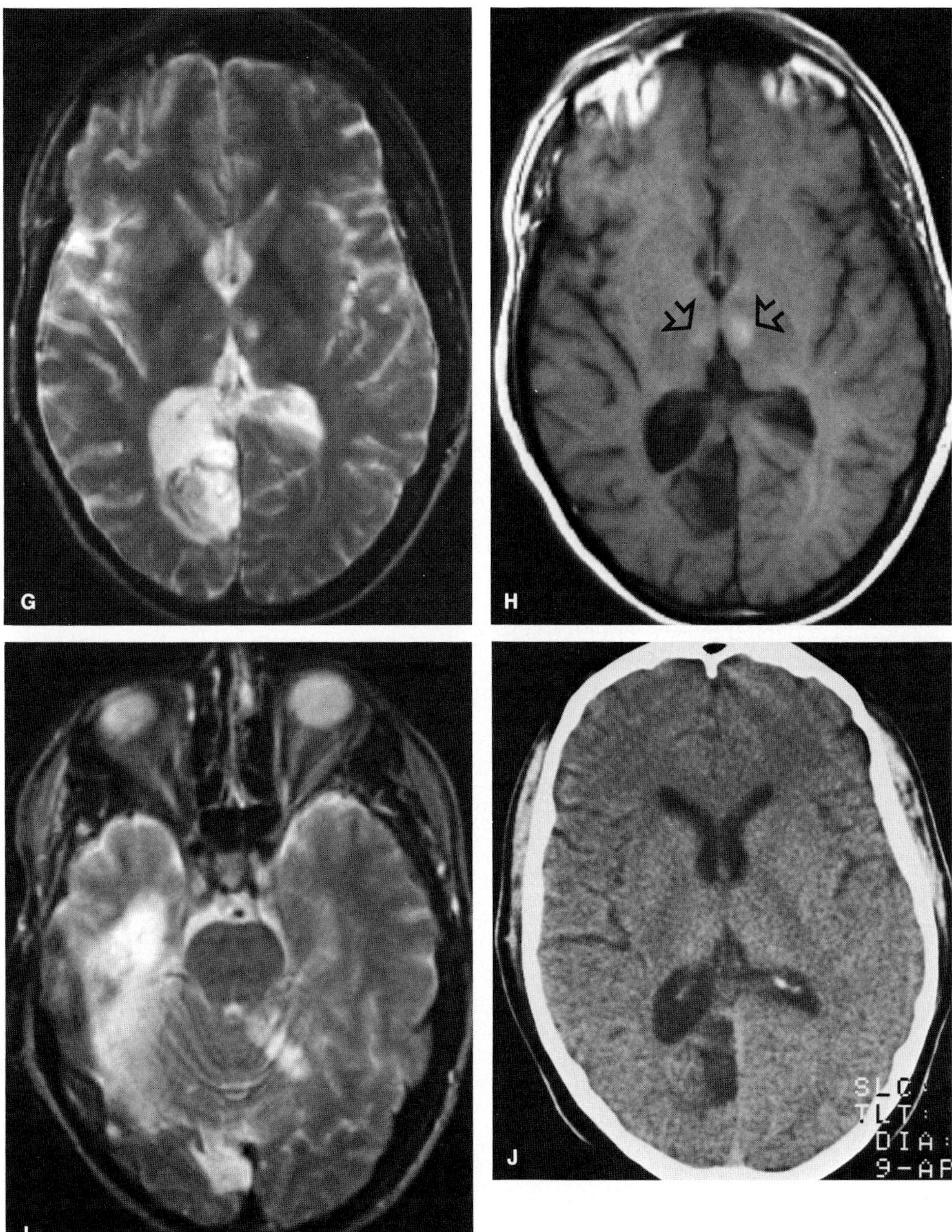

HISTORY

A 49-year-old man with malignant hypertension who collapsed and was unresponsive at work 2 days before the initial MR examination. He was hospitalized, underwent anticoagulation, and was discharged with blood pressure controlled. The patient presented 2 weeks later with an acute change in balance and ambulation, with MR performed within 48 hours of symptom onset. Echocardiography revealed a small membranous ventriculoseptal defect.

FINDINGS

Precontrast T1-weighted (*A to C*) and T2-weighted (*D to F*) images reveal encephalomalacia (*arrows*) in the vascular territory of right PICA and posterior cerebral artery (PCA), consistent with old infarcts. Abnormal high signal intensity is noted in the thalami bilaterally (*curved arrows in F*) on the T2-weighted scan, without corresponding abnormality on the T1-weighted scan, consistent with an acute or subacute infarct. No enhancement was noted postcontrast (*images not shown*).

(*G*) Two weeks later, the thalamic abnormalities appear smaller in size on the T2-weighted scan. (*H*) The precontrast T1-weighted scan reveals petechial hemorrhage (*open arrows*). Abnormal contrast enhancement was also noted (*images not shown*). (*I*) A new abnormality in the vascular territory of the left superior cerebellar artery is well demonstrated on the T2-weighted scan. (*J*) CT revealed only the old right PCA infarct.

DIAGNOSIS

Hemorrhagic subacute bilateral thalamic infarction, acute left superior cerebellar artery infarction, old right PICA infarction, old right PCA infarction

DISCUSSION

Although cerebral infarction is typically characterized by low signal intensity on T1-weighted images and high signal intensity on T2-weighted images, hyperintensity on T1-weighted images can be noted.[1] This finding is most frequent with cortical lesions, both in the cerebrum and in the cerebellum, where a rich collateral circulation exists owing to leptomeningeal anastomoses. In such lesions, a temporal pattern of change has been noted at high field (1.5 T), with T2 hypointensity and T1 isointensity initially, progressing to T2 isointensity and T1 hyperintensity, and subsequently to T2 hypointensity and T1 isointensity. These changes are compatible with the known temporal evolution of blood products in the brain. The extent of petechial hemorrhage seen in brain infarction is influenced both by the recanalization of occluded vessels and the degree of collateral circulation.

In the case presented, risk factors for cerebral infarction include a congenital septal defect, which could lead to paradoxic emboli, and hypertension, with accompanying exaggerated atherosclerosis.

Clinical References

1. Nabatame H, Fujimoto N, Nakamura K, et al. High intensity areas on noncontrast T1 weighted MR images in cerebral infarction. J Comput Assist Tomogr 1990;14:521–526.

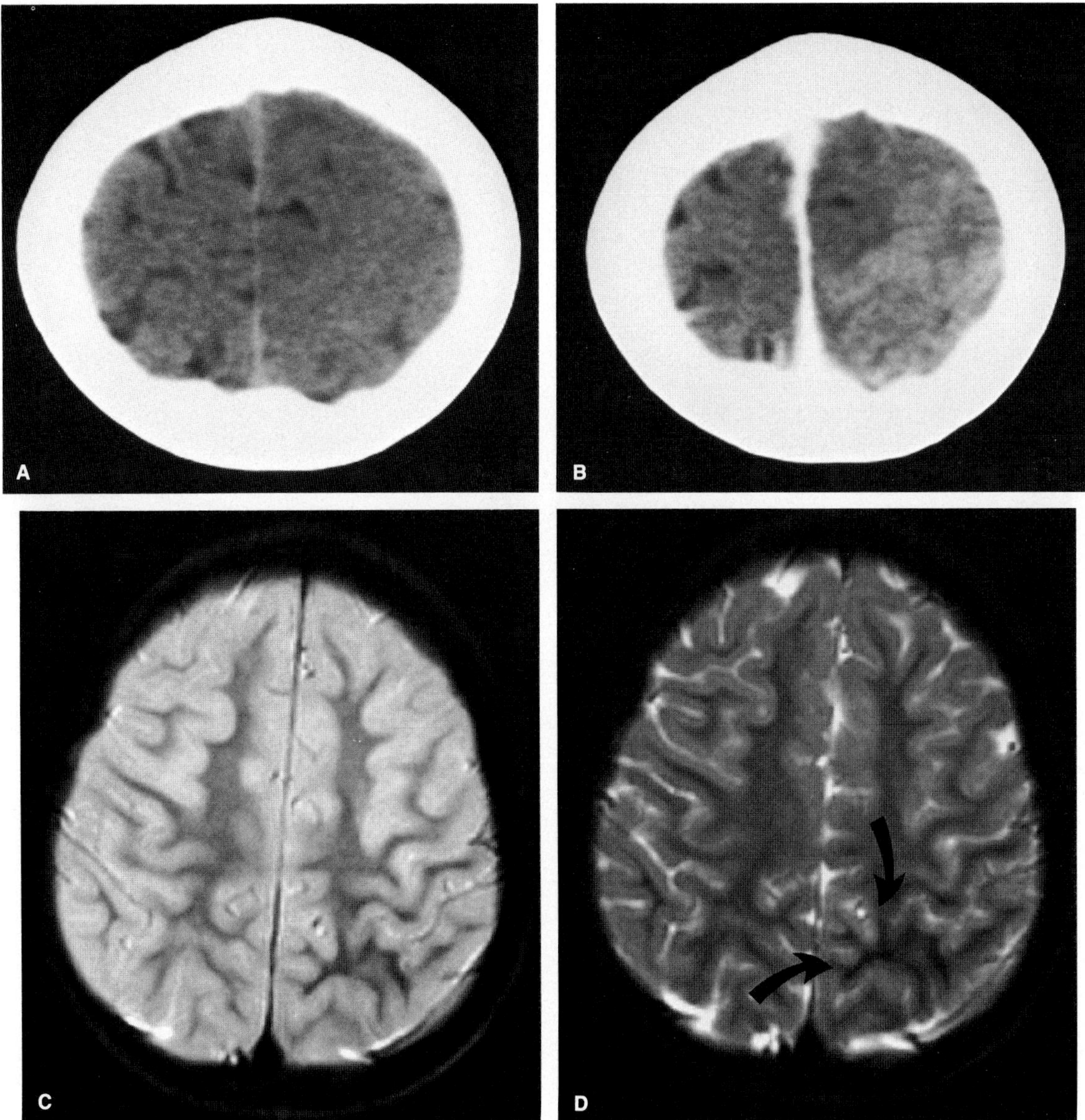

HISTORY

A 6-year-old child after chemotherapy and cranial irradiation for acute lymphocytic leukemia. She now presents with seizures and right-sided weakness.

FINDINGS

(*A*) Precontrast CT reveals effacement of the sulci on the left at the vertex. (*B*) On postcontrast CT, there is a suggestion of gyrallike enhancement also on the left. No abnormalities were seen on other sections. Prospectively, the question of an infarct was raised. MR with both moderate (TE = 45 msec) (*C*) and heavy (TE = 90 msec) (*D*) T2 weighting reveals only subtle hypointensity (*curved arrows in D*) in the left posterior white matter, suggesting the presence of deoxyhemoglobin. This hypointensity was noted throughout the white matter in the left occipital lobe (*images not shown*). (*E*) The precontrast T1-weighted image demonstrates sulcal effacement posteriorly on the left, with a subtle loss in gray–white matter differentiation (*open arrow*). (*F*) On the postcontrast T1-weighted image there is abnormal heterogeneous enhancement (*arrows*), moderate in degree and not strictly gyriform in location, in this region. This abnormal enhancement was present in much of the PCA distribution on the left (*additional levels not shown*), with extension into the watershed distribution between the posterior and middle cerebral arteries.

One week later, the T2-weighted examination was unchanged (*images not shown*). (*G*) The precontrast T1-weighted image again demonstrates loss of cortical sulci (gyral effacement) on the left posteriorly, with greater

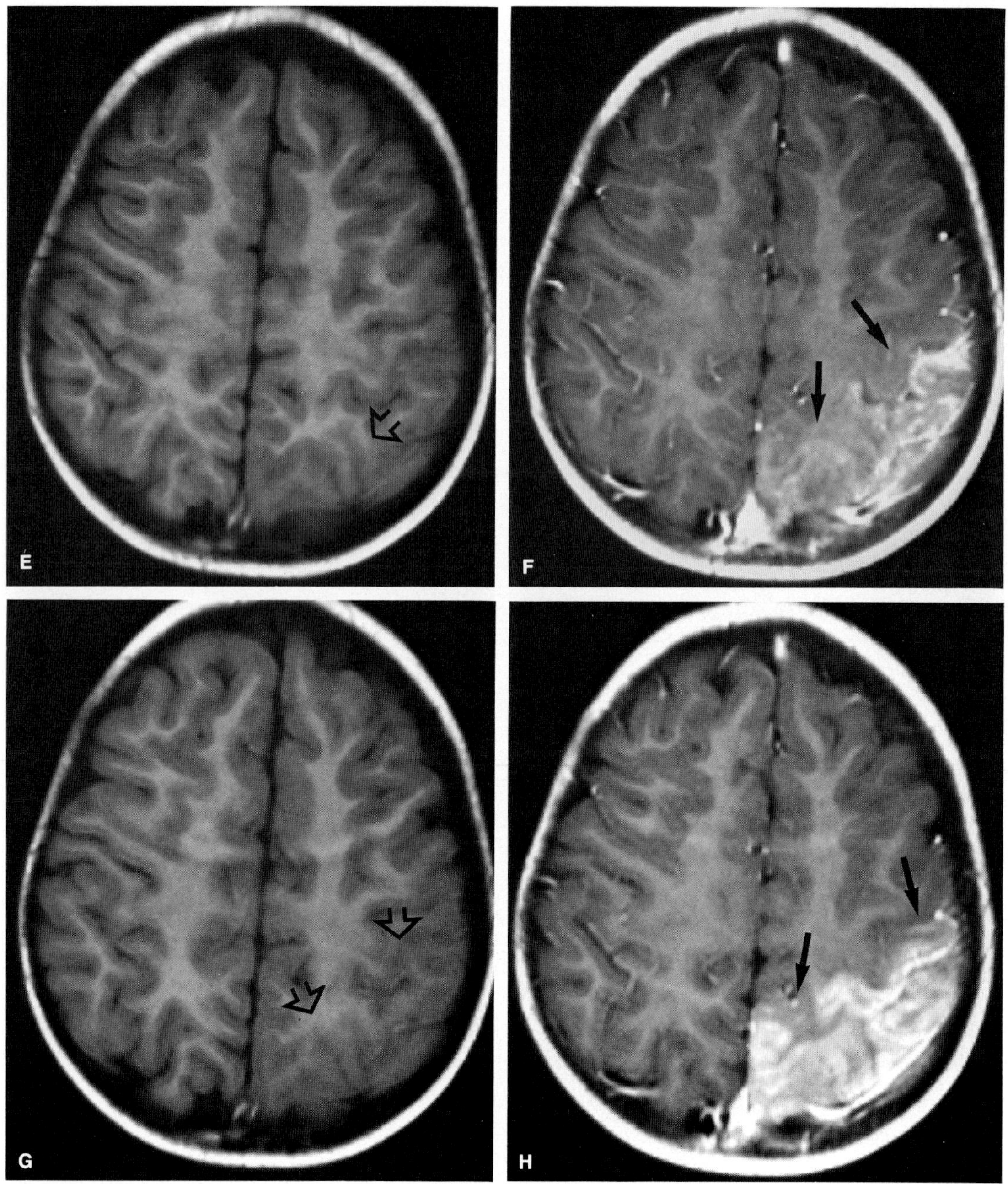

loss of gray–white matter differentiation (*open arrows*) as compared with the previous examination. (*H*) The abnormal enhancement on the postcontrast image is now more intense, definitely gyriform in nature, and more extensive (*arrows*). The region of tissue involved is now well defined, extending from the falx medially to the cortex laterally. Additional images (*not shown*) demonstrated prominent abnormal enhancement in the entire left PCA distribution, together with involvement of the watershed and posterior and middle cerebral artery territories.

DIAGNOSIS

Infarction in the left posterior and middle cerebral artery territories, with abnormal iron deposition in the subcortical white matter

DISCUSSION

The case presented demonstrates the presence of iron in subcortical white matter (not in cortical gray matter) as more typically seen in subacute hemorrhagic infarction. We have seen this appearance in a number of cases, and specifically in the pediatric population. Although it is likely that the presence of iron correlates with petechial hemorrhage, it is also possible that this is unrelated to hemorrhage and represents a nonspecific brain response to injury, as a result of the interruption of transport mechanisms or direct cell injury.[1]

Contrast enhancement following IV administration of a gadolinium chelate can also be used to identify subacute infarction, as in this case. The extent of involvement often becomes more clear by imaging in the late subacute time period, rather than in the earlier course, with blood–brain barrier disruption progressing and thus becoming more distinctly outlined by contrast enhancement.

Disorders of either cranial blood vessels or the cardiovascular system can lead to cerebral artery thrombosis and brain infarction. By far the most common cause of thrombosis is atherosclerosis. However, inflammatory blood vessel disorders can also predispose a patient to thrombus formation. In the case presented, radiation therapy, which is known to cause blood vessel damage, is presumed to be the major predisposing factor.

MR Technique

In cerebral infarction, it is particularly important to acquire images sensitive to magnetic susceptibility to demonstrate the presence of deoxyhemoglobin and hemosiderin. Suitable scan types include many T2-weighted SE and GRE techniques.

With respect to detection of abnormal contrast enhancement, delayed imaging (30 to 60 minutes after injection) can be of value. Subacute cerebral infarction (with disruption of the blood–brain barrier) is one of the few brain conditions in which enhancement is typically more intense on delayed scans.

Pitfalls in Image Interpretation

Although vasogenic edema can be an important clue to the diagnosis of an acute or subacute infarct, it may not be present, as illustrated in the current case. Standard SE MR techniques have also been shown to be insensitive to cytotoxic edema, an early histologic finding in cerebral infarction, which precedes vasogenic edema. Images should be closely inspected for sulcal effacement (in the absence of signal intensity changes), an indirect sign of gyral swelling and thus cytotoxic edema.

Clinical References

1. Cross PA, Atlas SW, Grossman RI. MR evaluation of brain iron in children with cerebral infarction. AJNR 1990; 11:341–348.

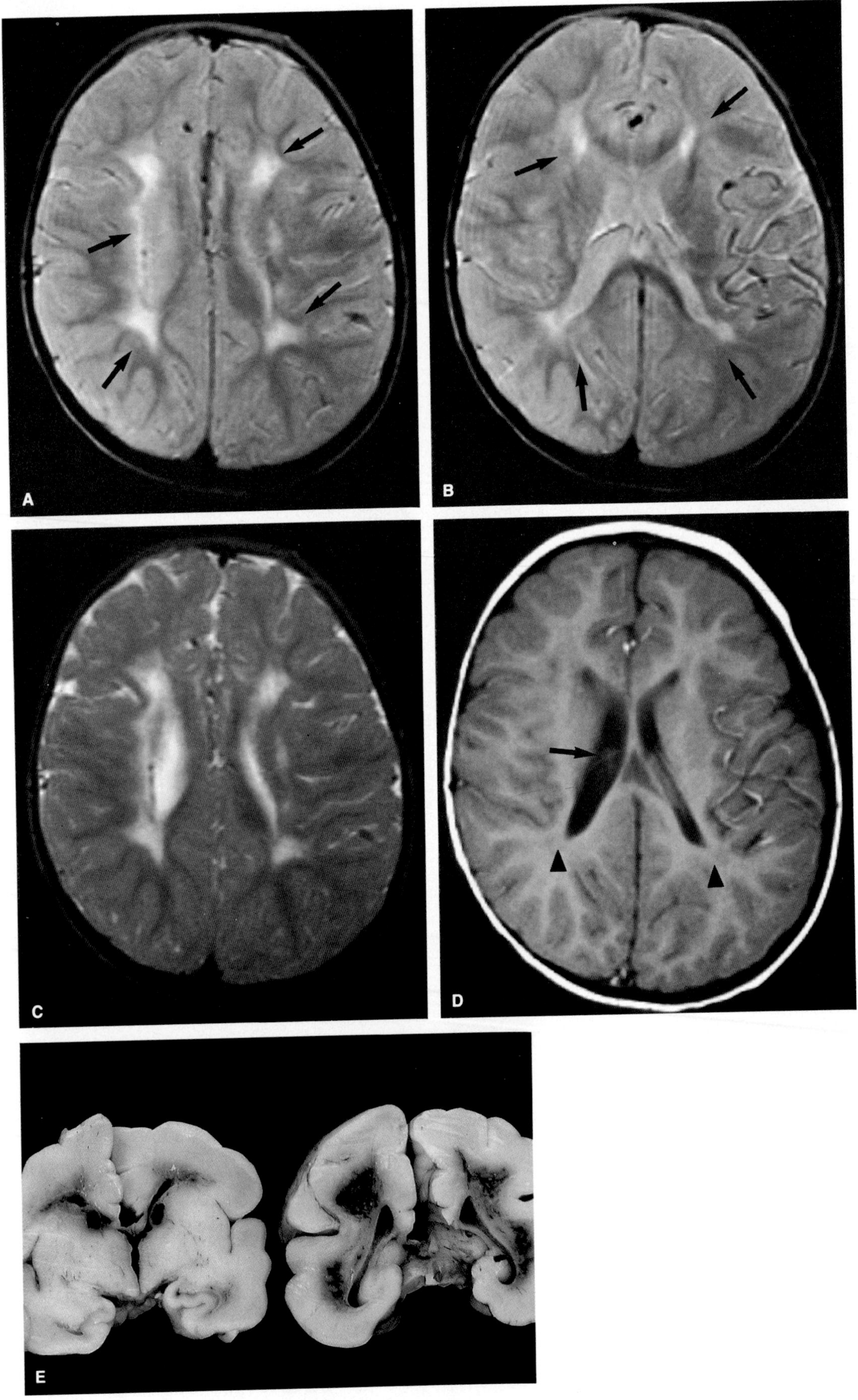
A
B
C
D
E

HISTORY

A 17-month-old infant, born prematurely, now with paraparesis and abnormal vision

FINDINGS

(*A and B*) Intermediate T2-weighted axial images demonstrate abnormal increased signal intensity within the periventricular white matter (*arrows*). (*C*) The abnormal white matter has approximately the same signal intensity as CSF on the heavily T2-weighted axial image. The amount of periventricular white matter is decreased. (*D*) This is best illustrated on the T1-weighted axial image where the gray matter of the insular cortex lies almost directly adjacent to the ventricular atria (*arrowheads*), indicating loss of white matter volume in the peritrigonal regions. There is also abnormal dilatation of the body of the right lateral ventricle (*arrow*).

DIAGNOSIS

Periventricular leukomalacia (PVL)

DISCUSSION

Infarction of the white matter adjacent to the lateral ventricles of a premature infant's brain is known as periventricular leukomalacia.[1] PVL usually occurs in infants with a birth weight of less than 1500 g or a gestational age of less than 35 weeks who have respiratory distress syndrome. Autoregulation of cerebral blood flow is not fully developed in the immature brain, and PVL is the result of a hypoxic-ischemic insult that causes hypoperfusion of the white matter in the watershed areas of arterial supply. The areas most commonly affected are adjacent to the trigone and frontal horn of the lateral ventricle. These locations account for the neurologic sequelae of PVL, which include spastic diplegia or quadriplegia (cerebral palsy), and cortical blindness.[2] Severely affected patients are mentally retarded.

Ultrasonography remains the primary imaging modality for the diagnosis of the early stages of PVL, which appears initially as an increase in periventricular echoes.[1] MR is useful in evaluating PVL in its later gliotic stages. Its ability to depict myelin gives MR a unique advantage over other imaging modalities. The MR findings in end-stage PVL include the characteristic triad of abnormally increased signal intensity on T2-weighted images in the periventricular white matter representing gliosis and demyelination, decreased quantity of periventricular white matter, and ex vacuo enlargement of the lateral ventricles adjacent to the abnormal white matter.[3]

MR Technique

The periventricular gliosis associated with PVL is best depicted as high signal intensity on intermediate T2-weighted images, where the signal intensity of CSF is moderate. Periventricular gliosis and CSF can have similar signal intensity on heavily T2-weighted images, making differentiation difficult.

Pitfalls in Image Interpretation

Normal unmyelinated white matter in the peritrigonal regions of children has mildly increased signal intensity on T2-weighted images and should not be mistaken for PVL.

Pathologic Correlate

(*E*) Coronal view of a gross specimen shows abnormal infarcted periventricular white matter. In patients who survive the ischemic insult, there is subsequent development of gliosis and atrophy in the infarcted white matter.

Clinical References

1. Wilson D, Steiner R. Periventricular leukomalacia: evaluation with MR imaging. Radiology 1986;160:507–511.
2. Flodmark O, Lupton B, Li D, et al. MR imaging of periventricular leukomalacia in childhood. AJR 1989;152:583–590.
3. Baker L, Stevenson D, Enzmann D. End-stage periventricular leukomalacia: MR evaluation. Radiology 1988;168:809–815.

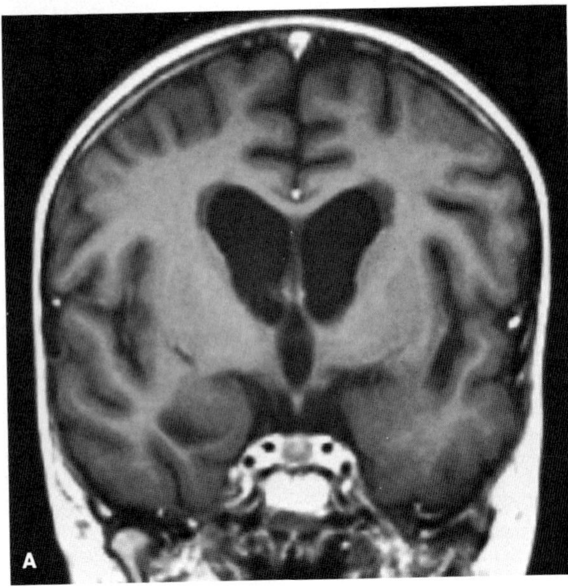

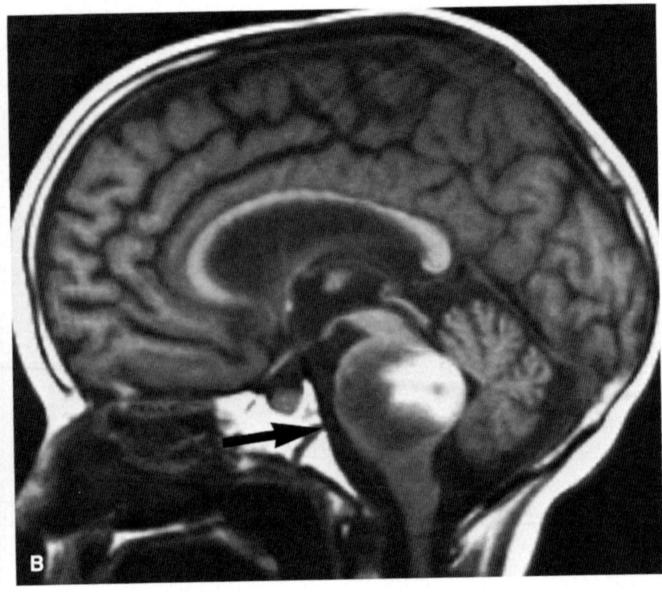

HISTORY

Brain stem glioma in a 5-year-old girl treated with radiation therapy

FINDINGS

Moderate dilatation of the lateral and third ventricles is present on coronal (*A*) and sagittal (*B*) T1-weighted and axial (*C and D*) T2-weighted images. (*B*) On the sagittal T1-weighted image, a large hemorrhagic brain stem glioma (*black arrow*) is identified causing ventricular obstruction at the superior aspect of the fourth ventricle. A thick smooth rim of periventricular white matter hyperintensity is identified surrounding the lateral ventricles on the first (*C*) and second (*D*) echoes of the axial T2-weighted sequence. This involves only the periventricular white matter and does not extend into the basal ganglia. (*E*) Ventricular size and periventricular signal intensity were normal on the axial T2-weighted image performed 45 days earlier. At that time, there was no obstruction to CSF flow.

DIAGNOSIS

Obstructive hydrocephalus with transependymal resorption of CSF

DISCUSSION

Any tumor encroaching on the fourth ventricle or cerebral aqueduct can lead to obstructive hydrocephalus. In children, this is most commonly due to cystic astrocytoma or medulloblastoma. Brain stem gliomas are also known to cause obstructive hydrocephalus.

In most instances, hydrocephalus develops secondary to decreased CSF absorption and at some point the CSF pressure is elevated. The latter may or may not be maintained, depending on compensatory mechanisms.[1]

Transependymal resorption of CSF is a common finding in acute obstructive hydrocephalus. Fluid is forced out of the ventricles into the periventricular white matter by increased CSF pressure. This results in a smooth thick rim of periventricular hyperintensity (on T2-weighted images) surrounding the lateral ventricles. This hyperintensity does not extend into the gray matter of the basal ganglia.[2]

The smooth thick rim of periventricular hyperintensity (characteristic of transependymal resorption of CSF) must be differentiated from mild periventricular hyperintensity (PVH), ischemic-gliotic disease, demyelinating processes and radiation white matter injury. Mild PVH is a common MR finding and is usually unassociated with intracranial pathology. Hyperintense foci adjacent to the frontal horns of the lateral ventricles are particularly common in ischemic disease. In multiple sclerosis, periventricular involvement is typically patchy. Radiation-induced brain injury results in diffuse and confluent white matter lesions that are scalloped laterally and extend to the cortical gray matter.[3,4]

MR Technique

The intermediate T2-weighted echo allows better differentiation of hyperintense periventricular abnormalities from CSF within the ventricular system.

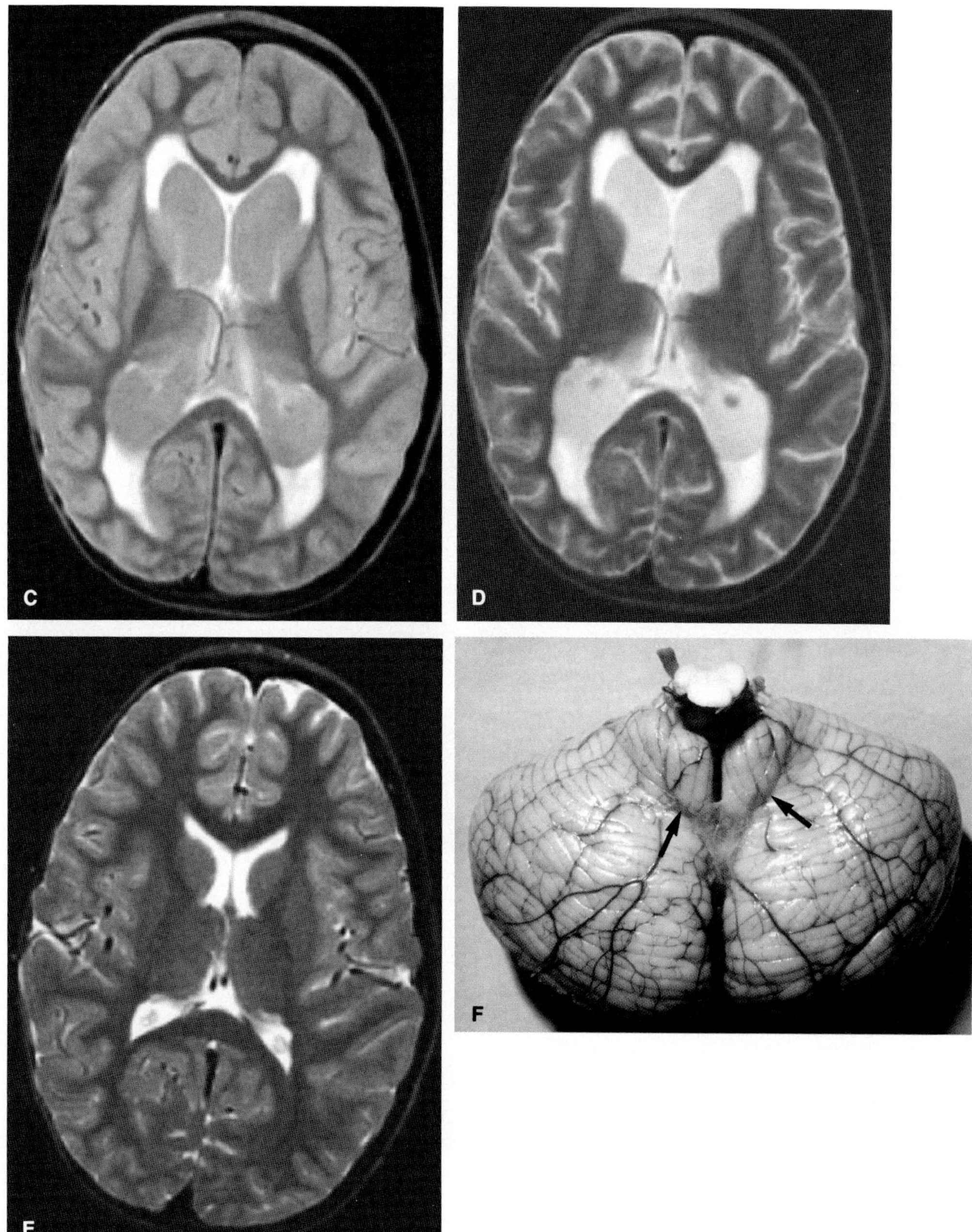

Pitfalls in Image Interpretations

Mild PVH on T2-weighted sequences is a common nonspecific finding and does not indicate significant intracranial pathology.

Pathologic Correlate

F shows the gross appearance of cerebellar tonsillar herniation (*arrows*) with the brain viewed from below. As in the MR case presented, a brain stem glioma was present (*not illustrated*), with death due to hydrocephalus and obstruction of the cerebral aqueduct. Tonsillar herniation through the foramen magnum leads to compression of the medulla oblongata, with resultant dysfunction of the centers that control respiration and cardiac rhythm. Tonsillar herniation is usually a dramatic event clinically, with poor prognosis. Lumbar puncture in the setting of an unrecognized posterior fossa lesion, or in the presence of obstructive hydrocephalus, is a known precipitating factor.

Clinical References

1. Davis RL, Robertson DM. Textbook of neuropathology. Baltimore, Williams & Wilkins, 1991:184–187.
2. Zimmerman RD, Fleming CA, Lee BCP, et al. Periventricular hyperintensity as seen by magnetic resonance: prevalence and significance. AJNR 1986;7:13–20.
3. Dooms GC, Hecht SH, Brant-Zawadzki M, et al. Brain radiation lesions: MR imaging. Radiology 1986;158:149–155.
4. Hecht-Leavitt C, Grossman RI, Curran SJ, et al. MR of brain radiation injury: experimental studies in cats. AJNR 1987; 8:427–431.

(F *courtesy of Daron G. Davis, MD.*)

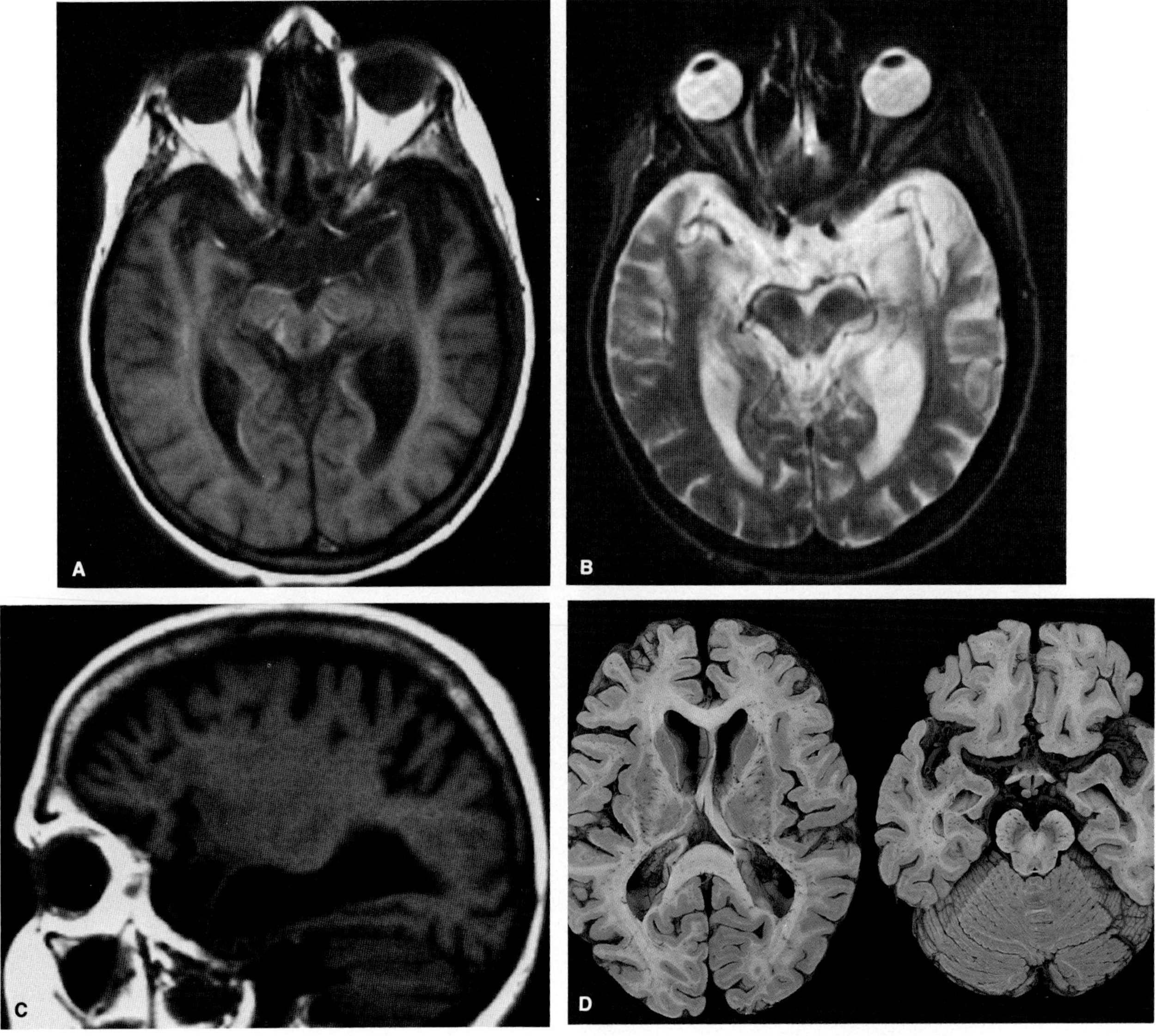

HISTORY

A 69-year-old woman with worsening dementia

FINDINGS

Marked temporal lobe and generalized cortical atrophy is identified on axial T1-weighted (*A*) and T2-weighted (*B*) images. (*C*) The right parasagittal T1-weighted image again shows marked temporal lobe atrophy. The ventricles are moderately enlarged. No abnormal enhancement was noted (*images not shown*).

DIAGNOSIS

Alzheimer's disease (AD)

DISCUSSION

Alzheimer's disease is the most common cause of dementia. In most patients it is sporadic, but there is a familial association in up to 10% of patients. There is a slight female preponderance. There is a smooth exponential increase in disease incidence after the age of 40 years. Brain weights in AD are significantly decreased below normal for age.[1]

Several metabolic and structural studies have implicated the temporal lobes and especially the hippocampus in the pathogenesis of AD.[2] On imaging studies, AD patients demonstrate greater severity of temporal lobe atrophy.[3] The absence of temporal lobe atrophy excludes AD with a high degree of specificity (95%).[2] The presence of temporal lobe atrophy does not necessarily indicate AD since a significant percentage of normal patients do show temporal lobe atrophy.

There is diffuse gray matter loss in AD, with the temporal lobes showing the greatest loss. No significant decrease in the relative volume of white matter is seen in these patients.

The major histologic lesions found in AD are the flame-shaped Alzheimer's neurofibrillary tangle, the neuritic (senile) plaque, the Hirano body, and granulovacuolar degeneration of Simchowicz. None of these lesions are specific, since each can be found in nondemented brains of middle- and older-age patients, as well as in a variety of other conditions.

Pathologic Correlate

(*D*) Two axial sections of a brain from a patient with AD demonstrate widening of the sulci and ventricular dilatation, reflecting cortical atrophy. The loss of brain substance is accentuated in the temporal lobes. Gross atrophy is not always apparent, despite abundant histologic changes.

Clinical References

1. Davis RL, Robertson DM. Textbook of neuropathology. Baltimore, Williams & Wilkins, 1991:909–911.
2. George AE, deLeon MJ, Stylopoulos LA, et al. CT diagnostic features of Alzheimer disease: importance of the choroidal/hippocampal fissure complex. AJNR 1990;11:101–107.
3. Rusinek H, de Leon MJ, George AE, et al. Alzheimer disease: measuring loss of cerebral gray matter with MR imaging. Radiology 1991;178:109–114.

(D *from Okazaki H, Scheithauer B. Slide atlas of neuropathology. New York, Gower Medical Publishing, 1988. By permission of Mayo Foundation.)*

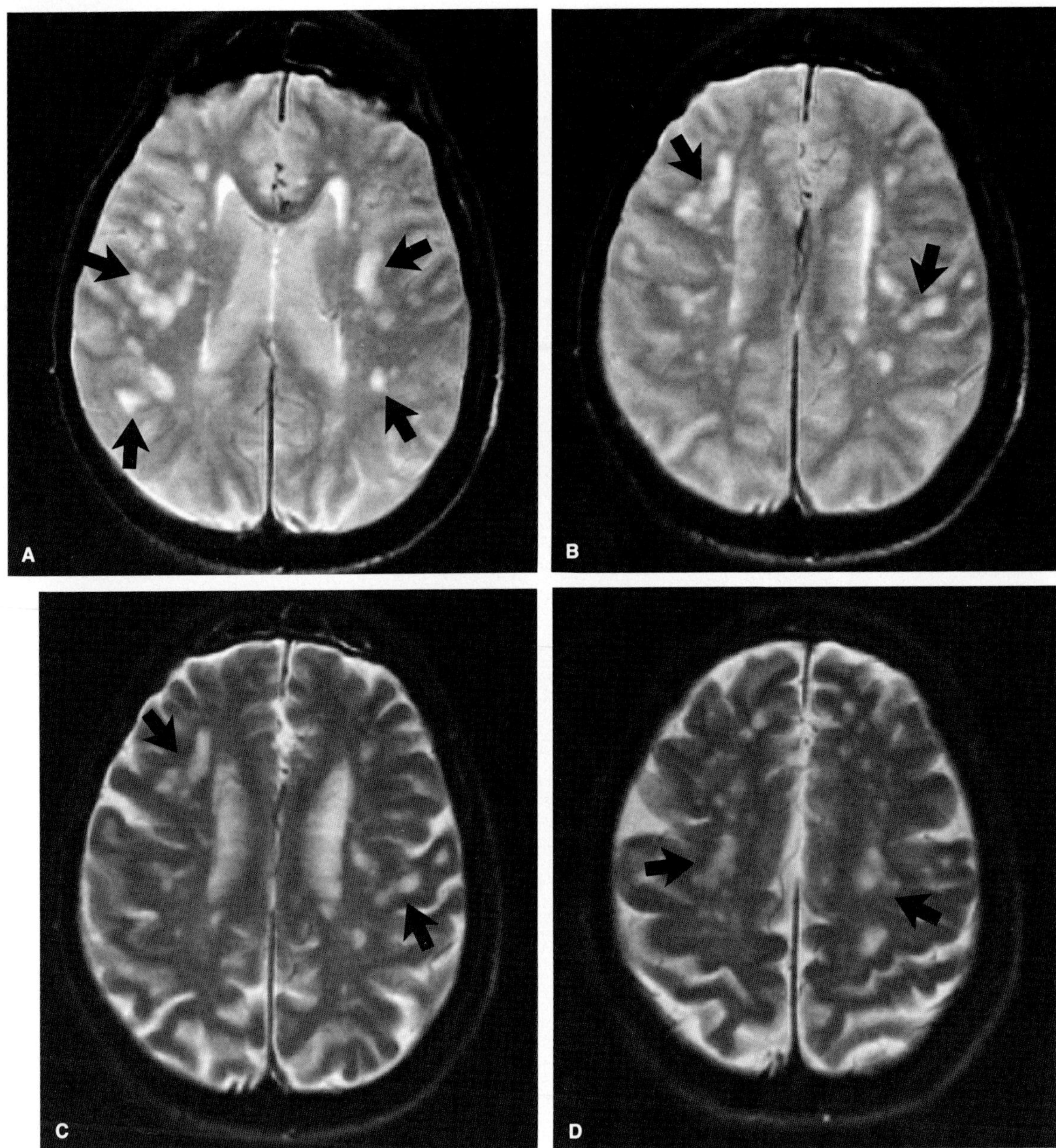

HISTORY

A 72-year-old man with multiple medical problems

FINDINGS

First (*A and B*) and second (*C and D*) echoes of the axial T2-weighted sequence depict numerous foci (*black arrows*) of increased signal intensity in the white matter (primarily the subcortical white matter). These abnormalities extend into the centrum semiovale. Most demonstrate signal intensity greater than that of CSF on the intermediate weighted T2 sequence (*A and B*). Smooth frontal horn capping is identified on the lower two sections. (*E*) Axial T1-weighted image (at the anatomic level corresponding to *B* and *C*) shows no discrete lesions. Note the poor gray–white matter contrast on both T1- and T2-weighted images. No abnormal contrast enhancement was noted (*images not shown*).

DIAGNOSIS

Severe ischemic gliotic disease (deep white matter ischemia)

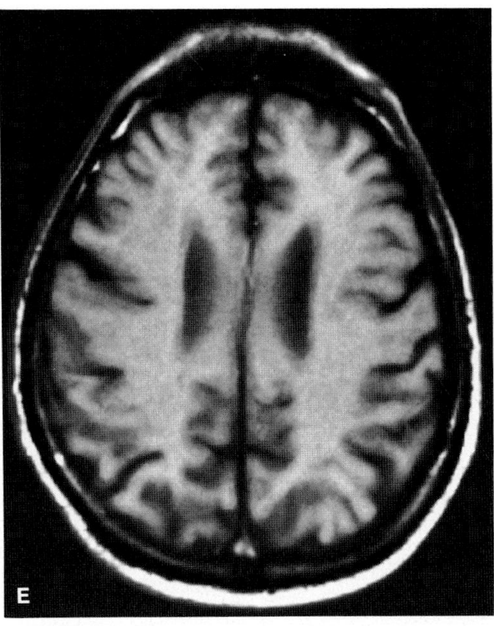

DISCUSSION

Approximately 30% of neurologically normal individuals over 60 years of age have focal white matter abnormalities on MR imaging studies. Foci of increased signal intensity on T2-weighted images in the subcortical and periventricular white matter and the centrum semiovale, as well as capping of the lateral ventricles, are findings commonly seen with aging. These abnormalities are better delineated by MR than CT.

Pathologic correlation has shown that these white matter lesions correspond to areas of necrosis, small infarcts, diffuse white matter demyelination, astroglial proliferation, and arteriolosclerosis. Two mechanisms may be involved in the production of these lesions; both have a common denominator: ischemia. Chronic, sustained arterial hypertension induces changes in the penetrating arterioles (ie, arteriolosclerosis) that may result in permeability alterations and occlusive phenomena; both changes, fluid exudation and decreased blood flow, would cause many of the lesions described. Alternatively, multiple hypotensive events could cause local tissue changes at the arterial border zone that exists in the periventricular white matter.[2]

Pitfalls in Image Interpretation

Ischemic gliotic disease must be differentiated from a demyelinating process, such as multiple sclerosis, and radiation changes. Although all these entities involve white matter, patchy relatively symmetric involvement of deep white matter (and, in particular, the white matter somewhat peripheral to the ventricular system) is characteristic of ischemic gliotic disease.

Clinical References

1. George AE, de Leon MJ, Kalnin A, et al. Leukoencephalopathy in normal and pathologic aging. 2. MRI of brain lucencies. AJNR 1986;7:567–570.
2. Davis RL and Robertson DM. Textbook of neuropathology. Baltimore, Williams & Wilkins, 1991:677–679.

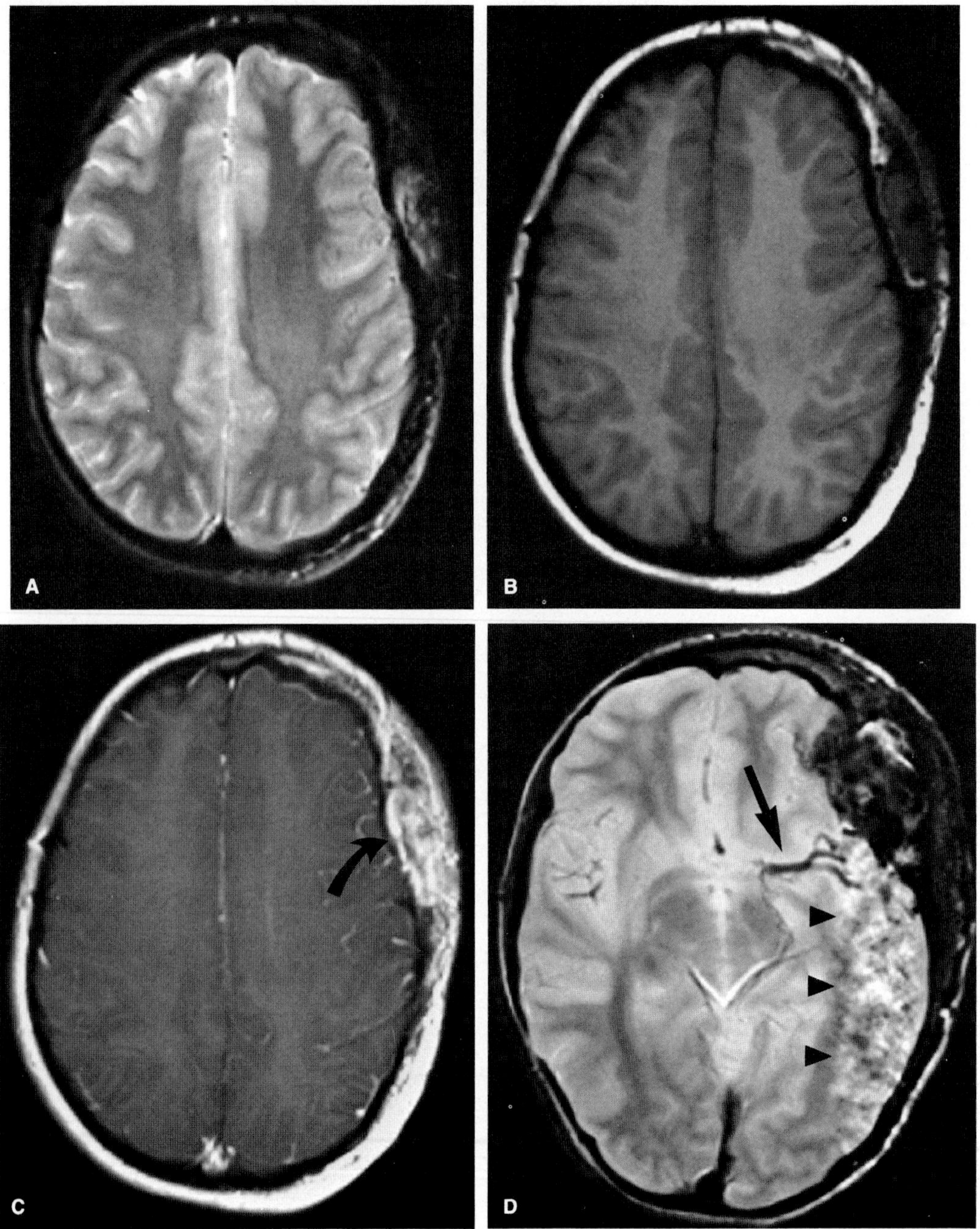

HISTORY

A 15-year-old girl with facial swelling, pain, and proptosis, all on the left side

FINDINGS

Axial T2-weighted (TE = 90 msec) (*A*) and T1-weighted (*B*) scans demonstrate an expansile intradiploic mass just superior to the lateral ventricles, which shows, relative to normal marrow, slight hyperintensity on *A* and hypointensity on *B*. (*C*) On the postcontrast T1-weighted scan, there is marked enhancement (*curved arrow*). At a lower level, on the first (TE = 45 msec) (*D*) and second (TE = 90 msec) (*E*) echoes of the T2-weighted examination, the middle cerebral artery branches (*arrow in D*) on the left appear enlarged and a prominent pulsation artifact (*arrowheads in D*) can be noted. The latter originates from the same expansile lesion, which is of low signal intensity ("flow void") at this level and can be noted to involve both the frontal and temporal bones. (*F*) The lesion demonstrates mixed isointensity and hyperintensity (a result also of flow phenomena) on the corresponding T1-

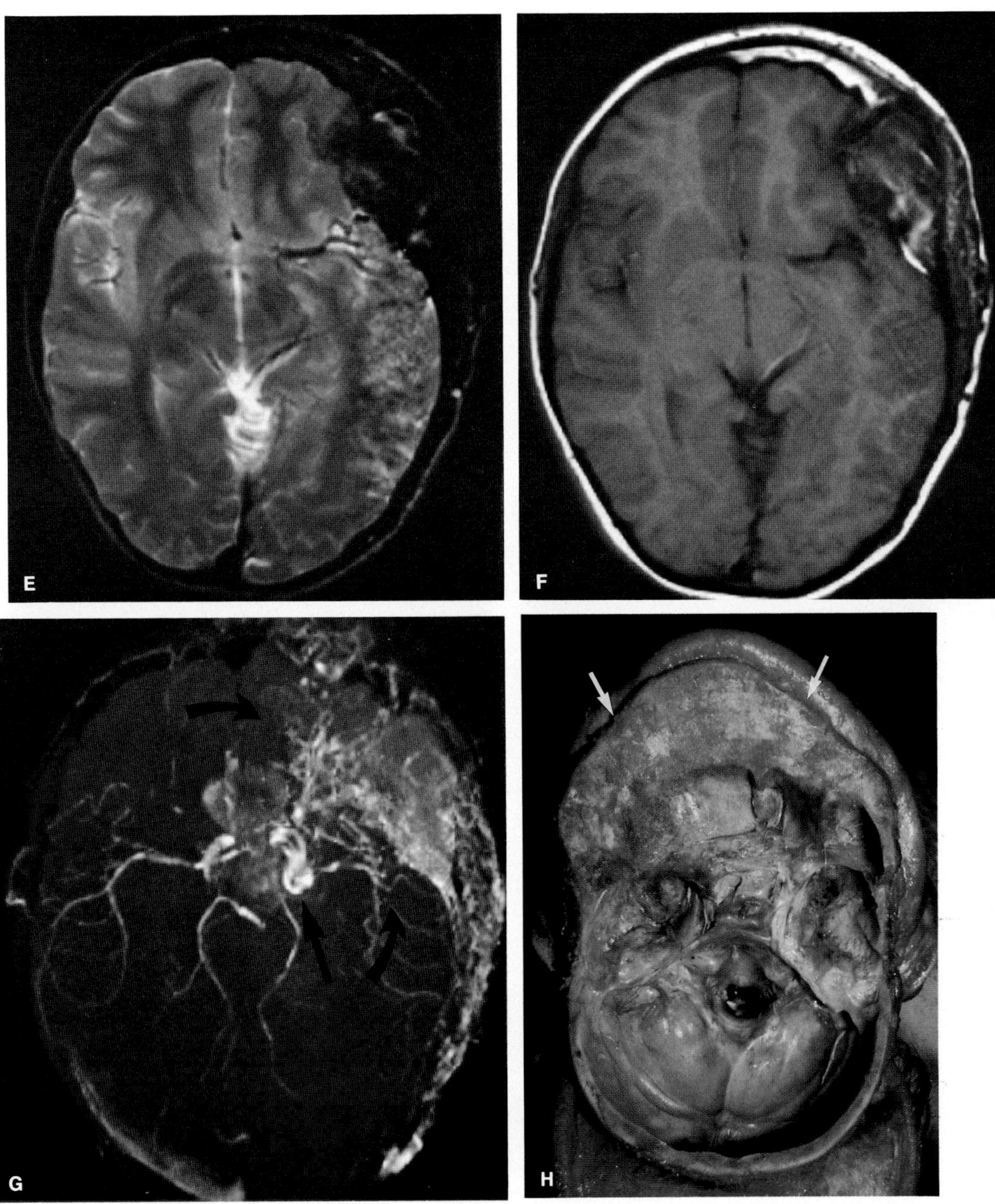

weighted section. (*G*) On the maximum intensity projection from a 3D TOF MRA, the marked vascularity (*curved arrows*) of the lesion is evident. The left cavernous carotid artery (*arrow*) is also seen to be enlarged, and multiple large draining veins (*open arrow*) are noted.

DIAGNOSIS

Fibrous dysplasia

DISCUSSION

On MR, fibrous dysplasia has sharply defined borders, with low signal intensity on T1-weighted scans and variable signal intensity (intermediate to high, with inhomogeneity common) on T2-weighted scans.[1] The lesions are well vascularized, with numerous small vessels centrally and large peripheral sinusoids.[2] The degree of vascularity in this case, however, is unusual.

Fibrous dysplasia is a developmental skeletal anomaly that may be monostotic or polyostotic in nature. The presence of fibrous dysplasia (usually polyostotic) with endocrine dysfunction—typically precocious puberty in a female—and cutaneous pigmentation is referred to as the McCune-Albright syndrome. Involvement of the skull or facial bones occurs in 10% to 25% of patients with monostotic disease, and 50% of patients with polyostotic disease. The globe may be displaced because of involvement of orbital bones. The lesion may be lucent or sclerotic on plain film. Hazy ("ground-glass") lucent lesions of the facial or skull bones are typically also expansile, with widening of the diploic space.

Pitfalls in Image Interpretation

The MR appearance of fibrous dysplasia is not specific for the underlying histology, with the differential diagnosis including many other entities, in particular Paget's disease and metastatic disease.

Pathologic Correlate

(*H*) Fibrous dysplasia (*white arrows*) in a different patient is illustrated by the appearance on gross examination of skull involvement (primarily frontal bone). The normal cancellous bone of the marrow space is replaced by a gritty rubbery tissue. Although not well seen in this instance, the endosteal surface is often scalloped. The grittiness is due to irregular bone spicules imbedded in the fibrous tissue.

Clinical References

1. Norris MA, Kaplan PA, Pathria M, Greenway G. Fibrous dysplasia: magnetic resonance imaging appearance at 1.5 tesla. Clin Imaging 1990;14:211–215.
2. Utz JA, Kransdorf MJ, Jelinek JS, et al. MR appearance of fibrous dysplasia. J Comput Assist Tomogr 1989;13:845–851.

(H *courtesy of Daron G. Davis, MD.*)

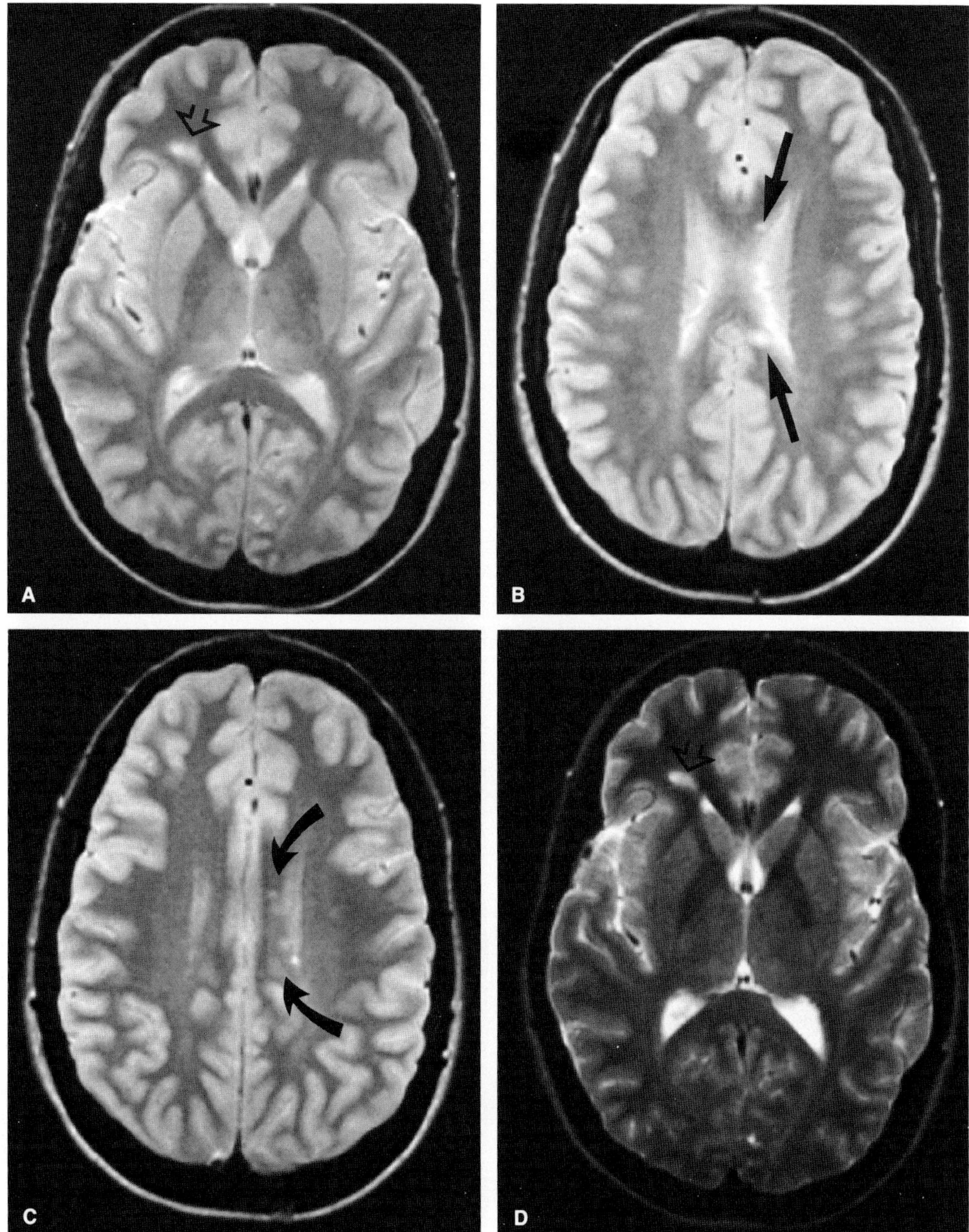

HISTORY

An 18-year-old woman with new onset of left lower extremity paresthesia 7 days before admission, which progressed to include the left upper extremity. On day 4 after onset, abnormal sensation developed in the right lower extremity. Reflexes and motor strength were normal. Visual and brain stem evoked potentials were also normal. The CSF was abnormal, with moderate mononuclear pleocytosis (40 cells/μL) and a slight elevation of total protein

FINDINGS

Axial SE scans are presented at three anatomic levels with intermediate T2 weighting (TE = 45 msec) (*A to C*), heavy T2 weighting (TE = 90 msec) (*D to F*), and T1 weighting (TE = 10 msec) (*G to I*). In the right frontal white matter, a large (1-cm) punctate abnormality is well seen on both T2- and T1-weighted scans (*open arrows in A, D, and G*). This demonstrated uniform enhancement postcontrast (*image not illustrated*). At the level of the lateral ventricles, at least four periventricular lesions can be noted on

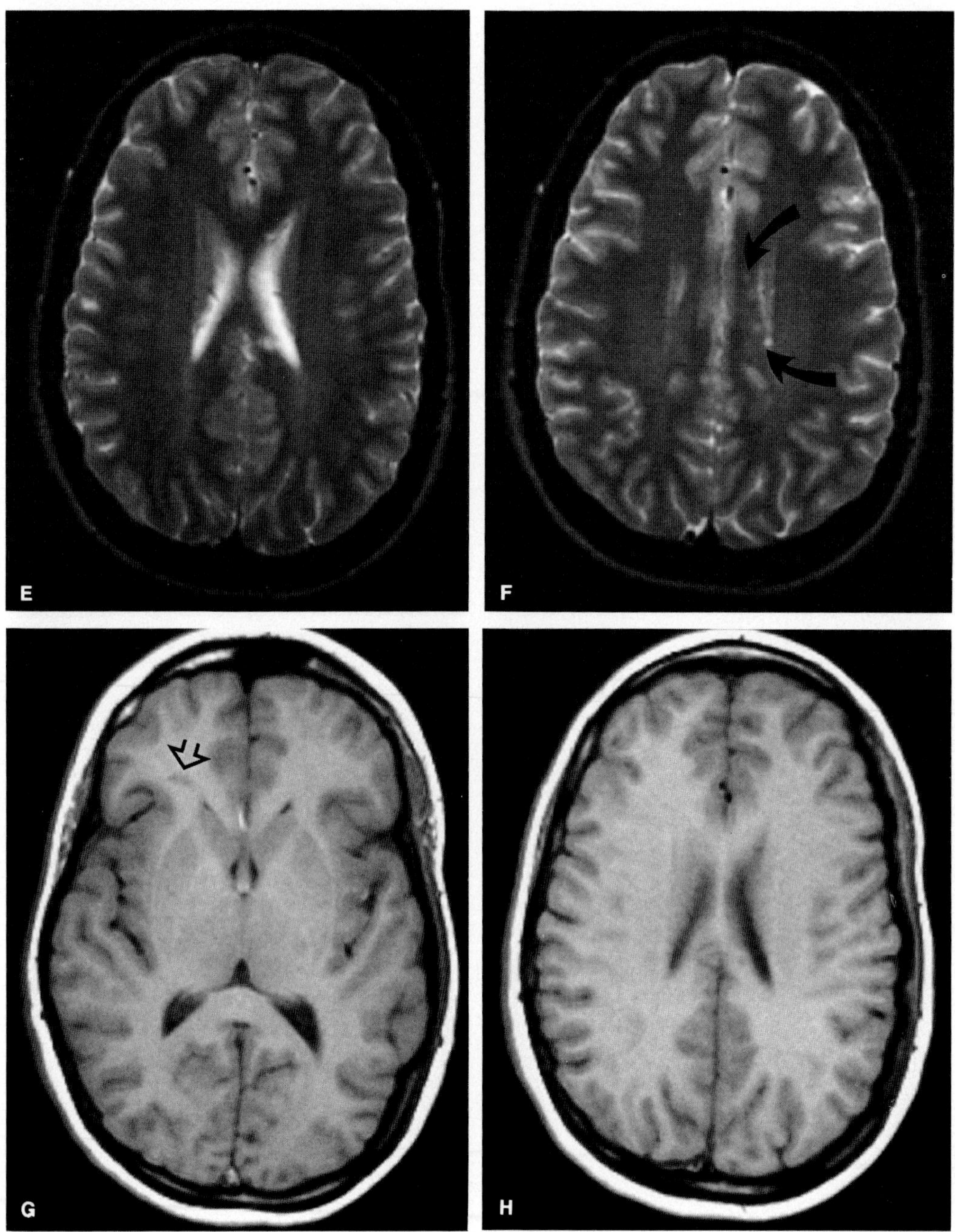

the first echo of the T2-weighted examination (*arrows in B*), with only two of these well seen on the second echo (*E*) and only one noted on the T1-weighted examination (*H*). The largest and most posterior of these also demonstrated contrast enhancement (*image not illustrated*). Immediately above the ventricular system, additional lesions are noted on the T2-weighted examination (*curved arrows in C and F*), which are not well visualized on the corresponding T1-weighted image (*I*). (*J and K*) On sagittal imaging with intermediate T2 weighting (TE=45 msec), both the callosal (*arrows in J*) and frontal (*open arrow in K*) lesions are well seen. A large enhancing cord lesion was also noted at the C2 level on the cervical spine MR examination (*not illustrated*).

DIAGNOSIS

Multiple sclerosis (MS)

DISCUSSION

MR is without question markedly superior to x-ray CT for the detection of lesions in MS. At this time, MR is the imaging modality of choice for diagnosis of MS. In an early study (1984) of 33 MS patients diagnosed with both CT and MR, CT was positive in only 15 of 33 patients while MR was positive in all.[1] Milder involvement of the brain by MS was typically not detectable on CT. The ab-

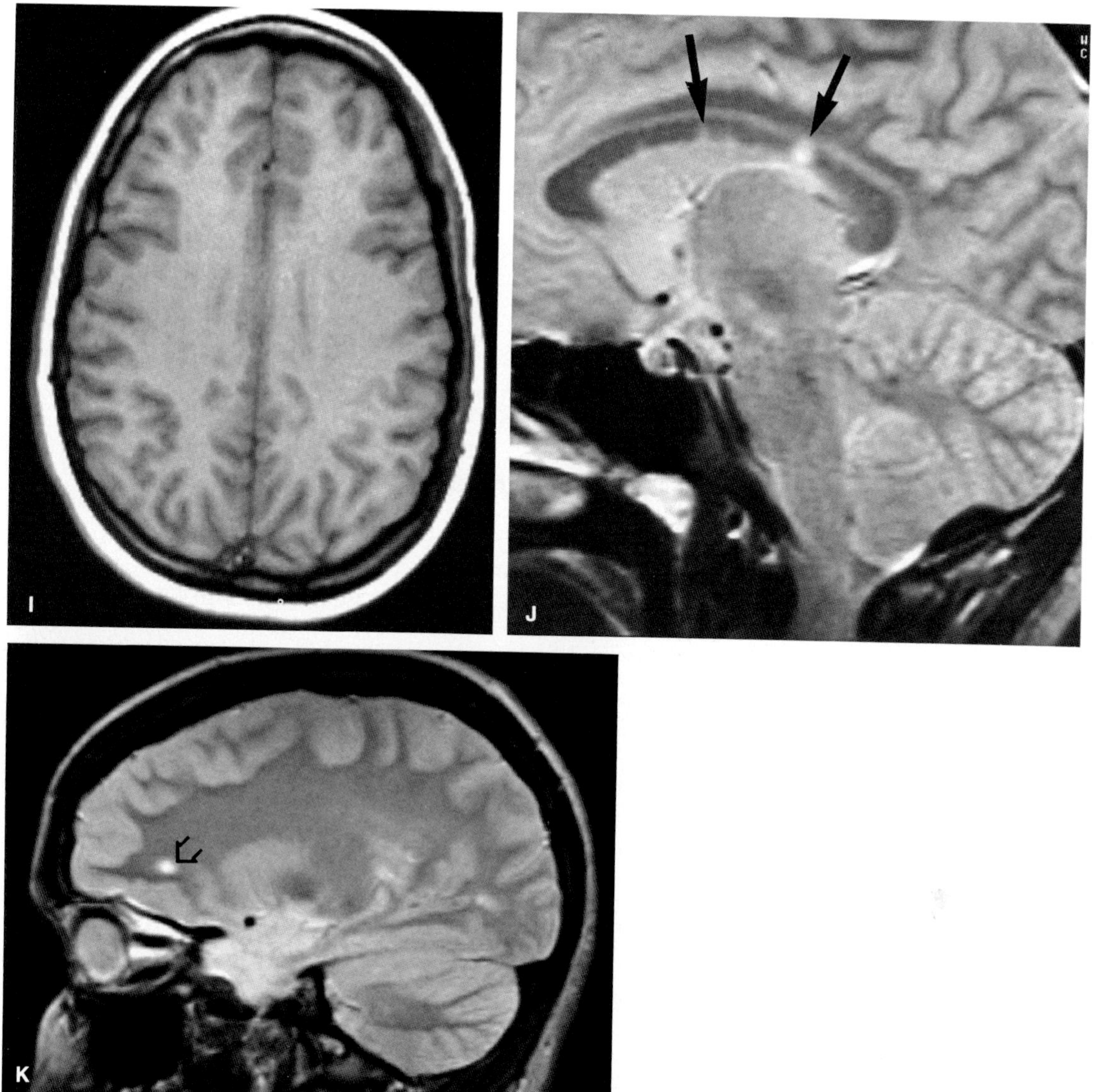

normalities noted on MR were also consistently more extensive than that seen on CT. MS lesions are well depicted on both proton density weighted and T2-weighted scans, with mild T2 weighting (TE = 40 to 50 msec) recommended for best overall lesion detection. Lesions adjacent to CSF in either the subarachnoid space or ventricular system can be obscured on more heavily T2-weighted scans because of the hyperintense signal from CSF. For example, in the case presented, four lesions can be noted in the corpus callosum on the intermediate T2-weighted scan (*B*), with at least two of these lesions no longer visible on the heavily T2-weighted image (*E*). T1-weighted images are typically inferior for detection of disease, unless both heavy T1 weighting is employed (eg, with inversion recovery technique) and the lesions themselves are surrounded completely by normal white matter. MS plaques demonstrate a wide range of abnormal relaxation times,[2] possibly due to differences in composition (eg, edema versus gliosis). Both the T1 and T2 relaxation times of *normal-appearing* white matter in MS are also higher than that of controls, possibly owing to the presence of microscopic disease involvement, although this abnormality cannot be typically demonstrated with confidence on visual inspection of the images.[3]

In early cases of MS, such as that presented, characteristic lesions must be carefully sought in the MR examination. The presence of three or more discrete punctate abnormalities, in a characteristic location such as the immediate periventricular white matter, corpus callosum, or brain stem, together with a compatible clinical history, permits diagnosis. The frontal white matter lesion in the clinical case presented is nonspecific for MS, whereas the callosal and periventricular lesions are characteristic. MS is principally a disease of white matter, with gray matter involvement seen both in smaller lesions at the tips of gyri (which spill over into gray matter) and in the caudate nucleus, globus pallidus, putamen, thalamus, and dentate nucleus. Contrast enhancement need not be present, with most plaques representing chronic lesions (without enhancement). Clinical symptoms can be principally due to spinal cord involvement, as in the present case, with the head MR examination serving for disease diagnosis.

The initial clinical presentation in MS may be that of sensory involvement without other definite findings. Evoked potentials may be normal. CSF findings include a slight to moderate mononuclear pleocytosis (30% of cases) and slightly elevated total protein (40% of cases). The presence of oligoclonal bands in the CSF is a more specific finding for MS. Two thirds of patients have onset between 20 and 40 years of age, with the incidence of disease higher in women (1.7:1). Although the etiology of the disease remains unclear, there is an increasing risk of disease with higher latitude, suggesting an environmental factor. Remission and relapse, with focal involvement of the brain, optic nerves, or spinal cord, are characteristic.

MR Technique

SE technique with intermediate T2 weighting (TE = 40 to 50 msec) is recommended for best overall brain lesion detection in MS.

Pitfalls in Image Interpretation

A head MR examination with negative findings does not completely rule out the possibility of MS, although it makes the diagnosis much less likely. Cases have been reported with a normal MR head examination, presumably because of either very early disease or dominant spinal cord involvement. If the MR head examination is normal in a patient with clinical evidence suggesting MS, MR of the spinal cord, and in particular the cervical cord, is recommended.

Clinical References

1. Runge VM, Price AC, Kirshner HS, et al. Magnetic resonance imaging of multiple sclerosis: a study of pulse-technique efficacy. AJR 1984;143:1015–1026.
2. Larsson HB, Frederiksen J, Kjaer L, et al. In vivo determination of T1 and T2 in the brain of patients with severe but stable multiple sclerosis. Magn Reson Med 1988;7:43–55.
3. Miller DH, Johnson G, Tofts PS, et al. Precise relaxation time measurements of normal-appearing white matter in inflammatory central nervous system disease. Magn Reson Med 1989;11:331–336.

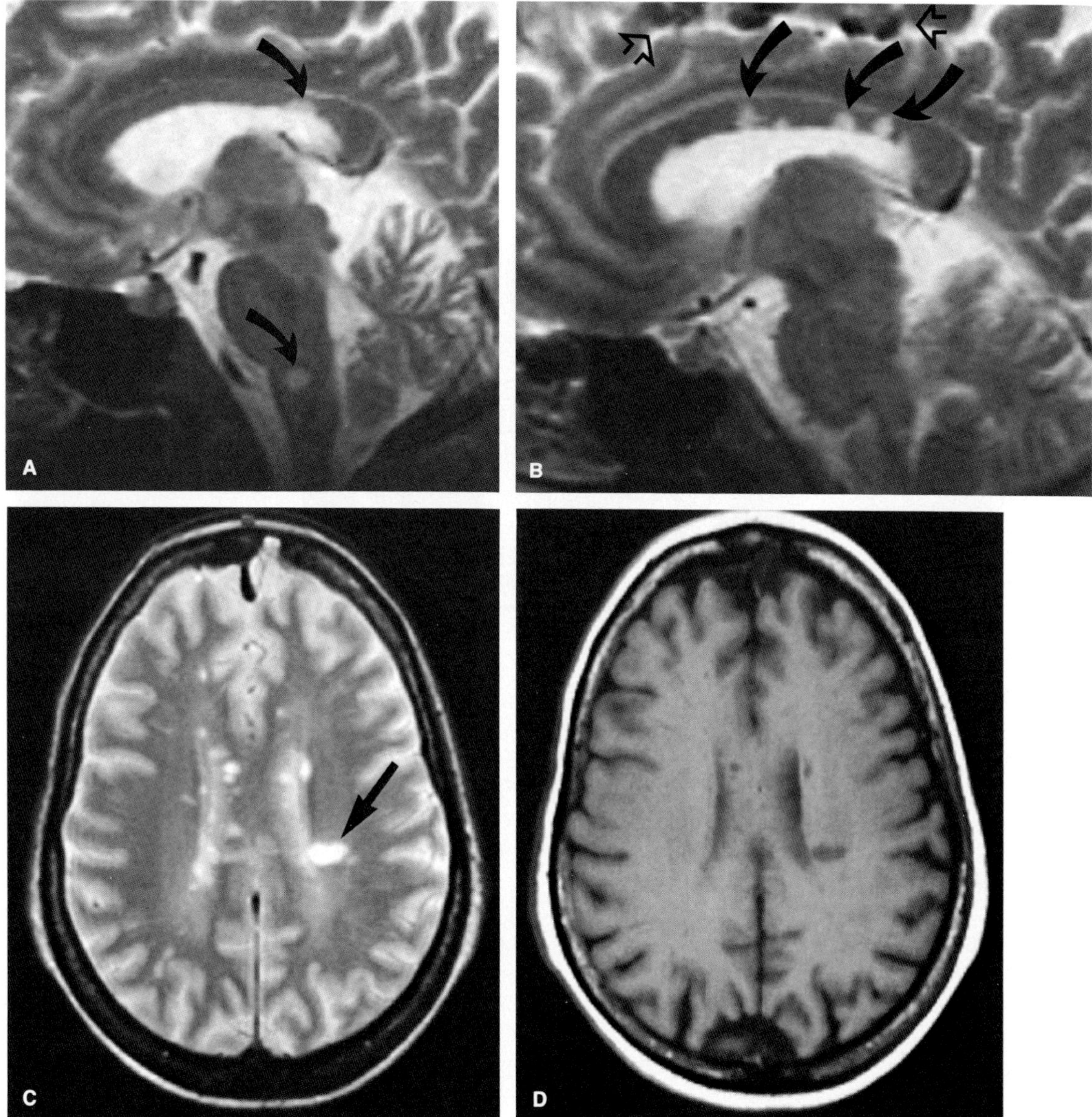

HISTORY

A 50-year-old woman with a 1-month history of tingling and burning first in the right foot, which subsequently spread up the right leg, and later in the left leg. She became unable to walk, although recently symptoms have abated slightly. MR was obtained. Subsequent tests included a brain stem auditory evoked potential, which was normal, and CSF for oligoclonal bands, which was positive.

FINDINGS

Midline (*A*) and parasagittal (*B*) thin-section (4-mm) T2-weighted images (TE = 90 msec) reveal a 0.5-mm–diameter lesion in the medulla as well as multiple callosal lesions (*curved arrows*). The latter are remarkable in that they involve the inner surface of the corpus callosum and appear to radiate toward the periphery. (*C*) An axial 4-mm section with intermediate T2 weighting (TE = 45 msec) depicts multiple punctate periventricular white matter and callosal lesions with asymmetric involvement of the right and left brain. One lesion in particular is ovoid in appearance (*arrow*). Comparison of precontrast (*D*) and postcontrast (*E*) 4-mm T1-weighted axial images reveals that several lesions enhance (*arrows in E*), although the majority do not. Some plaques enhance subtly, some intensely, some in part, some in whole. Incidental note is made of dense falx calcification (*open arrows in B*) and mild cortical atrophy (*D and E*).

DIAGNOSIS

Multiple sclerosis (active disease)

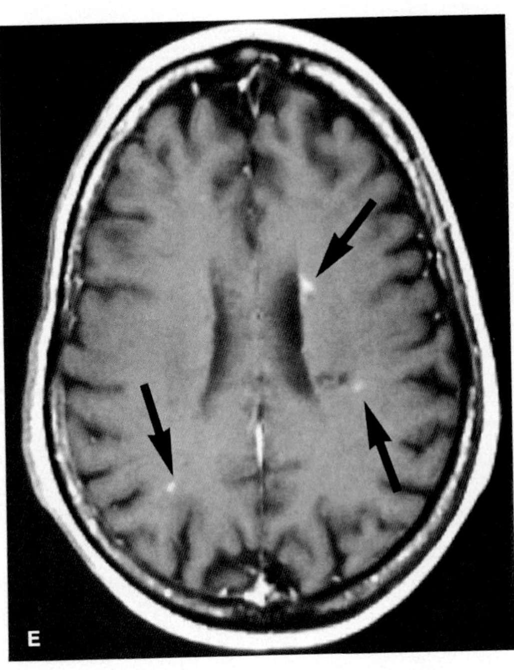

DISCUSSION

It was elected to start the patient on high-dose IV methylprednisolone (Solu-Medrol), with subsequent tapering. By day 3, there was improvement in both lower extremity strength and gait.

Gadolinium chelate–enhanced MR is more sensitive than high–iodine-dose CT for demonstration of active multiple sclerosis (MS) lesions with disruption of the blood–brain barrier.[1] Enhancement is best demonstrated on immediate postcontrast scans. Serial MR studies have demonstrated that most enhancing lesions are asymptomatic, with persistence of enhancement in only 12 of 54 lesions by 3 to 5 weeks and in no lesions by 6 months.[2] Most importantly, blood–brain barrier disruption as reflected by contrast enhancement appears to be a consistent marker of *new* MS lesions, with significant implications for monitoring of therapeutic trials. Contrast-enhanced MR specifically also appears more sensitive for the determination of clinical disease activity than clinical examination.[3]

In a recent study of MS patients undergoing high-dose IV methylprednisolone therapy,[4] the suppression of lesion enhancement (as depicted by MR) appears to correlate with clinical improvement. Temporal studies have also examined the characteristic change in size of new lesions (on unenhanced T2-weighted imaging), with maximum diameter achieved by approximately 4 weeks, followed by gradual shrinkage.[5] The typical scattering of small, punctate white matter lesions in chronic disease thus likely represents the accumulated residua of many active episodes and lesions.

In the interest of shortening examination, a 192 × 256* matrix was used for both the sagittal and axial T2-weighted sequences in this case. Given a TR of 2500 msec and a single data acquisition, the scan time was thus shortened from 12.8 minutes (for a 256 × 256 matrix) to 8 minutes. Since the field-of-view (FOV) was not changed, the S/N also improved by 15% (there is more tissue and thus greater S/N in each voxel of the 192 × 256 matrix image). Two compromises are made with the use of a reduced imaging matrix. First, in-plane spatial resolution suffers. In this instance with an FOV of 25 cm, a 256 × 256 matrix has a pixel resolution of 1 × 1 mm as compared with 1.3 × 1 mm with a 192 × 256 matrix. This difference is subtle and often not appreciable clinically. Of possible greater concern is the second compromise, the presence of an increased Gibbs phenomenon, or truncation artifacts. This occurs because of the finite number of spatial frequencies used in image sampling. In MR head imaging, the thin line of subcutaneous fat often produces such artifacts, which become less noticeable as the matrix size is increased, for example, from a 192 × 256 to a 256 × 256 matrix. The effect is also diminished as T2 weighting increases, which reduces the signal intensity of fat and thus the sharpness of the edge or interface between fat and adjacent tissue. Truncation lines are difficult to see on the 90-msec (*A and B*), as compared with the 45-msec, T2-weighted images. Given

**Number of phase encoding versus number of frequency encoding or readout steps.*

the decrease in scan time and the increase in S/N (important because of the use of thin sections), the increased truncation artifacts appear to be an acceptable compromise.

Thin-section (4 mm, 30% gap) T2-weighted imaging was used in both the sagittal and axial planes. Early clinical MR experience proved that the use of thin sections substantially increased lesion detection in patients with small, low-contrast lesions[6]—specifically diseases like MS. For detection of such lesions, partial volume effects are critical and minimized with thin slices. Sagittal sections are particularly important for the visualization of MS lesions in the periventricular region and corpus callosum. In one study of 50 MS patients using T2-weighted SE technique, 858 lesions were noted in axial imaging as compared with 1196 in sagittal imaging.[7] Axial imaging, however, proved superior for detection of brain stem lesions. The differences in lesion detection according to imaging plane can be explained by partial volume effects, the orientation of certain anatomic structures (eg, the corpus callosum), and the longer diameter of MS lesions in the axial plane. Of perhaps even greater significance, in 3 patients, lesions were detected only on sagittal imaging. Detection of corpus callosal lesions *characteristic* of MS, which specifically involve the inferior aspect of the corpus callosum with radiation from the ventricular surface, is optimal on sagittal imaging. In this manner, sagittal T2-weighted imaging also appears to improve the specificity of MR for the diagnosis of MS and the differentiation of MS from other periventricular white matter diseases.[8] Although long TE (90 msec) images are illustrated in the case presented, the prior discussion pertains in particular to detection of lesions on mildly T2-weighted images where CSF is isointense with normal brain. A standardized protocol for MR head examinations, when MS is a clinical question, is thus strongly recommended. This should include both sagittal and axial thin-section mild and moderately T2-weighted images. Both greater lesion detectability and improved clinical correlation with patient disability and function have been demonstrated[9] with the use of a standardized protocol.

Clinical References

1. Grossman RI, Gonzalez-Scarano F, Atlas SW, et al. Multiple sclerosis: gadolinium enhancement in MR imaging. Radiology 1986;161:721–725.
2. Miller DH, Rudge P, Johnson G, et al. Serial gadolinium enhanced magnetic resonance imaging in multiple sclerosis. Brain 1988;111:927–939.
3. Grossman RI, Braffman BH, Brorson JR, et al. Multiple sclerosis: serial study of gadolinium-enhanced MR imaging. Radiology 1988;169:117–122.
4. Burnham JA, Wright RR, Dreisbach J, Murray RS. The effect of high-dose steroids on MRI gadolinium enhancement in acute demyelinating lesions. Neurology 1991;41:1349–1354.
5. Willoughby EW, Grochowski E, Li DK, et al. Serial magnetic resonance scanning in multiple sclerosis: a second prospective study in relapsing patients. Ann Neurol 1989; 25:43–49.
6. Bradley WG, Glenn BJ. The effect of variation in slice thickness and interslice gap on MR lesion detection. AJNR 1987;8:1057–1062.
7. Wilms G, Marchal G, Kersschot E, et al. Axial vs sagittal T2-weighted brain MR images in the evaluation of multiple sclerosis. J Comput Assist Tomogr 1991;15:359–364.
8. Gean-Marton AD, Vezina LG, Marton KI, et al. Abnormal corpus callosum: a sensitive and specific indicator of multiple sclerosis. Radiology 1991;180:215–221.
9. Truyen L, Gheuens J, Van de Vyver FL, et al. Improved correlation of magnetic resonance imaging (MRI) with clinical status in multiple sclerosis (MS) by use of an extensive standardized imaging protocol. J Neurol Sci 1990;96:173–182.

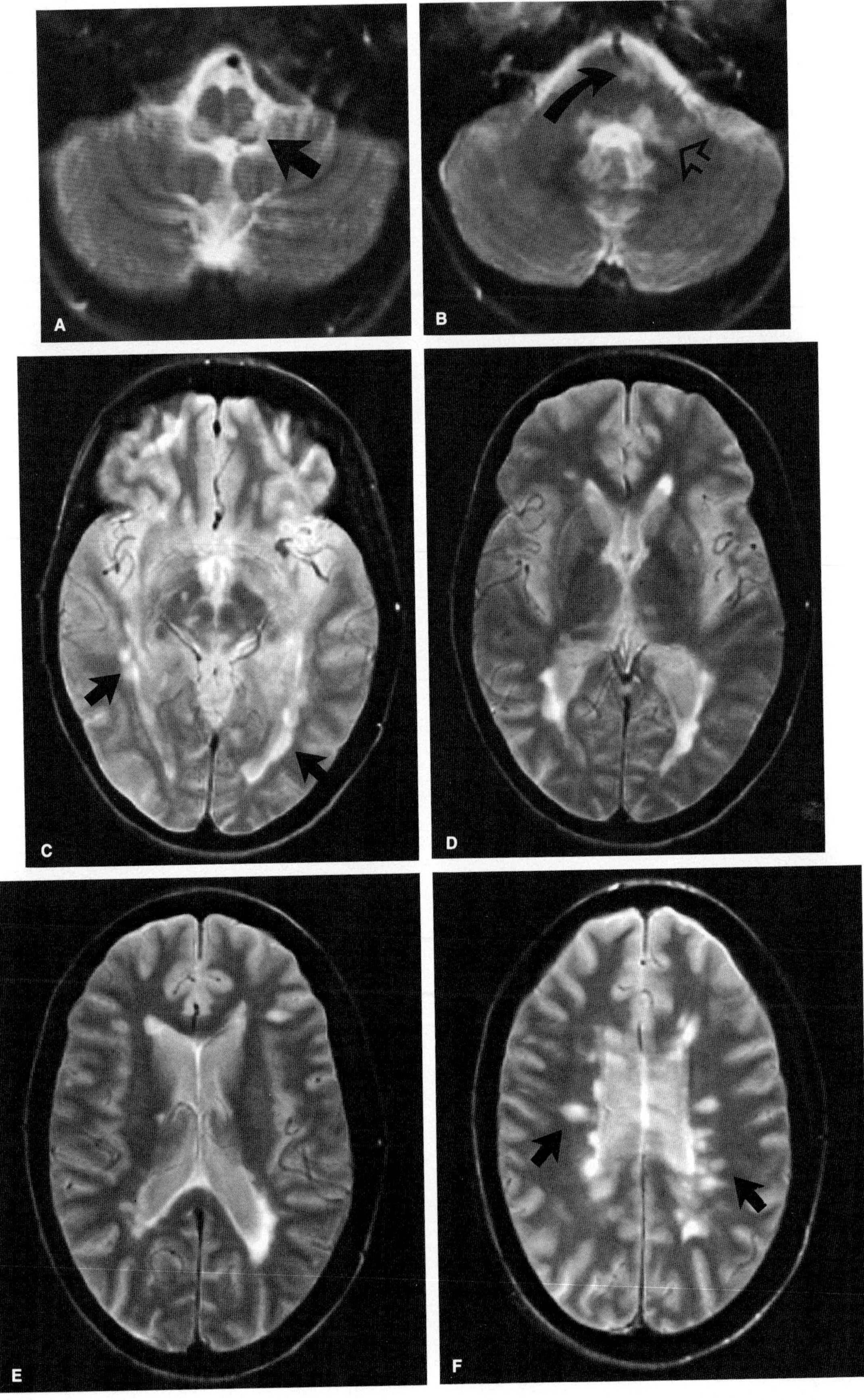
A
B
C
D
E
F

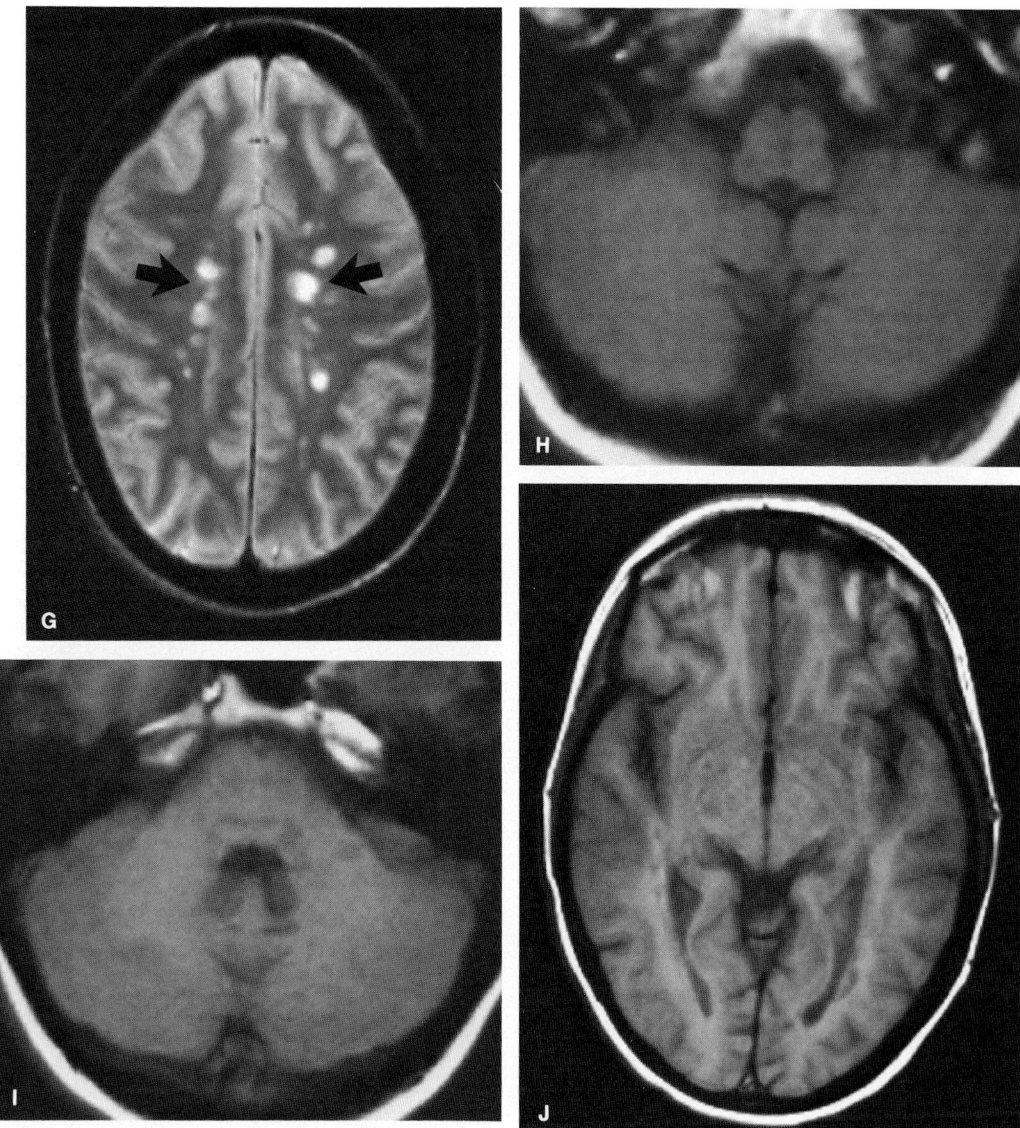

HISTORY

Two patients, a man and a woman, both 38 years old. Each has intermittent weakness and numbness of both the upper and lower extremities, as well as problems with balance

FINDINGS

Axial T2-weighted (*A and B:* TE = 90 msec; *C to G:* TE = 45 msec) and corresponding T1-weighted (*H to N*) images, as well as sagittal T1-weighted images (*O and P*), are presented from the MR examination of the first patient. On the T2-weighted images, which best depict the full extent of disease, multiple punctate high-signal-intensity lesions are noted. These are located primarily in white matter. Lesions can be specifically identified in the medulla (*arrow in A*), pons (*curved arrow in B*), middle cerebellar peduncle (*open arrow in B*), and in the immediate periventricular white matter, in particular, adjacent to the occipital horns (*arrows in C*) and lateral ventricles (*arrows in F and G*). The disease involvement adjacent to the ventricular atria is somewhat confluent in nature, particularly on the left. Many of these lesions can be identified on the T1-weighted scans, with abnormal low signal intensity relative to surrounding normal white matter. In reality, however, only the periventricular and supraventricular lesions are well seen on T1-weighted images. Certain lesions also seem to have a slightly hyperintense border (*curved arrows in M and N*) on T1-weighted images, an appearance characteristic of this disease. Sagittal T1-weighted images (*O and P*) identify lesions in both the corpus callosum (*arrows in O*), which involve specifically the inner surface of this structure, and immediate periventricular white matter (*curved arrows in P*).

In the second patient, similar punctate abnormalities

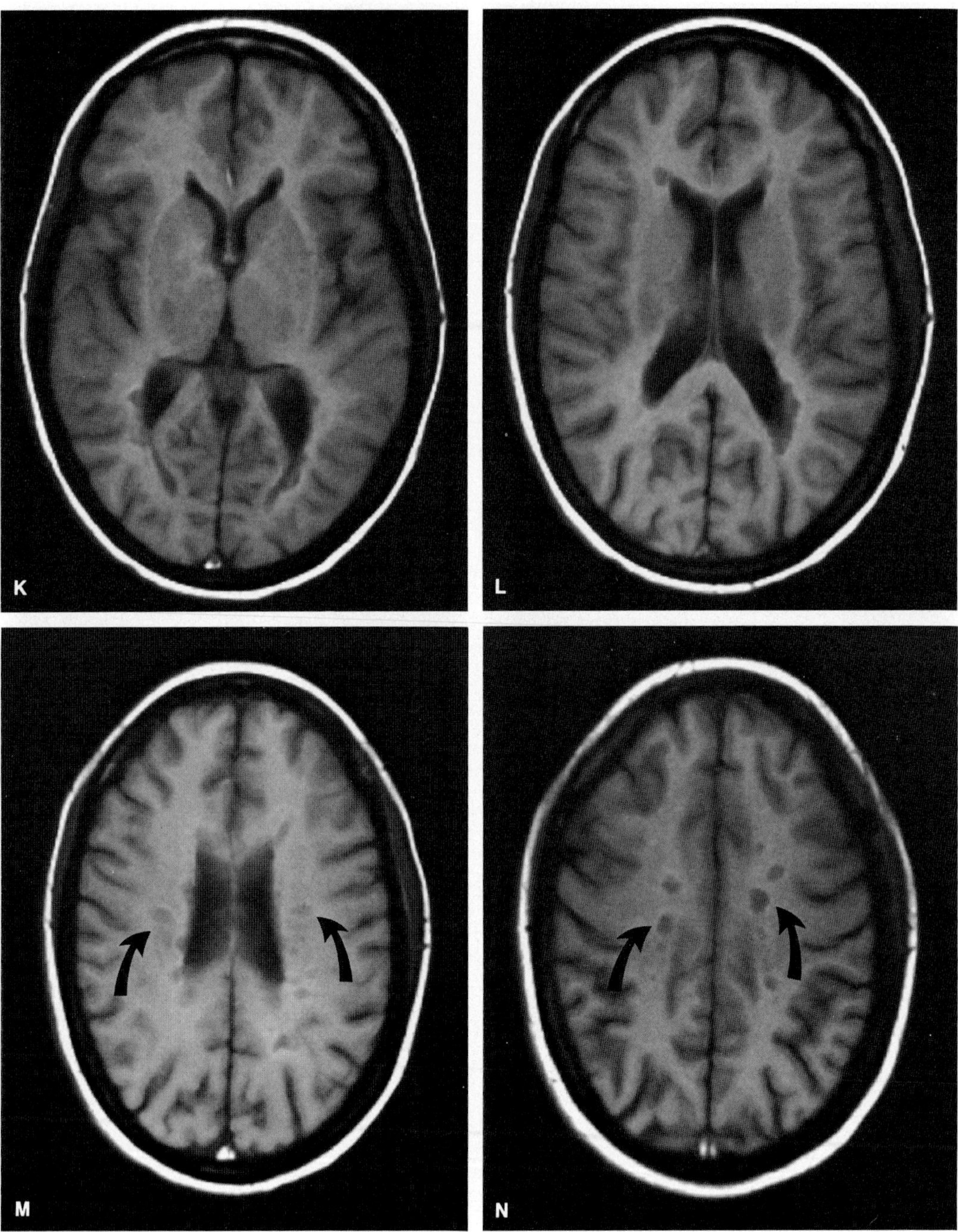

are identified, on both the first (TE = 45 msec) (*Q*) and second (TE = 90 msec) (*R*) echo of the T2-weighted examination, adjacent to the temporal horns (*arrows in Q*). The specific relation of these lesions relative to the temporal horns is difficult to ascertain on the first echo of the T2-weighted examination (*Q*), since CSF is isointense with gray matter. On *R,* however, the immediate periventricular nature of the lesions is well seen. (*S*) Both lesions (*arrows*) appear hypointense to white matter on the corresponding T1-weighted image.

In both patients, all the MR images depicted are precontrast, with no abnormal enhancement noted on the postcontrast examinations (*not shown*).

DIAGNOSIS

Multiple sclerosis (MS)

DISCUSSION

The most well known criteria for clinical disease classification in MS is that of McAlpine.[1] In "definite" disease, a history of transient neurologic symptoms characteristic specifically of MS is present, together with one or more documented relapses. In "probable" MS, there is a history of one or more disease attacks, with clinical evidence

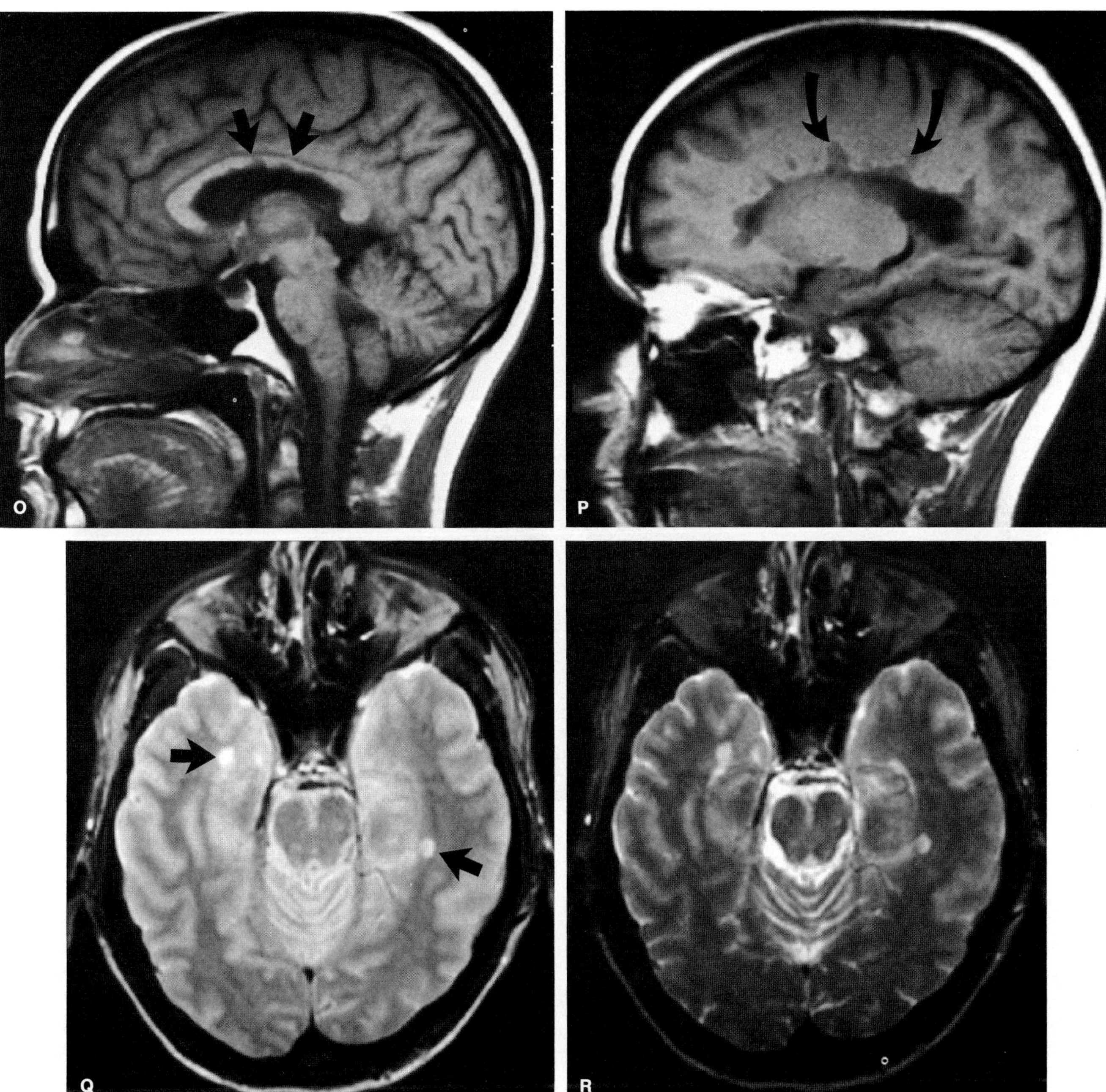

of multiple lesions during the original attack. In "possible" MS, the history is similar to that of "probable" disease, but there are unusual features or a paucity of findings. This category also includes patients with progressive paraplegia in early middle age without evidence of remission, in whom other possible causes of paralysis have been ruled out, including spondylosis, motor neuron disease, and spinal cord tumor. A more rigid diagnostic criterion has been described by Schumacher and colleagues[2] for use in therapeutic trials. This criterion was created specifically for the identification of clinically definite MS. By history or examination, there must be evidence of two or more separate CNS lesions. Clinical signs must be those of white matter involvement. Two episodes must have occurred lasting at least 24 hours in duration and separated by at least 1 month. Arbitrary age limits were also set for between 10 and 50 years.

The ability of MR to correctly predict the diagnosis of MS in suspect patients was examined in a recent prospective 2-year study.[3] In patients who had developed clinically definite MS on follow-up, the initial MR was strongly suggestive of MS in 84%. Of those patients with clinically definite MS, 95% had at least one abnormality characteristic of MS on the original MR. MR was shown to

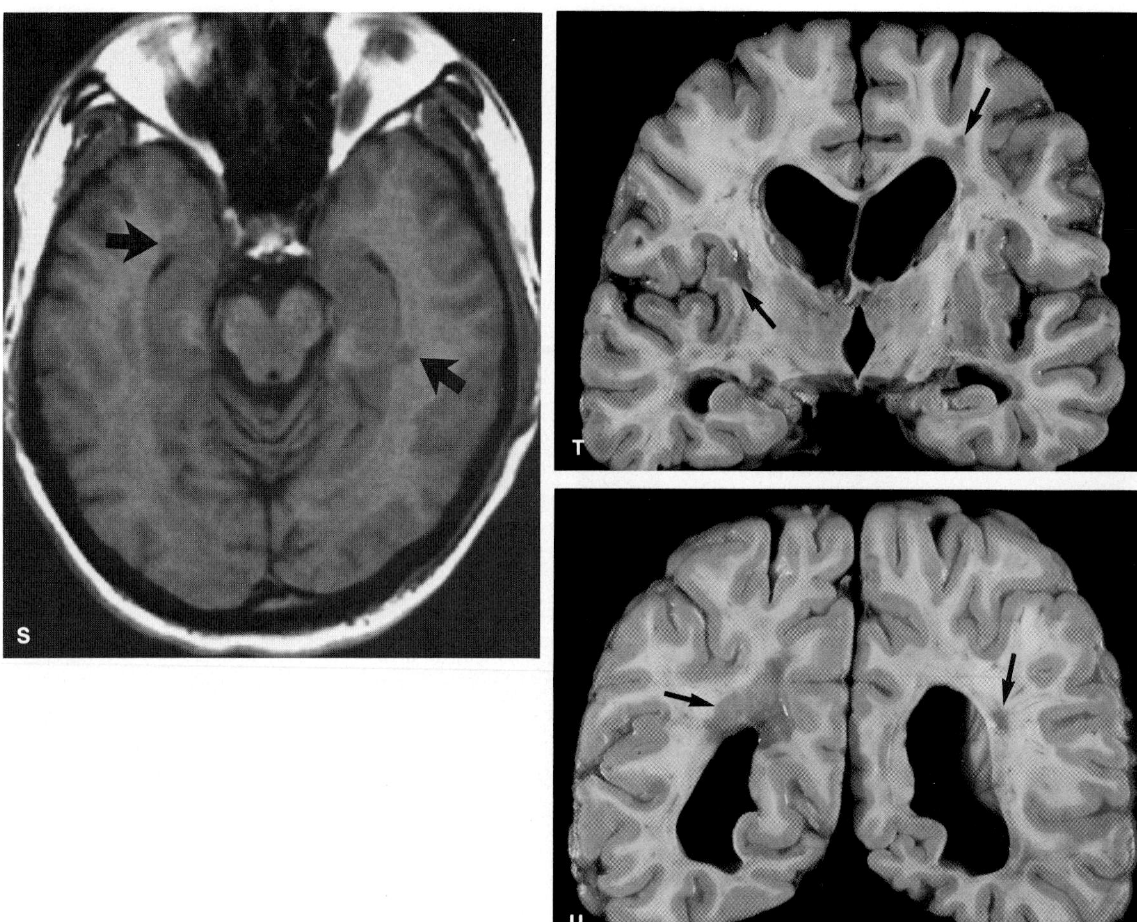

be the best paraclinical test for the detection of MS and for predicting the diagnosis of clinically definite MS. The sensitivity of MR was greater than that of CSF oligoclonal bands, visual evoked potentials, somatosensory evoked potentials, and CT.

Serial study of patients with chronic progressive MS[4] has demonstrated evidence of active lesions in 51%, despite disease inactivity by clinical assessment. These results suggest that the clinical evolution of MS, from a disease of relapses and remissions to that of chronic progression, does not represent a fundamental change in the disease process. Serial MR also proved in this study to be much more sensitive in the detection of disease activity than clinical examination.

A greater number of MS plaques can be visualized in the brain by MR than even by gross pathologic examination.[5] However, T2-weighted scans may fail to detect lesions in certain parts of the brain, particularly the cerebral cortex, thalamus, and hindbrain. Partial volume effects can make such lesions difficult to identify. The cases examined fell into two distinct groups, one in which there was good correlation between histologic examination and MR, and the second in which extensive signal intensity abnormalities were noted on MR, but only small plaques were seen on histologic examination. Changes in vascular permeability, seen in both active and chronic plaques, could account for the extensive abnormalities observed on MR in the latter group. In three cases, both the head MR and gross pathologic examination of the brain were negative for the presence of disease, emphasizing the importance of imaging the cervical spine.

Pitfalls in Image Interpretation

Although the MR images in the case presented should be considered diagnostic for MS, many other diseases can mimic this pattern and should be considered in the differential diagnosis. The most common dilemma is the differentiation of ischemic or gliotic lesions in deep white matter from MS. Such lesions tend to be symmetric in distribution and are often confluent, unlike MS plaques.[6] Despite the experience of the interpreter, incidental periventricular white matter foci can be misinterpreted as MS plaques.[7] However, MR does carry a high degree of specificity if clinical information is available, particularly age and sex. The location of lesions can aid in disease differentiation, with MS plaques predominantly in the subependymal region. Vascular white matter lesions, however, tend to occur in the watershed region between the superficial middle cerebral artery branches and deep perforating long medullary vessels. Infratentorial lesions are also much more common in MS.

Although both vascular lesions and MS plaques are best identified on T2-weighted images, and somewhat indistinguishable, T1-weighted images may aid in differentiation.[8] MS plaques, as illustrated in this case, tend to be hypointense on T1-weighted images, with a more or less distinct border. Ischemic or gliotic foci tend not to be well visualized on T1-weighted images. Cavitated lacunar infarcts or large, dilated perivascular spaces could, however, be confused on T1-weighted images with MS plaques.

When isolated or multiple periventricular lesions are seen on MR, other differential diagnostic considerations include neurosarcoidosis, primary CNS lymphoma, acute disseminated encephalomyelitis, and neurobrucellosis. Cases of systemic lupus erythematosus with multiple white matter lesions mimicking MS have also been described. In this instance, however, the lesions typically do not involve the immediate periventricular white matter.

Pathologic Correlate

(*T and U*) Two coronal postmortem brain sections from a different patient with MS are presented for comparison. There is ventriculomegaly. Multiple large lesions (*arrows*), which vary in shape and size and show a predilection for the periventricular area, are noted in the white matter. These "plaques" are brown or gray in coloration, due to demyelination.

Clinical References

1. McAlpine's multiple sclerosis, 2nd ed. Mathews WB, ed. New York, Churchill Livingstone, 1991:189–193.
2. Schumacher GA, Beebe G, Kibler RF, et al. Problems of experimental trials of therapy in multiple sclerosis. Ann NY Acad Sci 1965;122:552–568.
3. Lee KH, Hashimoto SA, Hooge JP, et al. Magnetic resonance imaging of the head in the diagnosis of multiple sclerosis: a prospective 2-year follow-up with comparison of clinical evaluation, evoked potentials, oligoclonal banding, and CT. Neurology 1991;41:657–660.
4. Koopmans RA, Li DKB, Oger JJF, et al. Chronic progressive multiple sclerosis: serial magnetic resonance brain imaging over six months. Ann Neurol 1989;26:248–256.
5. Newcombe J, Hawkins CP, Henderson CL, et al. Histopathology of multiple sclerosis lesions detected by magnetic resonance imaging in unfixed postmortem central nervous system tissue. Brain 1991;114:1013–1023.
6. Runge VM, Price AC, Kirshner HS, et al. The evaluation of multiple sclerosis by magnetic resonance imaging. Radiographics 1986;6:203–212.
7. Yetkin FZ, Haughton VM, Papke RA, et al. Multiple sclerosis: specificity of MR for diagnosis. Radiology 1991;178:447–451.
8. Uhlenbrock D, Sehlen S. The value of T1-weighted images in the differentiation between MS, white matter lesions, and subcortical arteriosclerotic encephalopathy (SAE). Neuroradiology 1989;31:203–212.

(T *and* U *courtesy of Daron G. Davis, MD.*)

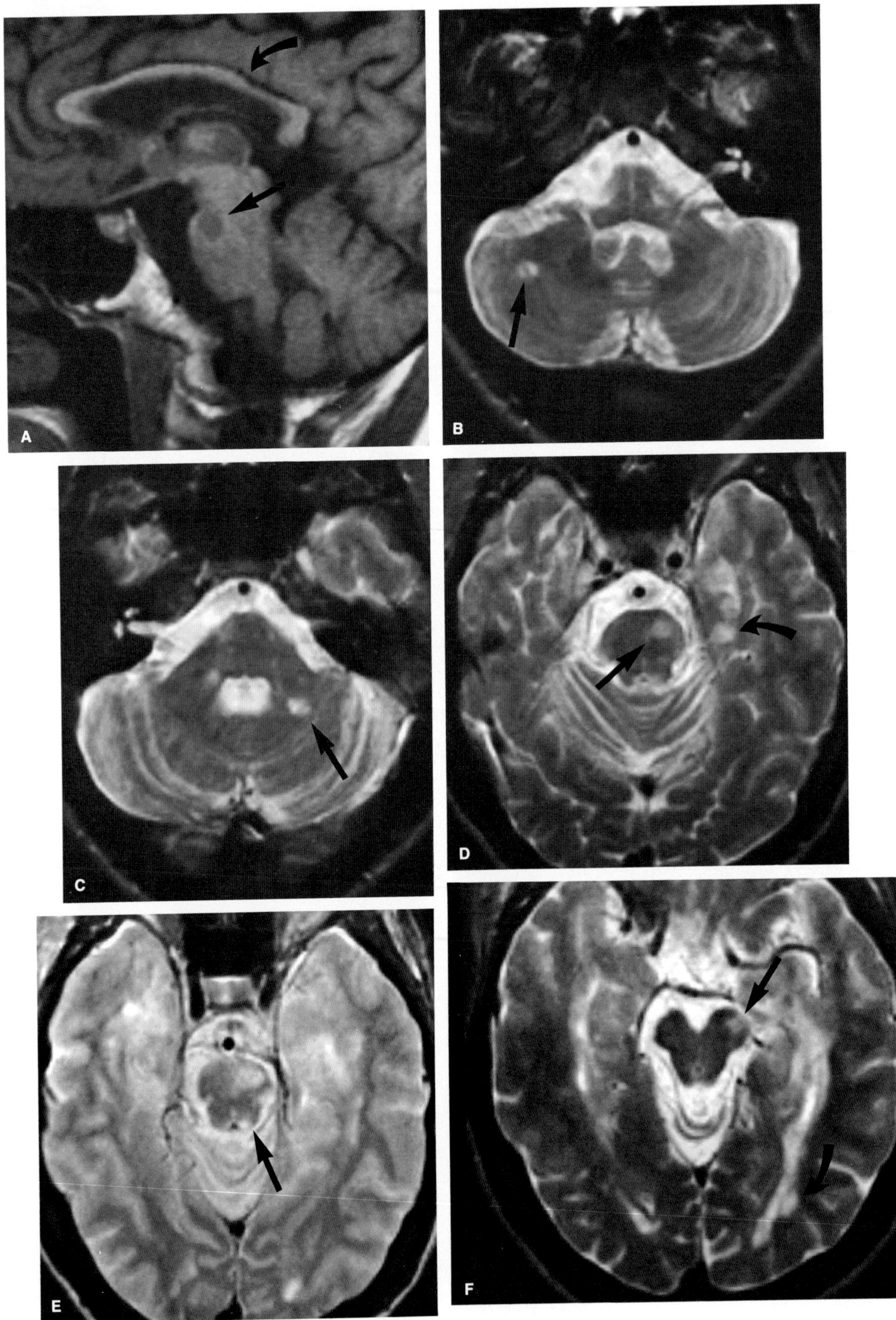
A
B
C
D
E
F

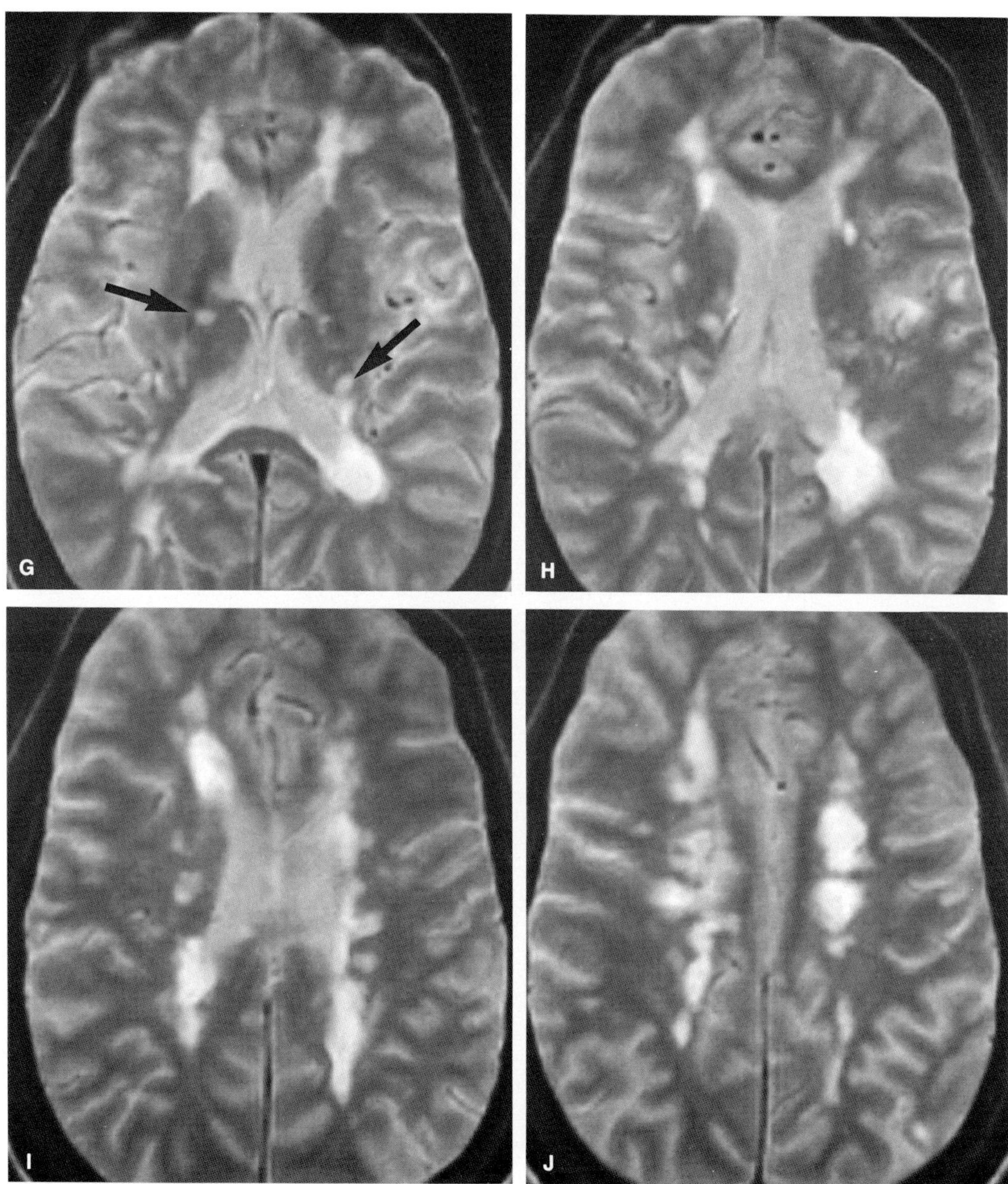

HISTORY

A 32-year-old woman with a 10-year history of disability. The patient initially presented with fatigue and unsteadiness. Clinical exacerbation of disease led to two previous hospital admissions. Ataxia of all extremities was noted 3 years before the current admission, with the patient becoming wheelchair-bound 1 year later. The patient now presents with increasing numbness of the extremities and urinary incontinence. However, neurologic examination does not reveal evidence of a new focal brain lesion.

FINDINGS

(*A*) Thinning of the corpus callosum (*curved arrow*) and a pontine lesion (*arrow*) can be noted on this midline sagittal T1-weighted image. (*B to K*) T2-weighted axial images (*B to D, F:* TE=90 msec; *E, G to K:* TE=45 msec) reveal multiple bilateral, predominantly punctate lesions in an asymmetric distribution (right versus left), principally involving white matter. Lesions are noted in the following specific regions (this list is not all-inclusive): right cerebellar hemisphere (*arrow in B*), middle cerebellar peduncle (*arrow in C*), pons (*arrow in D*),

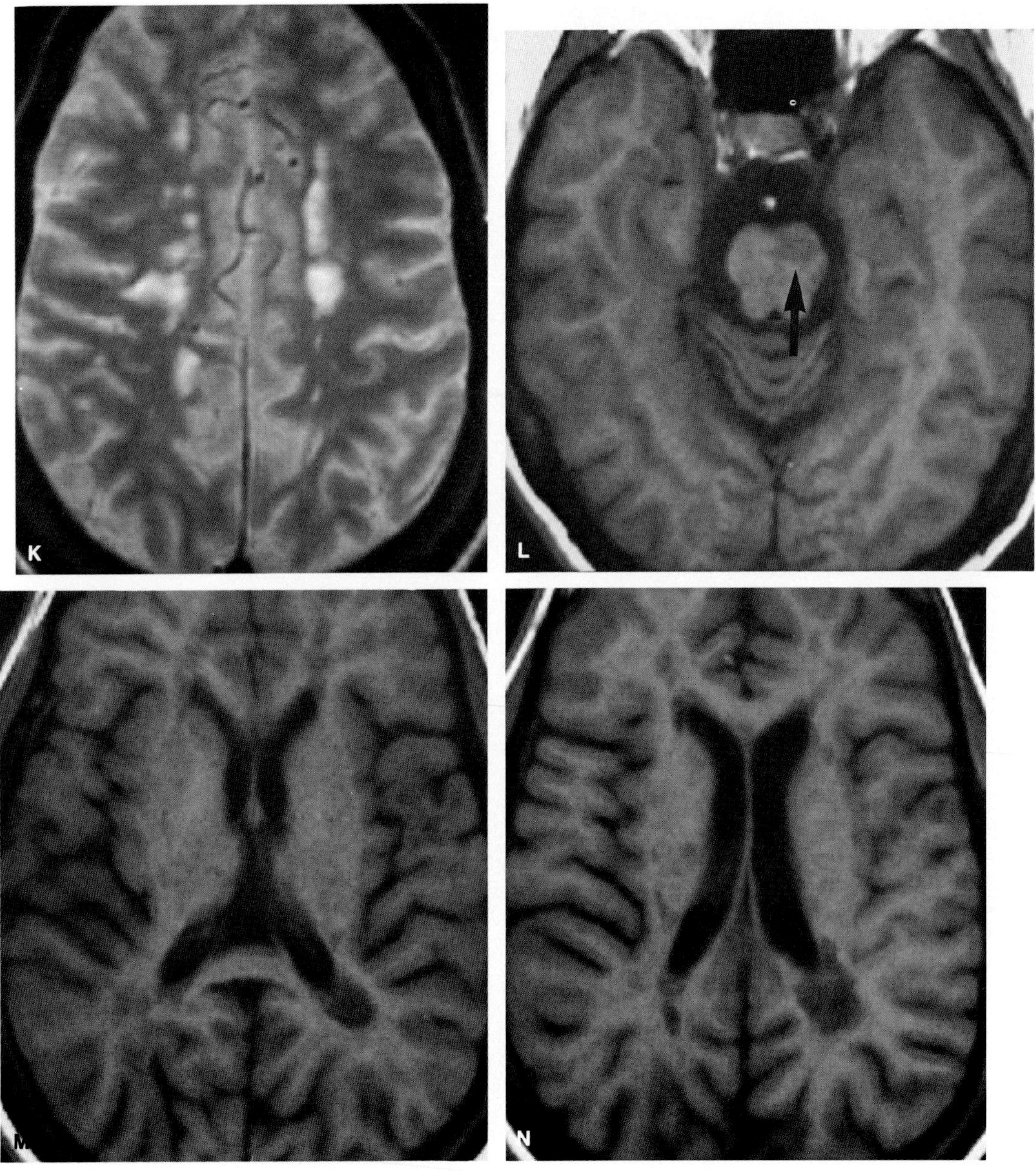

temporal lobe (immediately adjacent to the temporal horn [*curved arrow in D*]), left superior colliculus (*arrow in E*), left cerebral peduncle (*arrow in F*), left occipital lobe (immediately adjacent to the occipital horn [*curved arrow in F*]), and internal capsule (*arrows in G*). The periventricular white matter and centrum semiovale (*H to K*) are involved by a very large number of lesions. Because of the large number of plaques immediately adjacent to the lateral ventricles, the disease appears in part confluent in this region. The scan with intermediate T2 weighting (TE = 45 msec) best depicted lesions adjacent to CSF spaces (*E and G to K*) and is thus illustrated in these instances. There is a generalized loss in contrast between gray and white matter on the T2-weighted images.

(*L to Q*) Some of the lesions can be noted on the T1-weighted precontrast examination, as low-signal-intensity abnormalities compared with surrounding normal brain, in particular, the pontine and periventricular abnormalities. However, lesion recognition is best on the T2-weighted examination. The pontine lesion (*arrow in L*) in particular is poorly visualized on the T1-weighted examination, with only slightly lower signal intensity as compared with surrounding brain. Mild diffuse cortical atrophy is also seen on the T1-weighted sequences. No abnormal enhancement was noted on postcontrast T1-weighted scans (*not shown*).

DIAGNOSIS

Multiple sclerosis (chronic disease)

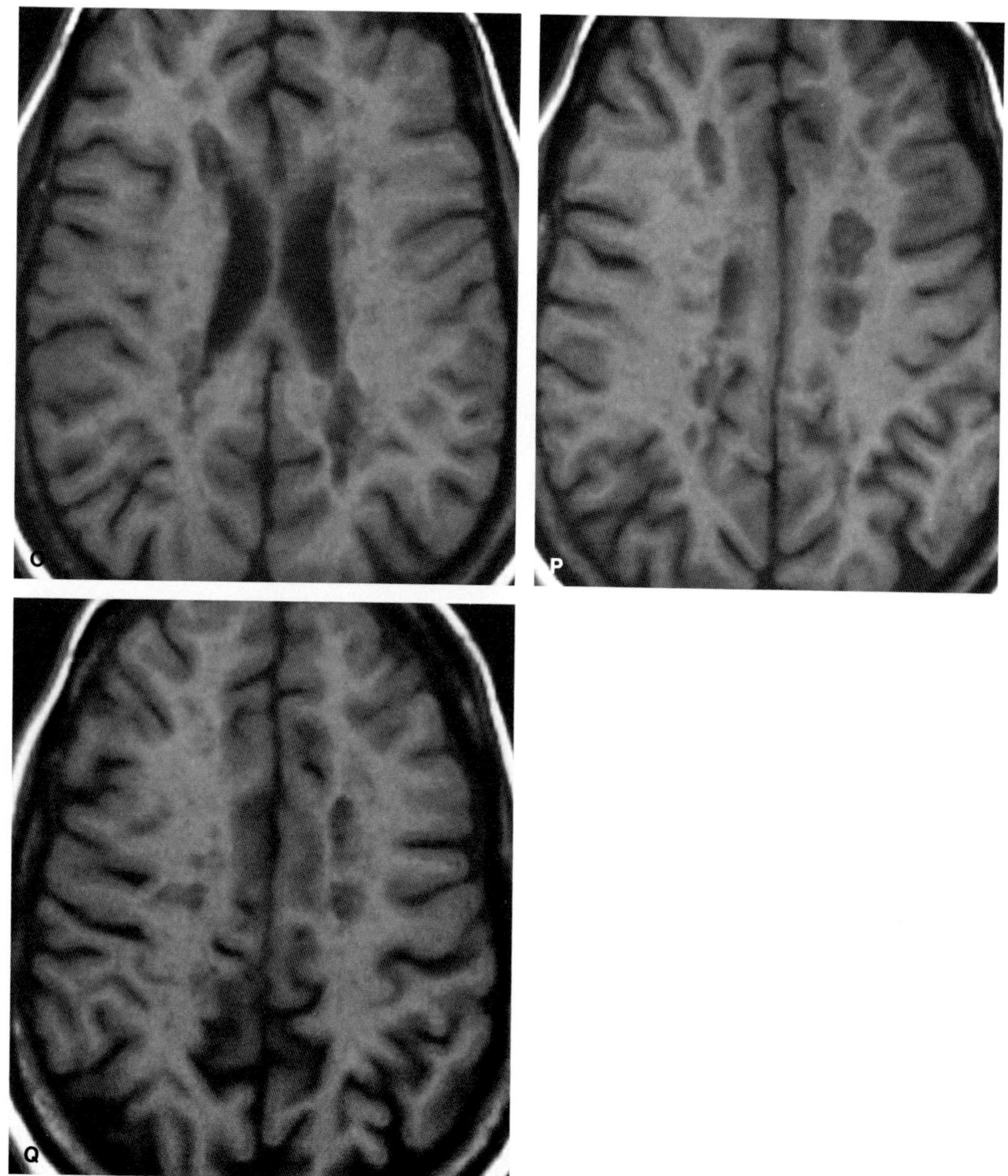

DISCUSSION

In chronic MS, multiple plaques (often confluent) can be noted in the immediate periventricular white matter, brain stem, and spinal cord. Diffuse brain atrophy and ventricular enlargement (with thinning of the corpus callosum) are common. Individual lesions are small (1 to 2 cm), with larger plaques due to confluent disease.

The clinical symptoms noted in this patient are characteristic of MS. Weakness and numbness are the presenting complaints in about half of patients. Involvement of the extremities varies from poor control to spasticity and ataxia. Bladder dysfunction (hesitation, frequency, urgency, and incontinence) occurs with spinal cord involvement. The absence of lesion contrast enhancement in this patient is consistent with the neurologic findings.

The specific sites of involvement described in this case all represent areas commonly involved by plaques in MS, but also include sites typically not involved with ischemic white matter disease. Perhaps the only exception to this is the periventricular, internal capsule, and supraventricular involvement, although the punctate nature of the lesions and asymmetry in distribution (from side to side) are clues to the nature of the disease in this patient. The loss of gray–white matter contrast on the T2-weighted examination is a nonspecific sign of diffuse disease, although common in MS. Regardless, given the patient's age, ischemic white matter disease should be considered of extremely low likelihood in the differential diagnosis.

Recurrent inflammatory episodes may be the prelude to the irreversible demyelination and gliosis seen in chronic MS.[1] In chronic progressive MS, a subcategory of disease with fulminant and unremitting progression, greater confluency of lesions and higher numbers of infratentorial plaques have been demonstrated on MR.[2]

The occurrence of relapses is the most characteristic clinical feature of MS. Relapses vary greatly in site of involvement, frequency, duration, severity, and residual dysfunction. The most common form of disease is relapsing (for 10 to 20 years), followed by insidious progression.

Pitfalls in Image Interpretation

Long-standing ischemic white matter disease and chronic MS can appear similar on MR. Patient age (young), asymmetry (right versus left hemisphere) of disease, and characteristic areas of involvement (which are not commonly seen with ischemic disease, ie, cervical cord, cerebellar hemispheres, middle cerebellar peduncle, colliculi, and temporal lobe) improve the certainty with which a diagnosis of MS can be made.

Clinical References

1. Koopmans RA, Li DK, Oger JJ, et al. The lesion of multiple sclerosis: imaging of acute and chronic stages. Neurology 1989;39:959–963.
2. Koopman RA, Li DK, Grochowski E, et al. Benign versus chronic progressive multiple sclerosis: magnetic resonance imaging features. Ann Neurol 1989;25:74–81.

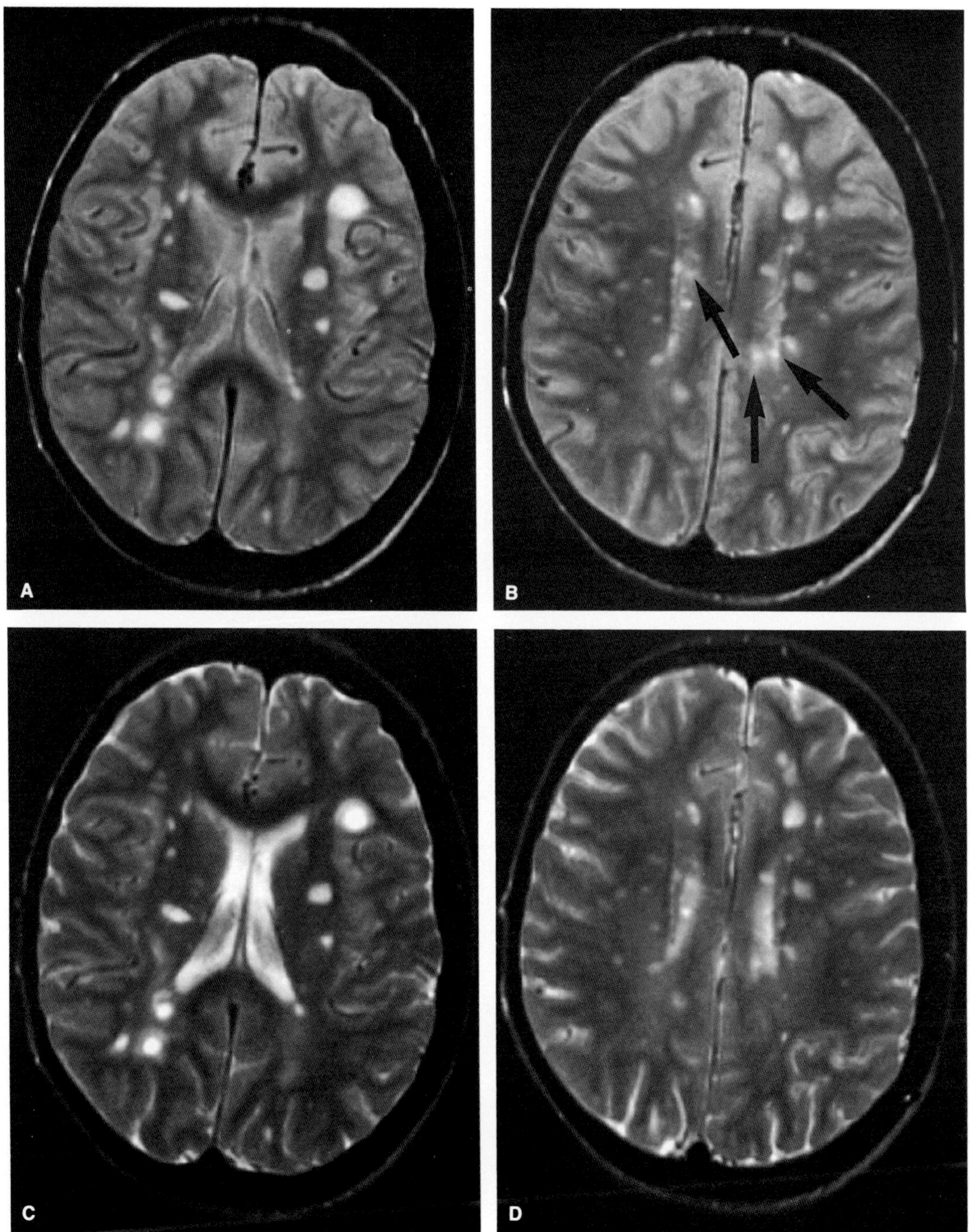

HISTORY

A 14-year-old girl with recent onset of diplopia (due to right abducens paresis), which resolved by follow-up ophthalmologic examination at 4 months

FINDINGS

Multiple, bilateral, punctate white matter abnormalities are noted in an asymmetric periventricular white matter distribution, with high signal intensity on T2-weighted (*A*

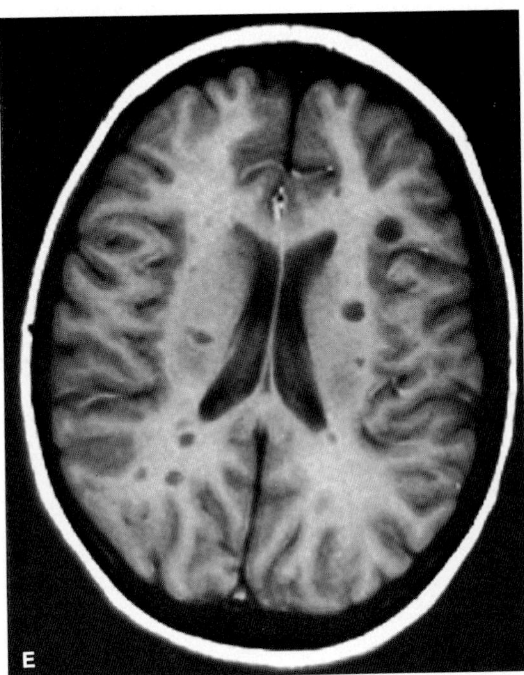

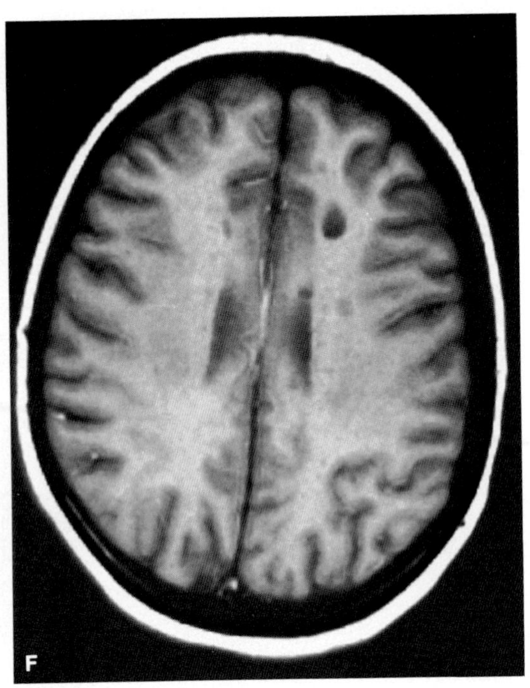

and B: TE=45 msec; *C and D:* TE=90 msec) and low signal intensity on T1-weighted (*E and F*) examinations. Lesions (*arrows in B*) which are immediately adjacent to the ventricular system are better depicted on the first echo of the T2-weighted examination, where CSF is isointense with normal brain. Infratentorial lesions (*not illustrated*) were also noted, specifically in the medulla, pons, middle cerebellar peduncle, and cerebellar hemisphere.

DIAGNOSIS

Multiple sclerosis (MS) in childhood

DISCUSSION

In pediatric MS, the distribution and appearance of lesions are similar to that found in the adult form of the disease.[1] Symptoms and clinical course do not appear to differ from adult disease in most of these children. MR is more sensitive than multimodal evoked potentials for confirmation of diagnosis in childhood MS.

The clinical presentation of pediatric MS is highly variable, with acute findings of retrobulbar optic neuritis, transverse myelitis, or cerebellitis common.[2] Ocular manifestations of MS (in the general population) include unilateral optic neuritis, uveitis, decreased vision, nystagmus, internuclear ophthalmoplegia, and diplopia. In a study of 21 children presenting with optic neuritis, 9 (8 were girls) subsequently developed MS.[3]

MR Technique

Thin-section (4 to 5 mm) axial and sagittal first echo (TE=20 to 45 msec) T2-weighted examinations applied with motion compensation techniques such as GMR (gradient moment refocusing) are recommended for lesion detection and follow-up examinations.[4]

Pitfalls in Image Interpretation

Multiple sclerosis in childhood must be differentiated from acute disseminated encephalomyelitis, which can present on MR with similar asymmetric and multifocal white matter lesions.

Clinical References

1. Scaioli V, Rumi V, Cimino C, Angelini L. Childhood multiple sclerosis (MS): multimodal evoked potentials (EP) and magnetic resonance imaging (MRI)—comparative study. Neuropediatrics 1991;22:15–33.
2. Boutin B, Esquivel E, Mayer M, et al. Multiple sclerosis in childhood: report of clinical and paraclinical features in 19 cases. Neuropediatrics 1988;19:118–123.
3. Riikonen R, Donner M, Erkkila H. Optic neuritis in children and its relationship to multiple sclerosis: a clinical study of 21 children. Dev Med Child Neurol 1988;30:349–359.
4. Ebner F, Millner MM, Justich E. Multiple sclerosis in children: value of serial MR studies to monitor patients. AJNR 1990;11:1023–1027.

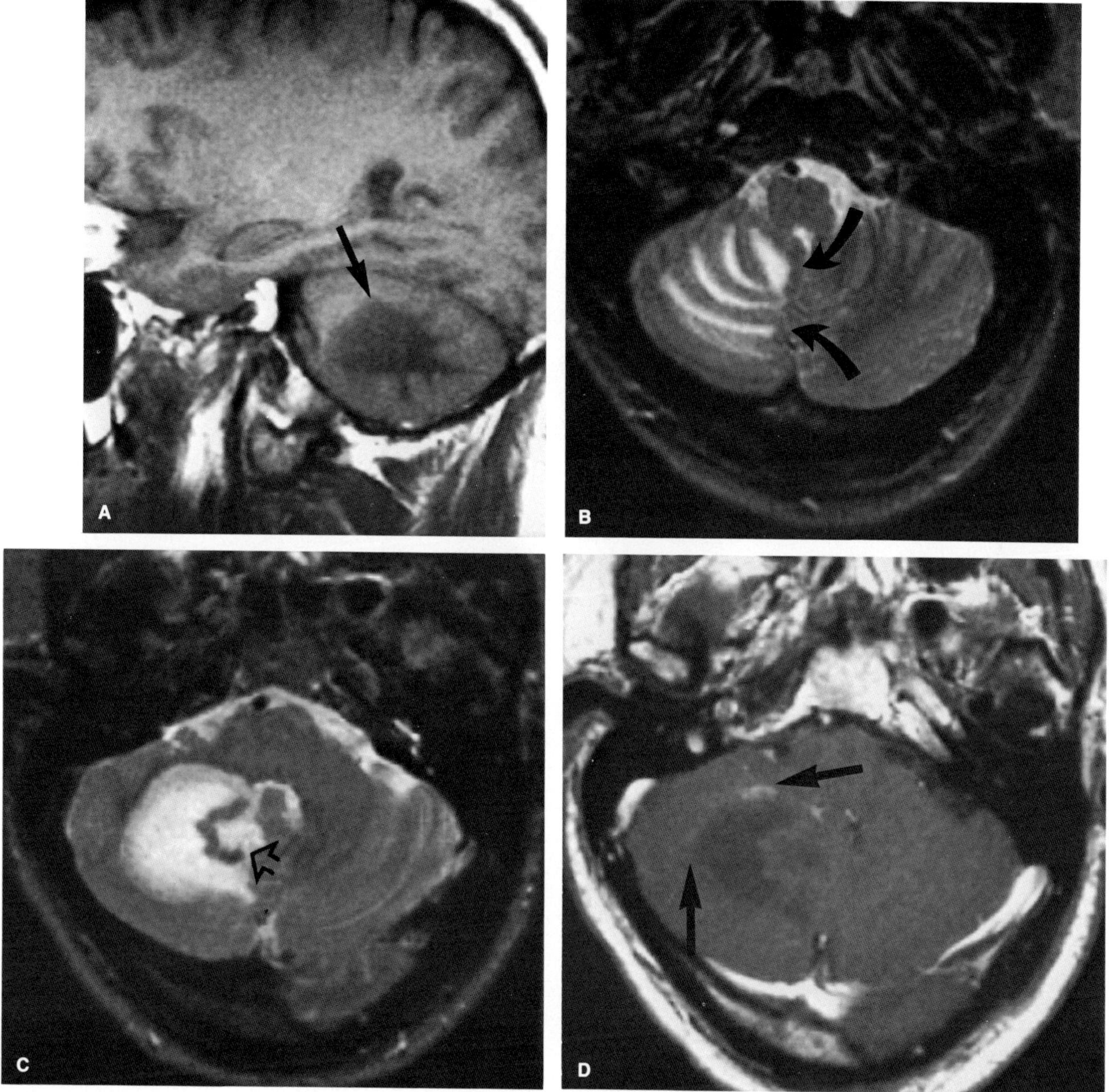

HISTORY

A 36-year-old man with new onset, over 1 week, of right-sided weakness, difficulty in walking, and slurred speech

FINDINGS

(*A*) An off-midline sagittal T1-weighted image reveals an abnormality (*arrow*) in the right cerebellum, confined principally to white matter and in a nonvascular distribution. (*B and C*) Axial T2-weighted images (TE = 90 msec) also show this lesion to involve principally white matter, with extension into the right middle cerebellar peduncle. On the more caudal image, edema is noted tracking in white matter (*curved arrows in B*). The dentate nucleus (*open arrow in C*) is surrounded by abnormal hyperintensity on the T2-weighted scan. There is slight mass effect, revealed by mild torquing of the medulla and obliteration of the right lateral dorsal recess. (*D*) The postcontrast T1-weighted image corresponding to *C* also demonstrates the mass and peripheral white matter edema, with faint rim enhancement (*arrows in D*). On images (*not shown*) adjacent anatomically to *D,* peripheral enhancement was further noted, in an apparent concentric distribution. Of significance, no other

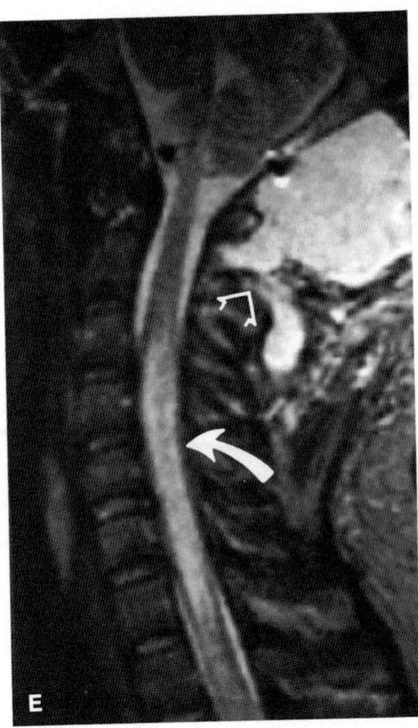

brain abnormalities were detected, even in retrospect. Following biopsy of the cerebellar lesion (with the diagnosis established pathologically), a cervical spine MR was performed. (*E*) A single midline sagittal T2-weighted (TE = 90 msec) image demonstrates a large postoperative pseudomeningocele (*open white arrow*) and extensive spinal cord expansion with central abnormal hyperintensity extending from C3 to C7 (*curved white arrow*). The T2-weighted thoracic spine MR (*not shown*) revealed multiple additional cord lesions.

DIAGNOSIS

Multiple sclerosis—large (giant) plaque

DISCUSSION

The presentation of multiple sclerosis (MS) on CT as a single, unusually large lesion with mass effect and peripheral ring enhancement, mimicking tumor, has been described.[1] The lack of mass effect has been reported (on CT) as a differential diagnostic criterion for MS lesions; however, mass effect may occur with large plaques. Contrast enhancement is associated with acute lesions and active demyelination.

The improved sensitivity of MR for delineation of MS plaques has led to greater confidence in diagnosis. A second literature report[2] describes a single case with a large solitary enhancing lesion on CT, with diagnosis possible by MR because of the presence of additional lesions in the centrum semiovale and periventricular white matter. Unfortunately, although likely to be quite rare and not previously reported, a patient such as that illustrated can present with a solitary MS plaque even on MR. Clinical symptoms in the current patient are consistent with a cerebellar lesion but nonspecific with regard to differential diagnosis. Cerebellar peduncle and hemispheric lesions (the latter when extensive) cause ataxia and mild ipsilateral extremity weakness. Lesions that involve either the superior cerebellar peduncle or the dentate nucleus cause the most severe symptoms. Cerebellar lesions also commonly lead to speech disorders, including slowing and slurring. The spinal cord lesions noted in the present case represent additional MS plaques.

Pitfalls in Image Interpretation

The differential diagnosis for a large, solitary enhancing lesion with mass effect on MR should include primary neoplasm, metastatic disease, infection, and (although likely to be extremely rare) MS.

Clinical References

1. Nelson MJ, Miller SL, McLain LW Jr, Gold LH. Case report: multiple sclerosis—large plaque causing mass effect and ring sign. J Comput Assist Tomogr 1981;5:892–894.
2. Knapik JR, Galloway DC. Atypical CT pattern in multiple sclerosis. South Med J 1987;80:777–779.

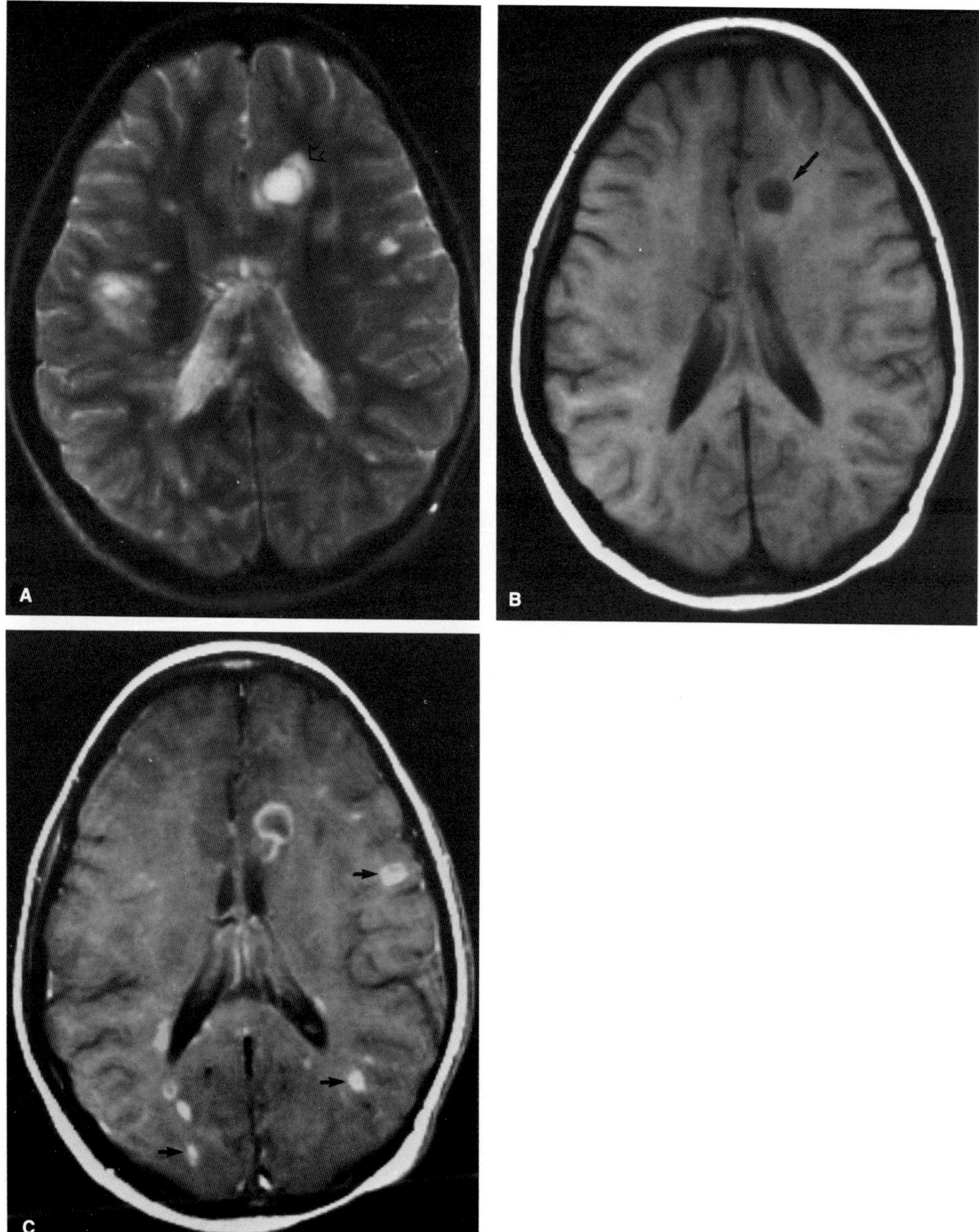

HISTORY

Two patients, both children who presented with headaches and ataxia, 1 to 2 weeks after a viral illness

FINDINGS

Patient 1: (*A*) The precontrast T2-weighted scan (TR/TE = 3000/90) reveals multiple white matter abnormalities, predominantly in peripheral and deep white matter (but specifically not periventricular). The most anterior lesion is exerting some mass effect and has a thin halo of surrounding edema (*open arrow*). (*B*) On the precontrast T1-weighted scan, only the largest lesion is well identified (*arrow*). (*C*) The postcontrast T1-weighted scan shows multiple abnormal enhancing foci (*small arrows*). Enhancement marks almost every lesion noted on the T2-weighted scan, with multiple additional abnormalities noted only on the postcontrast scan.

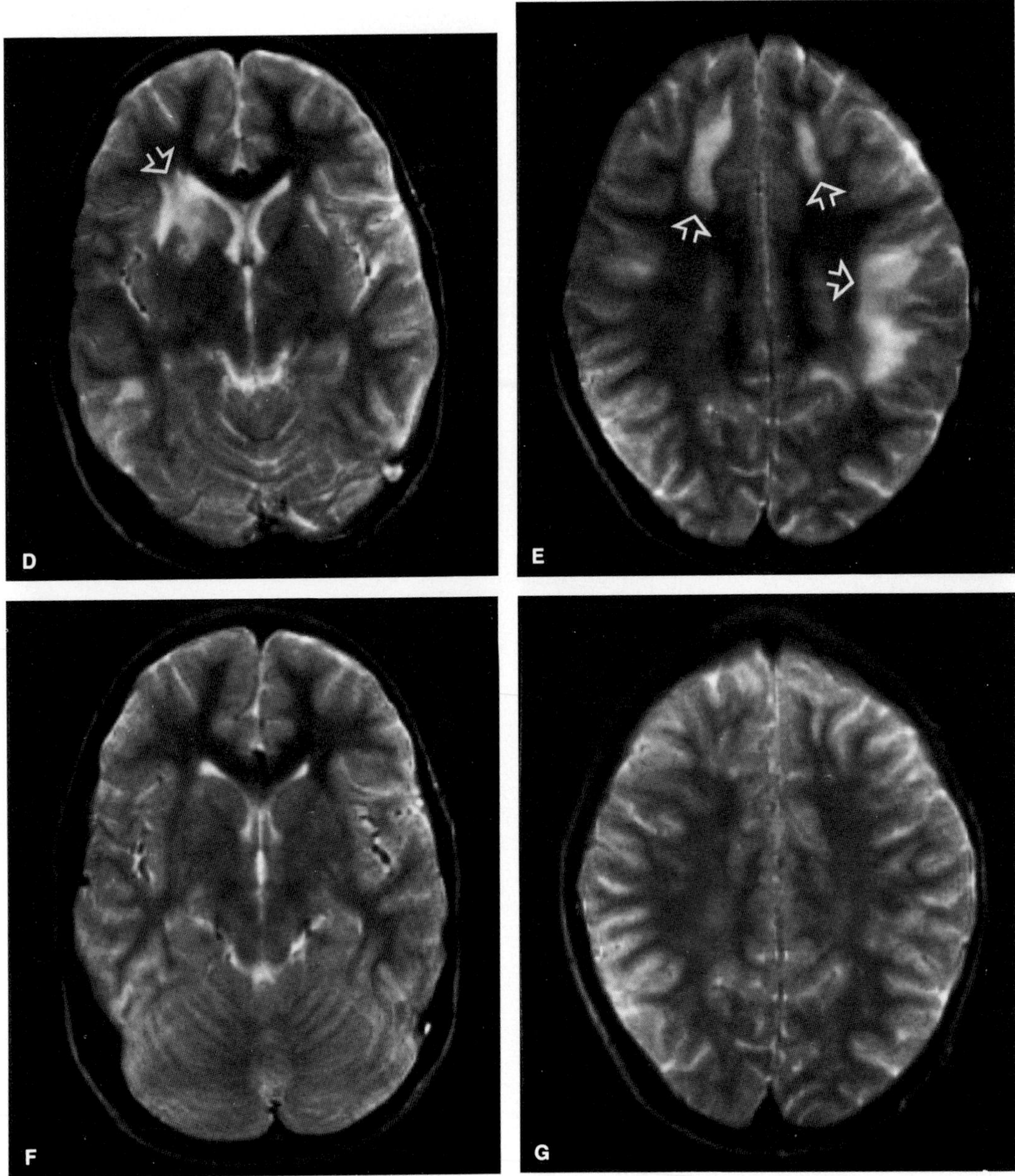

Patient 2: (*D and E*) T2-weighted scans (TR/TE = 3000/90) at two anatomic levels reveal multiple, ill-defined high-signal-intensity abnormalities (*open arrows*). These predominantly involve white matter, with disease involvement extending to the gray–white matter junction. *D and E* are scans made 1 month after the patient's initial presentation. (*F and G*) At 2 months after onset, the follow-up T2-weighted MR examination is essentially normal.

DIAGNOSIS

Acute disseminated encephalomyelitis

DISCUSSION

Acute disseminated encephalomyelitis is an inflammatory and demyelinating disease of white matter, typically seen in children, which can occur following viral illness or vaccination. Clinical manifestations include confusion, somnolence, convulsions, headache, fever, ataxia, and in more severe cases, coma. Despite widespread neurologic abnormalities, CT may be normal.[1] MR demonstrates multifocal white matter lesions in the cerebrum, cerebellum, and brain stem. Lesion resolution can be noted on MR with successful treatment (high-dose steroids), in parallel with clinical improvement. Some patients, however, are left with persistent abnormality, noted on MR.

Because acute disseminated encephalomyelitis is typically a monophasic illness, one might anticipate that all lesions would enhance in the acute phase. A recent case report,[2] however, suggests that both enhancing and nonenhancing lesions may be noted in the same patient.

Acute disseminated encephalomyelitis can occur shortly after viral infection (primarily measles, rubella, chickenpox, and smallpox, and rarely with mumps and rubella), following vaccination (against rabies, smallpox, and tetanus), and occasionally without known preceding illness or event. Mortality and long-term morbidity are substantial. Following acute recovery, a child may be left with permanent neurologic disability, including mental retardation and epilepsy. However, the disability seen during the acute stage of the disease is out of all proportion with permanent damage. The disease is characterized pathologically by perivenular demyelination and inflammation, presumably the result of an immune-mediated reaction rather than direct viral infection. An animal model of acute disseminated encephalomyelitis exists, experimental allergic encephalomyelitis, which is produced by inoculation with sterile brain tissue and adjuvants.

The incidence of acute disseminated encephalomyelitis has markedly declined in the last 15 years, presumably because of widespread vaccination against measles (previously the single major postviral cause of this disease, with an incidence as high as 1:800 cases of measles) and discontinuation of smallpox vaccination.

Pitfalls in Image Interpretation

The MR appearance of acute disseminated encephalomyelitis, with multifocal white matter lesions, can be indistinguishable from multiple sclerosis.[3] Follow-up scans may be useful for distinction of these two diseases, with resolution of many lesions noted in time in acute disseminated encephalomyelitis, and the appearance of new lesions described to be rare.

Although experience is limited, it has been noted that lesions in acute disseminated encephalomyelitis tend, unlike those in multiple sclerosis, not to have distinct borders (they may appear "fluffy"), do not occur commonly in the immediate periventricular white matter, and are frequently located peripherally—adjacent to the gray–white matter junction.

Clinical References

1. Dunn V, Bale JR, Zimmerman RA, et al. MRI in children with postinfectious disseminated encephalomyelitis. Magn Reson Imaging 1986;4:25–32.
2. Caldemeyer KS, Harris TM, Smith RR, Edwards MK. Gadolinium enhancement in acute disseminated encephalomyelitis. J Comput Assist Tomogr 1991;15:673–675.
3. Kesselring J, Miller DH, Robb SA, et al. Acute disseminated encephalomyelitis: MRI findings and the distinction from multiple sclerosis. Brain 1990;113:291–302.

*(*A *to* C *from Runge VM. Magnetic resonance imaging: clinical principles. Philadelphia, JB Lippincott, 1992;* D *through* G *from Runge VM. Clinical magnetic resonance imaging. Philadelphia, JB Lippincott, 1990.)*

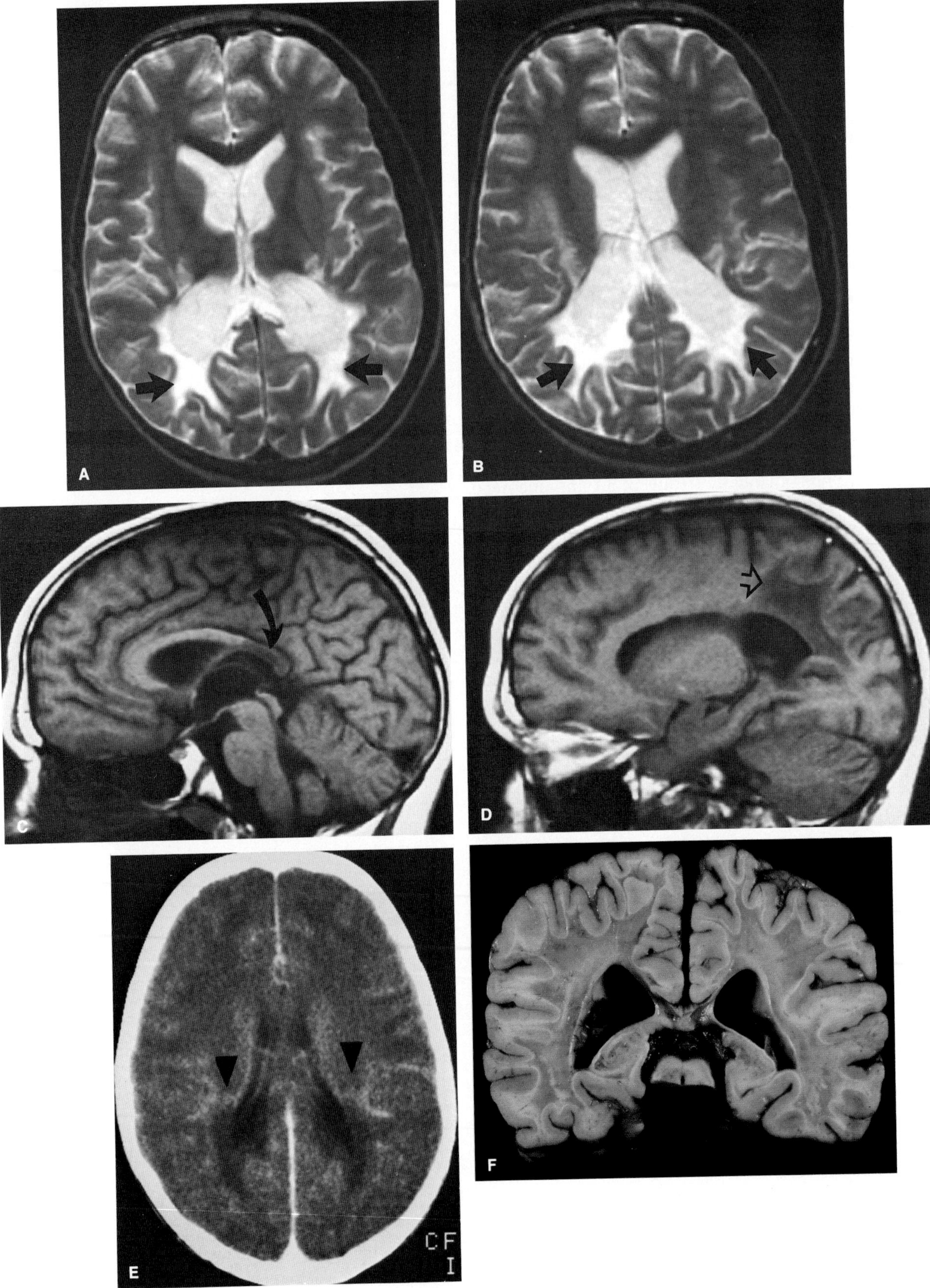
A
B
C
D
E
CF
I
F

HISTORY

A 15-year-old boy with impaired vision, hearing loss, and intellectual decline

FINDINGS

(*A and B*) Axial T2-weighted scans demonstrate abnormal hyperintensity in the peritrigonal white matter (*arrows*). (*C and D*) Sagittal T1-weighted scans show involvement of both the splenium (*curved arrow in C*) of the corpus callosum and the parietooccipital white matter (*open arrow in D*) as reflected by abnormal hypointensity. (*E*) Contrast-enhanced CT, obtained 1 year before MR, demonstrates mild enhancement (*arrowheads*) along the anterior margin of the involved white matter.

DIAGNOSIS

Adrenoleukodystrophy

DISCUSSION

Early in disease progression, adrenoleukodystrophy is characterized by signal intensity abnormalities (low on T1- and high on T2-weighted scans) on MR and hypodensity on CT in the white matter of the parietooccipital region and splenium of the corpus callosum.[1] Contrast enhancement following gadolinium chelate injection can be demonstrated at the leading edge of lesions, consistent with blood–brain barrier disruption and active demyelination. Follow-up examinations demonstrate posterior-to-anterior disease progression.[2] MR is the imaging technique of choice for detection of demyelination in the visual pathway (lateral geniculate body, Meyer's loop, and optic radiation), auditory pathway (lateral lemniscus and medial geniculate body), and motor systems.[3] Brain lesions can be demonstrated by MR in asymptomatic patients before neurologic deterioration.[4] MR may prove critical for the institution of effective therapy in the future because of its ability to detect early white matter lesions in neurologically asymptomatic patients and to follow disease progression.[5] Atypical patterns of white matter involvement (frontal region or asymmetric involvement) have been described.

Childhood adrenoleukodystrophy (the most common form of X-linked adrenoleukodystrophy) is characterized by the development of adrenal insufficiency and progressive multifocal demyelination of the CNS. The defective gene has been localized to the Xq28 region of the X chromosome. There is impaired degradation of saturated very-long-chain fatty acids, with diagnosis based on detection of their increased concentrations in plasma or fibroblasts. Age of onset ranges from 5 to 14 years, with rapid neurologic deterioration (mean of 2 years between first neurologic symptoms and vegetative state) followed by death. Successful bone marrow transplantation has recently been reported in one patient, with reversal of symptoms and disappearance of multifocal brain lesions on MR.[6]

MR Technique

IV gadolinium chelate administration permits demonstration of active inflammation along the advancing disease margin.

Pathologic Correlate

(*F*) Coronal section of gross pathologic specimen of adrenoleukodystrophy is shown. In this instance, there is severe involvement of the periatrial white matter, which is darker than normal and shrunken following formalin fixation. Ventricular dilatation is also present. The corpus callosum and fornix are frequently involved, in addition to the centrum semiovale. Lesions are typically symmetric posteriorly, but involvement of the frontal lobes may be asymmetric. Involvement of cerebellar white matter may also be present.

Clinical References

1. Romero C, Dietemann JL, Kurtz D, et al. Adrenoleukodystrophy: value of contrast-enhanced MR imaging. J Neuroradiol 1990;17:267–276.
2. Jenson ME, Sawyer RW, Braun IF, Rizzo WB. MR imaging appearance of childhood adrenoleukodystrophy with auditory, visual, and motor pathway involvement. Radiographics 1990;10:53–66.
3. Kumar AJ, Rosenbaum AE, Naidu S, et al. Adrenoleukodystrophy: correlating MR imaging with CT. Radiology 1987; 165:497–504.
4. Pasco A, Kalifa G, Sarrazin JL, et al. Contribution of MRI to the diagnosis of cerebral lesions of adrenoleukodystrophy. Pediatr Radiol 1991;21:161–163.
5. Aubourg P, Sellier N, Chaussain JL, Kalifa G. MRI detects cerebral involvement in neurologically asymptomatic patients with adrenoleukodystrophy. Neurology 1989;39: 1619–1621.
6. Aubourg P, Blanche S, Jambaque I, et al. Reversal of early neurologic and neuroradiologic manifestations of X-linked adrenoleukodystrophy by bone marrow transplantation. New Engl J Med 1990;322:1860–1866.

(F *courtesy of Daron G. Davis, MD.*)

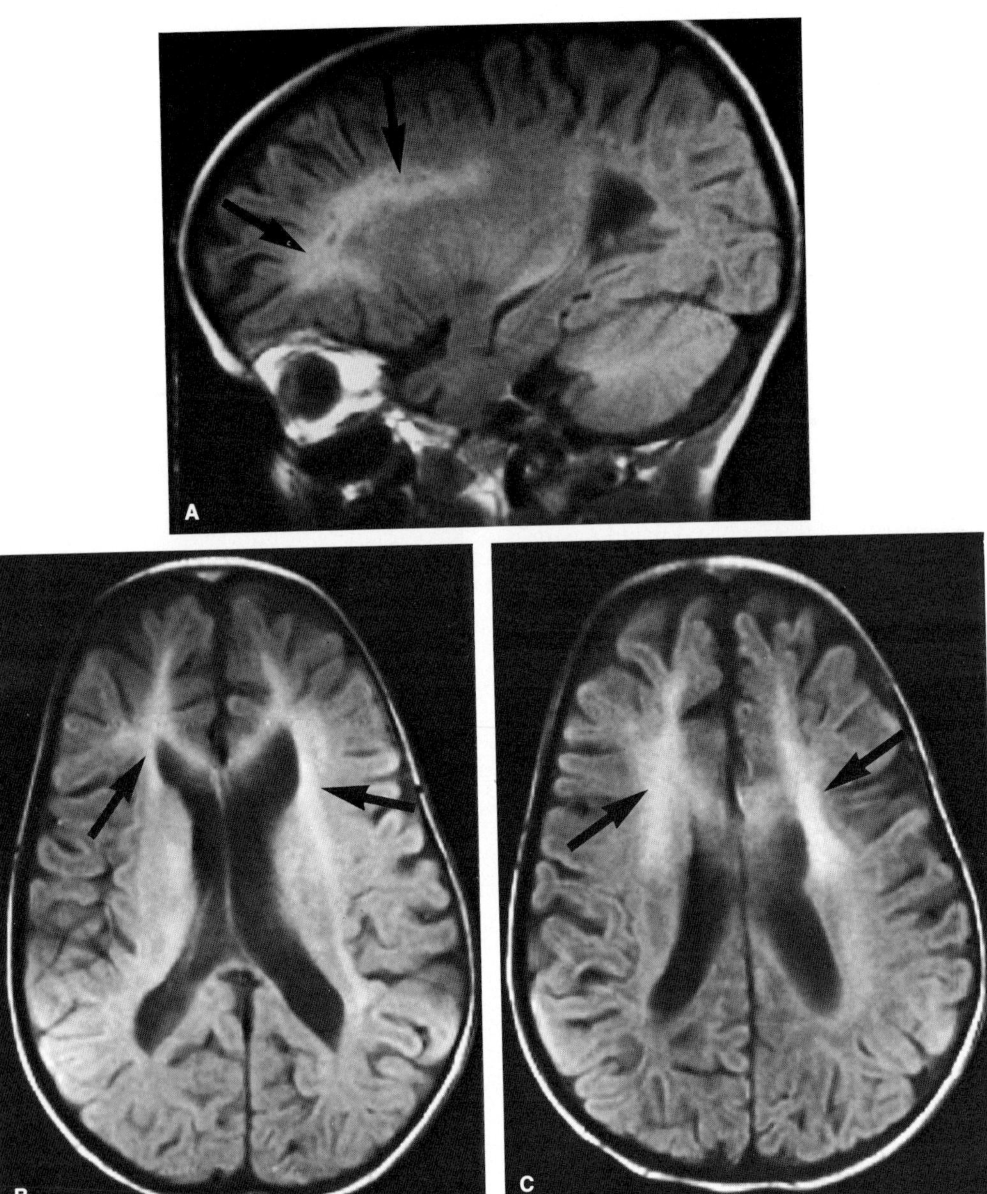

HISTORY

A blind 4-year-old child with progressive weakness and severe learning disability

FINDINGS

Sagittal (*A*) and axial (*B and C*) T1-weighted images reveal macrocephaly, cortical atrophy, and ventriculomegaly. Anteriorly, the central white matter (*arrows in A to C*) appears of normal intensity (hyperintense relative to gray matter). Both posteriorly and peripherally, the signal intensity of white matter is abnormal for age. (*D and E*) On T2-weighted images (TR/TE = 3000/90), there is diffuse white matter abnormality (*small arrows*), with the white matter hyperintense relative to gray matter, with sparing anteriorly. The signal intensity of the internal and external capsules (*curved arrows in D*) is also abnormal.

DIAGNOSIS

Canavan's disease

DISCUSSION

Canavan's disease is an autosomal recessive leukodystrophy presenting in the first 6 months of life with hypotonia, developmental regression, cortical blindness, and

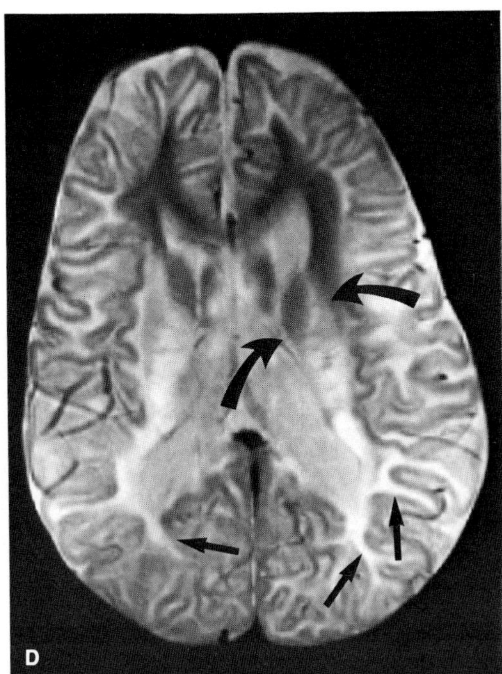

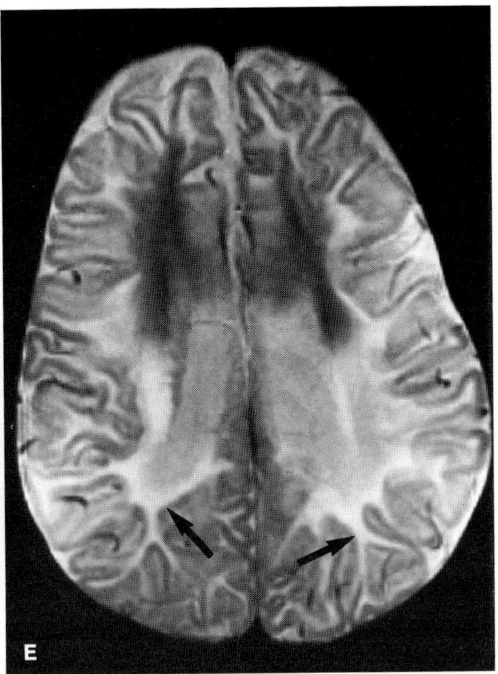

macrocephaly. There is progressive spasticity, with death usually by midchildhood. Differentiation on the basis of clinical findings from other dysmyelinating disorders, with the exception of Alexander's disease, is usually not difficult.[1]

Abnormal symmetric white matter hyperintensity on T2-weighted images is noted in Canavan's disease, with occasional sparing of the internal and external capsules, corpus callosum, and deep cerebellar white matter.[2] There may also be some sparing of central white matter. Involvement of central gray matter has been reported. Severe cortical atrophy and ventriculomegaly are late findings. However, the findings on MR in Canavan's disease are nonspecific, and similar to that of other dysmyelinating disorders.

A deficiency of the enzyme aspartoacylase has been reported in brain tissue and skin fibroblast cultures of patients with Canavan's disease, together with very high levels of *N*-acetylaspartate (NAA) in brain, blood, and urine—findings not seen with other leukodystrophies. Elevated NAA/Cr (Cr, creatine plus phosphocreatine) and NAA/Cho (Cho, choline-containing compounds) ratios have been reported in CD using localized ^{1}H NMR spectroscopy.[3] With the increasing availability of MR spectroscopy, it may be possible in the future to confirm the diagnosis of Canavan's disease by spectroscopic means, immediately after observation of typical white matter abnormalities by MR imaging.

Pitfalls in Image Interpretation

The normal MR appearance of white matter in the neonate and infant is different from that in the adult, with white matter hyperintense relative to gray matter on T2-weighted scans. Patient age must be carefully considered in the diagnostic evaluation of MR scans to prevent confusion between the appearance of normal brain maturation and that of a dysmyelinating disorder.

Clinical References

1. McAdams HP, Geyer CA, Done SL, et al. CT and MR imaging of Canavan disease. AJNR 1990;11:397–399.
2. Brismar J, Brismar G, Gascon G, Ozand P. Canavan disease: CT and MR imaging of the brain. AJNR 1990;11:805–810.
3. Austin SJ, Connelly A, Gadian DG, et al. Localized ^{1}H NMR spectroscopy in Canavan's disease: a report of two cases. Magn Reson Med 1991;19:439–445.

(C and E from Runge VM. Magnetic resonance imaging: clinical principles. Philadelphia, JB Lippincott, 1992.)

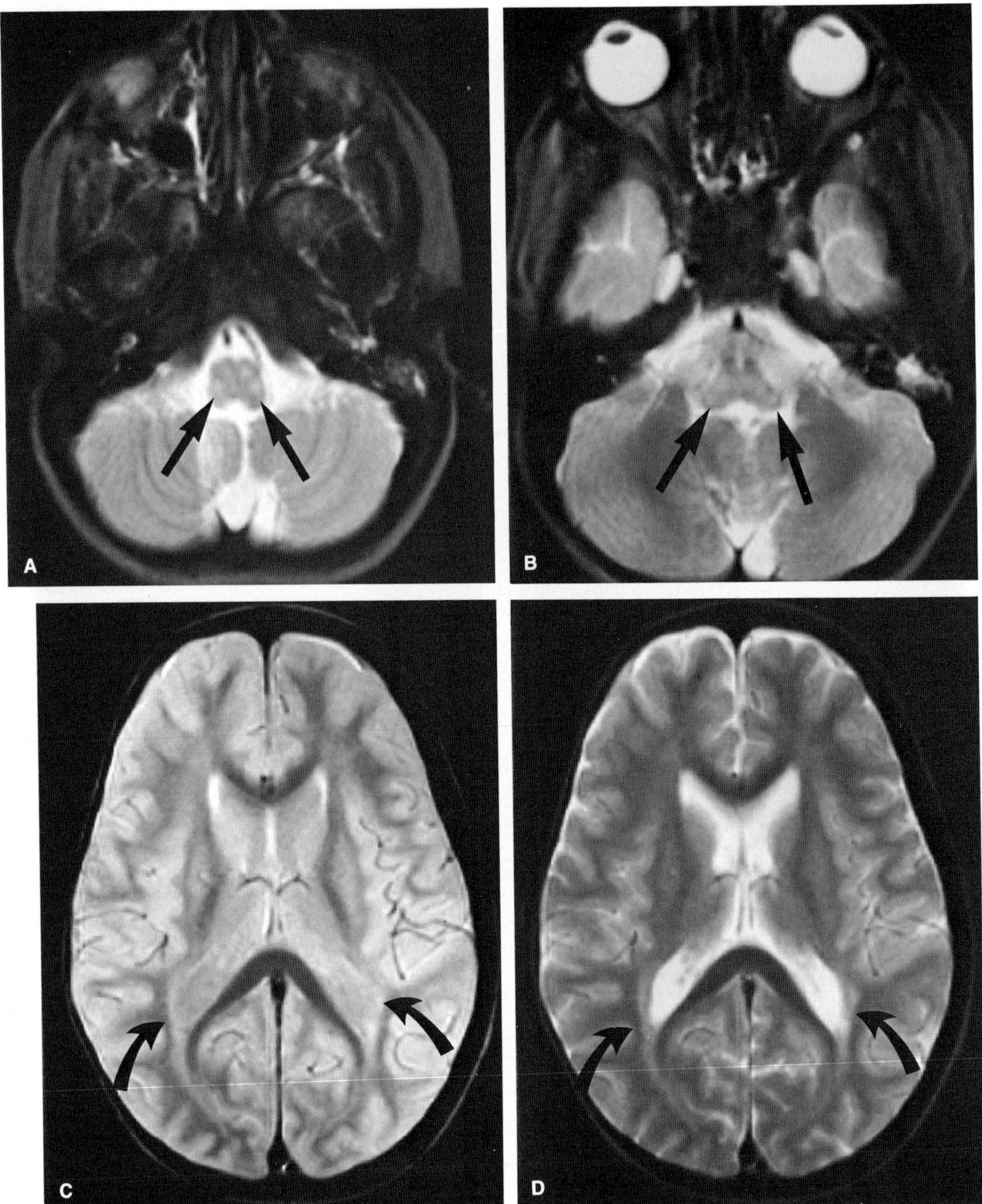

HISTORY

A 3-year-old boy with deteriorating physical mobility and generalized weakness

FINDINGS

(*A and B*) Consecutive axial images through the brain stem demonstrate abnormal increased signal intensity in the brain stem (*arrows*) on these axial T2-weighted images. Incidental note is made of inflammatory changes in the left mastoid air cells. Increased signal intensity is present in the optic radiations (*curved arrows*) on the first (*C*) and second (*D*) echoes of the T2-weighted sequence. The T1-weighted images were normal (*not shown*).

DIAGNOSIS

Leigh's disease

DISCUSSION

Leigh's disease, also known as subacute necrotizing encephalomyelopathy (SNE), is a rare neurodegenerative disorder that usually affects infants and children but that occasionally has an adult onset.[1] Feeding difficulties and psychomotor retardation often arise during the first 2 years of life. Death usually occurs within 4 years of symptom onset. The metabolic defect involves cerebral inhibition of ATP-TPP (thiamine pyrophosphate) phosphoryl transferase, which catalyzes a reaction resulting in thiamine triphosphate (TTP). The mitochondrial enzyme deficiencies in this disease include pyruvate carboxylase, pyruvate dehydrogenase, and cytochrome C oxidase deficiencies. It is a familial disease that is transmitted as an autosomal recessive trait. Laboratory findings consist of metabolic acidosis with elevated lactate and pyruvate concentrations in the blood and CSF.[2]

The clinical presentation varies, but most children are normal at birth. At presentation the disease manifests itself as multiple neurologic deficits including ataxia, hypotonia, nystagmus, bulbar paresis, visual disturbances, abnormal ocular movement, and regressive psychomotor development. Pathologic findings include symmetric areas of necrosis in the putamen, thalamus, medulla, subcortical white matter, hypothalamus, dentate nuclei, cerebellum, visual system, and posterior column of the spinal cord. The mamillary bodies are rarely involved.

On MR, symmetric lesions of increased signal intensity on T2-weighted images are seen in various locations, most commonly the brain stem (tegmentum), spinal cord, basal ganglia, and optic pathways. In the basal ganglia, the putamen in particular is often involved.

Pitfalls in Image Interpretation

The distribution of lesions in Leigh's disease is similar to Wernicke's encephalopathy, except for sparing of the mamillary bodies in Leigh's disease. The differential diagnosis of diseases having basal ganglia involvement that present in childhood include various toxic conditions such as carbon monoxide poisoning, cyanide poisoning, Wilson's disease, Hallervorden-Spatz disease and a rare complication of viral encephalitis.[3]

Clinical References

1. Davis PC, Hoffman JC, Braun IF, et al. MR of Leigh's disease (subacute necrotizing encephalomyelopathy). AJNR 1987; 8:71–75.
2. Mirowitz SA, Sartor K, Prensky AJ, et al. Neurodegenerative diseases of childhood: MR and CT evaluation. J Comput Assist Tomogr 1991;15:210–222.
3. Medina L, Chi TL, DeVivo DC, et al. MR findings in patients with subacute necrotizing encephalomyelopathy (Leigh syndrome): correlation with biochemical defect. AJR 1990; 154:1269–1274.
4. Geyer CA, Sartor KJ, Prensky AJ, et al. Leigh disease (subacute necrotizing encephalomyelopathy). J Comput Assist Tomogr 1988;12:40–44.

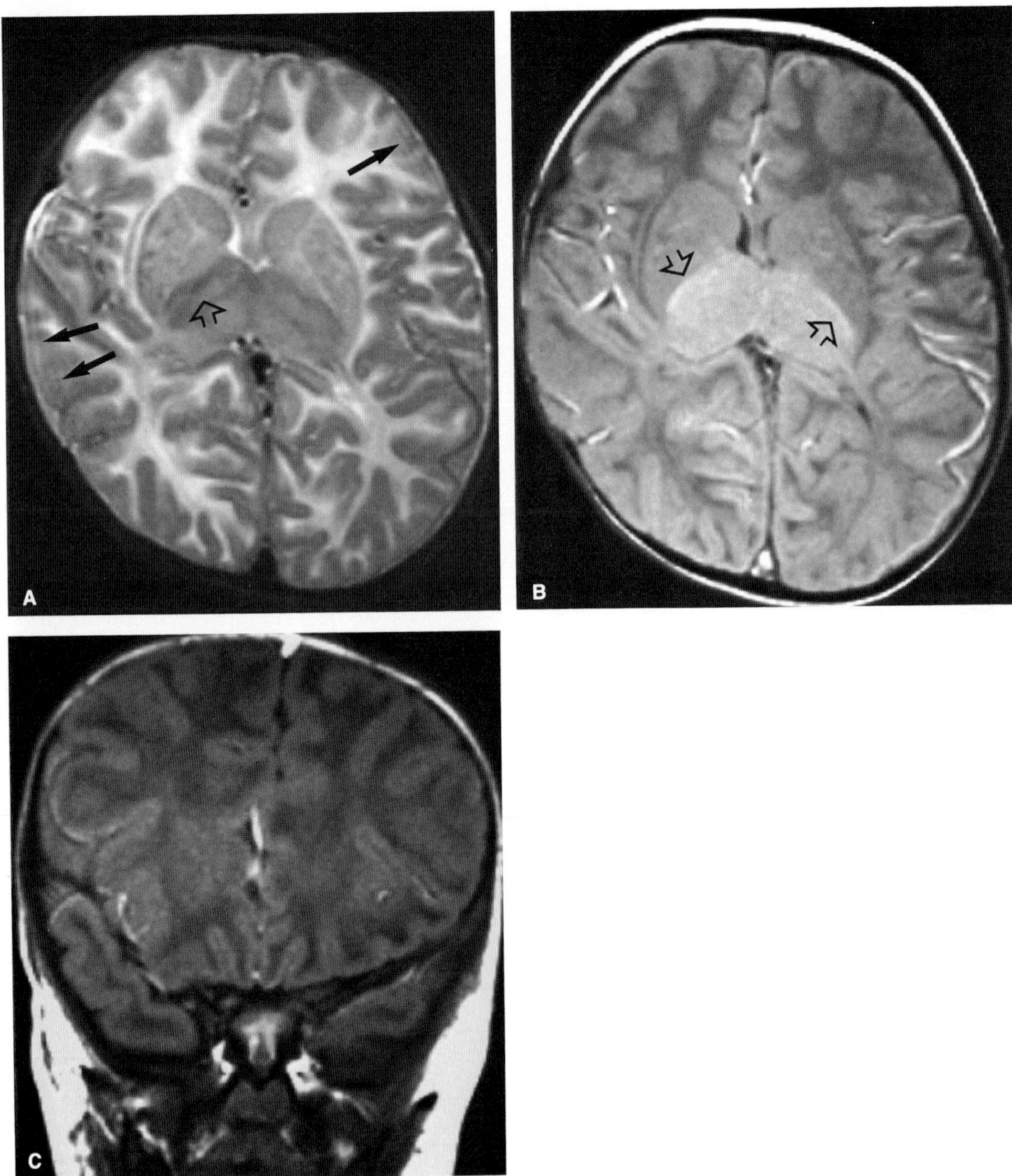

HISTORY

An 11-month-old infant with cessation of normal development at 3 months of age and subsequent regression. The patient cannot sit, roll over, or raise her head. On physical examination, there is hepatosplenomegaly.

FINDINGS

(*A*) On the T2-weighted (TR/TE = 3500/90) axial scan, the white matter is diffusely abnormal with marked hyperintensity. Axial (*B*) and coronal (*C*) T1-weighted images confirm this finding, with the white matter of diffuse abnormal hypointensity. There is apparent normal myelination of only the posterior limb of the internal capsule (*open arrows in A and B*). Truncation lines (also known as Gibbs artifact; *arrows in A*) are prominent on the axial T2-weighted image (*A*) because of the use of a reduced number (192) of phase encoding lines.

DIAGNOSIS

G_{M1} gangliosidosis

DISCUSSION

The inherited metabolic diseases are generally restricted to those that are genetic, progressive, and largely neurologic, with a demonstrable or presumed inborn error of metabolism. Most are disorders of lysosomes, although those involving mitochondria and peroxisomes are known. The inherited metabolic diseases are traditionally categorized into storage diseases, leukodystrophies, and other miscellaneous conditions. The storage diseases are subdivided into four groups: lipidoses, mucopolysaccharidoses, mucolipidoses, and glycogenoses. Major sphingolipidoses (lipidoses) include Gaucher's, Niemann-Pick, Krabbe's, metachromatic leukodystrophy, Fabry's, G_{M1} gangliosidosis, and Tay-Sachs disease. The mucopolysaccharidoses include Hurler's, Scheie's, Hunter's, Sanfilippo's, Morquio's, and Sly's syndromes.

G_{M1} gangliosidosis is characterized by accumulation of G_{M1} ganglioside in nerve tissue.[1] In addition to this substance, neutral glycolipids, glycosaminoglycans, and oligosaccharides also accumulate in both neural and extraneural tissue. These are all the result of low activity of the enzyme G_{M1}-β-galactosidase A, which metabolizes G_{M1} to G_{M2}. As with most metabolic diseases, the pattern of inheritance is autosomal recessive. Type 1 (demonstrated in this patient) is the most severe form and is often clinically demonstrable from birth, with poor appetite, hypotonia, and decreased activity. Rapid deterioration occurs, with death common during the second year (the patient died 2 months after the current examination). Neuronal loss, axon degeneration with myelin loss, and astrogliosis are prominent pathologically. A closely related disease is Tay-Sachs, a G_{M2} gangliosidosis (with deficiency of the enzyme that catabolizes G_{M2} to G_{M3}, and thus abnormal accumulation of G_{M2} ganglioside).

Pitfalls in Image Interpretation

The inherited metabolic diseases on imaging can have two somewhat disparate appearances,[2] cerebral atrophy and diffuse white matter abnormality (abnormal signal intensity on MR and hypodensity on CT). The latter should not be confused in the infant with delayed myelination. Knowledge of the normal evolution of myelinization and the relative appearance of gray and white matter on MR is essential for correct diagnosis.

Clinical References

1. Becker LE, Yates AJ. Inherited metabolic disease. In: Davis RI, Robertson DM, eds. Textbook of neuropathology, 2nd ed. Baltimore, Williams & Wilkins, 1991:331–427.
2. Wende S, Ludwig B, Kishikawa T, et al. The value of CT in diagnosis and prognosis of different inborn neurodegenerative disorders in childhood. J Neurol 1984;231:57–70.

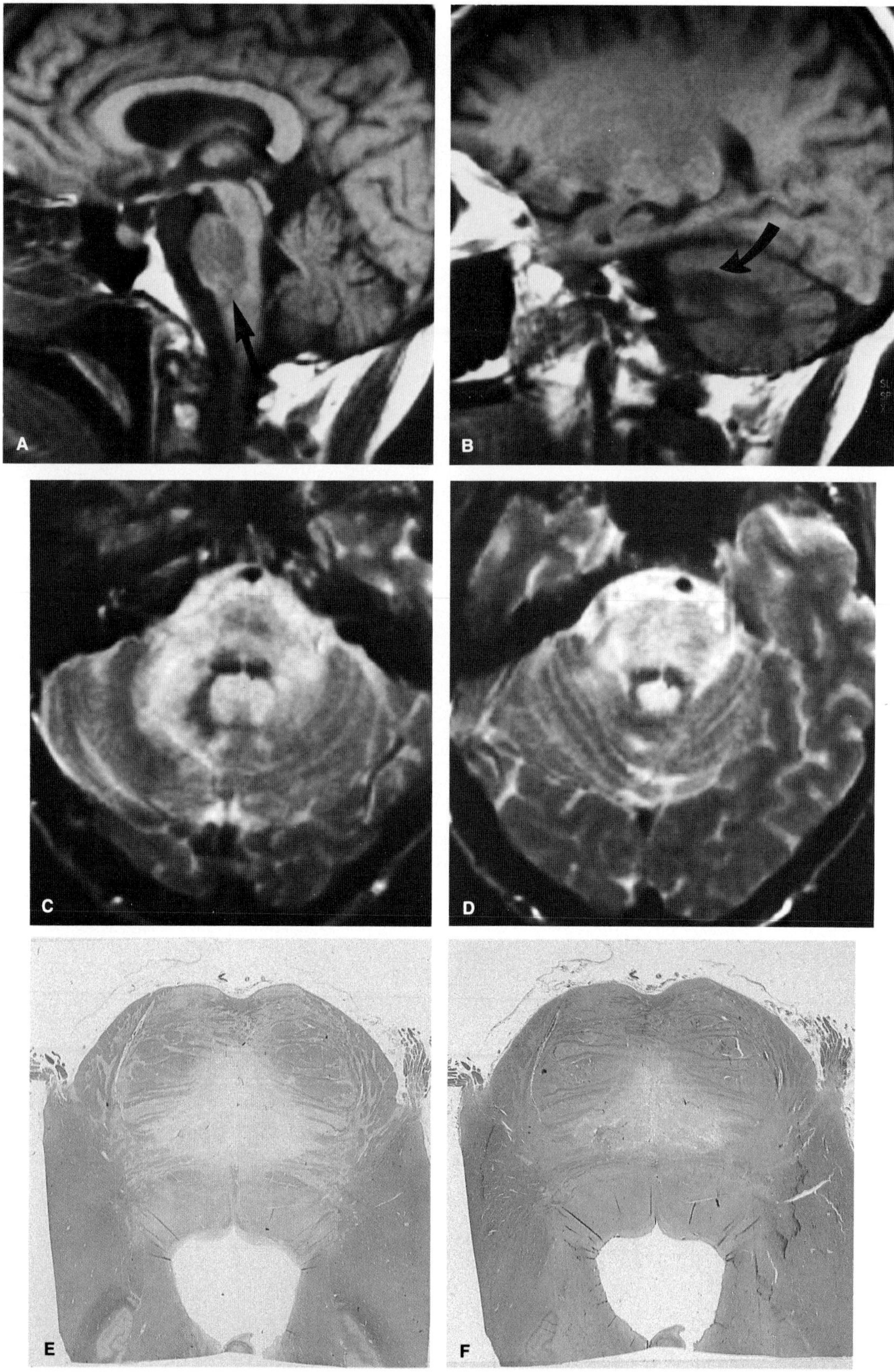
A
B
C
D
E
F

HISTORY

A 52-year-old chronic alcoholic with recent onset of lethargy. MR was requested when the patient became quadriplegic after rapid correction of profound hyponatremia.

FINDINGS

(*A and B*) Sagittal T1-weighted scans demonstrate abnormal decreased signal intensity in the pons (*arrow in A*) and cerebellar peduncles (*curved arrow in B*). (*C and D*) There is abnormal high signal intensity in the corresponding anatomic location on axial T2-weighted scans.

DIAGNOSIS

Central pontine myelinolysis

DISCUSSION

In central pontine myelinolysis, there is symmetric destruction of myelin sheaths, which appears to start from the median raphe of the pons. The lesion can involve part or all of the base of the pons, with contiguous spread into the dorsal pons (tegmentum) and superiorly into the mesencephalon (midbrain) reported. The etiology is believed to be an osmotic injury, secondary to rapid correction of severe chronic hyponatremia. Clinical studies with MR have demonstrated the development of pontine lesions in patients with rapid correction of serum sodium concentration.[1] A history of alcoholism and malnutrition is common. Clinically, there is rapid progression of corticospinal and corticobulbar symptoms, with flaccid quadriplegia and facial, pharyngeal, and glottal paralysis. Recovery is variable.

In 12 patients with central pontine myelinolysis by clinical or neuropathologic criteria, CT was positive in only 1 case (and that retrospectively), with MR positive in all cases.[2] Persistence of a lesion in the pons, presumably corresponding to gliosis, has been documented in some cases following resolution of symptoms.[3] Resolution of the lesion has also been documented with clinical recovery.[4]

Pitfalls in Image Interpretation

The abnormalities on T1- (low signal intensity) and T2- (high signal intensity) weighted images in central pontine myelinolysis are not disease specific. Involvement of the pons by infarction, metastasis, glioma, multiple sclerosis, or radiation changes can mimic central pontine myelinolysis.[2]

Pathologic Correlate

(*E and F*) On histologic section, central pontine myelinolysis demonstrates a characteristic triangular appearance. The area of involvement appears blue in *E* and pink in *F* because of a difference in vital stains. More extensive lesions, round in appearance, can also occur. Axonal damage is not unusual, in addition to myelinolysis.

Clinical References

1. Brunner JE, Redmond JM, Haggar AM, et al. Central pontine myelinolysis and pontine lesions after rapid correction of hyponatremia: a prospective MRI study. Ann Neurol 1990; 27:61–66.
2. Miller GM, Baker HL, Okazaki H, Whisnant JP. Central pontine myelinolysis and its imitators: MR findings. Radiology 1988;168:795–802.
3. Thompson PD, Miller D, Gledhill RF, Rossor MN. Magnetic resonance imaging in central pontine myelinolysis. J Neurol Neurosurg Psychiatry 1989;52:675–677.
4. Ragland RL, Duffis AW, Gendelman S, et al. Central pontine myelinolysis with clinical recovery: MR documentation. J Comput Assist Tomogr 1989;13:316–318.

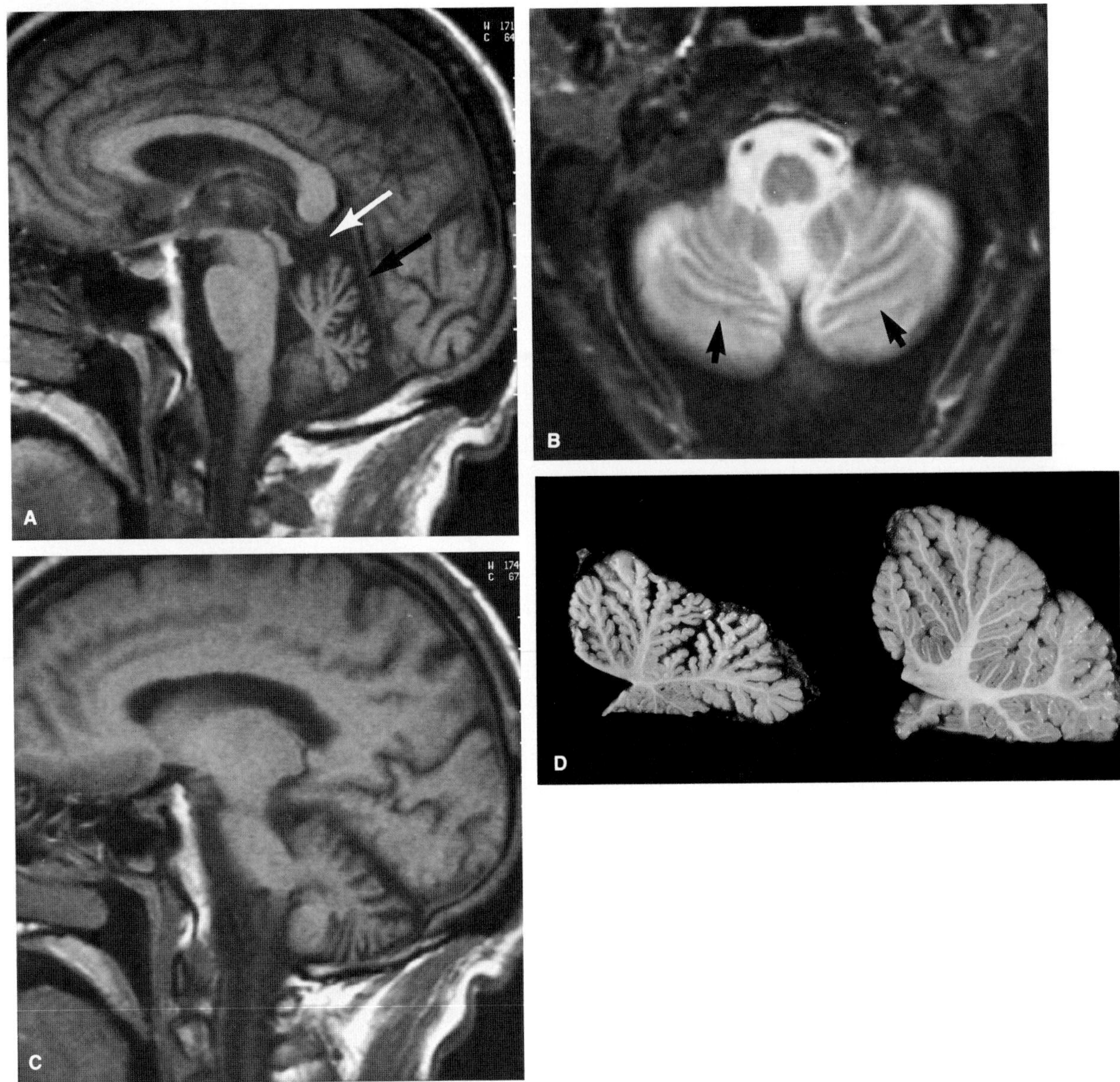

HISTORY

A 57-year-old alcoholic with ataxia

FINDINGS

(*A*) The midline T1-weighted sagittal image demonstrates the folia of the cerebellar vermis (*arrow*) to be atrophic, and the interfolial sulci are enlarged. The supracerebellar cistern (*white arrow*) is larger than normal. The T2-weighted axial image (*B*) and a T1-weighted sagittal image (*C*) through the right cerebellar hemisphere show that the cerebellar hemispheres are also atrophic, with enlarged sulci (*small arrows in B*). The degree of atrophy of the cerebellum is much greater than that of the supratentorial cerebrum.

DIAGNOSIS

Cerebellar degenerative disease (alcoholic)

DISCUSSION

Degeneration and atrophy of the cerebellar vermis and hemispheres occur in up to 40% of individuals with chronic alcoholism.[1] Alcoholic cerebellar degeneration is the most common form of chronic cerebellar disease.[1] Signs and symptoms of cerebellar degeneration include a broad-based staggering gait, truncal instability, ataxia, and impaired heel-to-toe walking. However, only about 50% of patients with radiographic or pathologic evidence of cerebellar degeneration associated with alcoholism have symptoms or abnormal neurologic examinations.

Patients who show both radiologic and clinical signs of cerebellar degeneration generally have a longer history of drinking, more severe cerebral atrophy, and more profound neuropsychologic impairment than those who are asymptomatic.[1]

MR is superior to CT for evaluation of the posterior fossa because of superior contrast, the ability to scan in multiple planes, and the lack of beam hardening artifacts from bony structures. Atrophy of the cerebellar vermis is best seen on midline sagittal images, and is manifested by enlarged sulci between the folia. Usually, the rostral vermis is most severely affected. Atrophy of the cerebellar hemispheres can also be evaluated by sagittal images, although the contrast between the widened cerebellar sulci and the normal cerebellar tissue is best seen on T2-weighted axial images. T2-weighted sagittal images are not normally routinely acquired when evaluating the posterior fossa.

The exact cause of alcoholic cerebellar degeneration is not known, although it has been attributed to both the direct toxic effects of alcohol and to thiamine deficiency, which is common in alcoholics. In severely affected areas, there is loss of Purkinje cells and granular cells, and atrophy of the molecular layer.[1] Atrophy of the cerebellum is not reversible, although clinical improvement commonly occurs with abstinence from alcohol. This is in contrast to alcoholism-induced cerebral atrophy, which is rapidly reversible with abstinence, primarily because of rehydration caused by the increase in alcohol-inhibited antidiuretic hormone.[2]

Pitfalls in Image Interpretation

Olivopontocerebellar degeneration and cerebelloolivary degeneration are primary forms of cerebellar degeneration that may be either familial or sporadic and can cause cerebellar atrophy in nonalcoholics. Olivary atrophy, which is not typically seen in alcoholism-induced cerebellar atrophy, is a hallmark of both of these entities.

Pathologic Correlate

D compares the gross specimen (sagittal section) of the cerebellar vermis from an alcoholic patient (*left*) with that from a normal patient (*right*). The vermis from the alcoholic patient is diffusely atrophic, with both the gray and white matter affected.

Clinical References

1. Hillbom M, Muuronen A, Holm L, et al. The clinical versus radiological diagnosis of alcoholic cerebellar degeneration. J Neurol Sci 1986;73:45–53.
2. Schroth G, Naegele T, Klose U, et al. Reversible brain shrinkage in abstinent alcoholics, measured by MRI. Neuroradiology, 1988;30:385–389.

(F *courtesy of Daron G. Davis, MD.*)

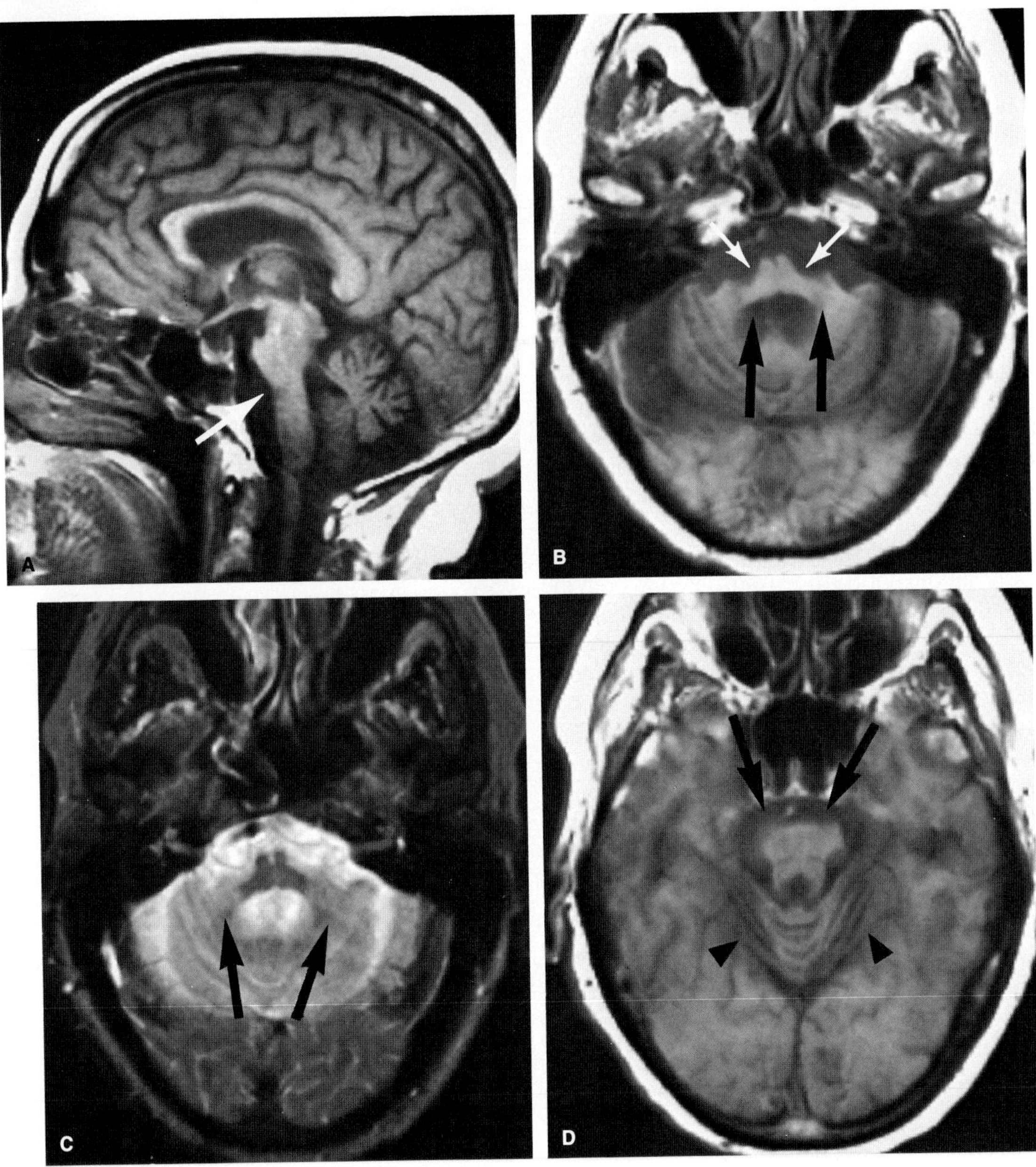

HISTORY

A 72-year-old with ataxia

FINDINGS

(*A*) On the T1-weighted midline sagittal image the pons is severely atrophied and flattened at the pontomedullary junction (*white arrow*). There is mild atrophy of the cerebellar vermis. (*B*) The T1-weighted axial image at the level of the medulla demonstrates loss of the normal olivary bulge bilaterally (*small white arrows*) and atrophy of the middle cerebellar peduncles bilaterally (*black arrows*). The sulci of the cerebellar hemispheres are widened. (*C*) The T2-weighted axial image at the same level reveals abnormally increased signal intensity in the middle cerebellar peduncles (*black arrows*) at their junction with the white matter of the cerebellum. (*D*) Flattening of the ventral pons (*arrows*) and widening of the cerebellar hemispheric sulci (*arrowheads*) are also seen on a T1-weighted axial image at the level of the pons. (*E*) The cerebral hemispheres are not atrophic, as seen on the T1-weighted axial image through the bodies of the lateral ventricles.

DIAGNOSIS

Olivopontocerebellar degeneration

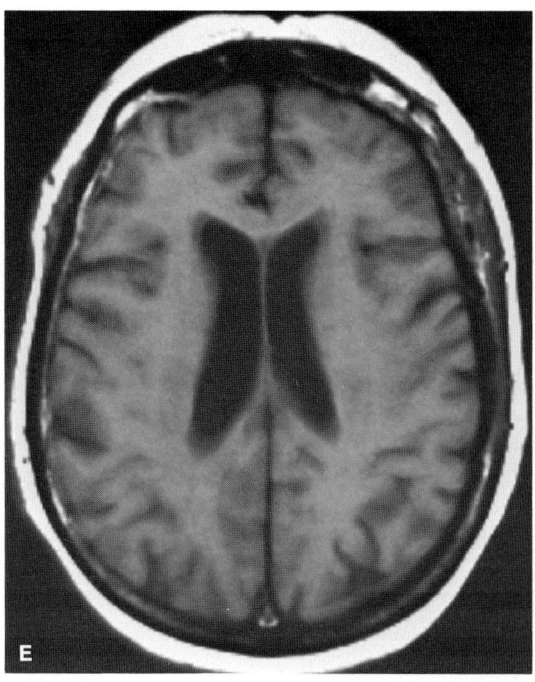

DISCUSSION

Olivopontocerebellar degeneration is a primary CNS disease characterized by atrophy of the pons, middle cerebellar peduncles, and cerebellar hemispheres.[1] Patients with olivopontocerebellar degeneration present with ataxia, initially in the lower extremities, and then in the upper extremities. Most cases occur between the first and fifth decades of life, but it may be seen at any age. Both sporadic and familial cases have been reported.

The degeneration in olivopontocerebellar degeneration is caused by myelin sheath loss and gliosis in the pontocerebellar pathways, and neuronal loss in the pons, cerebellar hemispheres, and olives. Pontine nuclei are the primary centers of degeneration in olivopontocerebellar degeneration. There is subsequent anterograde degeneration of pontocerebellar fibers which originate in these abnormal nuclei. These axons have a transverse course in the pons and then travel to the Purkinje cells in the cerebellar cortex by way of the middle cerebellar peduncles. As a result of the cerebellar cortical atrophy, there is retrograde degeneration of the inferior olives that communicate with the cerebellum by way of axons traveling in the inferior cerebellar peduncles.

The radiographic demonstration of atrophy in the proper structures (pons, middle cerebellar peduncles, cerebellum, and olives) is essential in establishing the diagnosis of olivopontocerebellar degeneration.[1] On MR, selective flattening of the pons, and cerebellar atrophy are well seen on sagittal images. Loss of the normal bulge of the olives is best seen on axial images. Gliosis in the olives, transverse pontine fibers, middle cerebellar peduncles, and cerebellum appears as abnormal high signal intensity on intermediate and heavily T2-weighted images.

Clinical References

1. Savoiardo M, Strada L, Girotti F, et al. Olivopontocerebellar atrophy: MR diagnosis and relationship to multisystem atrophy. Radiology 1990;174:693–696.

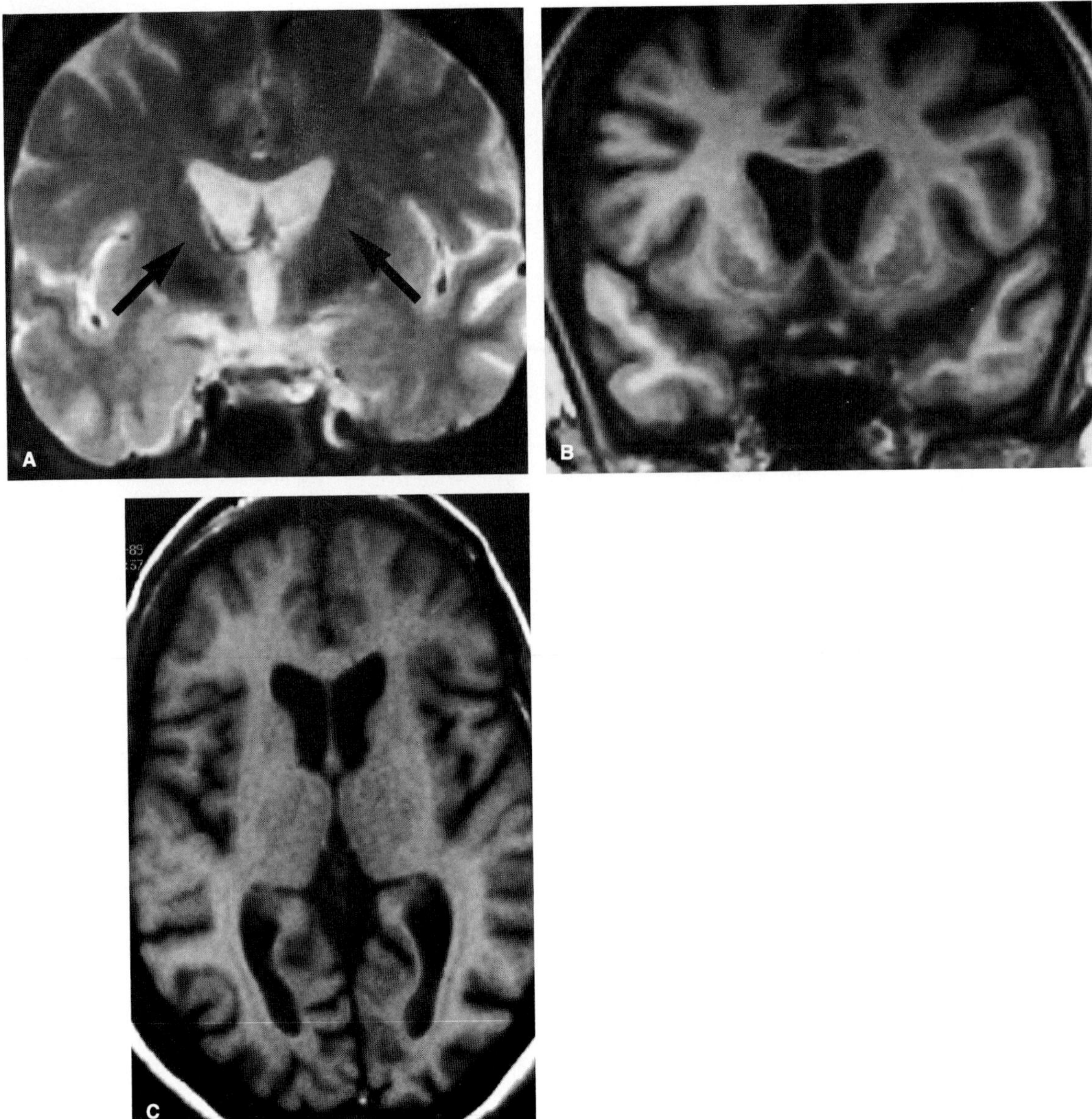

HISTORY

A 54-year-old man with progressive dementia and choreoathetosis

FINDINGS

A decrease in size of the caudate nuclei (*arrows in A*) can be noted on both coronal T1- and T2-weighted (*A and B*) and axial T1-weighted (*C*) images. There is also mild cortical atrophy and ventriculomegaly.

DIAGNOSIS

Huntington's disease

DISCUSSION

MR is superior to CT for demonstration of the morphologic changes in Huntington's disease.[1] Profound degeneration with volume loss occurs in the corpus striatum (which consists of both the caudate nucleus and putamen), followed in time by cortical atrophy. Abnormalities have also been noted in the thalamus and mesial temporal lobe, possibly playing a role in memory loss.[2]

Huntington's disease is a progressive degenerative disorder of the basal ganglia with autosomal dominant inheritance. The defective gene has been localized to chromosome 4. A test is now available using DNA linkage analysis for the identification of individuals carrying the defective gene (who will eventually manifest the disease). Pathophysiologically, there is premature death of certain neurons. The disease is typically manifested in the fourth through sixth decades of life, with a characteristic movement disorder (choreoathetosis) and progressive dementia.

MR Technique

Thin-section axial and coronal images with sufficient contrast (either T1 or T2) to differentiate gray and white matter improve assessment of the corpus striatum. 3D T1-weighted GRE techniques (FLASH or MP-RAGE) are recommended for improved multiplanar depiction and greater accuracy in volume measurements.

Clinical References

1. Simmons JT, Pastakia B, Chase TN, Shults CW. Magnetic resonance imaging in Huntington disease. AJNR 1986;7:25–28.
2. Jernigan TL, Salmon DP, Butters N, Hesselink JR. Cerebral structure on MRI. Part II. Specific changes in Alzheimer's and Huntington's diseases. Biol Psychiatry 1991;29:68–81.

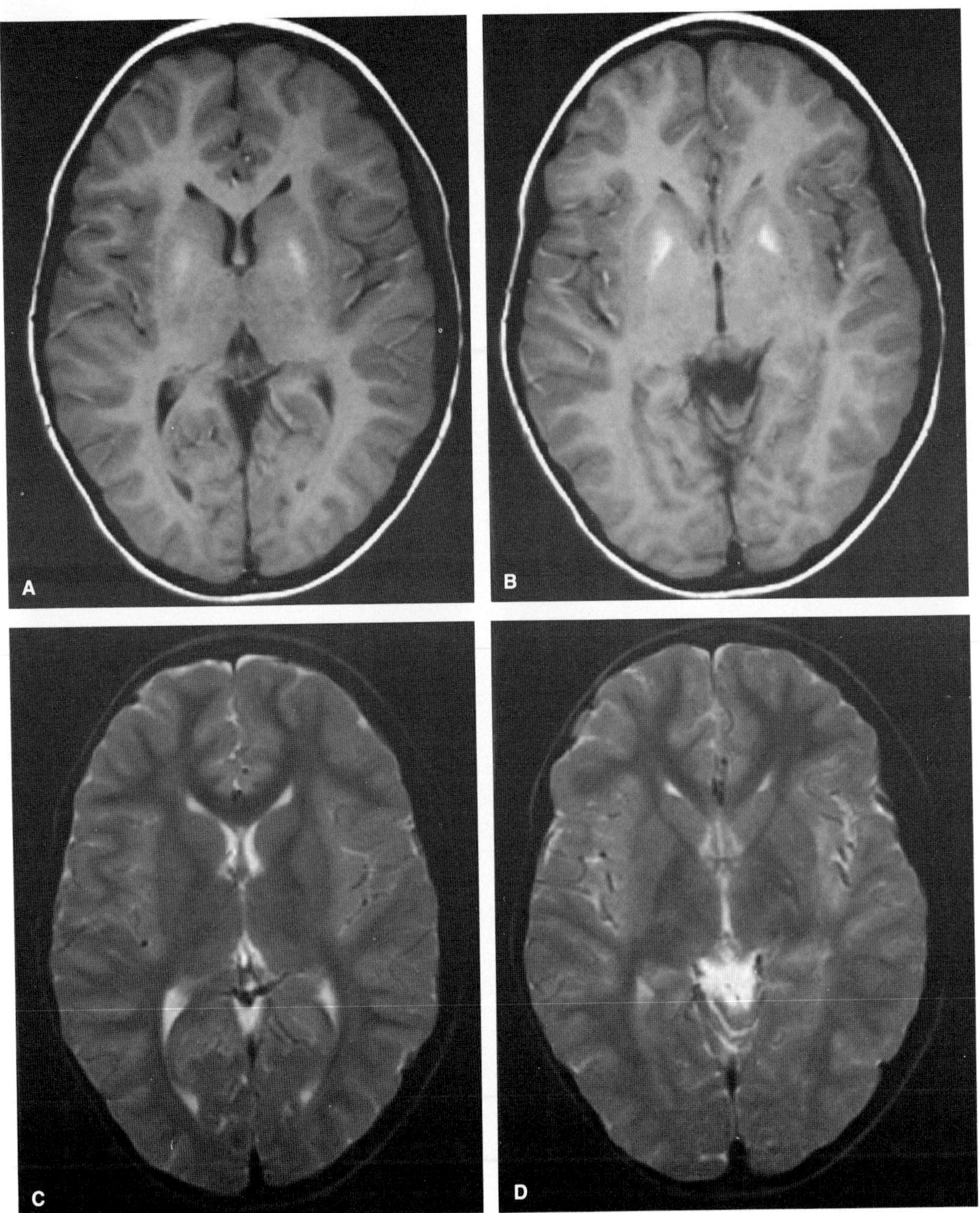

HISTORY

A 10-year-old boy with difficulty walking

FINDINGS

(*A and B*) Hyperintensity is identified in the globus pallidus on contiguous axial T1-weighted images. No abnormal contrast enhancement was noted (*images not shown*). (*C and D*) The lentiform nuclei (globus pallidus and putamen) are of normal signal intensity on the corresponding axial T2-weighted images.

DIAGNOSIS

Hallervorden-Spatz disease (HSD)

DISCUSSION

HSD is a rare metabolic disorder characterized by progression of gait impairment, rigidity of all limbs, slowing of voluntary movements, dystonic posturing, choreoathetosis, dysarthria, dysphasia, optic nerve atrophy, retinal degeneration, and mental deterioration.[1] Its onset is generally in late childhood or early adolescence.[2] No biochemical test is available to make the diagnosis of HSD.[3] Familial occurrence (autosomal recessive) has been reported in about half of cases.

Iron is normally found in the globus pallidus, substantia nigra, and red nuclei in adults, but only trace amounts are present at birth.[4] Ferrokinetic studies in patients with HSD demonstrate iron deposition in the basal ganglia. The neuropathologic changes include bilateral, destructive lesions of the globus pallidus (especially their internal segment) and pars reticulata of the substantia nigra, variable amounts of gliosis, iron deposits, loss of myelinated fibers, and swollen axonal "spheroids."

The globus pallidus can have a variable appearance on T2-weighted images in this disease. Hyperintensity, hypointensity, and mixed signal intensity of this nucleus on T2-weighted images have been described. The "eye of the tiger" sign has been described, which is a targetlike configuration with a peripheral hypointense ring and central hyperintensity.[5] Older patients (greater than 20 years) tended to have greater hypointensity of the globus pallidus than younger patients. Little has been written concerning the T1 appearance of the globus pallidus in HSD.

Pitfalls in Image Interpretation

The differential diagnosis of hyperintense basal ganglia on precontrast T1-weighted images, without accompanying T2-weighted changes, includes patients receiving total parenteral nutrition.[6] The symmetric abnormal hyperintensity on T2-weighted images in such patients is thought to be related either to deposition of paramagnetic trace elements, such as manganese, or to associated gliosis.

Clinical References

1. Gallucci M, Cardona F, Arachi M, et al. Follow-up MR studies in Hallervorden-Spatz disease. J Comput Assist Tomogr 1989;14:118–120.
2. Ambrosetto P, Nonni R, Bacci A, et al. Late onset familial Hallervorden-Spatz disease: MR finding in two sisters. AJNR 1992;13:394–396.
3. Tanfani G, Mascalchi M, Dal Pozzo GC, et al. MR imaging in a case of Hallervorden-Spatz disease. J Comput Assist Tomogr 1987;11:1157–1158.
4. Schaffert DA, Johnsen SD, Johnson PC, Drayer BP. Magnetic resonance imaging in pathologically proven Hallervorden-Spatz disease. Neurology 1989;39:440–442.
5. Sethi KD, Adams RJ, Loring DW, et al. Hallervorden-Spatz syndrome: clinical and magnetic resonance imaging correlations. Ann Neurol 1988;24:692–694.
6. Mirowitz SA, Westrich TJ, Hirsh JD. Hyperintense basal ganglia on T1-weighted MR images in patients receiving parenteral nutrition. Radiology 1991;181:117–120.

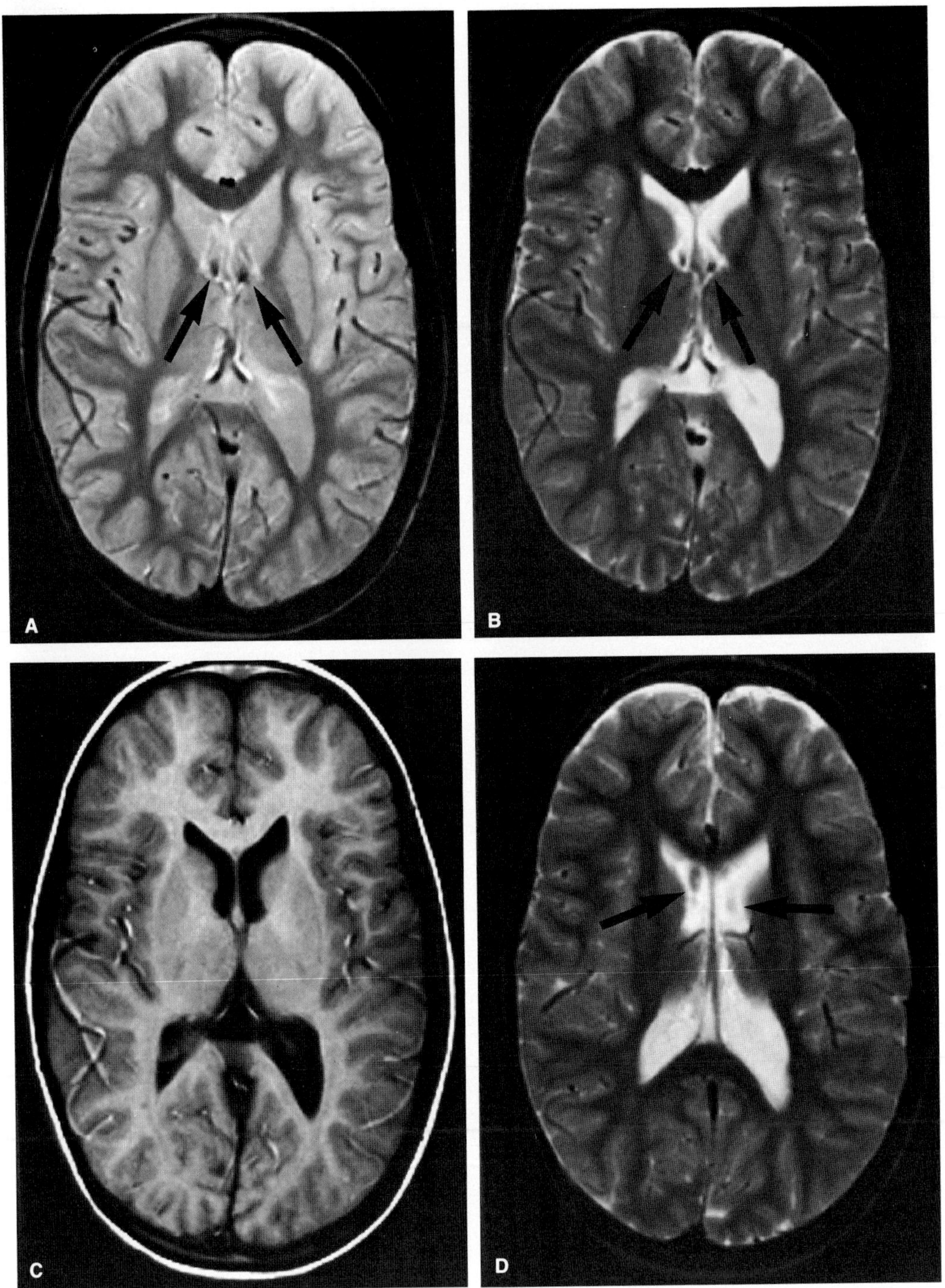

HISTORY

Noncontributory

FINDINGS

Bilateral symmetric intraventricular lesions of decreased signal intensity (*arrows in A and B*) are identified in the frontal horns of the lateral ventricles just superior to the foramen of Monro on the first (*A*) and second (*B*) echoes of the axial T2-weighted sequence. (*C*) Axial T1-weighted image is normal. (*D*) At a position just superior to this level these low intensity lesions (*arrows*) appear to extend anteriorly into the lateral ventricles on an axial T2-weighted image (TE = 90 msec). No abnormal contrast enhancement was noted (*images not shown*).

DIAGNOSIS

CSF flow phenomena

DISCUSSION

Cerebrospinal fluid production within the ventricular system and CSF resorption by the arachnoid villi (located over the convexity) result in bulk CSF flow from within the ventricular system to outside the ventricular system. CSF flow is pulsatile and is related to the cardiac cycle. A vascular-driven movement of the entire brain results in pumping of the CSF. This is secondary to an arterial pulse wave transmitted from the aortic root through the vascular system into the cerebral vasculature. This pulse wave is then transmitted to the CSF, resulting in pressure variations within the CSF.[1] Expansion of the brain occurs during systole, forcing CSF downward; the brain relaxes during diastole and CSF flows superiorly.[2,3]

A flow void within the cerebral aqueduct is a common finding on MR imaging. Pulsatile or turbulent flow is noted in the lateral ventricles typically only adjacent to the foramen of Monro.

Pitfalls in Image Interpretation

CSF flow phenomena can produce intraventricular signal loss, which should be recognized as such and not mistaken for a space occupying lesion.

Clinical References

1. Quencer RM, Donovan Post MJ, Hinks RS. Cine MR in the evaluation of normal and abnormal CSF flow: intracranial and intraspinal studies. Neuroradiology 1990;32:371–391.
2. Feinberg DA, Mark AS. Human brain motion and cerebrospinal fluid circulation demonstrated with MR velocity imaging. Radiology 1987;163:793–799.
3. Levy LM, Chiro GD. MR phase imaging and cerebrospinal fluid flow in the head and spine. Neuroradiology 1990; 32:399–406.

CHAPTER
THREE

Face, Mastoids, and Neck

Val M. Runge
Robert A. Garneau
Mitchell A. Brack

Magnetic Resonance Imaging of the Brain,
edited by Val M. Runge.
J. B. Lippincott Company, Philadelphia © 1994.

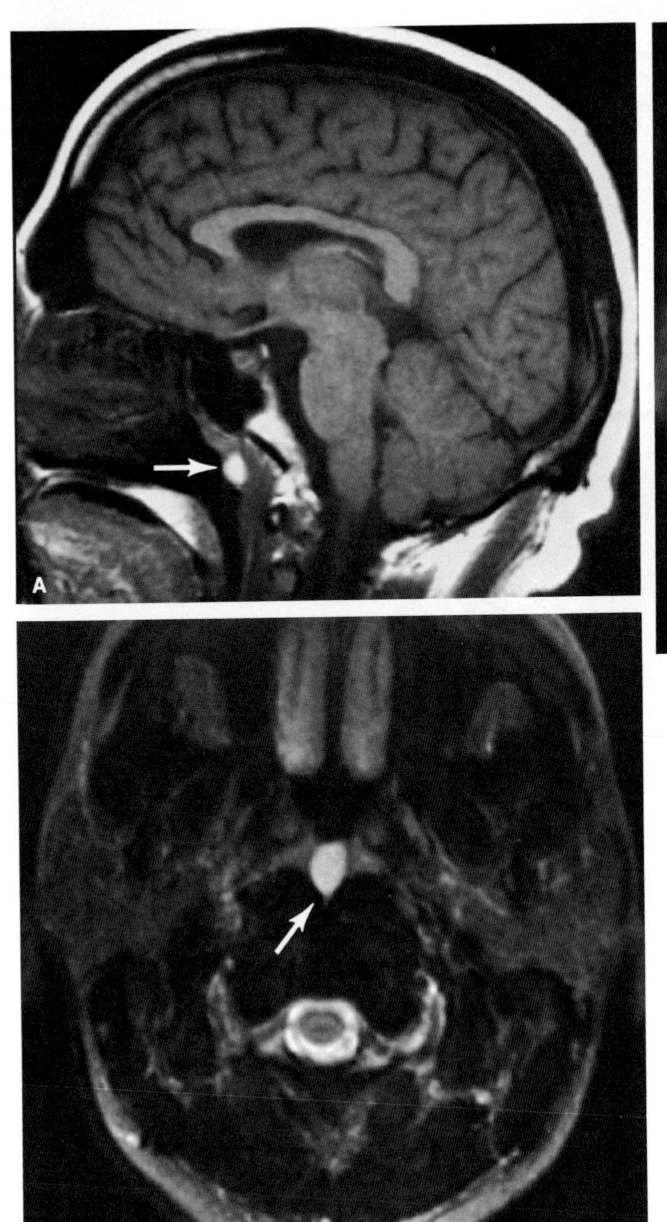
A
C

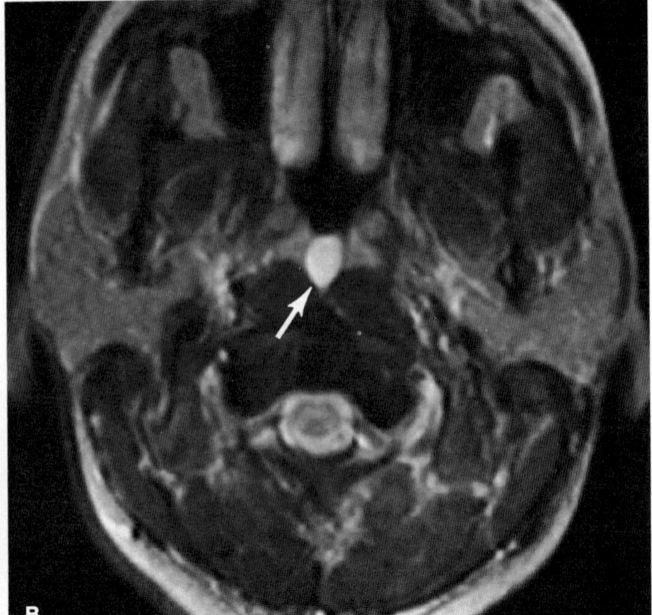
B

HISTORY

Noncontributory

FINDINGS

(*A*) A small round lesion (*white arrow*) of increased signal intensity on the sagittal T1-weighted image is identified in the midline in the posterior nasopharyngeal recess. No contrast enhancement was noted (*images not shown*). This lesion (*white arrow*) is hyperintense on the first (TE=45 msec) (*B*) and second (TE=90 msec) (*D*) echoes of the axial T2-weighted examination.

DIAGNOSIS

Thornwaldt cyst

DISCUSSION

Thornwaldt cyst is an incidental finding that presents as a midline nasopharyngeal, nonenhancing mass. This cyst arises from the notochordal remnant in the posterior nasopharyngeal vault and is lined by respiratory epithelium.[1] It can communicate with the nasopharyngeal lumen and typically is less than 3 cm in diameter, is smooth surfaced, and does not result in bony erosion.[2] Thornwaldt cyst is usually asymptomatic but can result in persistent nasopharyngeal drainage, headache, and an unpleasant taste. It occurs in all age groups, and has an approximate incidence of 4% in autopsy series.

Thornwaldt cysts present as oval, well-circumscribed, high-signal-intensity masses in the posterior nasopharynx on T2-weighted images. These lesions are usually of slightly increased signal intensity on T1-weighted images, but the signal intensity can vary from hyperintense to hypointense on T1-weighted images.

Pitfalls in Image Interpretation

A pharyngeal abscess is usually located in the posterior pharyngeal wall, but pain and systemic symptoms bring this lesion to attention.

Clinical References

1. Ford WJ, Brooks BS, Gammal TE. Thornwaldt cyst: an incidental MR diagnosis. AJNR 1987;8:922–933.
2. Potter GD, Bryan RN, Hanafee WN, et al. Disorders of the head and neck: syllabus (3rd series). Chicago, FH Young, 1985;334–335.

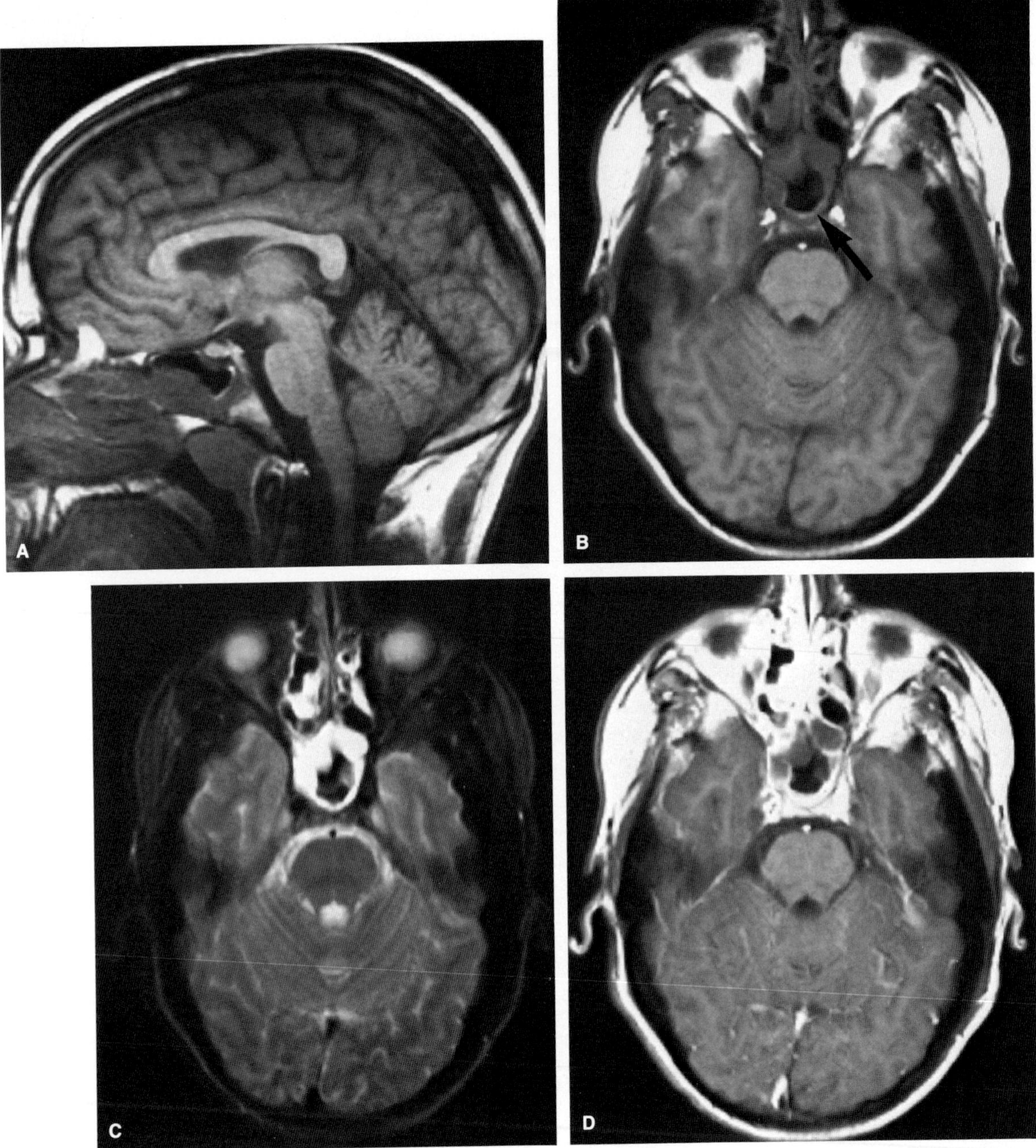

HISTORY

Noncontributory

FINDINGS

Abnormal hypointense soft tissue is seen at the periphery of the sphenoid sinus (*arrow in B*) on sagittal (*A*) and axial (*B*) T1-weighted images. The posterior ethmoid air cells also contain abnormal hypointense soft tissue. (*C*) This material is of marked hyperintensity on the axial T2-weighted image. (*D*) Rim enhancement of this material is demonstrated on the axial T1-weighted image postcontrast.

DIAGNOSIS

Mucosal membrane thickening

DISCUSSION

Paranasal sinus disease is seen as an incidental finding in as many as 40% of patients referred for head MR because of suspected intracranial pathology. The maxillary and ethmoid sinuses are affected most commonly with 27% and 26% abnormal, respectively. The frontal and sphenoid sinuses are affected far less frequently, showing abnormality in only 5% of studies. Similar findings have also been reported by CT.[1]

A positive culture of sinus aspirate is likely if the thickness of the sinus mucosal membrane is 5 mm or greater in adults, or 4 mm or greater in children. The predominant organisms include *Streptococcus pneumoniae, Branhamella catarrhalis,* and nontypable *Haemophilus influenzae.* Viruses such as adenovirus and parainfluenza have also been recovered in paranasal sinus aspirates.[2]

Paranasal sinuses develop during gestation. The maxillary and ethmoid sinuses are pneumatized in the neonatal and early infantile period. The sphenoid sinus does not pneumatize until 2 to 3 years of age and the frontal sinuses do not become distinct from the ethmoid air cells and reach their adult appearance until approximately 6 years of age.[3]

Pitfalls in Image Interpretation

A small retention cyst can be difficult to differentiate from focal mucosal membrane thickening.

Clinical References

1. Cooke LD, Hadley DM. MRI of the paranasal sinuses: incidental abnormalities and their relationship to symptoms. J Laryngol Otol 1991;105:278–281.
2. Wald ER. Sinusitis in children. Pediatr Infect Dis J 1988; 7:150–153.
3. Siegel JD. Diagnosis and management of acute sinusitis in children. Pediatr Infect Dis J 1987;6:95–99.

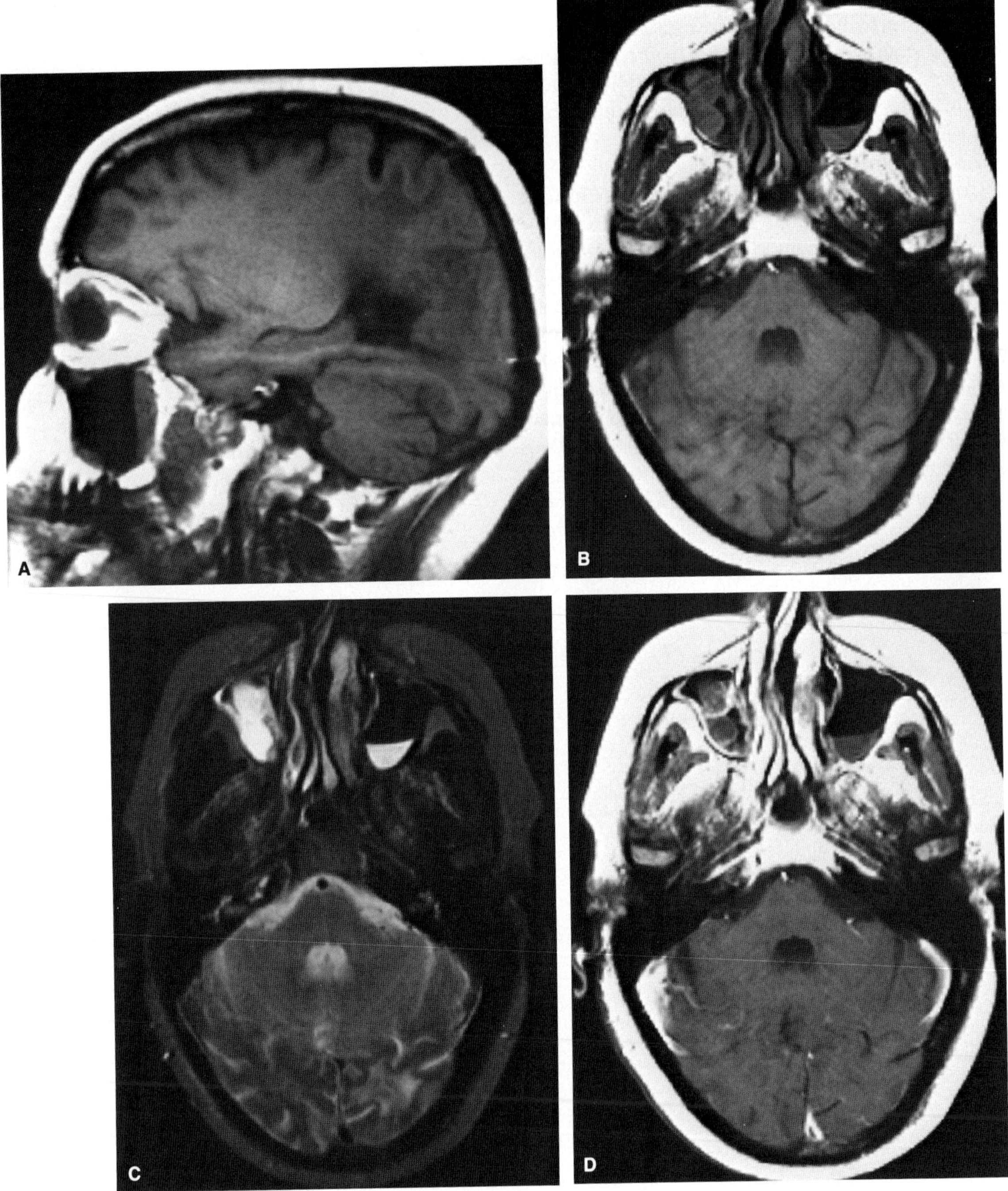

HISTORY

Noncontributory

FINDINGS

An anterior signal void, separated from the posterior dependent portion of the left maxillary sinus by a straight, smooth interface, is identified on sagittal (*A*) and axial (*B*) T1-weighted images. The dependent portion of the left maxillary sinus demonstrates mild hypointensity on *A* and *B* and marked hyperintensity on the axial T2-weighted image (*C*). (*D*) The peripheral margins of this dependent fluid collection enhance on the axial T1-weighted image postcontrast.

DIAGNOSIS

Air-fluid level (left maxillary sinus)

DISCUSSION

Almost all acute, and the majority of chronic, paranasal sinus inflammatory disease has increased signal intensity on T2-weighted images. This hyperintensity is secondary to increased water content. The signal intensity of paranasal sinus inflammatory disease on T1-weighted images is more variable and depends not only on water content but also on the protein content of the fluid within the sinus. Increasing the amount of proteinaceous material in a fluid collection results in shortening of the T1 relaxation time and thus increases the signal intensity on T1-weighted images.[1]

The diagnosis of acute sinusitis can only be made radiologically if an air-fluid level is demonstrated by MR, CT, or plain films. The maxillary sinus is most commonly involved.[2] Normal sinus function is dependent on patent ostia, ciliary function, and mucus production. Any condition that interferes with any one of these functions increases the risk of developing a sinus infection. The high incidence of sinusitis in patients with cystic fibrosis is attributed to the increased viscosity of mucus produced by these patients. A fluid culture obtained by sinus puncture is the only definitive test for determining the etiology of sinus infections. Throat and nasopharyngeal cultures do not correlate well with cultures of aspirated sinus fluid.[3]

The most common complications of sinusitis are orbital and intracranial infections, which are more common in children than adults. Preseptal cellulitis and orbital cellulitis are the most common complications seen in children.

Pitfalls in Image Interpretation

A retention cyst can mimic the appearance of an air–fluid level when viewed in only one anatomic plane.

Clinical References

1. Shapiro MD, Som PM. MRI of the paranasal sinuses and nasal cavity. Radiol Clin North Am 1989;27:447–475.
2. Harnsberger HR. Head and neck imaging. Handbooks in radiology. Chicago, Year Book Medical Publishers, 1990:
3. Siegel JD. Diagnosis and management of acute sinusitis in children. Pediatr Infect Dis J 1987;6:95–99.

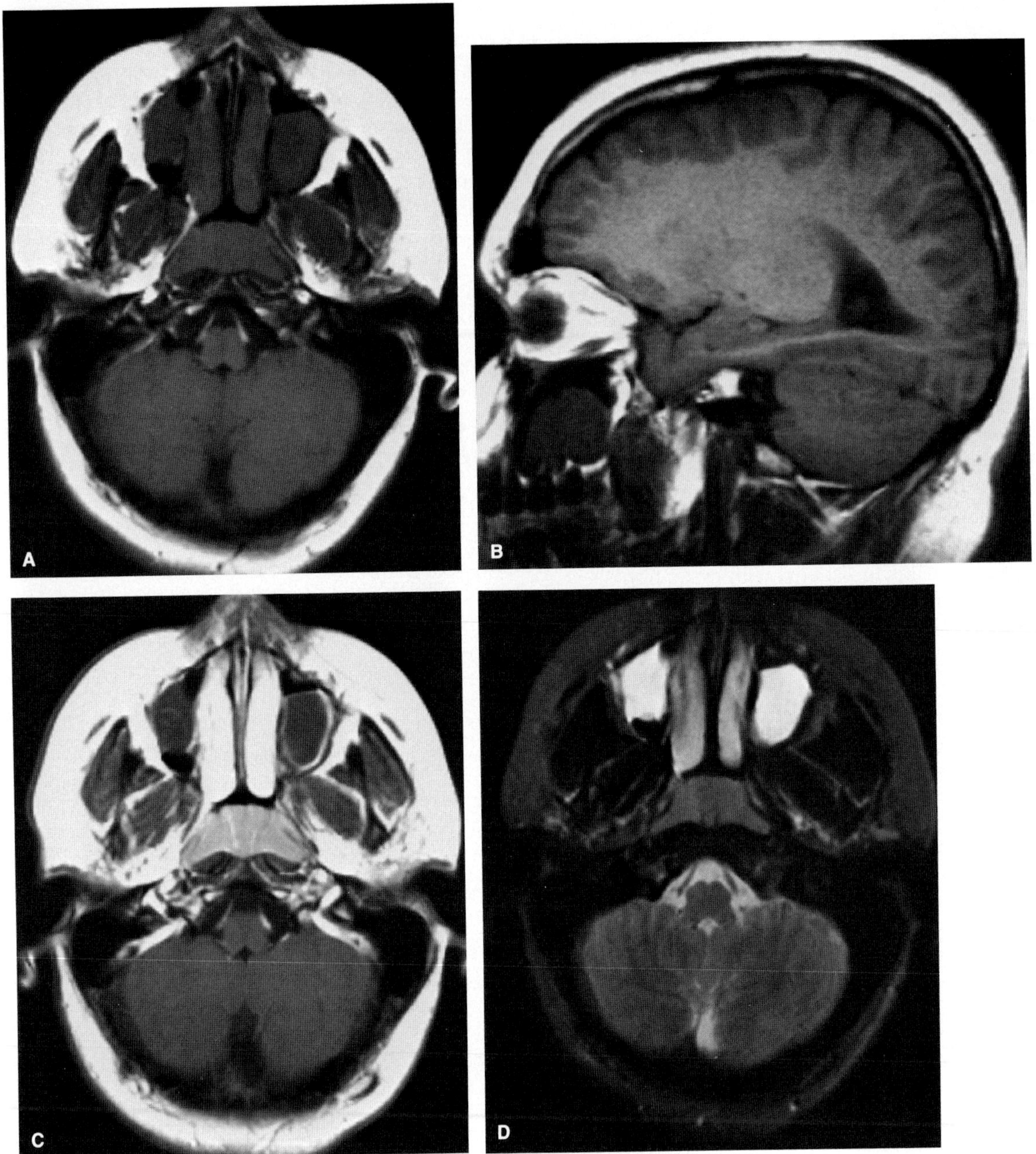

HISTORY

Noncontributory

FINDINGS

Patient 1: (*A*) Soft tissue intensity masses are identified in the right and left maxillary sinuses on the axial T1-weighted image. (*B*) The left parasagittal T1-weighted image reveals the mass in the left maxillary sinus to be oval in shape, with a broad base along the inferior surface of the sinus. (*C*) Postcontrast axial T1-weighted image shows intense peripheral enhancement of the left maxillary sinus mass and subtle peripheral enhancement of the right maxillary sinus mass. (*D*) Both masses are hyperintense on the axial T2-weighted image.

Patient 2: (*E*) On the axial T2-weighted image, abnormal soft tissue with intermediate signal intensity is seen invading the walls of the right maxillary sinus, right sphenoid wing, and right cavernous sinus. Hyperintense signal intensity (representing obstructive inflammatory changes) is identified within both maxillary sinuses.

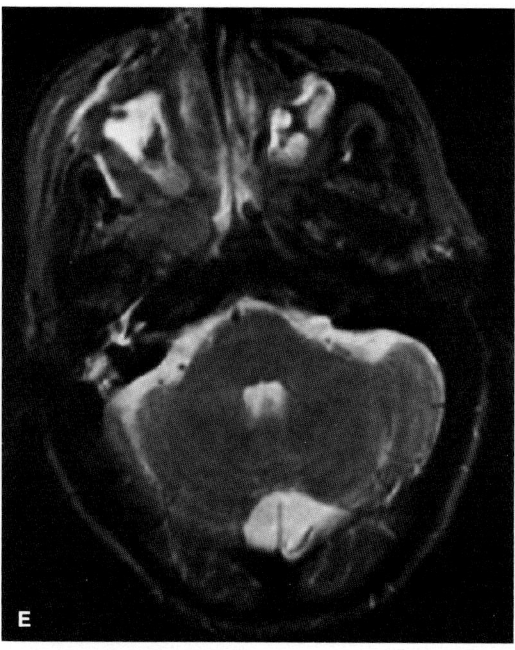

DIAGNOSIS

Patient 1: Bilateral maxillary sinus retention cysts

Patient 2: Squamous cell carcinoma with obstructive maxillary sinus inflammatory disease

DISCUSSION

It is important to differentiate paranasal and nasal inflammatory changes from sinonasal tumors. On T2-weighted images, inflammatory disease presents as very high signal intensity, whereas most (90% to 95%) tumors have an intermediate signal intensity (*as seen in E*). Approximately 80% of these tumors are squamous cell carcinoma. Minor salivary gland tumors are the next most frequent group of neoplasms occurring in this region. The most common sinonasal tumors that have a high T2 signal intensity are minor salivary gland tumors such as mucoepidermoid carcinomas (which contain mucin and serous material). Tumors other than minor salivary gland tumors that can have increased signal intensity on T2-weighted images include neuromas and inverted papillomas. Inflammatory tissue is characterized by interstitial edema, serous fluid, and mucous secretions, all of which have long T2 relaxation times. Thus, mucosal thickening, retention cysts, polyps, and mucoceles usually have very high signal intensity on T2-weighted images.[1,2]

The mucous retention cyst is a benign, self-limiting mass (it ruptures spontaneously), which is rarely symptomatic. These cysts result from accumulation of mucus within the soft tissue lining of the sinus secondary to ductal obstruction of a gland within the lining. They have a round or oval configuration and are based along the wall of a sinus.[3] The maxillary sinus is the most frequently affected.

Clinical References

1. Som PM, Shapiro MD, Biller HF, et al. Sinonasal tumors and inflammatory tissues: differentiation with MR imaging. Radiology 1988;167:803–808.
2. Shapiro MD, Som PM. MRI of the paranasal sinuses and nasal cavity. Radiol Clin North Am 1989;27:447–475.
3. Ruprecht A, Batniji S, El-Neweihi E. Mucous retention cyst of the maxillary sinus. Oral Surg Oral Med Oral Pathol 1986;62:728–731.

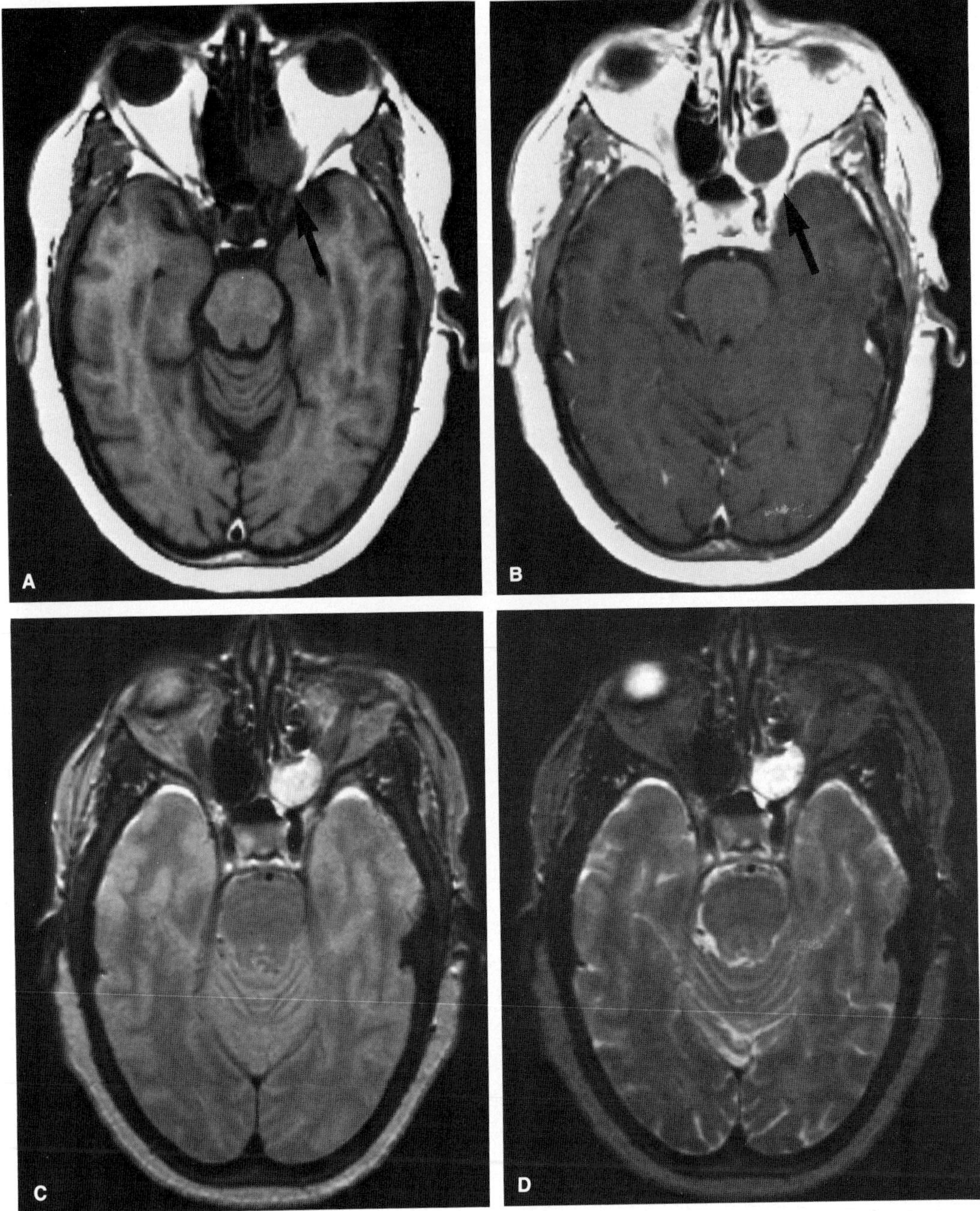

HISTORY

A 36-year-old man with hearing loss

FINDINGS

A round, low-signal-intensity expansile mass (*arrows*) is identified within a posterior ethmoid air cell on precontrast (*A*) and postcontrast (*B*) T1-weighted images. (*B*) Peripheral enhancement of this mass is noted postcontrast. The lesion is of increased signal intensity on the first (*C*) and second (*D*) echoes of the T2-weighted examination.

DIAGNOSIS

Mucocele

DISCUSSION

Mucoceles are common cystic expansile lesions involving the paranasal sinuses. Approximately 60% occur in the frontal sinuses, 30% in the ethmoid sinuses, with lesions less common in the maxillary and sphenoid sinuses.[1] The anterior ethmoid air cells are more frequently affected than the posterior.[2] Mucoceles are benign, slow-growing masses that develop secondary to obstruction of the sinus ostium. They are lined by secretory respiratory columnar epithelium. As the mucosa secretes mucoid fluid, the mass enlarges slowly, expanding and eroding adjacent bony structures. A history of sinus disease, allergies, or trauma is elicited in many of these patients.

MR demonstrates mucoceles as well-defined, expansile paranasal sinus lesions that have variable signal intensity depending on fluid content. Mucoceles can be hyperintense on both T1- and T2-weighted sequences, low signal intensity on T1-weighted sequences, and high signal intensity on T2-weighted sequences, or low signal intensity on both T1- and T2-weighted sequences.[3] Increased signal intensity on T1-weighted images is compatible with proteinaceous fluid resulting in more efficient T1 relaxation. As a mucocele ages, the relative water content of the secretions decreases, resulting in increased protein content.[4] Low-signal-intensity mucoceles have been reported with fungal infections, particularly allergic aspergillus sinusitis.

Pitfalls in Image Interpretation

The variable signal characteristics of paranasal sinus mucoceles should not lead to confusion if greater emphasis is placed on the morphologic features of these lesions.

Clinical References

1. Flanders AE, Rao VM. Paranasal sinus mucocele: unusual MR manifestations at 1.5T. Magn Reson Imaging 1989; 7:333–337.
2. Schwaighofer BW, Sobel DF, Klein MV, et al. Mucocele of the anterior cliniod process: CT and MR findings. J Comput Assist Tomogr 1989;13:501–501.
3. Van Tassel P, Lee Y, Jing B, et al. Mucoceles of the paranasal sinuses: MR imaging with CT correlation. AJR 1989;153:407–412.
4. Weissman JL, Tabor EK, Curtain HD. Magnetic resonance imaging of the paranasal sinuses. Top Magn Reson Imaging 1990;2:27–38.

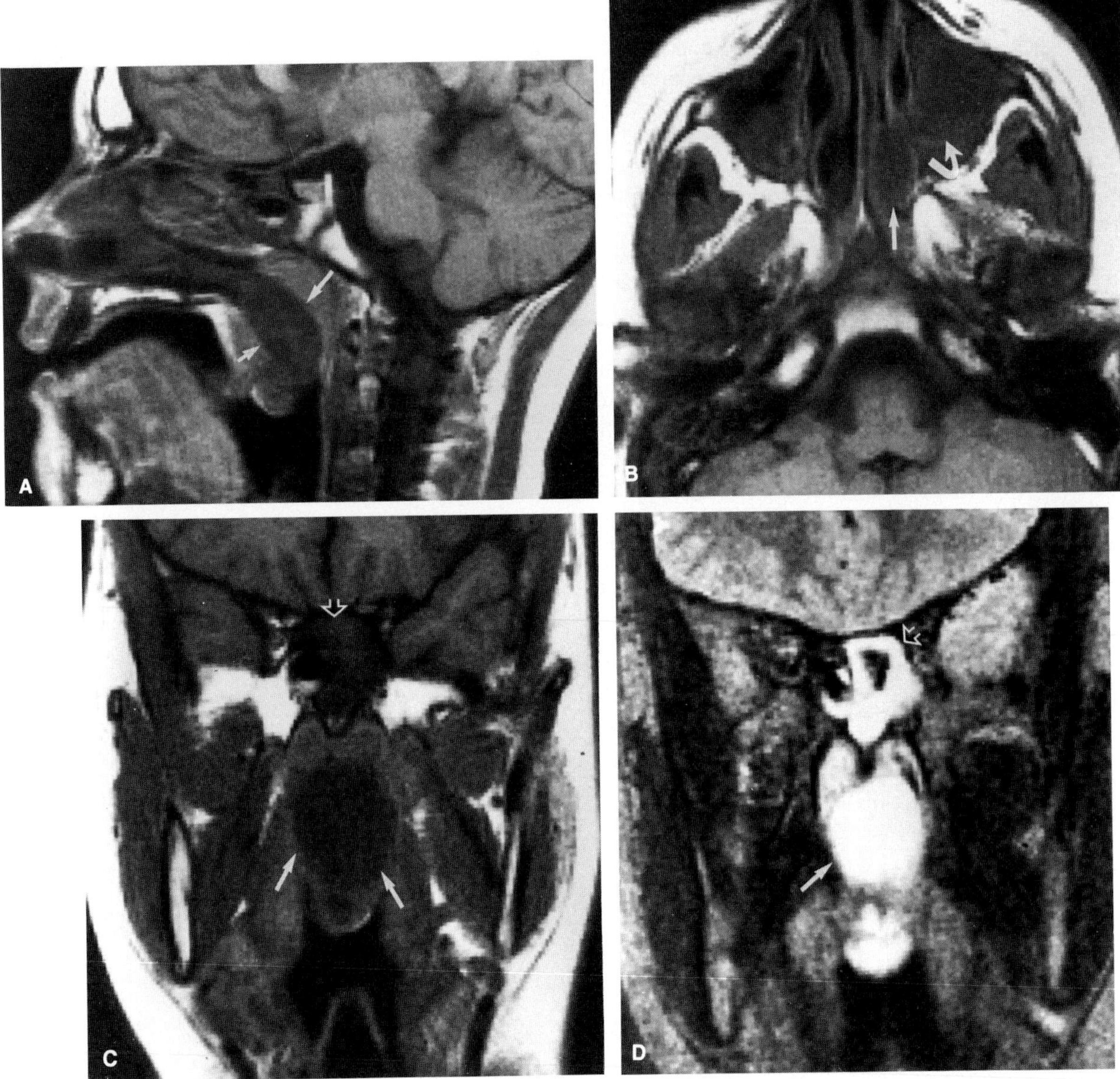

HISTORY

An adolescent with opacification of the left maxillary sinus and obliteration of the nasopharynx on conventional x-ray films

FINDINGS

Sagittal (*A*), axial (*B*), and coronal (*C*) T1-weighted images demonstrate a polypoid soft tissue mass (*arrows*), which originates in the maxillary sinus (*curved arrow in B*) and fills the nasopharyngeal airway. Retained secretions and mucosal thickening are noted in the sphenoid sinus (*open arrows in C and D*), also with low signal intensity on the T1-weighted scan and high signal intensity on the T2-weighted scan (*D*). By signal intensity characteristics alone, the sphenoid sinus disease and the polypoid mass (*arrow in D*) cannot be differented.

DIAGNOSIS

Antrochoanal polyp

DISCUSSION

Antrochoanal polyps represent approximately 5% of all nasal polyps and are more common in children. Nasal polyps in general can be of either allergic or inflammatory origin. The antrochoanal polyp arises in the maxillary antrum, expands the ostium, and extends into the nasal cavity along the choana. Bilateral disease is not uncommon. Clinically, this entity can be mimicked by other less benign lesions including juvenile angiofibroma, meningoencephalocele, and nasopharyngeal malignancy. On the basis of surgical exploration, it has been suggested that choanal polyps arise from a cyst within the lining of the sinus wall, which progressively expands.[1]

Current treatment for an antrochoanal polyp is by surgical resection of the nasal portion, with or without the antral portion.[2] Endoscopic surgery, with complete removal of the lesion, can now be performed as an outpatient procedure.

Pitfalls in Image Interpretation

Acute maxillary sinusitis, in rare instances, can mimic the appearance of an antrochoanal polyp. In such instances, the inflamed, swollen, redundant mucosa can prolapse through a widened sinus ostium into the nasal cavity. Fortunately, clinical management is similar.[3] In rare instances, a polyp may arise from the sphenoid sinus (sphenochoanal), with differentiation from an antrochoanal polyp important for surgical planning.[4]

Clinical References

1. Berg O, Carenfelt C, Silfversward C, Sobin A. Origin of the choanal polyp. Arch Otolaryngol Head Neck Surg 1988; 114:1270–1271.
2. Kamel R. Endoscopic transnasal surgery in antrochoanal polyp. Arch Otolaryngol Head Neck Surg 1990;116:841–843.
3. Nino-Murcia M, Rao VM, Mikaelian DO, Som P. Acute sinusitis mimicking antrochoanal polyp. AJNR 1986;7:513–516.
4. Wissman JL, Tabor EK, Curtin HD. Sphenochoanal polyps: evaluation with CT and MR imaging. Radiology 1991; 178:145–148.

*(*A *through* D *from Runge VM. Clinical magnetic resonance imaging. Philadelphia, JB Lippincott, 1990.)*

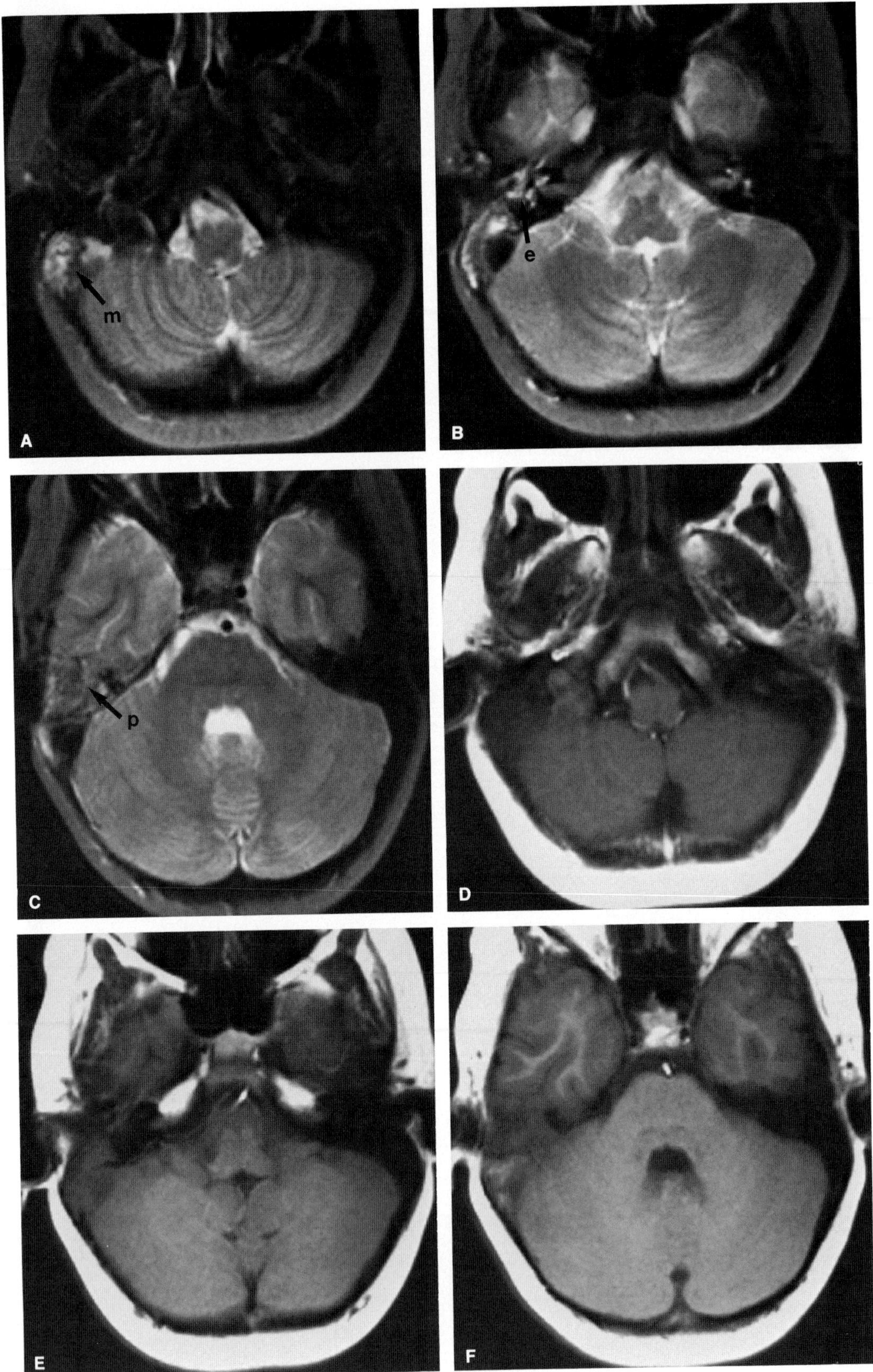
m
e
p
A
B
C
D
E
F

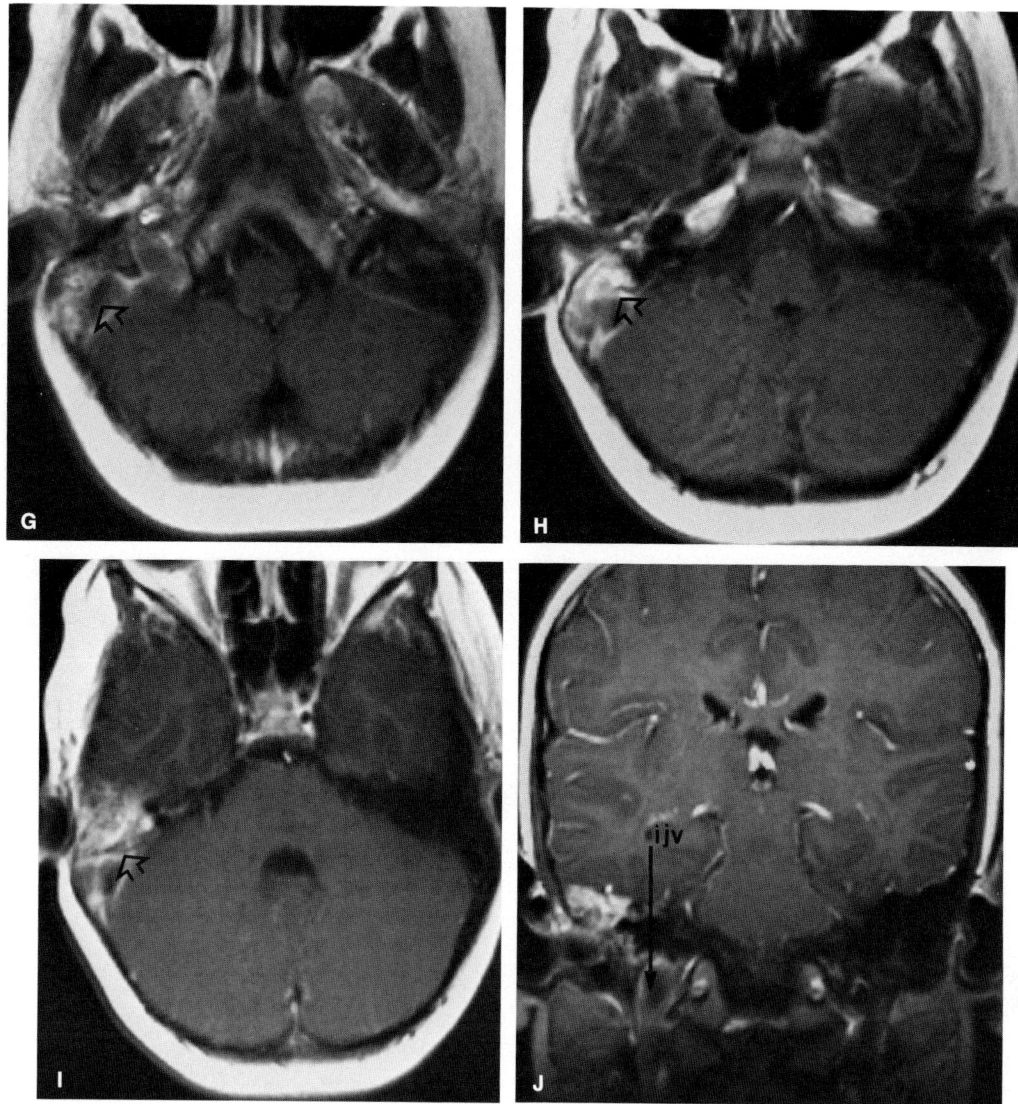

HISTORY

A 7-year-old boy with right earache, nausea, vomiting, and low-grade fever. Physical examination reveals a right sixth nerve palsy and an erythematous right tympanic membrane.

FINDINGS

(*A to C*) On the precontrast T2-weighted axial examination, there is abnormal mixed signal intensity in the right mastoid (m *in A*), middle ear (e *in B*), and petrous bone (p *in C*). (*D to F*) The precontrast T1-weighted axial examination at the same levels confirms the presence of abnormal soft tissue. (*G to I*) Postcontrast, on the axial examination, these regions demonstrate abnormal enhancement (*open arrows*). The right transverse and sigmoid sinuses, however, remain unopacified. (*J to M*) Occlusion of the right transverse sinus (ts), sigmoid sinus (ss), jugular bulb (jb), and internal jugular vein (ijv) is confirmed on the coronal postcontrast examination. These venous channels remain unopacified postcontrast, with enhancement of only the vessel wall. (*N*) Bone windows from a CT examination of the same date reveal opacification of the right mastoid air cells, but no definite bony erosion. On follow-up MR 10 days later, there is abnormal hyperintensity (*curved arrows*) on both the T2-weighted (*O*) and T1-weighted (*P*) images precontrast in the right transverse sinus, consistent with evolution of the thrombus from principally deoxyhemoglobin to methemoglobin. Repeat examination 1 month later demonstrated recanalization (*not shown*).

DIAGNOSIS

Mastoiditis, with secondary transverse and sigmoid sinus thrombosis

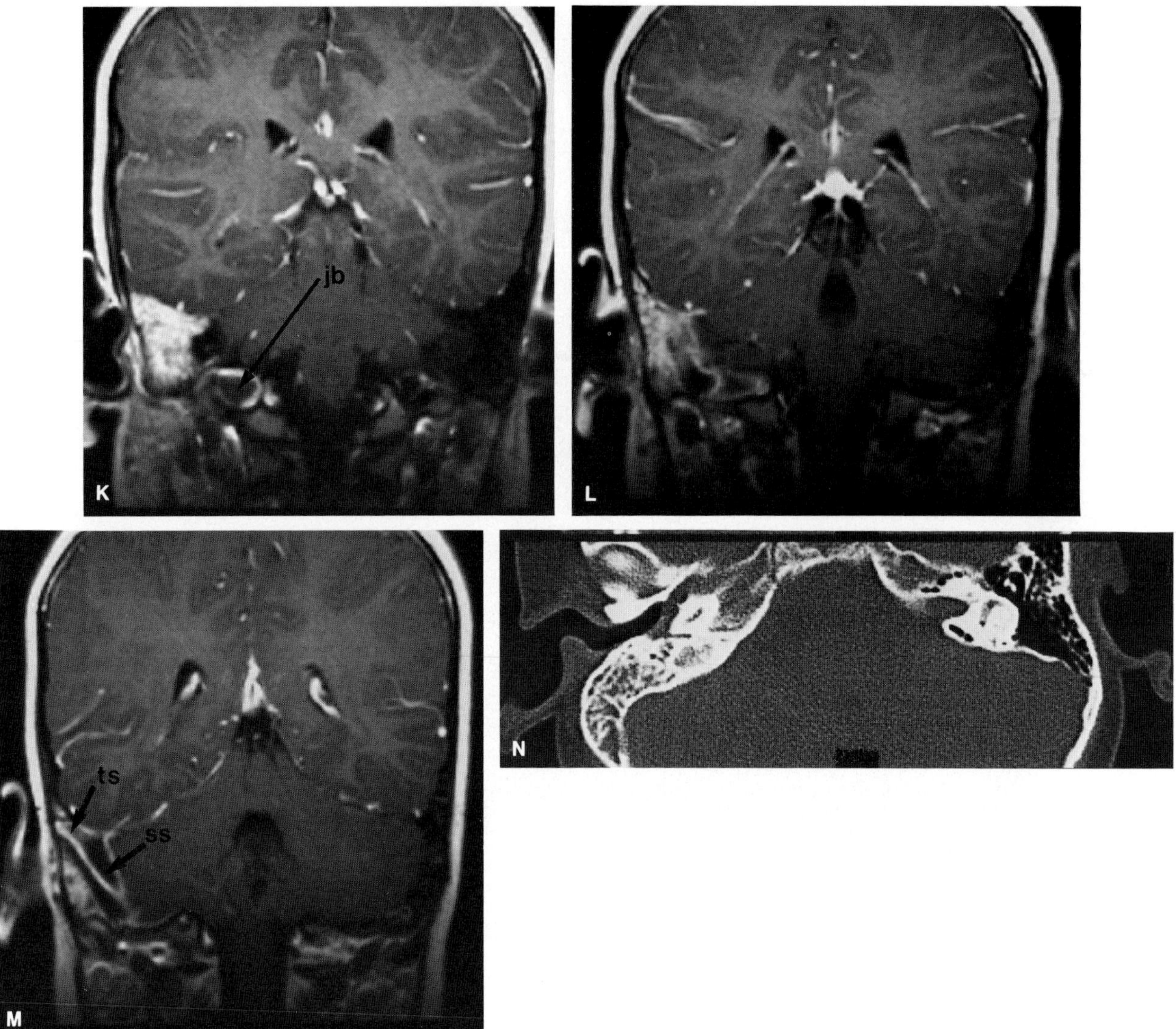

DISCUSSION

Acute otitis media is most commonly viral in origin, secondary to upper respiratory tract infection. Bacterial disease is most often caused by *Streptococcus pneumoniae* or *Haemophilus influenzae.* Treatment is with antibiotics. Persistent infection may necessitate myringotomy with tube placement. There is direct continuity between the middle ear cavity and the mastoid air cells, a simple route for spread of infection. Extracranial complications of otitis media and mastoiditis include hearing loss, paralysis of the ipsilateral facial nerve (due to labyrinthitis), and paralysis of the ipsilateral sixth cranial nerve (due to involvement of the petrous apex). Intracranial complications include meningitis, abscess (brain or epidural), sinus thrombosis, and hydrocephalus. The dural venous structure most commonly effected in otologic infection is the sigmoid sinus.[1]

Although incidental mastoid sinus disease is commonly seen on MR, the prominent soft tissue involvement and degree of enhancement in the present case favor active infection. The secondary finding of dural thrombosis confirms this diagnosis. Septic thrombosis of the transverse and sigmoid sinuses is a highly lethal condition, with clinical signs at presentation often subtle.[2] Contrast-enhanced MR demonstrates soft-tissue signal intensity thrombus surrounded by an enhancing dural sinus wall, a distinctive appearance which permits diagnosis. Although CT can also be diagnostic, enhanced MR appears more sensitive.

In the case presented, treatment included myringotomy with tube placement, intravenous (IV) antibiotics, and anticoagulation with IV heparin.

MR Technique

The transverse sinus can be assessed for patency by MR venography, phase imaging, GRE imaging, or acqui-

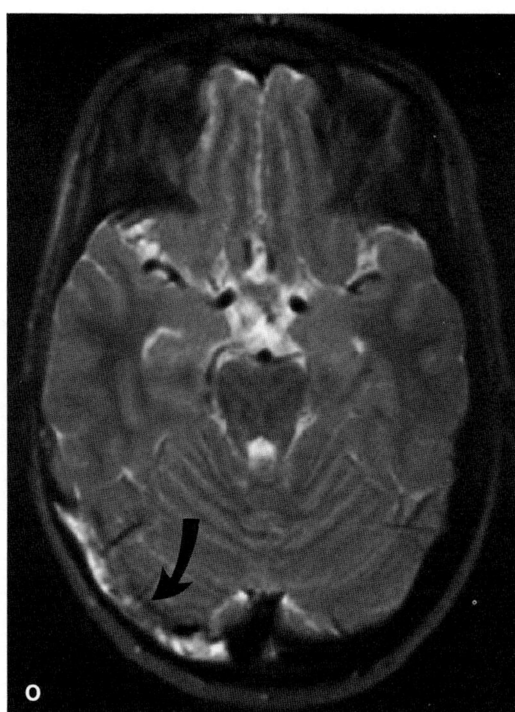

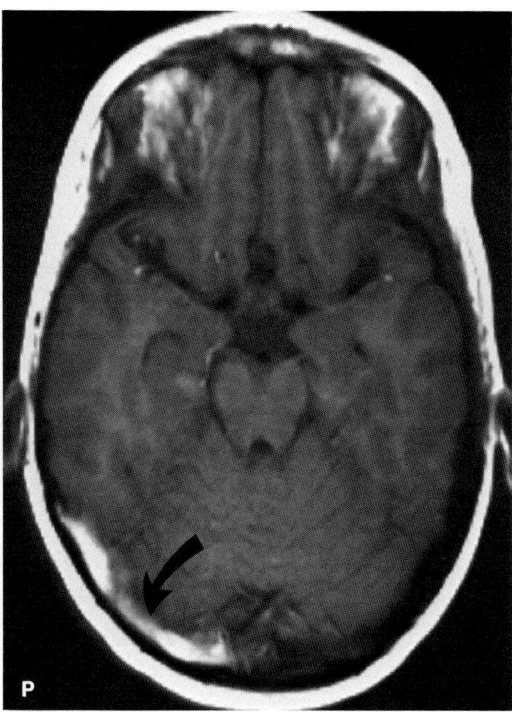

sition of conventional MR images with the sinus displayed in cross section. In the latter case, comparison of two planes (coronal and sagittal) is recommended to confirm that the observed change in signal intensity is due to occlusion and not flow-related phenomena. The appearance of sinus thrombosis on IV contrast-enhanced MR (using a gadolinium-chelate) is also distinct and can be used for diagnosis, as in the present case.

Pitfalls in Image Interpretation

Venous sinus thrombosis may appear as either abnormal high or low signal intensity on both T1- and T2-weighted MR images, depending on the temporal evolution of clot and hemoglobin products. The axial plane is particularly poor for evaluation of the transverse sinus because of the possibility of partial volume effects.

Clinical References

1. Doyle KJ, Jackler RK. Otogenic cavernous sinus thrombosis. Otolaryngol Head Neck Surg 1991;104:873–877.
2. Fritsch MH, Miyamoto RT , Wood TL. Sigmoid sinus thrombosis diagnosis by contrasted MRI scanning. Otolaryngol Head Neck Surg 1990;103:451–456.

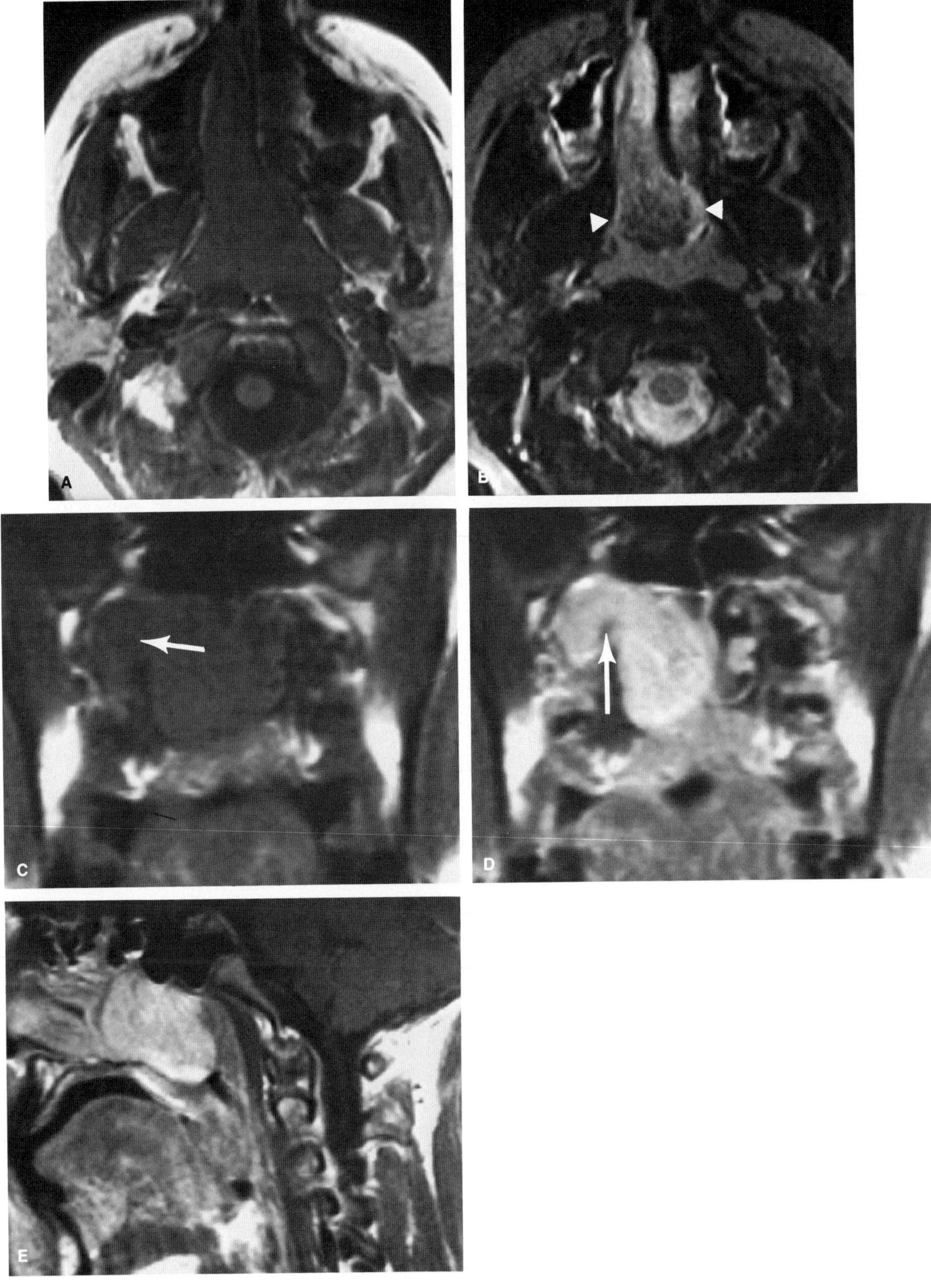
A
B
C
D
E

HISTORY

A 13-year-old boy with frequent epistaxis

FINDINGS

(*A*) The T1-weighted axial image demonstrates abnormal soft tissue intensity completely filling the nasal passages and nasopharynx. (*B*) On the T2-weighted axial image, a discrete heterogeneous, predominantly low-signal-intensity mass (*white arrowheads*) can be separated from the high-signal-intensity edematous mucosal tissue in the right nasal passage and lymphoid tissue in the posterior nasopharynx. There are multiple subtle signal voids within the mass, representing flow within vessels. Abnormal soft tissue expands the right pterygopalatine fossa (*white arrow*) a finding well shown on both precontrast (*C*) and postcontrast (*D*) T1-weighted coronal images. The borders of the lesion are best delineated on postcontrast T1-weighted coronal (*D*) and sagittal (*E*) images. The enhancement of the lesion is intense, although heterogeneous, because of vessels within the mass.

DIAGNOSIS

Juvenile angiofibroma

DISCUSSION

Juvenile angiofibroma is a benign, nonencapsulated, locally invasive tumor found in the nasopharynx almost exclusively in adolescent males. The tumor is composed of angiomatous tissue in a fibrous stroma arising from a hamartomatous ectopic nidus of vascular tissue.[1] Growth of the tumor is stimulated by testosterone, accounting for the predominance in adolescent boys during puberty.[1] Patients usually present with recurrent epistaxis or nasal obstruction.

Juvenile angiofibromas arise in the region of the sphenopalatine foramen and pterygopalatine fossa, and spread contiguously by way of the normal fissures and foramina into the adjacent spaces of the skull. Extension into the nasopharynx and nasal cavities often causes nasal obstruction. Expansion of the pterygopalatine fossa and tumor extension into the infratemporal fossa is common.[1] Large tumors may even extend intracranially by way of the orbit and superior orbital fissure or along the lateral wall of the sphenoid sinus, making surgical resection difficult.[1]

Juvenile angiofibromas are highly vascular tumors that surgeons are reluctant to biopsy because of the risk of hemorrhage. The main feeding vessel is usually the internal maxillary artery, but additional arterial supply from many other vessels is common. MR is useful for initial diagnosis and for determining tumor extent. Juvenile angiofibromas are heterogeneous masses on MR with predominantly soft tissue signal intensity on T1-weighted images. Vascular flow voids are common, and cause predominantly low signal intensity on T2-weighted images.[2] These tumors enhance intensely after contrast infusion. Inflamed mucosa or retained secretions enhance to a lesser degree, and have a higher signal intensity on T2-weighted images, allowing differentiation from tumor.[2]

Pitfalls in Image Interpretation

The differential diagnosis for a nasopharyngeal mass in an adolescent boy includes antrochoanal polyp, and embryonal rhabdomyosarcoma. Antrochoanal polyps arise within the maxillary antrum, and have a homogeneous appearance on MR. Embryonal rhabdomyosarcomas are rare and usually invade the neck either directly or by lymph node metastases.[2]

Clinical References

1. Harrison D. The natural history, pathogenesis, and treatment of juvenile angiofibroma. Arch Otolaryngol Head Neck Surg 1987;113:936–942.
2. Lloyd G, Lund V, Phelps P, et al. Magnetic resonance imaging in the evaluation of nose and paranasal sinus disease. Br J Radiol 1987;60:957–968.

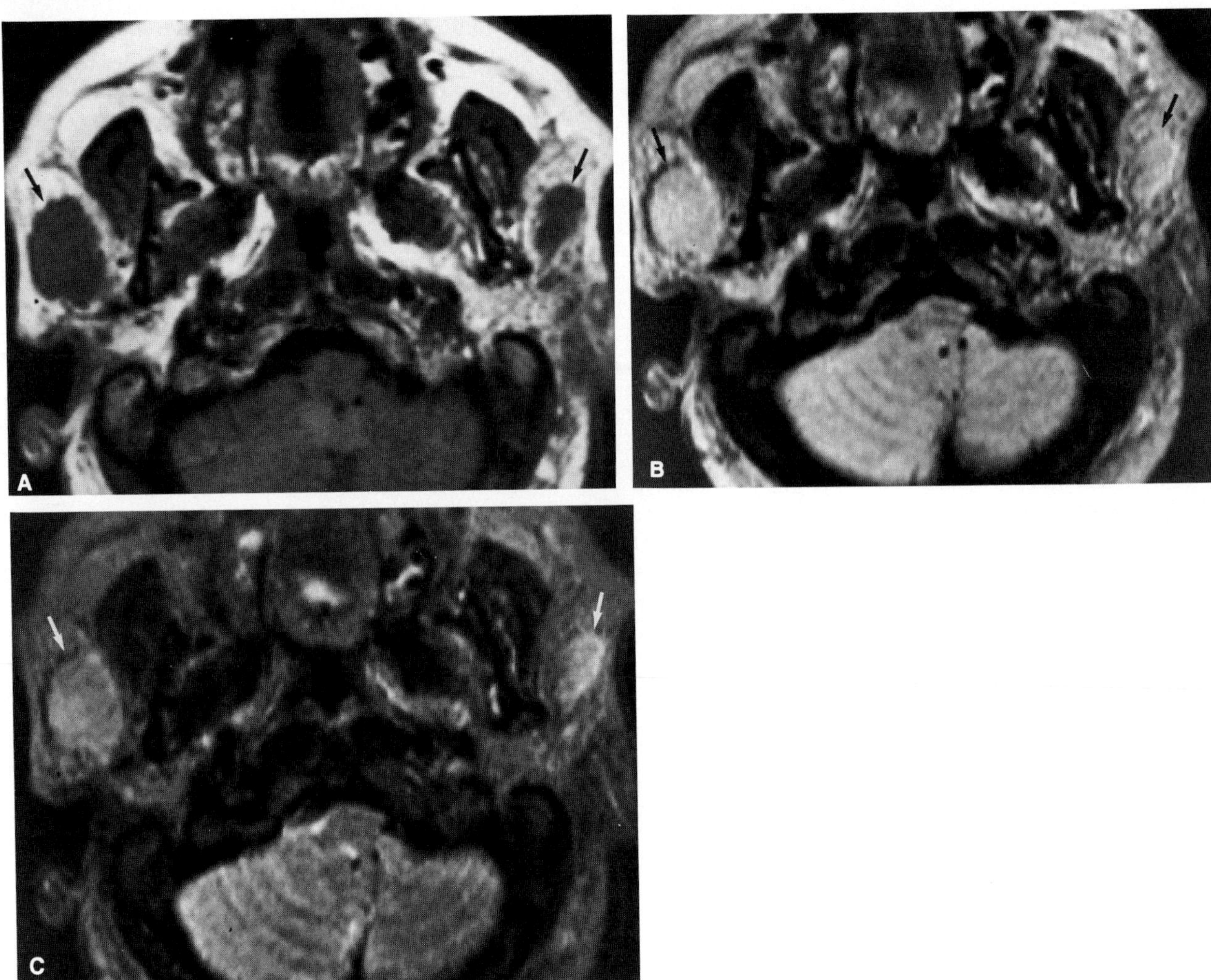

HISTORY

Bilateral facial swelling

FINDINGS

T1-weighted (*A*), proton density–weighted (*B*), and T2-weighted (TE = 90 msec) (*C*) images reveal soft tissue masses (*arrows*) in both parotid glands. These lesions are isointense with muscle on the T1-weighted scan, and slightly hyperintense on the heavily T2-weighted scan.

DIAGNOSIS

Lymphoma

DISCUSSION

Malignant lymphoma can present as a solitary mass within the parotid gland, indistinguishable from other more common lesions.[1] A specific subtype, monocytoid B-cell lymphoma, characteristically involves peripheral lymph nodes and has a propensity for intraparotid or periparotid nodes.

A recently described entity in acquired immunodeficiency syndrome (AIDS) is benign lymphoepithelial parotid neoplasm.[2,3] These lesions are often cystic (unlike the lesions shown in the current case), not uncommonly bilateral, and are accompanied by cervical adenopathy.

Pitfalls in Image Interpretation

The presence of bilateral or multiple parotid lesions favors the diagnosis of Warthin's tumor (papillary cystadenoma lymphomatosum), which is the second most common benign tumor of the parotid. Multiplicity of lesions, however, is also characteristic for metastases (including lymphoma). Metastatic disease commonly involves the parotid gland, presumably because of the presence of numerous intraparotid and periparotid lymph nodes.

Clinical References

1. Macht SD, Pett SD, Tsangaris NT. Non-Hodgkin lymphoma of the parotid gland: diagnosis, evaluation, and treatment. Ann Plast Surg 1979;2:37–41.
2. Holliday RA, Cohen WA, Schinella RA, et al. Benign lymphoepithelial parotid cysts and hyperplastic cervical adenopathy in AIDS-risk patients: a new CT appearance. Radiology 1988;168:439–441.
3. Kirshenbaum KJ, Nadimpalli SR, Friedman M, et al. Benign lymphoepithelial parotid tumors in AIDS patients: CT and MR findings in nine cases. AJNR 1991;12:271–274.

(A to C from Runge VM. Clinical magnetic resonance imaging. Philadelphia, JB Lippincott, 1990.)

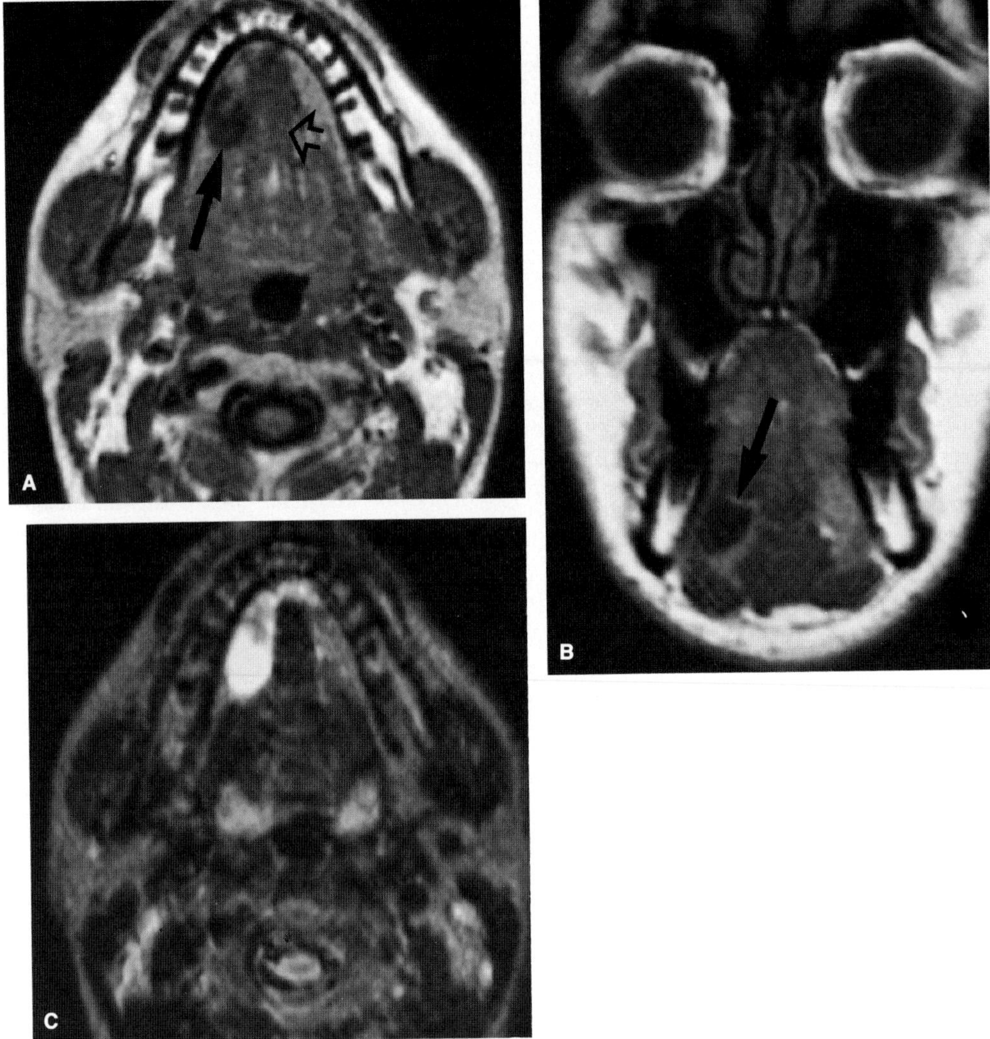

HISTORY

A 21-year-old with a nontender, fluctuant mass below the tongue on the right

FINDINGS

The T1-weighted axial (*A*) and coronal (*B*) images demonstrate a round, low-signal-intensity mass (*arrow*) in the floor of the mouth. The mass is located in the sublingual space, just lateral to the paired midline genioglossus muscles (*open arrow in A*). (*C*) The mass has homogeneous high signal intensity on the T2-weighted axial image. The lesion is well demarcated, has a thin rim, and does not extend beyond the sublingual space.

DIAGNOSIS

Ranula

DISCUSSION

Ranulas are benign mucous retention cysts resulting from an obstructed sublingual or minor salivary gland in the sublingual space.[1] There are two types of ranula: simple and plunging (or "diving"). A ranula is classified as simple if it is limited to the sublingual space, in which case it is confined by the capsule of the salivary gland from which it arose. Plunging ranulas arise in the sublingual space and extravasate into the submandibular or parapharyngeal space via herniation around or through the mylohyoid muscle.

Simple ranulas present as a mass lesion in the floor of the mouth, located in the lateral sublingual space separated from the midline by the genioglossus muscle. Infection or inflammation of a ranula is common and may result in pain. Complete surgical resection of a ranula and the associated obstructed salivary gland is necessary to prevent recurrence.

Ranulas are usually thin-walled, unilocular, homogeneous cystic lesions with low signal intensity on

T1-weighted images and high signal intensity on T2-weighted images.[2] Because of increased protein content, the signal intensity on T1-weighted images may be intermediate when a ranula is infected. Uncomplicated ranulas do not enhance. The periphery of an infected ranula may show mild enhancement.

Pitfalls in Image Interpretation

The differential diagnosis for a cystic mass in the floor of the mouth includes epidermoid, dermoid, hemangioma, lymphangioma, thyroglossal duct cyst, and necrotic node. An epidermoid may have an identical appearance to a ranula on MR. Dermoids are heterogenous. Hemangiomas and lymphangiomas enhance after contrast infusion. Thyroglossal duct cysts are located in the midline. Necrotic lymph nodes involved with metastatic squamous cell carcinoma have a thick enhancing wall and are usually accompanied by large primary oral tumors.[1]

Clinical References

1. Coit W, Harnsberger H, Osborn A, et al. Ranulas and their mimics: CT evaluation. Radiology 1987;163:211–216.
2. Mafee M, Campos M, Raju S, et al. Head and neck: high field magnetic resonance imaging versus computed tomography. Otolaryngol Clin North Am 1988;21:513–546.

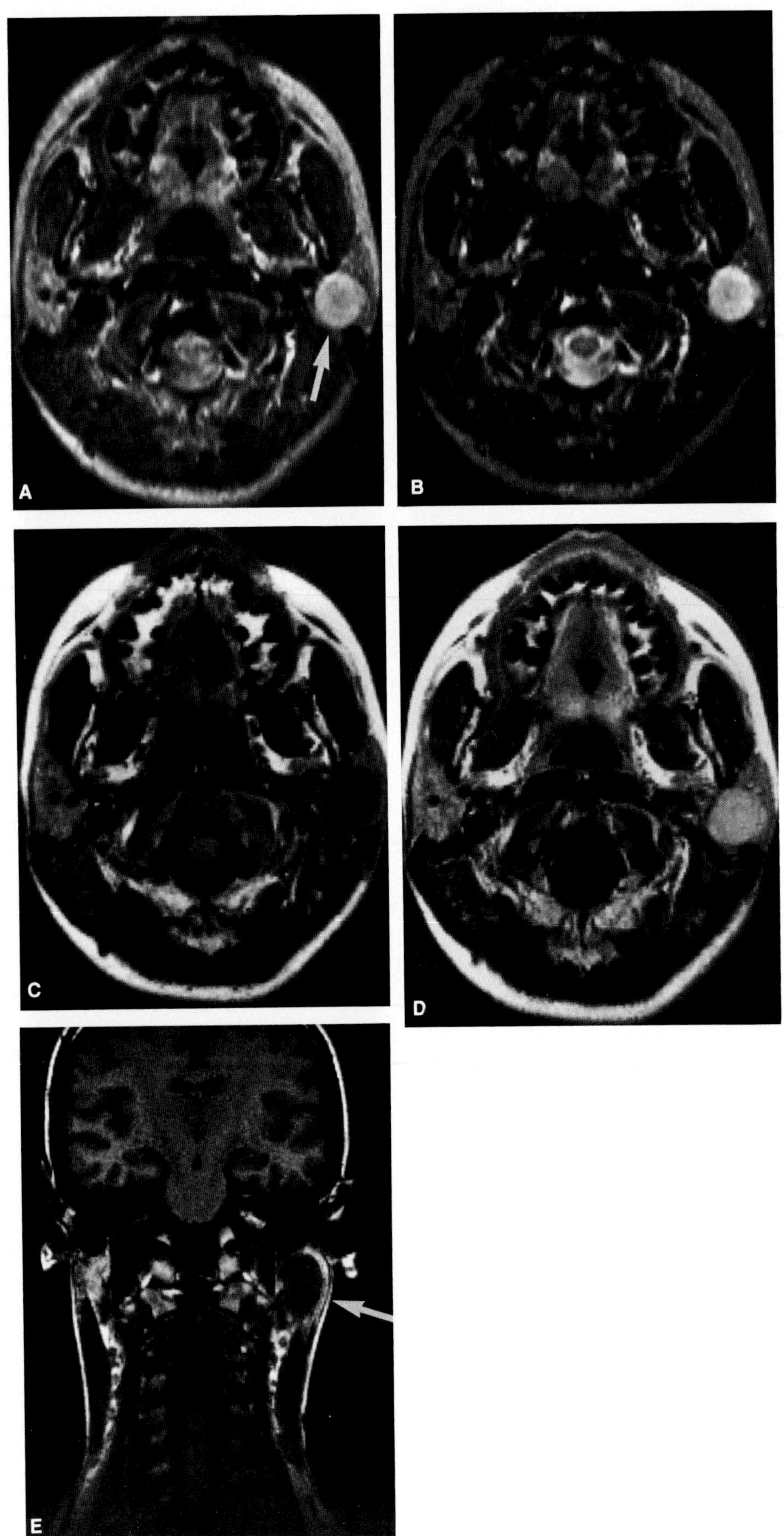

HISTORY

Left-sided retromandibular swelling

FINDINGS

On the first (*A*) and second (*B*) echoes of the T2-weighted examination, a high-signal-intensity mass (*arrow in A*) is demonstrated within the left parotid gland. The mass is homogeneous and smoothly marginated. Comparison of precontrast (*C*) and postcontrast (*D*) T1-weighted axial examinations reveals homogeneous enhancement. (*E*) The lesion (*arrow*) is also well demonstrated on the coronal T1-weighted precontrast image.

DIAGNOSIS

Pleomorphic adenoma

DISCUSSION

MR is superior to CT for the evaluation of parotid masses, permitting accurate differentiation between intraparotid lesions and neoplasms originating within the parapharyngeal space.[1] MR can also be used to demonstrate the relationship of a tumor to the facial nerve.[2] There is some correlation between MR appearance and histopathologic diagnosis, although definitive diagnosis requires biopsy.[3] Pleomorphic adenomas (benign mixed cell tumors) are predominantly homogeneous and smoothly marginated. Warthin's tumor (papillary cystadenoma lymphomatosum) can be strikingly heterogeneous, often with focal regions of hemorrhage, although this lesion is typically also well marginated. Malignancies and inflammatory masses are often accompanied by cervical lymphadenopathy. Infiltration of the subcutaneous fat and thickening of deep cervical fascia are features more characteristic of an inflammatory mass.

The terms *pleomorphic adenoma* and *benign mixed cell tumor* are used interchangeably to refer to a lesion made up of epidermoid and myoepithelial cells. This lesion, which can occur in any salivary gland, is the most common neoplasm of the parotid. Pleomorphic adenomas are benign, solitary, and characteristically ovoid in appearance.

Clinical References

1. Mandelblatt SM, Braun IF, Davis PC, et al. Parotid masses: MR imaging. Radiology 1987;163:411–414.
2. Teresi LM, Lufkin RB, Wortham DG, et al. Parotid masses: MR imaging. Radiology 1987;163:405–409.
3. Swartz JD, Rothman MI, Marlowe FI, Berger AS. MR imaging of parotid mass lesions: attempts at histopathologic differentiation. J Comput Assist Tomogr 1989;13:789–796.

(A to E from Runge VM. Clinical magnetic resonance imaging. Philadelphia, JB Lippincott, 1990.)

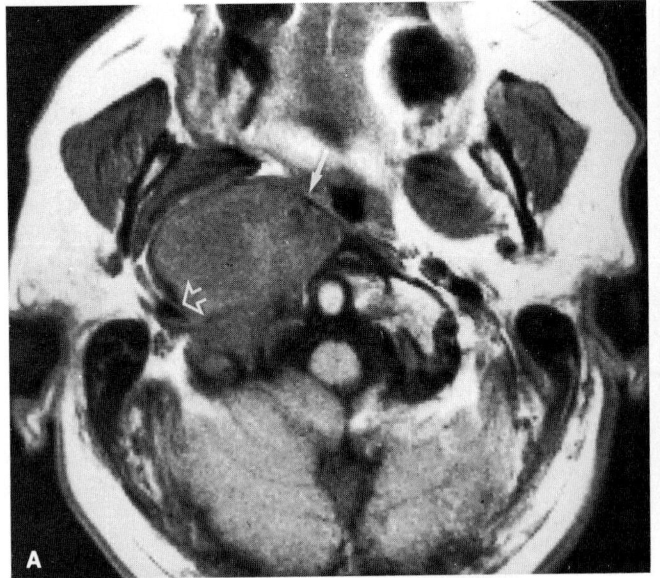

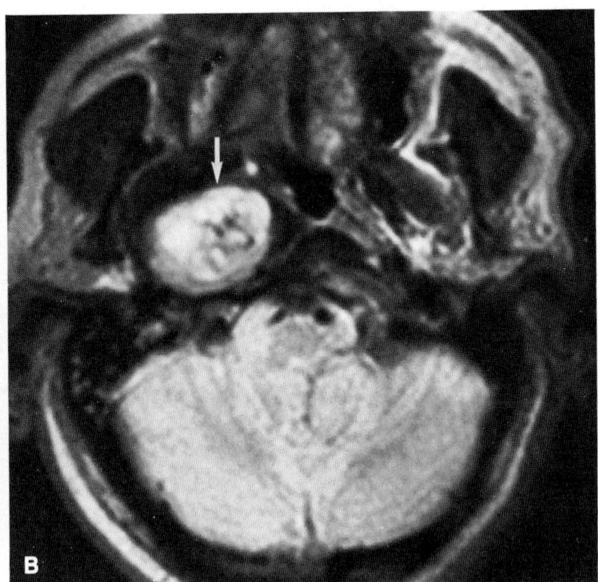

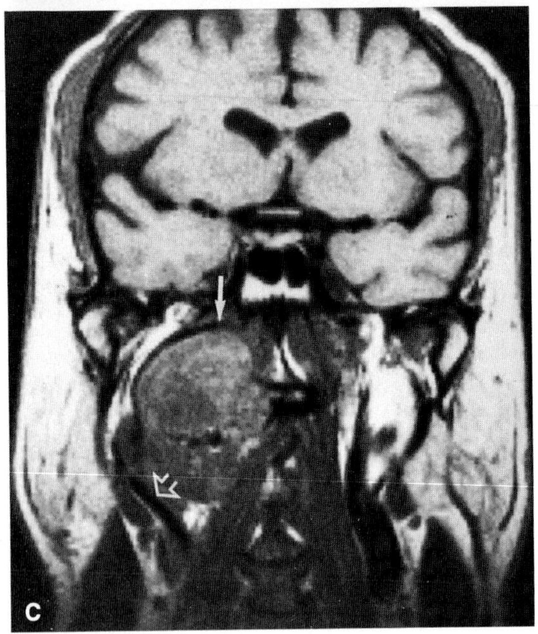

HISTORY

Recurrent otitis media, caused by obstruction of the right eustachian tube

FINDINGS

T1-weighted axial (*A*), T2-weighted axial (*B*), and T1-weighted coronal (*C*) images reveal a large soft tissue mass (*arrow*) at the skull base. The lesion encroaches upon the parapharyngeal space, and displaces the jugular vein and carotid artery (*open arrow*) posterolaterally. *A* also demonstrates destruction of the lateral mass of C1.

DIAGNOSIS

Schwannoma (of C1)

DISCUSSION

The infratemporal fossa is lateral to the nasopharynx and pterygopalatine fossa, and contains the lateral pterygoid muscle, a part of the medial pterygoid muscle, and the inferior section of the temporalis muscle. The fat plane that lies between the muscles of mastication (medial and lateral pterygoid, temporalis, and masseter muscles) and those of deglutition (pharyngeal constrictor and palatal muscles) defines the parapharyngeal space. Benign tumors of the nasopharynx and infratemporal fossa are rare, with the most common being juvenile angiofibroma. The differential diagnosis should also include benign tumors arising from adjacent regions, including the parapharyngeal space, carotid sheath, and temporal bone. Thus, paragangliomas, schwannomas, neurofibromas, tumors of salivary gland origin, and meningiomas should be considered. Squamous cell carcinoma is the most frequent malignant tumor of the nasopharynx.[1]

MR Technique

Fat suppression (*not illustrated*) can be employed, in particular on postcontrast T1- and precontrast T2-weighted images, for improved detection and delineation of head and neck lesions.[2]

Clinical References

1. Carter BL. Nasopharynx and infratemporal fossa. In: Valvassori GE, Buckingham RA, Carter BL, et al, eds. Head and neck imaging. New York, Thieme, 1988:235–250.
2. Tien RD, Hesselink JR, Chu PK, Szumowski J. Improved detection and delineation of head and neck lesions with fat suppression spin-echo MR imaging. AJNR 1991;12:19–24.

(A to C from Runge VM. Clinical magnetic resonance imaging. Philadelphia, JB Lippincott, 1990.)

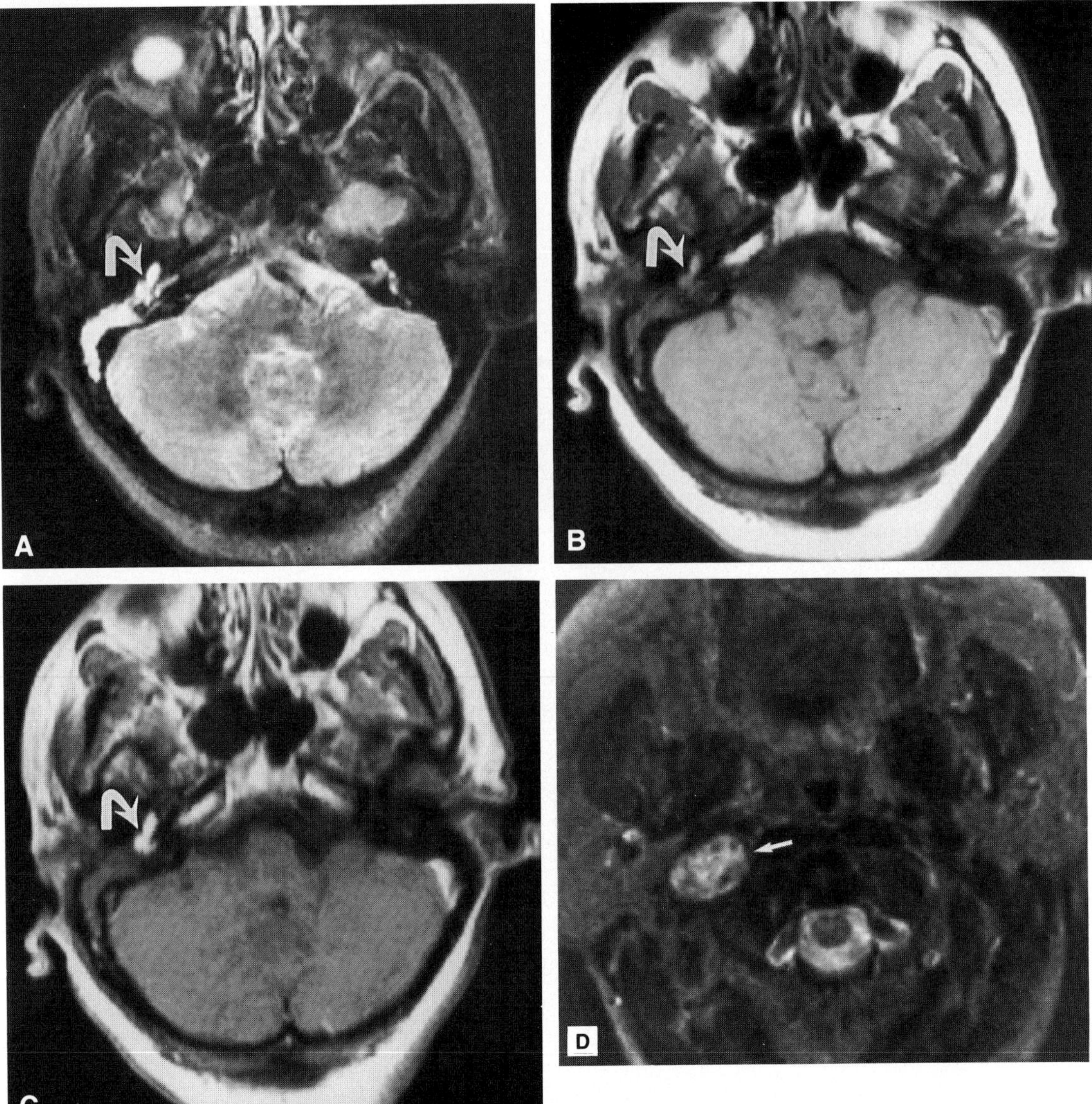

HISTORY

Three different patients, all with unilateral lower cranial nerve symptoms

FINDINGS

Patient 1: (*A*) On the T2-weighted (TR/TE = 3000/90) examination, a small, abnormal hyperintense mass (*curved arrow*) is noted in the right middle ear. There is opacification of the adjacent mastoid air cells. Comparison of precontrast (*B*) and postcontrast (*C*) T1-weighted scans reveals intense enhancement of this small soft tissue mass (*curved arrows*), but not of the adjacent air cell disease.

Patient 2: (*D*) The T2-weighted (TR/TE = 3000/90) examination reveals a soft tissue mass (*arrow*) with a distinctive "salt and pepper" signal intensity pattern. (*E*) Signal voids can also be demonstrated within the mass (*arrow*) on the axial T1-weighted image. (*F*) The coronal T1-weighted image demonstrates that the bulk of the mass (*arrow*) lies within the lumen of the internal jugular vein.

Patient 3: (*G*) On the T2-weighted (TR/TE = 3000/90) scan, a well-defined hyperintense mass is seen in the left parapharyngeal space. Comparison of precontrast (*H*) and postcontrast (*I*) T1-weighted images demonstrates marked lesion enhancement. Scattered foci of low signal intensity, compatible with either fibrosis or flow voids, can be seen within the mass on all pulse sequences.

DIAGNOSIS

Glomus tumor

1—Glomus tympanicum
2—Glomus jugulare
3—Glomus vagale

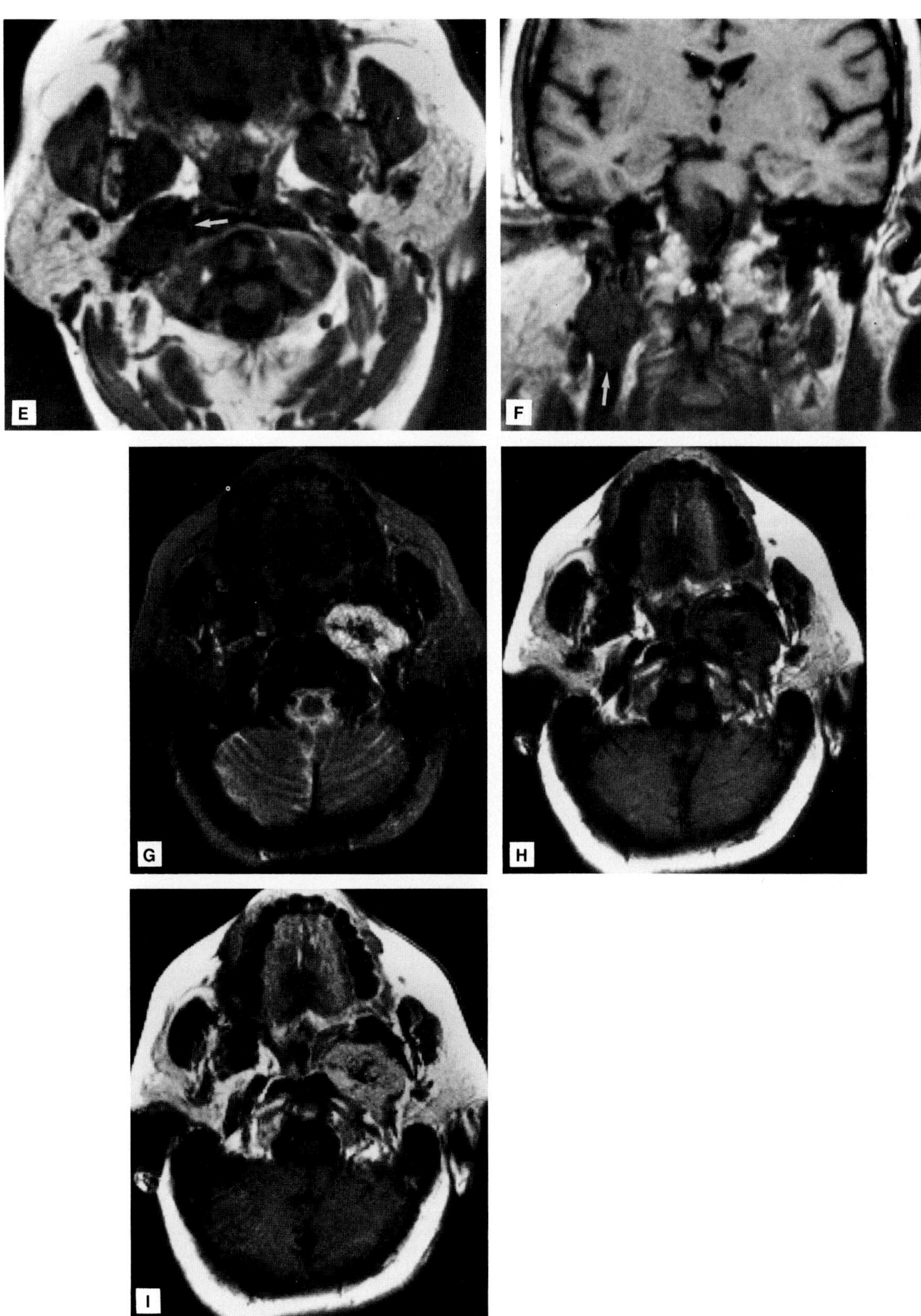
E
F
G
H
I

DISCUSSION

Glomus tumors, also called paragangliomas or chemodectomas, are slow-growing hypervascular neoplasms that arise from neural crest cell derivatives. In the head and neck region, common locations include the middle ear (glomus tympanicum), jugular fossa (glomus jugulare), inferior ganglion of the vagus nerve (glomus vagale), and carotid bifurcation (carotid body tumor). Conductive deafness may be observed with a tumor that involves the middle ear. Lesions in the jugular fossa encroach on and cause dysfunction of cranial nerves IX (glossopharyngeal), X (vagus), and XI (accessory).

Glomus tumors have a characteristic appearance on unenhanced MR, with lesions greater than 2 cm demonstrating a "salt and pepper" pattern.[1] Rapid vascular flow produces signal voids, which are interspersed with areas of higher signal intensity as a result of slow flow and tumor cells. MR is superior to CT for demonstrating the relation of a glomus tumor to carotid sheath vessels and adjacent intracranial structures. CT may, however, better demonstrate subtle osseous changes.

MR Technique

IV contrast enhancement is important for reliable detection of glomus tumors of less than 5 mm.[2] Measurement of the temporal enhancement pattern, by demonstration of immediate uptake (peak, approximately 150 seconds) and gradual washout, enables improved lesion differentiation from meningiomas and neuromas.

Clinical References

1. Olsen WL, Dillon WP, Kelly WM, et al. MR imaging of paragangliomas. AJR 1987;148:201–204.
2. Vogl T, Bruning R, Schedel H, et al. Paragangliomas of the jugular bulb and carotid body: MR imaging with short sequences and Gd-DTPA enhancement. AJR 1989;153:583–587.

(A *to* C *from Runge VM. Magnetic resonance imaging: clinical principles. Philadelphia, JB Lippincott, 1992;* D *to* I *from Runge VM. Clinical magnetic resonance imaging. Philadelphia, JB Lippincott, 1990.)*

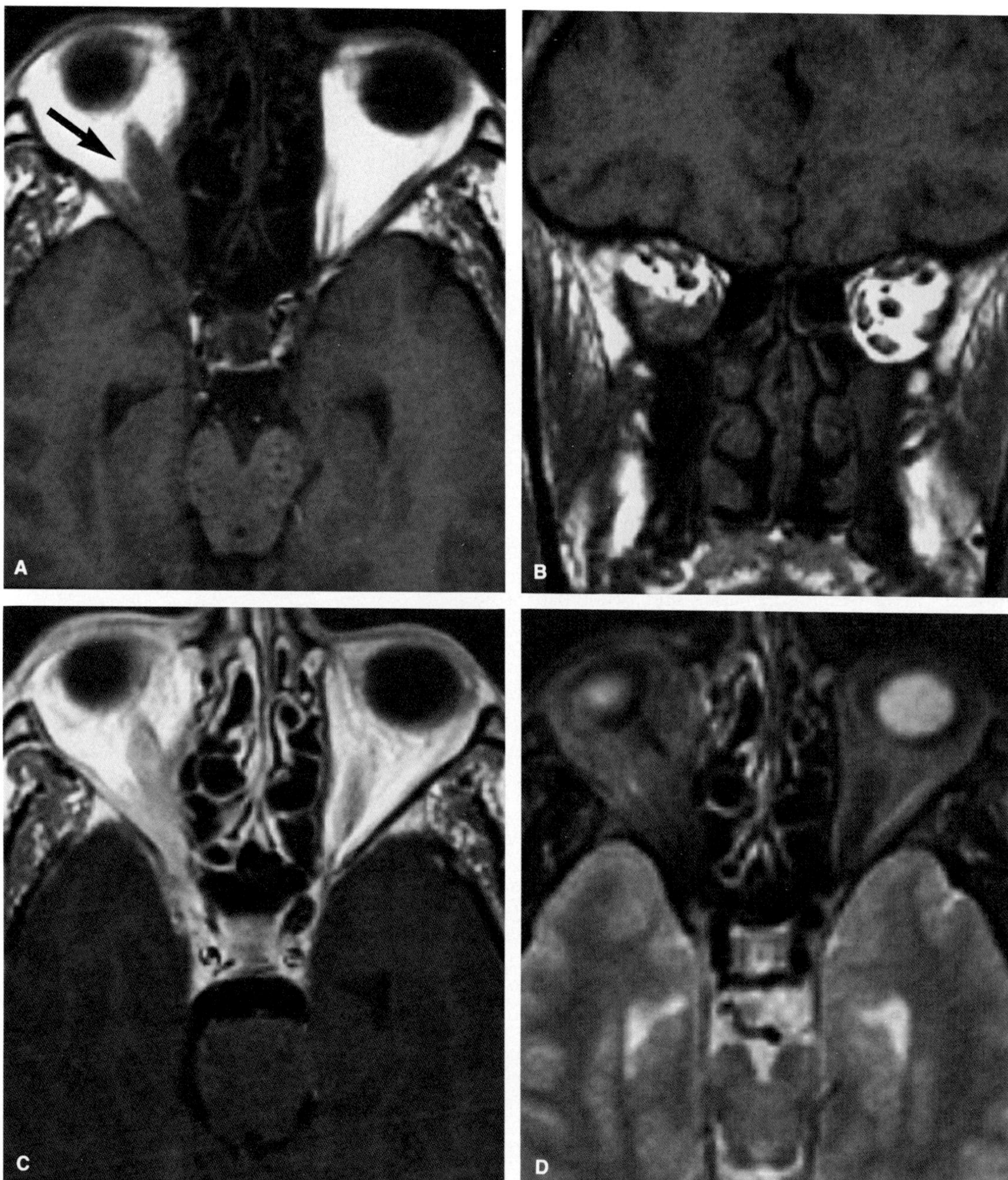

HISTORY

A 41-year-old with right proptosis, right inferior rectus palsy, and history of Wegener's granulomatosis

FINDINGS

(*A*) On the T1-weighted axial image there is thickening of the right inferior rectus muscle (*arrow*), and abnormal soft tissue in the right orbital apex. (*B*) The abnormal soft tissue intensity fills the inferior half of the orbit, and is inseparable from the inferior rectus muscle on the T1-weighted coronal image. (*C*) After IV contrast infusion there is enhancement of the abnormal soft tissue in the orbital apex on the T1-weighted axial image. (*D*) The abnormal soft tissue is isointense to orbital fat on the precontrast T2-weighted axial image. The left orbit is normal.

DIAGNOSIS

Orbital pseudotumor

DISCUSSION

Pseudotumor of the orbit is the most common cause of an intraorbital mass in an adult. It is a nongranulomatous inflammatory process that may affect all intraorbital soft tissues. Most cases are idiopathic, but pseudotumor can be associated with underlying diseases such as Wegener's granulomatosis, and collagen-vascular disorders. Patients often present with the classic clinical triad of pain, ophthalmoparesis, and proptosis, although pain may be absent or minimal.[1] Most cases are unilateral, but bilateral disease is not uncommon, especially when associated with an underlying condition.

Pseudutomor of the orbit may involve any or all of the intraorbital contents, and thus can have many different appearances on MR or CT. Enlargement of the extraocular muscles is most common, but the disease may also cause uveal-scleral thickening, a lacrimal mass, diffuse infiltration of orbital fat, or an irregular retrobulbar soft tissue mass,[2] as in this case. Orbital pseudotumor is isointense to muscle on T1-weighted images, and isointense to minimally hyperintense to orbital fat on T2-weighted images. This appearance allows differentiation from metastatic disease, which is hyperintense to fat on T2-weighted images. Orbital pseudotumor usually responds dramatically to steroid therapy, and the definitive diagnosis is often based on such a response, without biopsy confirmation.

MR Technique

Images of the orbit obtained with a surface coil can be substantially degraded by motion artifact. Therefore, patients should be instructed to keep their eyes open and fix their gaze in one direction for the entire scan time.[2]

Pitfalls in Image Interpretation

Lymphoma and myeloma may look exactly like pseudotumor on MR, both in disease distribution and signal intensity on both T1- and T2-weighted images. Differentiation from other benign entities such as sarcoidosis and myositis is also not possible with MR. Involvement of the tendinous insertions of the extraocular muscles is much more likely to occur with pseudotumor than with thyroid ophthalmopathy. Thyroid ophthalmopathy is bilateral in 95% of cases.

Clinical References

1. Atlas S, Grossman R, Savino P, et al. Surface coil MR of orbital pseudotumor. AJR 1987;148:803–808.
2. Atlas S. Magnetic resonance imaging of the orbit: current status. Magn Reson Q 1989;5:39–96.

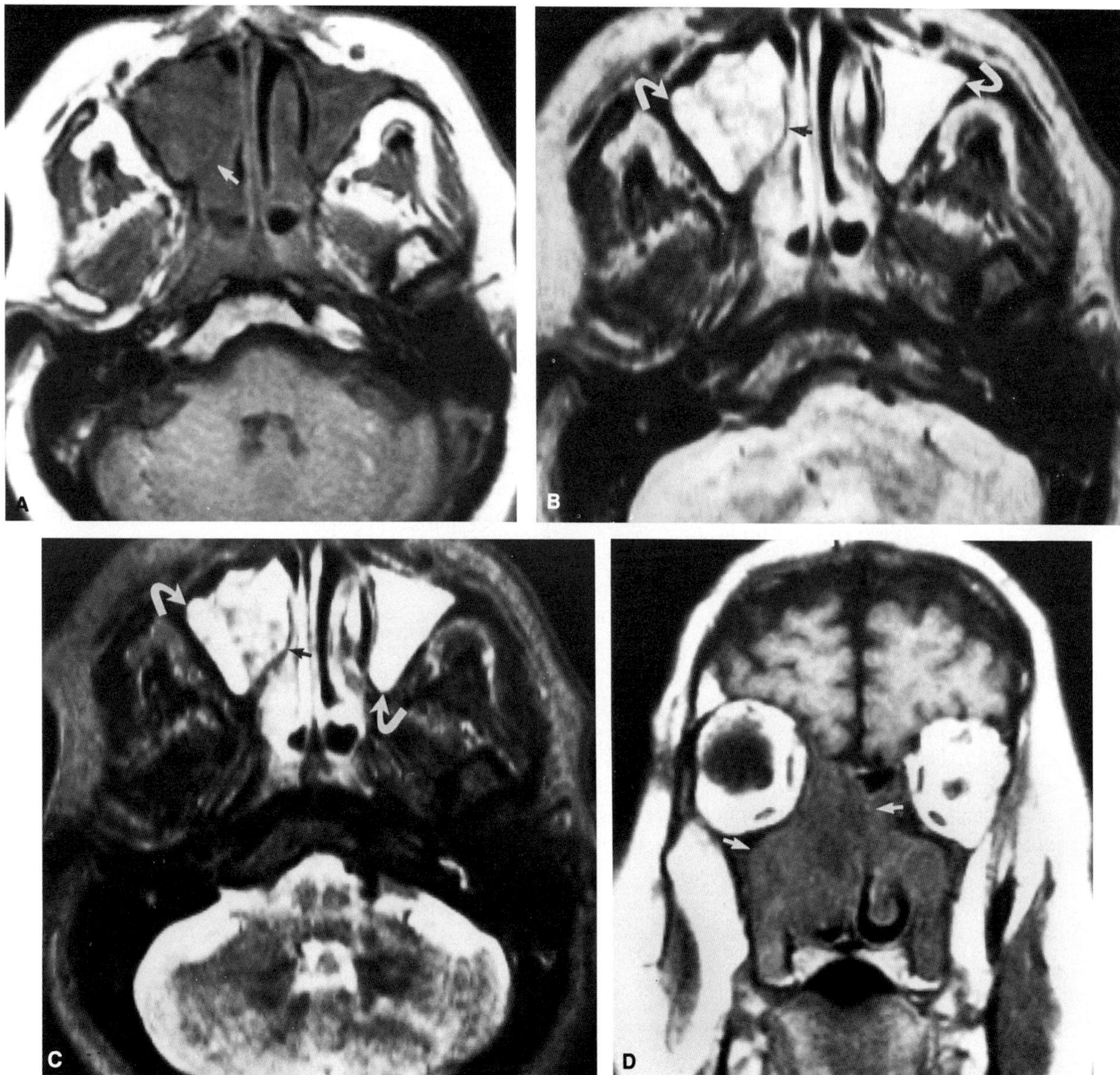

HISTORY

A 50-year-old man with right nasal obstruction

FINDINGS

(*A*) T1-weighted axial image demonstrates opacification of the maxillary sinuses bilaterally. There is expansion of the right maxillary sinus, and the soft tissue signal intensity (*arrow*) within the sinus cannot be separated from the right middle turbinate. Intermediate (*B*) and heavily (*C*) T2-weighted axial images demonstrate high-signal-intensity fluid (*curved white arrows*) in the left maxillary sinus and in the lateral part of the right maxillary sinus. Within the medial two thirds of the right maxillary sinus and in the right nasal passage there is heterogeneous signal intensity (*arrow*) suggesting a soft tissue mass, which is clearly separated from the high-signal-intensity fluid. (*D*) The superior extension of the mass (*short white arrows*) into the right ethmoid air cells is demonstrated on the T1-weighted coronal image. The mass extends between the right middle turbinate and right maxillary sinus with destruction of the lateral wall of the right nasal passage. The left middle turbinate is normal.

DIAGNOSIS

Inverted papilloma

DISCUSSION

An inverted papilloma is an uncommon benign tumor of the nasal fossa that has a characteristic histologic appearance. Histologically, this tumor shows inversion of the neoplastic epithelium into the underlying stroma, rather than exophytic growth outward such as that seen in squamous papillomas.[1] Thus, the name *inverted* papilloma. The peak incidence of inverted papillomas is in the fifth and sixth decades of life, although it has an age range from adolescence to the ninth decade.[1] There is a 2:1 male to female predominance. The etiology of inverted papilloma is unknown, although there is evidence of an association with the human papillomavirus.[1] Patients present with unilateral nasal obstruction, epistaxis, rhinorrhea, or secondary sinusitis.

Although inverted papillomas are benign, they are locally aggressive. The lesion usually arises from the lateral nasal wall in the region of the middle meatus and middle turbinate and grows slowly, extending into and eroding adjacent structures in the process. Inverted papillomas are unilateral, and most commonly destroy the lateral nasal wall with invasion of the maxillary sinus. The nasal septum may be bowed in the contralateral direction, and thinned, but is usually intact.[2] Advanced large tumors may extend into all of the ipsilateral sinuses, the orbit, the pterygopalatine fossa, and even the anterior cranial fossa.[2] Radiographic evaluation can be performed with CT or MR and is essential for treatment planning. MR is superior for distinguishing between a soft tissue mass and fluid in the nasal passages and sinuses. CT is superior for evaluation of bony destruction.

Inverted papillomas are associated with synchronous or subsequent nasal malignancy in up to half of cases.[1] Because of that, it has been suggested that there may be a continuous gradation of papilloma to carcinoma, although this is controversial.[1] The insinuating growth pattern of an inverted papilloma makes complete surgical resection difficult, and recurrence is common. The high recurrence rate and association with malignancy has led to more radical surgical approaches.[1]

Pitfalls in Image Interpretation

The radiographic appearance of an inverted papilloma is nonspecific. The differential diagnosis for a soft tissue tumor in the nasal passages of an adult includes the more common squamous cell carcinoma, adenocarcinoma, adenoid cystic carcinoma, and lymphoma.[2]

Clinical References

1. Lawson W, Le Benger J, Som P, et al. Inverted papilloma: an analysis of 87 cases. Laryngoscope 1989;99:1117–1124.
2. Momose K, Weber A, Goodman M, et al. Radiological aspects of inverted papilloma. Radiology 1980;134:73–79.

(A to D from Runge VM. Clinical magnetic resonance imaging. Philadelphia, JB Lippincott, 1990.)

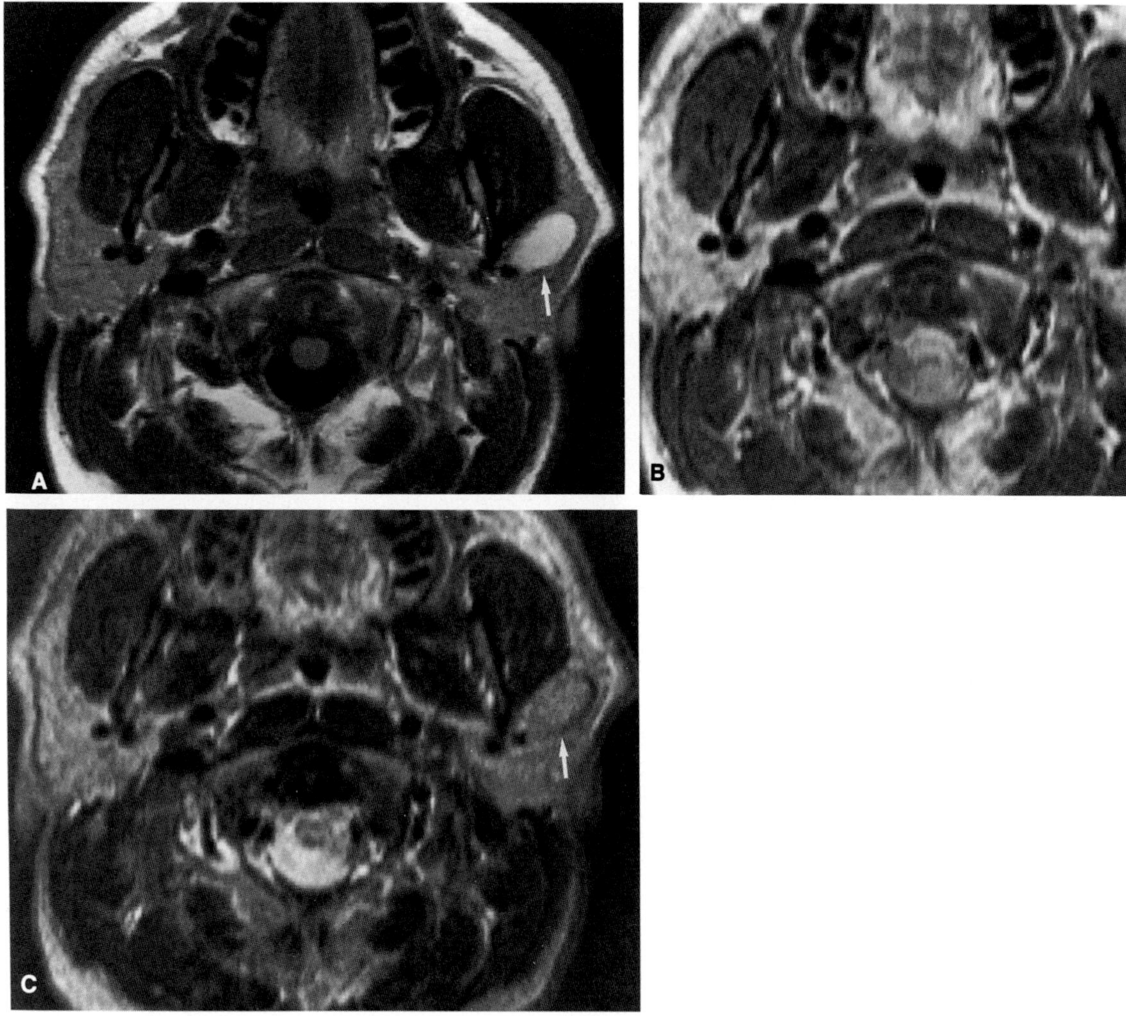

HISTORY

Physical examination reveals an asymptomatic, nontender cheek mass.

FINDINGS

On T1-weighted (*A*), proton density–weighted (*B*), and T2-weighted (*C*) images, a mass (*arrows*) is readily apparent within the left parotid gland, just anterior and lateral to the retromandibular vein. The signal intensity of this lesion parallels that of subcutaneous fat on all pulse sequences. On the proton density–weighted and T2-weighted images, which were performed with low bandwidth, a prominent chemical shift artifact can be seen as a low-signal-intensity interface between the mass (specifically its lateral margin) and the adjacent parotid gland.

DIAGNOSIS

Lipoma of the parotid gland

DISCUSSION

Although rare, lipomas should be considered in the differential diagnosis of tumors that involve the parotid gland.[1] Treatment is by surgical excision. Both MR and CT permit accurate preoperative diagnosis.

Most salivary gland neoplasms are benign or low grade, with high-grade tumors uncommon. Lesions that arise from the superficial lobe of the parotid gland are likely to be benign. Conversely, lesions arising in the deep lobe, submandibular or sublingual glands, or minor salivary glands are more likely to be malignant. Rapid growth, pain, or facial nerve paralysis suggest malignancy. On MR, high-grade malignancies demonstrate poorly defined margins and, often, *low* signal intensity on T2-weighted images.[2] The most common benign epithelial neoplasms of the salivary glands are pleomorphic adenomas (benign mixed tumors) and Warthin's tumors. The most common low-grade neoplasms are mucoepidermoid and adenocystic carcinomas. High-grade neoplasms include undifferentiated carcinomas, adenocarcinomas, squamous cell carcinomas, and some mucoepidermoid carcinomas. Nonepithelial neoplasms include lipomas, hemangiomas, and neurogenic tumors.

Clinical References

1. Korentager R, Noyek AM, Chapnik JS, et al. Lipoma and liposarcoma of the parotid gland: high-resolution preoperative imaging diagnosis. Laryngoscope 1988;98:967–971.
2. Som PM, Biller HF. High-grade malignancies of the parotid gland: identification with MR imaging. Radiology 1989; 173:823–826.

(A to C from Runge VM. Clinical magnetic resonance imaging. Philadelphia, JB Lippincott, 1990.)

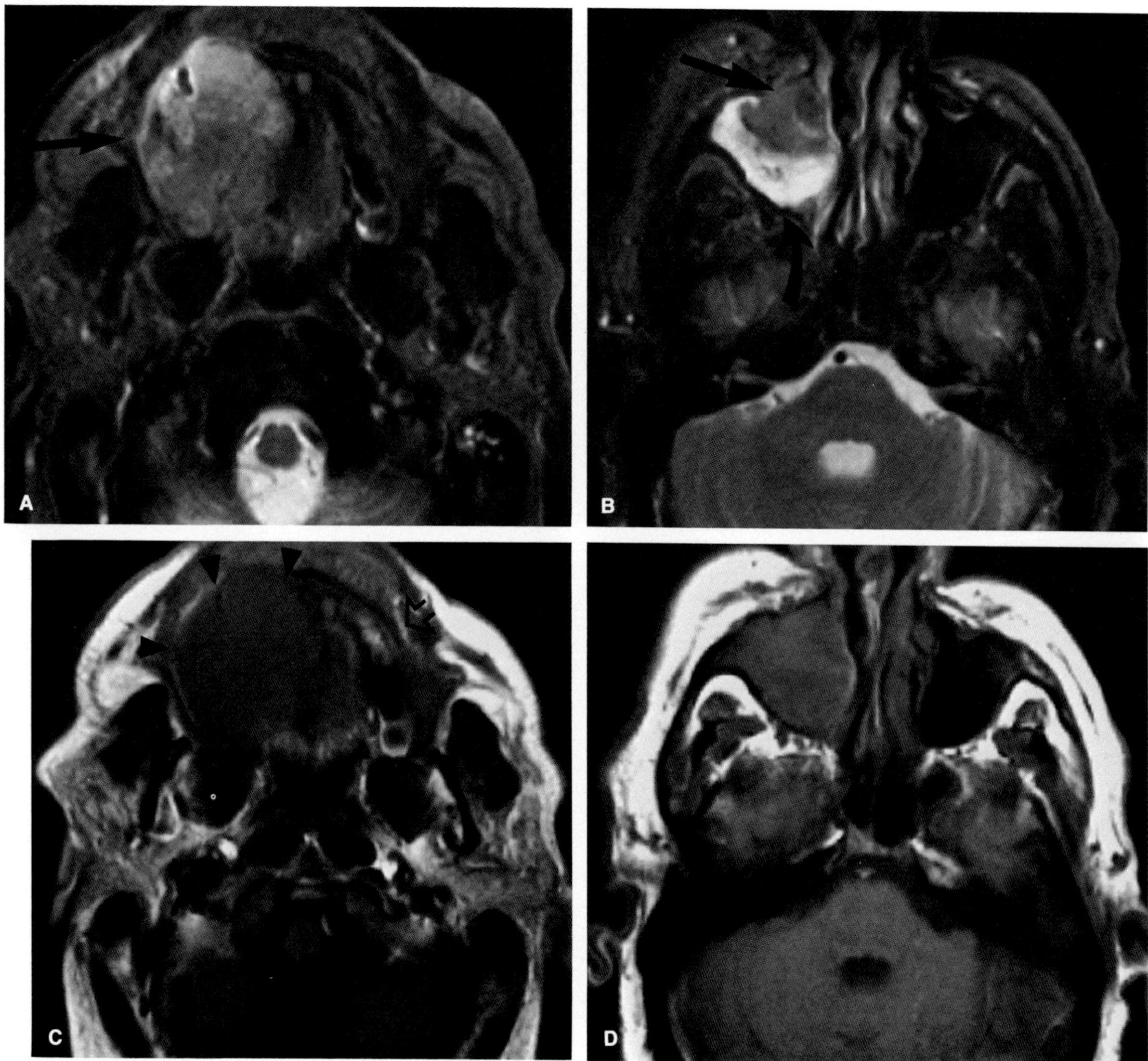

HISTORY

A 59-year-old man who presented 4 months before the present examination with an ulceration on the right alveolar ridge

FINDINGS

(*A and B*) A large soft tissue mass (*arrows*) is seen to occupy the right maxillary sinus on the T2-weighted scans. On the more superior section (*B*), fluid with marked hyperintensity (*curved arrow*) is also noted within the maxillary sinus. (*C and D*) The corresponding T1-weighted images show that the mass remains isointense with soft tissue. On the more inferior section (*C*) involvement of the right alveolar ridge (*arrowheads*) can be noted, which is particularly evident by comparison with the normal left side (*open arrow*). The posterior wall of the maxillary sinus is expanded but appears intact. By inspection of both axial (*C*) and coronal (*E*) T1-weighted images, involvement of both the hard and soft palate can be diagnosed. The coronal image also clearly demonstrates destruction of the floor and medial wall of the maxillary sinus.

DIAGNOSIS

Squamous cell carcinoma of the right maxillary sinus

DISCUSSION

The patient in this case was treated by complete surgical resection (radical maxillectomy) followed by radiation

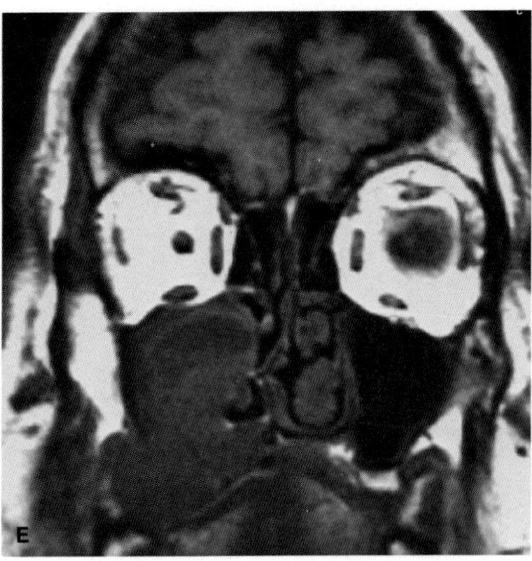

therapy. The symptoms of maxillary sinus carcinoma are similar to that of chronic sinusitis, often resulting in a delay in diagnosis. Common presenting symptoms include tissue swelling, nasal obstruction, nasal discharge, and epistaxis. CT and MR are used for early diagnosis and to determine tumor extent.[1] Malignant lesions in the paranasal sinuses can extend into adjacent areas, including the orbit, parapharyngeal space, and intracranial cavity. IV contrast administration using a gadolinium chelate can improve the delineation of intracranial extension.[2] However, unenhanced T2-weighted scans are often sufficient for determining disease extent.

Most sinonasal tumors have intermediate signal intensity on T2-weighted images, with only approximately 5% being hyperintense.[3] Inflammatory tissue in the sinuses consistently demonstrates marked hyperintensity on T2-weighted images. Thus, T2-weighted studies are often sufficient for differentiation of sinonasal tumors from inflammatory tissue. The multiplanar imaging capability of MR is particularly useful for identifying tumor margins.[4] The definition of cortical bone thinning and possible disruption remains superior by CT.

Squamous cell carcinoma accounts for more than 80% of all malignant tumors involving the paranasal sinuses and nasal cavity. Superior extension into the orbit may produce proptosis. Extension posteriorly into the pterygopalatine fossa portends a poor prognosis. Intracranial extension occurs by way of the cranial nerves. Metastasis to regional lymph nodes is relatively uncommon. In regard to tissue type, adenocarcinoma is substantially less common, with an increased incidence in woodworkers attributed to wood dust inhalation.

MR Technique

Imaging in all three planes (axial, sagittal, and coronal) improves depiction of lesion extent with tumors of the paranasal sinuses.

Pitfalls in Image Interpretation

Attention must be directed to the paranasal sinuses to rule out the presence of a soft tissue malignancy. Detection and correct diagnosis of tumors in this area is complicated by the prevalence of incidental inflammatory sinus disease.

Clinical References

1. Weber AL. Tumors of the paranasal sinuses. Otolaryngol Clin North Am 1988;21:439–454.
2. Van Tassel P, Lee YY. Gd-DTPA–enhanced MR for detecting intracranial extension of sinonasal malignancies. J Comput Assist Tomogr 1991;15:387–392.
3. Som PM, Shapiro MD, Biller HF, et al. Sinonasal tumors and inflammatory tissues: differentiation with MR imaging. Radiology 1988;167:803–808.
4. Weissman JL, Tabor EK, Curtin HD. Magnetic resonance imaging of the paranasal sinuses. Top Magn Reson Imaging 1990;2:27–38.

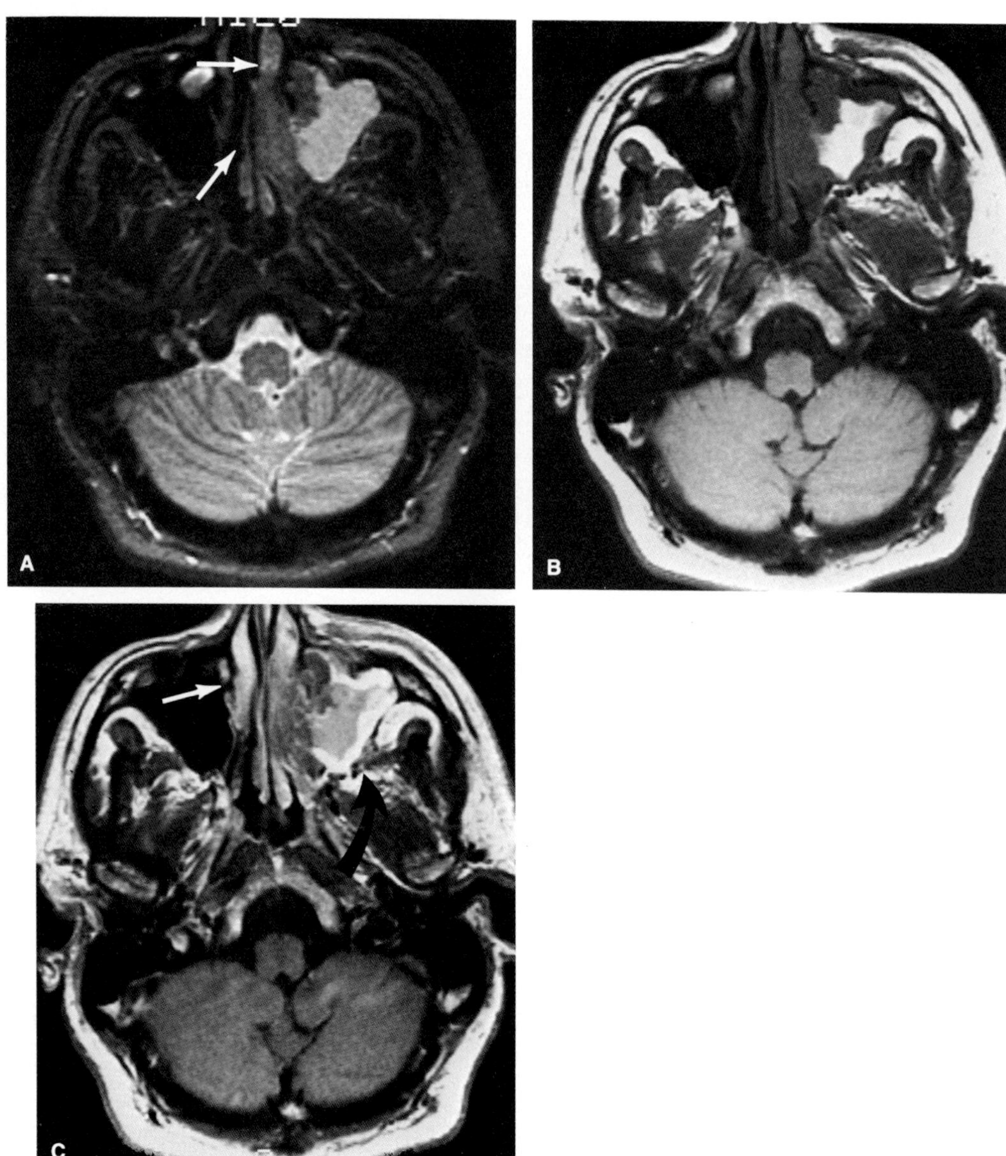

HISTORY

A 41-year-old patient with left proptosis

FINDINGS

(*A*) The axial T2-weighted (TE = 80 msec) scan reveals opacification of the left maxillary sinus by fluid and a soft tissue mass (*white arrows*) in the medial portion of the sinus and adjacent nasal cavity. By signal intensity characteristics alone, it is difficult to distinguish the mass in the nasal cavity from the normal turbinates. (*B*) Precontrast axial T1-weighted scan reveals the fluid within the maxillary sinus to be of high signal intensity (hemorrhagic). (*C*) On the postcontrast axial T1-weighted scan, inflammatory mucosal thickening (*curved arrow*) demonstrates the most substantial enhancement, followed by the turbinates (*white arrow*). This scan, unlike the T2-weighted image, permits differentiation between sinus fluid and mucosal thickening, as well as between the normal turbinates and the soft tissue mass. On precontrast (*D*) and postcontrast (*E*) coronal T1-weighted scans, involvement of both the maxillary and ethmoid sinuses is evident, with displacement of the contents of the left orbit. It is unclear whether the medial wall of the orbit (lamina papyracea) is destroyed or simply displaced. By comparison of the coronal precontrast and postcontrast images, it is evident that the mass (*arrows in E*) enhances (although to a lesser degree than the turbinates), since the lesion is lower in signal intensity than white matter precontrast, but isointense postcontrast.

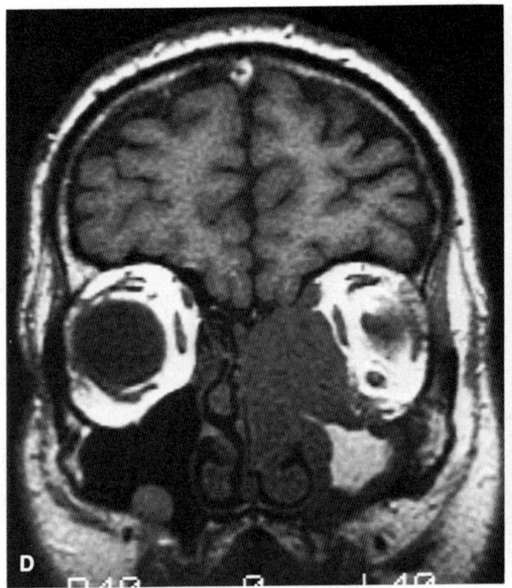

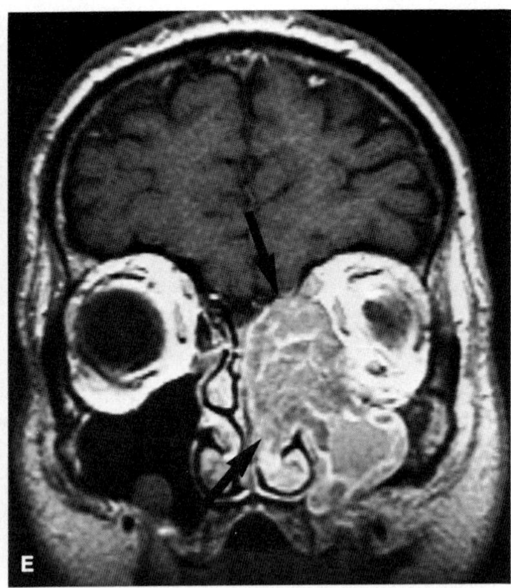

DIAGNOSIS

Rhabdomyosarcoma, involving the maxillary and ethmoid sinuses and nasal cavity

DISCUSSION

The most common malignancy in childhood in the head and neck region is rhabdomyosarcoma.[1] Although rhabdomyosarcomas are occasionally seen in the paranasal sinuses, these lesions are more common in the infratemporal fossa, orbit, and nasopharynx. CT and now MR are used for the determination of possible intracranial involvement, definition of tumor extent, and to monitor the results of therapy.

In the evaluation of head and neck tumors, MR has several advantages over CT. These include improved soft tissue contrast, the ability to acquire direct high-resolution multiplanar images, and the lack of ionizing radiation.[2] The drawbacks of MR include poor detection of subtle cortical bone abnormalities, degradation of image quality due to patient motion, and artifacts due to dental appliances. However, dental hardware commonly leads to more serious degradation of CT than MR images, with the effect of dental amalgam on MR being minimal.

MR Technique

IV contrast enhancement improves the depiction by MR of small normal anatomic details, particularly in the nasopharynx, as well as the detection of small tumors. In a recent study,[3] MR with IV contrast enhancement proved superior to CT in the study of tumors of the nasopharynx and adjacent areas, with the exception of tumors involving the maxillary sinus.

Pitfalls in Image Interpretation

Whenever malignancy is encountered in the paranasal sinuses or nasal cavity, the possibility of metastatic disease should be considered. Common primary sites include kidney, lung, and breast.

Clinical References

1. Latack JT, Hutchinson RJ, Heyn RM. Imaging of rhabdomyosarcomas of the head and neck. AJNR 1987;8:353–359.
2. Dillon WP. Magnetic resonance imaging of head and neck tumors. Cardiovasc Intervent Radiol 1986;8:275–282.
3. Vogl T, Dresel S, Bilaniuk LT, et al. Tumors of the nasopharynx and adjacent areas: MR imaging with Gd-DTPA. AJR 1990;154:585–592.

(A *through* E *courtesy of Mark Osborne, MD.*)

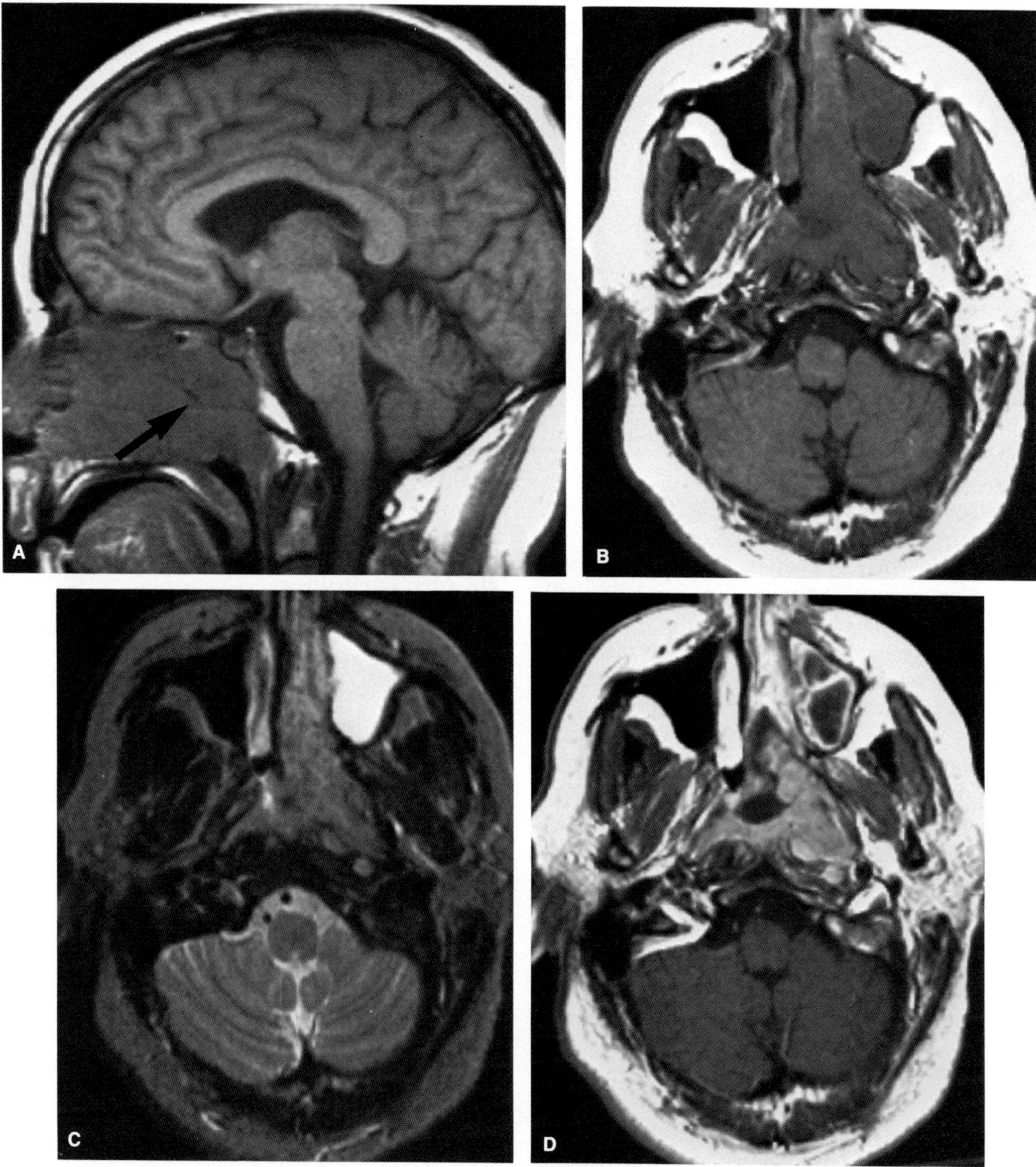

HISTORY

A 53-year-old male smoker

FINDINGS

A large, abnormal soft-tissue-intensity mass is identified in the posterior nasopharynx, extending anteriorly into the left nasal cavity on sagittal (*A*) and axial (*B*) T1-weighted and axial (*C*) T2-weighted images. The mass is invading and destroying the sphenoid sinus (*arrow in A*). There is obliteration of the fossa of Rosenmüller bilaterally and invasion of the pharyngeal mucosal space. A postobstructive fluid collection is present in the left maxillary sinus. (*D*) Moderate enhancement of the mass is seen on the axial T1-weighted image postcontrast. (*E*) A large lymph node is identified within the posterior triangle of the right neck (*arrow*) on the coronal T1-weighted image postcontrast. A smaller lymph node is present in the left neck (*arrowhead*).

DIAGNOSIS

Squamous cell carcinoma of the nasopharynx

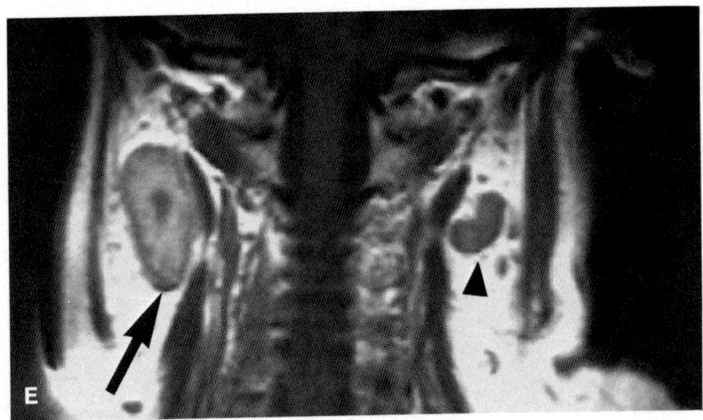

DISCUSSION

The nasopharynx is lined by squamous epithelial mucosa, and occupies the most superior extent of the gastrointestinal tract. The nasopharynx is demarcated from the oropharynx inferiorly by the soft palate. Minor salivary glands are present in both the oropharynx and nasopharynx, and are the origin of benign and malignant tumors. The eustachian tubes terminate within the nasopharynx in lateral cartilaginous structures, the torus tubarii. The fossae of Rosenmüller are lateral pharyngeal recesses formed by mucosal reflections over the longus colli and longus capitis muscles; they lie immediately posterior to the torus tubarii.

Squamous cell carcinoma represents approximately 80% of all epithelial carcinomas of the nasopharynx; adenocarcinoma makes up about 18%.[1] Squamous cell carcinoma can occur at any age but is most frequent in the middle-aged and elderly population. The clinical presentation is dependent on the location and size of the tumor. The most common presentation is asymptomatic enlargement of a cervical lymph node in either the internal jugular chain or the posterior triangle of the neck. The fossa of Rosenmüller is the most frequent site of origin of squamous cell carcinoma. On MR imaging, squamous cell carcinoma presents with focal mass effect on the fossa of Rosenmüller or invasion of the musculofascial planes around the levator and tensor palatini muscles.[2] Mastoid air cell and middle ear signal abnormality on the ipsilateral side is a common finding. Nasopharyngeal carcinoma is most frequently treated with radiation therapy.

MR Technique

Coronal imaging is the most useful plane in diagnosing skull base invasion.

Pitfalls in Image Interpretation

Normal adenoidal tissue is prominent in children and adolescents and occupies the superior and lateral recesses of the nasopharynx. Small tumors can be difficult to differentiate from adenoidal tissue, although benign adenoidal tissue never invades soft tissue planes deep to the mucosa.

Clinical References

1. Batsakis JG. Tumors of the head and neck: clinical and pathologic consideration, 2nd ed. Baltimore, Williams & Wilkins, 1979.
2. Silver AJ, Mawad M, Hilal S, et al. Computed tomography of the nasopharynx and related spaces. Radiology 1983; 147:725–731.
3. Som PM. Lymph nodes of the neck. Radiology 1987; 165:593–600.

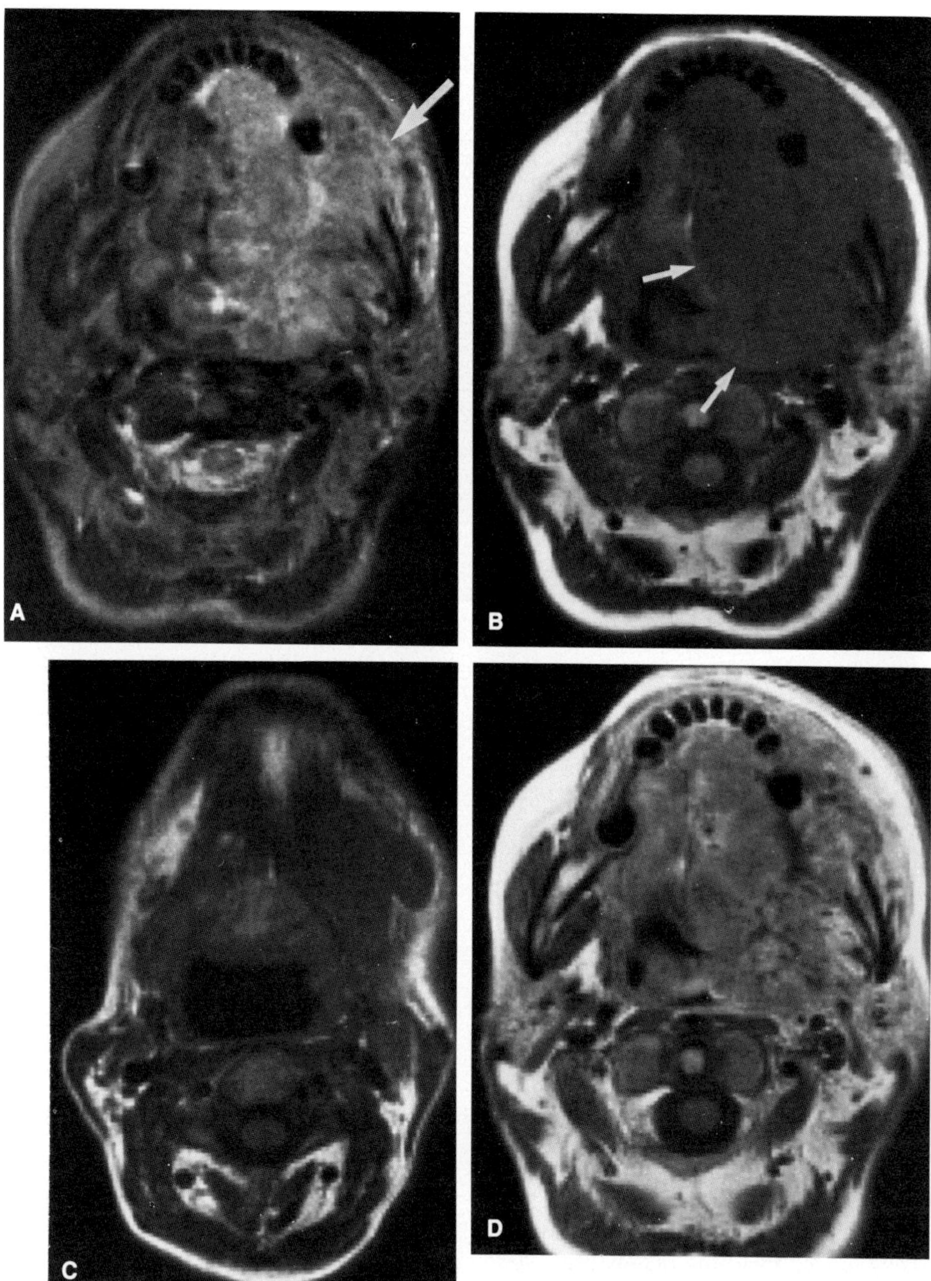

HISTORY

A 52-year-old with swelling of the left jaw

FINDINGS

(*A*) The T2-weighted axial image demonstrates an abnormal high-signal-intensity mass lesion involving the left half of the oral cavity extending from the anterior mandible to the posterior oropharynx. There is destruction of the left side of the mandible (*white arrow*) and extension of the lesion into the superficial soft tissues. (*B*) The multilobulated component of the mass projecting into the posterior oropharynx (*white arrows*) is well seen on the T1-weighted axial image. (*C*) Subcutaneous extent is seen on the T1-weighted axial image at a lower level. (*D and E*) Postcontrast T1-weighted axial images reveal marked lesion enhancement. However, differentiation of the mass from surrounding fat is superior on the precontrast images. An enlarged left jugulodigastric lymph node is also seen with peripheral enhancement (*open arrow in E*), findings consistent with central necrosis of a metastatic deposit.

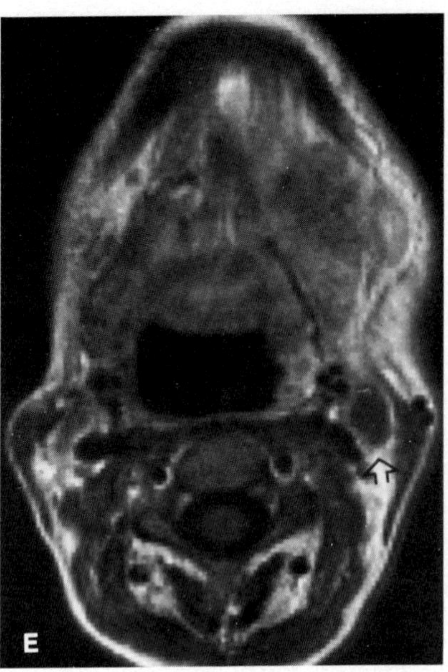

DIAGNOSIS

Squamous cell carcinoma of the oropharynx

DISCUSSION

Squamous cell carcinoma is the most common malignant tumor of the oral cavity and oropharynx, accounting for approximately 90%.[1] Malignant tumors of minor salivary gland origin, lymphoma, and other rare tumors account for the other 10%. The major risk factors for squamous cell carcinoma of the head and neck are tobacco and alcohol use. Smoking and chewing tobacco are both associated with malignancy.

MR is superior to CT for evaluation of the oral cavity and oropharynx because of its greater soft tissue contrast and multiplanar capabilities. Anatomic details are often best seen on coronal and sagittal images when studying the soft tissues of the neck and oral cavity. In addition, dental amalgam and the dense bone of the mandible do not cause artifact on MR as they do on CT. Multiplanar MR of the neck allows for accurate assessment of the local spread of the tumor and for improved detection of enlarged lymph nodes indicating distant metastases.

The signal intensity characteristics of a squamous cell carcinoma of the oropharynx are nonspecific. Lesions are usually hypointense to isointense to normal muscle on T1-weighted images and hyperintense on T2-weighted images. The use of IV contrast is often helpful in determining local tumor extension, although tumor–fat interfaces are more difficult to identify.[2]

Pitfalls in Image Interpretation

The role of MR in evaluation of the oral cavity and oropharynx is principally for directing surgical biopsy or for staging of a suspected malignancy. The findings in squamous cell carcinoma are nonspecific, and a histologic diagnosis cannot be made.

Clinical References

1. Lufkin R, Hanafee W. MRI of the head and neck. Magn Reson Imaging 1988;6:69–88.
2. Robinson J, Crawford S, Teresi L, et al. Extracranial lesions of the head and neck: preliminary experience with Gd-DTPA-enhanced MR imaging. Radiology 1989;172:165–170.

(A through E from Runge VM. Clinical magnetic resonance imaging. Philadelphia, JB Lippincott, 1990.)

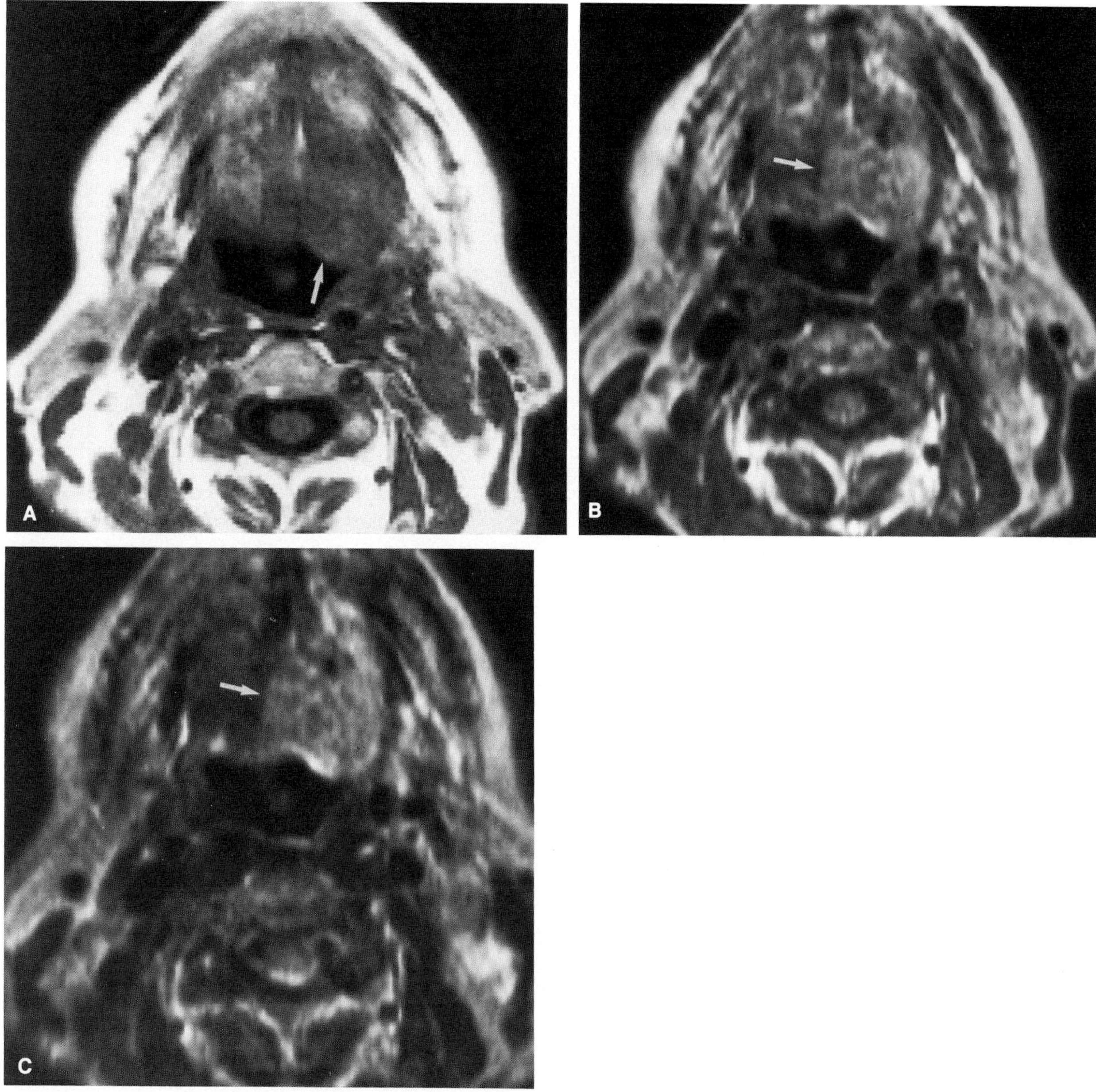

HISTORY

Tongue mass in a 50-year-old patient who chews tobacco

FINDINGS

(*A*) The T1-weighted axial image demonstrates asymmetry of the posterior tongue, with abnormal soft tissue extending posteriorly and obliterating the left glossopharyngeal fossa (*white arrow in A*). The mass extends slightly across the midline (*white arrows in B and C*) on the intermediate (*B*) and heavily (*C*) T2-weighted axial images. Abnormally enlarged lymph nodes are also present in the left jugular chain, located between the internal jugular vein and sternocleidomastoid muscle.

DIAGNOSIS

Squamous cell carcinoma of the tongue

DISCUSSION

The tongue is a common site of origin of squamous cell carcinoma of the oral cavity.[1] Like all squamous cell carcinomas of the oral cavity, malignancies of the tongue are associated with tobacco and alcohol use. Tumors that involve the anterior third of the tongue are usually detected clinically in their early stages and seldom require imaging studies. Carcinomas of the posterior tongue are less accessible clinically and are usually advanced when discovered; about 75% have nodal metastases at the time of initial examination. The lymphatic drainage of the posterior tongue is bilateral, and bilateral lymphadenopathy is not uncommon. The lateral portion of the posterior tongue is intimately associated with the glossopharyngeal sulcus and tonsillar bed, and tongue carcinomas have a propensity for direct extension into these structures. Squamous cell carcinomas of the oral cavity are frequently so extensive that determining the exact site of origin is impossible.

The tongue is a muscle and normally has low signal intensity on both T1- and T2-weighted images. Therefore, tumors involving the tongue are often best detected on T2-weighted images because of their high signal intensity. Asymmetry is also a clue in detecting tumors of the tongue, as it is in all pathology of the head and neck.

MR Technique

Anatomic details of midline structures such as the tongue are best evaluated with coronal images. The relation between abnormal lymph nodes, the jugular veins, and the sternocleidomastoid muscles is well depicted on coronal images.

Clinical References

1. Lufkin R, Hanafee W. MRI of the head and neck. Magn Reson Imaging 1988;6:69–88.

(A to C from Runge VM. Clinical magnetic resonance imaging. Philadelphia, JB Lippincott, 1990.)

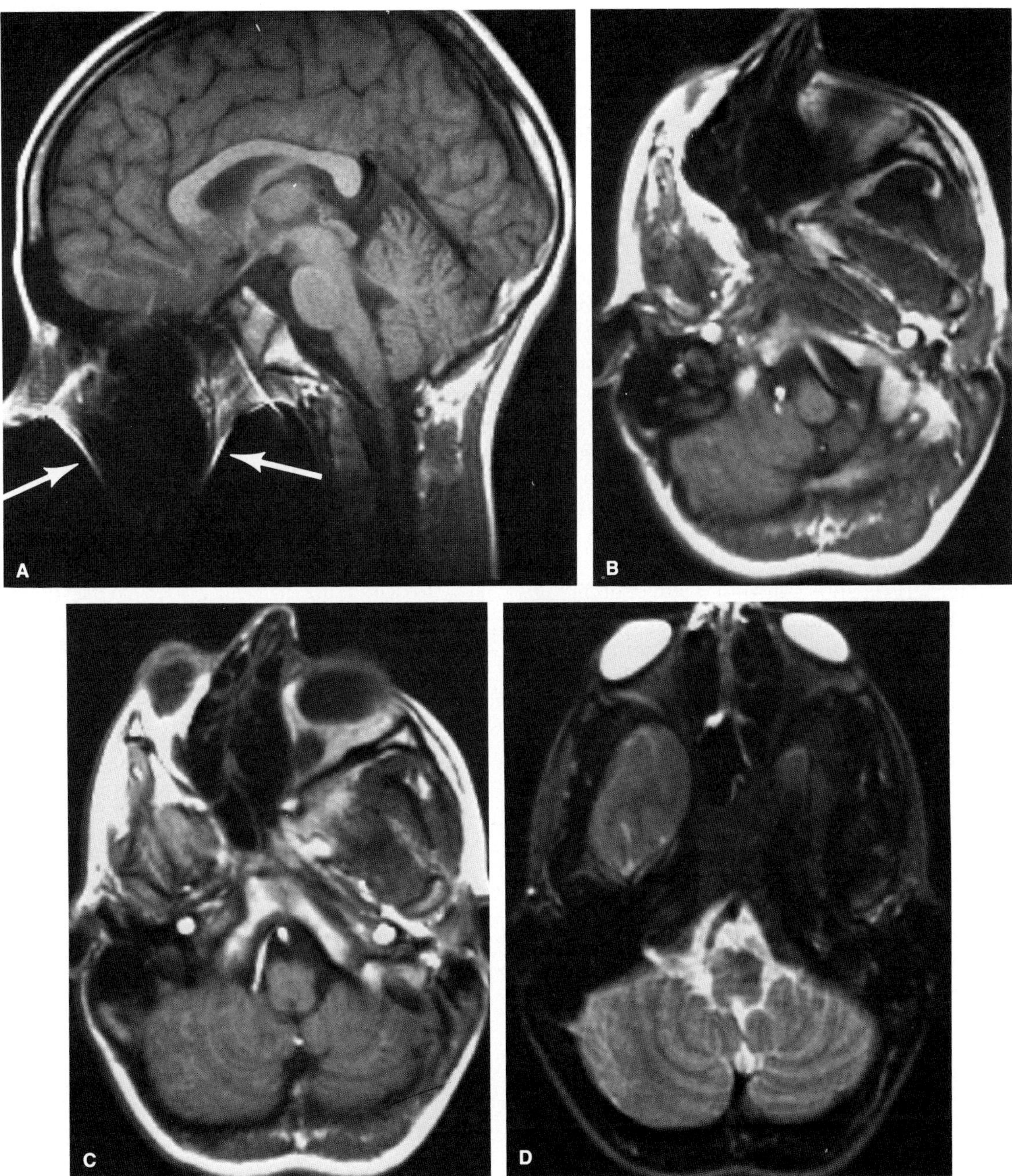

HISTORY

A 12-year-old boy with headaches

FINDINGS

(*A*) The T1-weighted sagittal image reveals a large area of signal void in the expected region of the nasal passages, palate, and oropharynx. The normal signal from these structures has been completely replaced by a black signal void. Along the edge of the signal void there is a band of high signal intensity (*white arrows*). (*B and C*) On the T1-weighted axial images through the base of the skull, there is distortion of the anterior portion of each image, a finding more marked on the lower image. The nasal passages are artifactually curved and the shape of each globe is artifactually distorted. (*D*) On the T2-weighted axial image, the middle cranial fossa is artifactually elongated in the anteroposterior direction, which is the frequency encoding direction. The shape of the globes is also distorted, but in a different manner than on the T1-weighted images, where the frequency encoding direction is from right to left.

DIAGNOSIS

Image artifact from dental braces

DISCUSSION

Ferromagnetic objects have a high magnetic susceptibility—that is, when they are placed in a constant applied magnetic field (such as an MR imager) they respond with an induced magnetic field that is as strong as or stronger than, and is in the same direction as, the applied constant magnetic field. Normal brain tissue is diamagnetic, and responds to a constant applied magnetic field with an induced magnetic field that is weakly opposed to the constant field. Thus, when a ferromagnetic material is present adjacent to the normal tissue of the head, a local gradient in magnetic field is produced with resultant distortion of images and creation of a "susceptibility" artifact.

The characteristic appearance of a susceptibility artifact caused by the presence of a ferromagnetic object in the magnetic field is a signal void with a surrounding band of high signal intensity.[1] The resultant local magnetic field inhomogeneity causes distortion (artifactual elongation) of the adjacent tissues. The geometric distortion occurs in the frequency encoding direction. This is seen in the case illustrated, where the elongation occurs along a different axis on the T1-weighted images compared with the T2-weighted images because of a difference in the specified frequency encoding direction for the two pulse sequences.

Dental crowns, dental braces, and dentures often contain ferromagnetic materials and cause significant susceptibility artifacts. Dental amalgam contains silver, tin, and mercury and does not produce such artifact.[1] Ferromagnetic surgical clips, shunt catheter ports, craniotomy wires, metal on clothing, and metallic fragments in the subcutaneous soft tissues (from metalworking accidents or gunshot wounds) also are common causes of local field distortions in MR. Susceptibility artifacts are also seen at the interface of the paranasal sinuses and the brain because of the large difference in magnetic susceptibility between air and soft tissue.

MR Technique

The amount of susceptibility artifact created by a ferromagnetic object is directly proportional to the strength of the magnetic field and inversely proportional to the strength of the magnetic gradient in the frequency encoding direction.[2] In general, susceptibility artifacts are greater at 1.5 T than at lower field strengths.

Clinical References

1. Bellon E, Haacke E, Coleman P, et al. MR artifacts: a review. AJR 1986;147:1271–1281.
2. Ludeke K, Roschmann P, Tischler R. Susceptibility artifacts in NMR imaging. Magn Reson Imaging 1985;3:329–343.

Index

Page numbers followed by *f* indicate figures; those followed by *t* indicate tables.

C

D

E

F

G

H

I

J

L

M

N

O

P